# Risk Factors and Therapy of Esophagus Cancer

Omer Engin
Editor

# Risk Factors and Therapy of Esophagus Cancer

Springer

*Editor*
Omer Engin
Department of Surgery
VM Medical Park Pendik Hospital
Istanbul, Türkiye

ISBN 978-3-031-47023-3 ISBN 978-3-031-47024-0 (eBook)
https://doi.org/10.1007/978-3-031-47024-0



This Springer imprint is published by the registered company Springer Nature Switzerland AG
The registered company address is: Gewerbestrasse 11, 6330 Cham, Switzerland

# Preface

Esophageal cancer is among the most common cancers. Due to the more widespread use of endoscopy, esophageal cancer is a disease that can be diagnosed early.

The esophagus is located in three different anatomical regions depending on its anatomical features. The esophagus lies in the cervical region, in the thorax, in the abdomen, and is adjacent to many important organs.

Accordingly, esophageal surgery requires a multidisciplinary approach. General surgery, ENT, thoracic surgery, and cardiovascular surgery can work together in the surgical treatment of esophageal cancer.

In metastases, orthopedics, neurosurgery, interventional radiology, and other branches can participate in the treatment process together. Medical oncologists and radiation oncologists also contribute to the treatment process in cancer treatment.

In our book, the main procedures that can be done from diagnosis to every stage of the treatment process are tried to be explained with a multidisciplinary approach.

The authors in our book are experienced specialist working actively in their fields and have made an effort to convey their knowledge and experience to the readers in our book.

We believe that our book will be useful to all physicians dealing with esophageal cancer.

Istanbul, Turkey　　　　Omer Engin

# Contents

# About the Editor

**Omer Engin, M.D.** is an Associate Professor of General Surgery in the Department of Surgery, VM Medical Park Pendik Hospital Istanbul, Turkey. Dr. Engin received his medical degree from Istanbul University Faculty of Medicine. He completed surgical training at the Ministry of Health Taksim Training and Research Hospital in Istanbul and then worked in training and research hospitals for many years, contributing to the training of many new general surgeons. Dr. Engin's special interests include in particular oncologic surgery, gastrointestinal surgery, and hepatopancreatobiliary surgery. He has authored numerous international research articles and congress proceedings and edited many books on general surgery. Dr. Engin is a member of various national and international surgical associations. As a person who enjoys research, he supports the principle of multidisciplinary work and is keen to share his experience and knowledge.

# Esophageal Cancer: A Comprehensive Overview

# 1

Omer Engin, Yalcin Burak Kara, and Ozhan Cetindag

In our book, we will provide information about esophageal cancer (EC) and the associated risk factors. We will also discuss about the multidisciplinary management of EC. It is extremely important to know the risk factors for EC. Although both curative medicine and preventive medicine are important, the latter can aid in lifestyle modifications of people with risk factors, thus reducing the risk of developing esophageal cancer. This makes preventive medicine far more important that curative medicine. Preventing esophageal cancer before it develops is extremely important both in terms of patient comfort and economic costs. After the development of EC, the cost of patient treatment is quite high. However, removing some of the risk factors for EC, from people at risk of the same, using some simple measures often incurs zero cost. In the period after the development of esophageal cancer, patient comfort may deteriorate, whereas eliminating risk factors may not lead to a deficiency in patient comfort. One of the most important duties of preventive medicine is to inform people about these risk factors and to take measures to reduce them [1].

Known and discussed risk factors include age, gender, lack of physical activity, tylosis, Plummer–Vinson syndrome, injury to the esophagus, history of certain other cancers, human papillomavirus (HPV) infection, gastroesophageal reflux disease (GERD), smoking, (Barrett's esophagus) obesity, alcohol consumption, bile reflux, achalasia, drinking hot liquids, minimal consumption of fruits and

O. Engin (✉)
Surgery Department, VM Medical Park Pendik Hospital, Istanbul, Türkiye

Y. B. Kara
Medicine Faculty, Surgery Department, Bahcesehir University, Medical Park Pendik Hospital, Istanbul, Turkey

O. Cetindag
Private Clinic, Izmir, Turkey



O. Engin (ed.), *Risk Factors and Therapy of Esophagus Cancer*,
https://doi.org/10.1007/978-3-031-47024-0_1

vegetables, and even radiation therapy. As can be seen, most of these are preventable risk factors. These issues will be explored in detail in the next chapters [2, 3].

The esophagus is shaped like a smooth muscular tube. The distance between the upper and lower sphincter is about 18–26 cm. The esophagus is collapsed between swallows, but the lumen expands and allows the swallowed substance to pass into the stomach, with the anterior posterior diameter expanding up to 2 cm and the lateral diameter up to 3 cm [4].

The esophagus consists of two different structures. In the proximal region, both striated muscles and smooth muscles are seen together, whereas, in the distal region, the esophageal wall is composed of smooth muscles [5].

In a cadaver study by Meyer et al., striated muscles were exclusively found in 4.1–5.6% of the proximal esophagus. In the distal region, in 54–62% of the esophagus, smooth muscles were exclusively detected. In the rest of the esophagus, the muscle structures were found to be mixed [6].

Chewed foods and drinks pass into the esophagus with the swallowing movement. The esophagus is not a motionless organ. The muscles in its wall contract and take part in the progression of the morsel and its transport to the stomach. With the swallowing movement, the upper esophageal sphincter relaxes and the bite passes into the esophagus. The bite first reaches the lower esophageal sphincter by peristaltic contractions and the lower esophageal sphincter relaxes, allowing the bite to pass into the stomach [7].

The bolus initiates the primary peristaltic movement in the esophagus. Primary peristalsis can be called bolus-induced esophageal contractions. Secondary peristalsis is known as distension-induced contractions. While the anterior part of the bolus relaxes with peristaltic movements, the posterior part of the bolus contracts and the bolus advances into the esophagus. Secondary peristaltic movements usually develop outside of swallowing. Local distention of the esophagus or the presence of a bolus of nutrients in the esophagus or refluxed contents from the stomach initiates secondary peristaltic movements. With secondary peristaltic contractions, the residual food in the esophagus is advanced into the stomach and the esophagus is cleaned. In the sitting position, the effect of gravity helps the bolus advance into the esophagus [7–10]. Tertiary contractions are non-propulsive, transient, and intermittent. They are often seen in older patients or in diseases such as achalasia [11, 12].

Cancer cells originating from the mucosa begin to grow and form a mass. At first, symptoms may not manifest. A tumor is detected incidentally at endoscopy of the upper gastrointestinal system (GIS) performed for other reasons. EC is most often diagnosed between the ages of 50 and 70 [13]. Frequently undergoing endoscopic examination and upper GIS endoscopy due to complaints such as reflux, gastritis, and peptic ulcer of the upper gastrointestinal tract may lead to early detection of esophageal cancer [14, 15].

The tumor in the lumen may grow and prevent the passage of the food bolus through the lumen. In this case, the patient begins to experience difficulty swallowing. Inhibition of the passage occurs with two ways:intraluminal mass effect of the tumor and invasion of the muscular layer. Patients can usually show the localization of the tumor by pointing at the place where they experience a feeling of being stuck [16].

Some patients may not visit the hospital out of fear, even if symptoms develop and they face difficulty in swallowing, which may lead to delay in diagnosis and treatment. Because of the feeling of being stuck when consuming solid foods, patients may turn to liquid foods or consume less food, which can lead to nutritional deficiencies and weight loss. The result of this is reflected in the laboratory values and findings such as anemia, decrease in protein values, etc.. If the obstruction has reached an advanced stage, then bad breath and regurgitation of recently eaten food may also be seen [17, 18].

In physical examination, palpation of the esophagus is not possible because the esophagus is located in the thorax. However, metastatic formations can be palpated. Cervical supraclavicular lymph nodes in the neck can be detected by palpation. In patients with metastases to the liver, metastatic masses can be found with physical examination. If pleural effusion develops due to a malignancy, then a decrease in breath sounds can be detected [19, 20].

Advanced presenting complaints of esophageal cancer include symptoms due to metastases. For example, in liver metastases, jaundice may develop with the compression of the metastatic masses on the biliary tract and icterus may be detected in the sclera. Ascites may develop due to fluid accumulation in the abdomen due to intra-abdominal metastases and abdominal distension may occur. Cardiological symptoms and respiratory distress due to cardiac and pleural metastases can be detected [21, 22].

The diagnosis may be made incidentally during examinations performed for another complaint or during examinations performed in people with swallowing difficulties. A tumoral mass in the esophagus can be seen on computed tomography (CT) scanning of the thorax performed for cough and lung- or thorax-related complaints. An esophageal tumor can be diagnosed during endoscopic procedures such as esophagogastroduodenoscopy due to complaints such as reflux and gastritis of the upper gastrointestinal tract. In patients with swallowing difficulties, more cause-oriented tests may be requested. For this purpose, esophagography, endoscopy, endoscopic ultrasonography (EUS), thoracic CT, or magnetic resonance imaging (MRI) can be used [23, 24].

With upper gastrointestinal endoscopy, it is possible to see a tumoral mass in the esophagus during endoscopy and collect biopsy samples for pathological diagnosis. In endoscopy, information can be obtained about the size of the tumor, whether it surrounds the lumen, the length of the segment it holds in the lumen, and whether it allows the passage of the endoscope. For example, a tumor in the esophagus that is 8 cm above the segment it holds in the lumen and does not allow the passage of the endoscope may indicate a poor prognosis. Endoscopic ultrasound provides extremely useful information about the spread of esophageal cancer into the inner lining of the esophageal wall, the muscular layer, and even to the outer layers of the wall [25–27].

The next step after diagnosis is choosing treatment. Again, imaging methods can help decide which treatment to undergo. Positron emission tomography (PET) is a highly effective imaging method to investigate the presence of distant metastases. Owing to radiological imaging methods, patients can choose to undergo either neoadjuvant chemoradiotherapy (CRT) or direct surgical treatment. These issues will be explained in detail in other chapters [28, 29].

In esophageal surgery, patient follow-up is extremely important to check whether the patient is facing any issues or problems owing to the complexity of the surgery. In the first postoperative days, blood tests and evaluation of parameters such as drain follow-up, fever, blood pressure, pulse, fluid intake and output, fluid electrolyte balance, acid–base balance, urine output, infection parameters in the blood, and oxygen saturation in the blood should be conducted and closely monitored [30, 31].

As the drain is placed in the cervical region, the patients should be followed to check whether there is anastomotic leakage. In anastomotic leakage, fluid matching the color of oral secretions may be encountered. The bacterial flora here is compatible with the oral flora. Underwater drainage is performed in patients with a thorax tube. Here, the fluid coming from the thoracic drain may be blood or fluid due to the fistula contents, as a result of bleeding that may occur in the postoperative period. Since anastomosis can be performed in the esophagus, colon, stomach, and small intestine, the secretion and bacterial flora of these organs can be investigated by analyzing the leaking fluid. Since pyloroplasty or other anastomoses can be performed in the abdomen, intra-abdominal drains can be used to follow up the complications that may develop as a result [32–34].

Oxygen saturation in the blood is important for patient follow-up. A decrease in oxygen saturation in the presence of pleural effusion and atelectasis or postoperative pneumonia in the postoperative period may be an indication of the presence of such complications. If the patient cannot breathe adequately due to pain, oxygen saturation may decrease. Painkillers can improve breathing [35, 36].

It is extremely important to monitor the fluid intake and output of the patient. If the patient's fluid intake is high but the output is less, then there may be a transition to the third space, and, in this case, blood pressure may decrease, the pulse rate may increase, and urine output may decrease. It is necessary to be careful about this. It is important to remember that a negative fluid balance can be seen in sepsis. Acid–base balance is also an important parameter that should be maintained during patient follow-up [37–39].

Hemogram follow-up can provide important information. High leukocyte levels may be due to surgical trauma in the postoperative period or may also increase secondary to infection. A low leukocyte count may be secondary to consumption due to sepsis or secondary to bone marrow depression. Platelet count is also one of the most affected parameters in sepsis-induced consumption, and platelet counts may decrease significantly in sepsis-induced consumption coagulopathy. In addition, elevations of leukocyte procalcitonin and C-reactive protein (CRP) may be among the early signs of fistula development [40, 41].

Combinations of chemotherapy, radiotherapy, and surgical treatment are used in the treatment, and the patient should be closely followed to check for complications that may occur [42, 43].

Lumen narrowing may develop in the advanced stages of esophageal cancer. In this case, a stent can be inserted to continue oral nutrition. Because the stent does not have peristaltic movements, large pieces of poorly chewed food may clog the stent. To prevent this, swallowing the bites by chewing them thoroughly and sitting upright while eating help the passage of the bite into the stomach. In addition, drinking water during meals may facilitate the passage of bites through the stent [44].

It is necessary to apply imaging methods at certain intervals in order to follow up with the treatment and to check whether there is tumor spread at all stages of the disease. Ultrasound tomography, magnetic resonance imaging, and PET/CT are all effective in evaluating the treatment process of the disease. These methods will be explored in detail in other chapters of this book [45].

## References

1. Marabotto E, Pellegatta G, Sheijani AD, Ziola S, Zentilin P, et al. Prevention strategies for esophageal cancer—An expert review. Cancers (Basel). 2021;13(9):2183. https://doi.org/10.3390/cancers13092183. PMID: 34062788; PMCID: PMC8125297.
2. Mayo Clinic. Esophageal cancer risk factors. 2024. https://www.mayoclinic.org/diseases-conditions/esophageal-cancer/symptoms-causes/syc-20356084.
3. American Cancer Society. Esophageal cancer risk factors. 2024. https://www.cancer.org/cancer/esophagus-cancer/causes-risks-prevention/risk-factors.html.
4. Kuo B, Urma D. Esophagus-anatomy and development. GI Motility; 2006.
5. Goyal RK, Chaudhury A. Physiology of normal esophageal motility. J Clin Gastroenterol. 2008;42(5):610–9. https://doi.org/10.1097/MCG.0b013e31816b444d. PMID: 18364578; PMCID: PMC2728598.
6. Meyer GW, Austin RM, Brady CE III, Castell DO. Muscle anatomy of the human esophagus. J Clin Gastroenterol. 1986;8(2):131–4.
7. Bajwa SA, Toro F, Kasi A. Physiology, esophagus. [Updated 2022 May 8]. In: StatPearls [Internet]. Treasure Island: StatPearls Publishing; 2022. https://www.ncbi.nlm.nih.gov/books/NBK519011/.
8. Paterson WG. Esophageal peristalsis. GI Motility; 2006.
9. Zifan A, Song HJ, Youn YH, Qiu X, Ledgerwood-Lee M, Mittal RK. Topographical plots of esophageal distension and contraction: effects of posture on esophageal peristalsis and bolus transport. Am J Physiol Gastrointest Liver Physiol. 2019;316(4):G519–26.
10. Pongpipatpaiboon K, Inamoto Y, Aihara K, Kagaya H, Shibata S, Mukaino M, et al. Thin liquid bolus volume alters pharyngeal swallowing: kinematic analysis using 3D dynamic CT. Dysphagia. 2022;37:1423–30.
11. Visaggi P, Ghisa M, Marabotto E, et al. Esophageal dysmotility in patients with eosinophilic esophagitis: pathogenesis, assessment tools, manometric characteristics, and clinical implications. Esophagus. 2023;20:29–38. https://doi.org/10.1007/s10388-022-00964-z.
12. Goyal RK. EndoFLIP topography: motor patterns in an obstructed esophagus. Gastroenterology. 2022;163(3):552–5.
13. Kollarova H, Machova L, Horakova D, Janoutova G, Janout V. Epidemiology of esophageal cancer—an overview article. Biomed Pap Med Fac Univ Palacky Olomouc Czech Repub. 2007;151:17.
14. Gao QY, Fang JY. Early esophageal cancer screening in China. Best Pract Res Clin Gastroenterol. 2015;29(6):885–93.
15. Yoshida S. Endoscopic diagnosis and treatment of early cancer in the alimentary tract. Digestion. 1998;59(5):502–8.

16. Koyama T, Umeoka S, Saga T, Watanabe G, Tamai K, Kobayashi A, et al. Evaluation of esophageal peristalsis in patients with esophageal tumors: initial experience with cine MR imaging. Magn Reson Med Sci. 2005;4(3):109–14.
17. Steenhagen E, van Vulpen JK, van Hillegersberg R, May AM, et al. Nutrition in peri-operative esophageal cancer management. Expert Rev Gastroenterol Hepatol. 2017;11(7):663–72.
18. Lagergren J, Lagergren P. Oesophageal cancer. BMJ. 2010;341:c6280.
19. van Overhagen H, Brakel K, Heijenbrok MW, van Kasteren JH, van de Moosdijk CN, Roldaan AC, et al. Metastases in supraclavicular lymph nodes in lung cancer: assessment with palpation, US, and CT. Radiology. 2004;232(1):75–80.
20. Fenton KN, Richardson JD. Diagnosis and management of malignant pleural effusions. Am J Surg. 1995;170(1):69–74.
21. Saha D, Majumder J, Chejara S, Har B, Pramanik S, et al. A rare presentation of carcinoma esophagus with scalp metastasis. Clin Cancer Investig J. 2015;4(5):655.
22. Tu Q, Bittencourt MDC, Cai H, Bastien C, Lemarie-Delaunay C, Bene MC, et al. Case report: detection and quantification of tumor cells in peripheral blood and ascitic fluid from a metastatic esophageal cancer patient using the CellSearch® technology. F1000Res. 2014;3:12.
23. Gollub MJ, Prowda JC. Primary melanoma of the esophagus: radiologic and clinical findings in six patients. Radiology. 1999;213(1):97–100.
24. Lee G, Hoseok I, Kim SJ, Jeong YJ, Kim IJ, Pak K, et al. Clinical implication of PET/MR imaging in preoperative esophageal cancer staging: comparison with PET/CT, endoscopic ultrasonography, and CT. J Nucl Med. 2014;55(8):1242–7.
25. Schena M, Battaglia AF, Munoz F. Esophageal cancer developed in a radiated field: can we reduce the risk of a poor prognosis cancer? J Thorac Dis. 2017;9(7):1767.
26. Welsh J, Settle SH, Amini A, Xiao L, Suzuki A, Hayashi Y, et al. Failure patterns in patients with esophageal cancer treated with definitive chemoradiation. Cancer. 2012;118(10):2632–40.
27. Zeybek A, Erdoğan A, Gülkesen KH, Ergin M, Sarper A, Dertsiz L, et al. Significance of tumor length as prognostic factor for esophageal cancer. Int Surg. 2013;98(3):234–40.
28. Hamai Y, Emi M, Ibuki Y, Murakami Y, Nishibuchi I, Nagata Y, et al. Predictions of pathological features and recurrence based on FDG-PET findings of esophageal squamous cell carcinoma after trimodal therapy. Ann Surg Oncol. 2020;27:4422–30.
29. Borggreve AS, Goense L, van Rossum PS, Heethuis SE, van Hillegersberg R, Lagendijk JJ, et al. Preoperative prediction of pathologic response to neoadjuvant chemoradiotherapy in patients with esophageal cancer using 18F-FDG PET/CT and DW-MRI: a prospective multicenter study. Int J Radiat Oncol Biol Phys. 2020;106(5):998–1009.
30. Akiyama Y, Sasaki A, Fujii Y, Fujisawa R, Sasaki N, Nikai H, et al. Efficacy of enhanced prehabilitation for patients with esophageal cancer undergoing esophagectomy. Esophagus. 2021;18:56–64.
31. Yu G, Chen G, Huang B, Shao W, Zeng G, et al. Effect of early enteral nutrition on postoperative nutritional status and immune function in elderly patients with esophageal cancer or cardiac cancer. Chin J Cancer Res. 2013;25(3):299.
32. Wang D, Xu L, Yang F, Wang Z, Sun H, Chen X, et al. The improved mediastinal drainage strategy for the enhanced recovery system after esophagectomy. Ann Thorac Surg. 2021;112(2):473–80.
33. Kato R, Makino T, Yamasaki M, Tanaka K, Miyazaki Y, Takahashi T, et al. Risk factors associated with increased drainage volumes of chest tubes after transthoracic esophagectomy for esophageal cancer. Surg Today. 2019;49:1058–65.
34. Yannopoulos P, Theodoridis P, Manes K. Esophagectomy without thoracotomy: 25 years of experience over 750 patients. Langenbecks Arch Surg. 2009;394:611–6.
35. Ramsay MA. Acute postoperative pain management. In: Baylor University Medical Center Proceedings. Taylor & Francis; 2000. p. 244–247.
36. Suzuki S. Oxygen administration for postoperative surgical patients: a narrative review. J Intensive Care. 2020;8(1):79.
37. Jacob M, Chappell D, Rehm M. The 'third space'—fact or fiction? Best Pract Res Clin Anaesthesiol. 2009;23(2):145–57.

38. Alsous F, Khamiees M, DeGirolamo A, Amoateng-Adjepong Y, et al. Negative fluid balance predicts survival in patients with septic shock. Chest. 2000;117(6):1749–54.
39. Besen BAMP, Taniguchi LU. Negative fluid balance in sepsis: when and how? Shock. 2017;47(1S):35–40.
40. Richter F, Mehdorn AS, Fedders T, Reichert B, Egberts JH, Becker T, et al. C-reactive protein as predictor for infectious complications after robotic and open esophagectomies. J Clin Med. 2022;11(19):5654.
41. Koyama K, Katayama S, Muronoi T, Tonai K, Goto Y, Koinuma T, et al. Time course of immature platelet count and its relation to thrombocytopenia and mortality in patients with sepsis. PLoS One. 2018;13(1):e0192064.
42. Kakeji Y, Oshikiri T, Takiguchi G, Kanaji S, Matsuda T, Nakamura T, et al. Multimodality approaches to control esophageal cancer: development of chemoradiotherapy, chemotherapy, and immunotherapy. Esophagus. 2021;18:25–32.
43. Egeland C, Bazancir LA, Bui NH, Baeksgaard L, Gehl J, Gögenur I, et al. Palliation of dysphagia in patients with non-curable esophageal cancer—a retrospective Danish study from a highly specialized center. Support Care Cancer. 2022;30:9029–38.
44. Guvenc E, Demirdoven BT, Engin O. Obstruction of the metallic esophageal stent in patients with esophageal cancer, oncologic emergency case report. Int J Oncotherapy. 2016;2(1). https://www.researchgate.net/publication/309847145_Page_1_Available_at_wwwijotin_1_Obstruction_of_the_metallic_esophageal_stent_in_patients_with_esophageal_cancer_oncologic_emergency_case_report. Accessed 12 June 2023.
45. Sun L, Su XH, Guan YS, Pan WM, Luo ZM, Wei JH, et al. Clinical usefulness of 18F-FDG PET/CT in the restaging of esophageal cancer after surgical resection and radiotherapy. World J Gastroenterol. 2009;15(15):1836.

# Esophageal Cancer Risk Factors

# 2

Yalcin Burak Kara and Omer Engin

## 2.1 Introduction

The eighth-most-common type of the cancer and the sixth leading cause of cancer deaths in the world is esophageal cancer. Two major histological types have been found: esophageal squamous cell carcinoma (ESCC) and esophageal adenocarcinoma (EAC). Other histological types of esophageal carcinomas are basal cell carcinomas, transitional cell carcinomas, and unspecified carcinomas. The distribution of esophageal cancer types throughout the world differs depending on the location. EAC is predominantly seen in the United States and other Western countries, whereas ESCC is predominantly seen in Eastern countries [1, 2].

The incidence rate of esophageal carcinoma in Eastern Asia is 12.2 per 100,000 people (the highest rate), whereas in Central America, the incidence rate is 0.98 per 100,000 (the lowest rate). When the risk rate is evaluated for the world population, it is 9.3 per 100,000. Globally, 5.3% of all cancer deaths are related to esophageal carcinoma. The cause of this high mortality rate is related to late diagnosis and distant metastasis at the time of diagnosis. Nearly 40% of patients have distant metastasis at the time of diagnosis. According to calculations of the estimated standardized mortality rate for all cancers by organ, the lungs (18.8 per 100,000) have the highest risk rate, followed by the breasts (13), the colorectum (8.9), the liver (8.5), the stomach (8.2), the prostate (7.6), the cervix uteri (6.9), and the esophagus (5.5) [1–5].

Esophageal cancer has a poor prognosis because of the late diagnosis time. The 5-year survival rate varies from 25.1% for a region-specific disease to 4.8% when in the distant metastasis condition. The estimated median survival time is 6 months

Y. B. Kara (✉)
Medicine Faculty, Department of General Surgery, Bahcesehir University, Istanbul, Turkey

Surgery Department, VM Medical Park Pendik Hospital, Istanbul, Turkey

O. Engin
Surgery Department, VM Medical Park Pendik Hospital, Istanbul, Türkiye


O. Engin (ed.), *Risk Factors and Therapy of Esophagus Cancer*,
https://doi.org/10.1007/978-3-031-47024-0_2

when under the distant metastasis condition, 13 months as a region-specific disease, and 30 months as a localized disease [2, 6].

## 2.2 Risk Factors

### 2.2.1 Age

According to the Globacan's (2018) data, in both sexes, lung cancer is the most commonly diagnosed cancer in the world. In men, the incidence rates of cancers are organized from highest to lowest as follows: lung (14.5%), prostate (13.5%), colorectum (10.9%), stomach (7.2%), liver (6.3%), bladder (4.5%), esophagus (4.2%), non-Hodgkin lymphoma (3.0%), kidney (2.7%), and leukemia (2.6%). In women, breast cancer is the most common (24.7%), followed by the following cancers: colorectum (9.5%), lung (8.4%), cervix uteri (6.6%), thyroid (5.1%), corpus uteri (4.4%), stomach (4.1%), ovary (3.4%), liver (2.8%), and non-Hodgkin lymphoma (2.6%). According to the Surveillance, Epidemiology, and End Results (SEER) database in the United States, the median age of cancer diagnosis is 66, usually between 65 and 75 years. The median ages of organ-specific cancer diagnoses are classified as follows: lung, 71 years; breast, 62; prostate, 66; pancreas, 70; colon, 67; bladder, 73; cervix, 50; and ovary, 63 [1].

The esophageal cancer risk rate increases as people age because carcinomas develop slowly with chronic irritation. In the United States, the average age of an esophageal carcinoma diagnosis is 68. According to the SEER database, the highest incidence rate is 24.9 per 100,000, for those aged 75 years and older. For ages between 65 and 74, the incidence rate is 20.3 per 100,000, and for ages between 50 and 64, the incidence rate is 8.0 per 100,000. The lowest incidence rate group is those aged between 20 and 49, whose risk rate is 0.3 per 100,000. The mortality rate increases with age, and the highest risk rate is nearly 25 per 100,000 for those aged 75 years and over [7].

Globally, the average age of esophageal carcinoma diagnosis varies: 65 for men and 74 for women in the United Kingdom, 63 in Malaysia, and 61 in China. In addition, patients under 40 years old have been diagnosed with esophageal carcinoma in Africa [7–9].

The routine use of an endoscopic screening program for patients aged 50 years and older is the best preventive method.

### 2.2.2 Sex

Esophageal cancer is predominantly seen in men rather than women. The risk rate for men is two to eight higher than that for women. Additionally, the mortality rate is higher in men (8.3 per 100,000) than in woman (3.0 per 100,000). That EAC is more commonly seen in men may be explained by the prevalence of abdominal obesity and gastroesophageal reflux disease in men, which is higher in men because of the hormone testosterone. In contrast, breastfeeding and the hormone estrogen, which is higher in women, have protective effects against EAC [2, 10, 11].

### 2.2.3 Race

Although ESCC is predominantly seen in black patients rather than white patients, EAC is more commonly seen in white patients rather than in black patients. Kubo and Corley demonstrated that the incidence rate of esophageal cancer for white men was two times higher than that for Hispanic men and four times higher than that for black men. Some studies have shown that the incidence of EAC development has dramatically increased in white men in the United States, whereas the incidence in the Asian population has tended not to increase [2, 5].

### 2.2.4 Family History

Some reports on the family histories of esophageal cancer disagree with one another. Studies from the United States, Italy, and Switzerland have suggested no relationship between family history and esophageal carcinoma. In contrast, studies from China have suggested that individuals who had a family history of ESCC from a first degree relative had double the risk rate of those who did not. This discrepancy could be related to different environmental factors, such as dietary habits and tobacco use [12, 13].

The individuals who had a family history of other cancers, such as lung, prostate, breast, cervix, oral, or pharyngeal cancer, face a higher risk of developing esophageal cancer. A family history of hiatal hernias may also increase the potential risk of developing EAC. Fanconi anemia, which is a genetic syndrome inherited from autosomal recessive genes, has been associated with a higher risk for developing esophageal cancer. Patients who had these genetic diseases or family histories should be enrolled in an endoscopic surveillance program, where they will be advised to avoid preventable risky behaviors that lead to the development of esophageal carcinoma, such as smoking and/or chewing tobacco and consuming alcohol [2, 14, 15].

### 2.2.5 Genetics

Various genomic defects or molecular changes may induce the development of esophageal carcinoma. Somatic mutations and the deletion or LOH in the p53 gene were associated with more than 83% of ESCC cases. The overexpression of CCND1 in 46.4% of cases, that of CDK4/CDK6 in 23.6% of cases, and that of MDM2 in 5.7% of cases were associated with the development of ESCC. The B cell translocation of gene 3, which works to promote cell-cycle progression, has been observed to decrease the gene's expression in EAC patients [16].

The inactivation of gene p16, aneuploidy, and LOH at chromosome 17 have been demonstrated as high risk factors for the development of esophageal carcinoma. Schulmann et al. suggested that the relationship between Barrett's esophagus/low-grade dysplasia and EAC is related to the hypermethylation of genes p16, RUNX3, and HPP1 [17].

The combination of LOH in 17p, LOH in 9p, and a DNA abnormality can be used to demonstrate a higher 10-year esophageal adenocarcinoma risk [2].

People who had these genetic defects or abnormalities should be recommended to enroll in an endoscopic surveillance program for early esophageal carcinoma detection. These biomarkers can be used to predict the chemo/radiotherapy response and survival rates of esophageal carcinoma and to determine its prognosis [12–15].

### 2.2.6 Obesity

Because of the increasing incidence of obesity in the Western world, the number of EAC cases has also increased. Several studies have shown a relationship between obesity and EAC [5].

Kubo and Corlet demonstrated that esophageal adenocarcinoma risk increases with increasing body mass index (BMI) values, especially BMI values above 25 kg/$m^2$, in both sexes. They also suggested that high BMI values increase esophageal adenocarcinoma risk [18].

A study from Australia demonstrated that individuals whose respective BMI values were over 40 kg/$m^2$ were in the group with the highest risk of developing EAC and were seven times more at risk than those with BMI values below 25 kg/$m^2$ [19].

The relationship between obesity and EAC might be explained by central obesity, which can cause increased intra-abdominal and intragastric pressure, potentially triggering gastroesophageal reflux. Higher levels of reflux could increase the risk of developing Barrett's esophagus [5, 20].

### 2.2.7 Gastroesophageal Reflux Disease

Gastroesophageal reflux symptoms are common, but the incidence of gastroesophageal reflux and that of esophageal carcinoma are not same. A Danish study suggested that individuals who had esophagitis were five times more at risk of developing esophageal carcinoma than healthy populations and that EAC is commonly associated with Barrett's esophagus [21].

Lagergren and colleagues demonstrated that individuals who experienced heartburn, regurgitation, or both at least once a week were eight times more at risk of developing EAC than those who did not and that those who experienced gastroesophageal reflux at nighttime were at an 11 times higher risk of developing EAC. The researchers suggested that if the frequency of symptoms increases, the risk rate of EAC also increases [22].

On the other hand, Solaymani Dodaran showed that no relationship exists between EAC and gastroesophageal reflux without esophagitis. Finally, 40% of patients with EAC have reflux symptoms [5].

If an individual has experienced gastroesophageal reflux disease symptoms for 5 years or longer and has at least two additional risk factors, enrolling them in a Barrett's esophagus screening program should be recommended. Additional risk factors are male sex, age greater than 50 years, white race, central obesity, a history of smoking tobacco, and a family history of Barrett's esophagus or esophageal carcinoma [21, 22].

### 2.2.8 Barrett's Esophagus

One of the well-known risk factors of EAC is Barrett's esophagus, which refers to the replacement of the normal squamous epithelium of the esophagus with a columnar epithelium. Barrett's esophagus is an acquired condition related to repeated esophageal mucosal damage. Patients who had Barrett's esophagus are at a 0.5–0.7% increased risk of developing EAC every year [23, 24].

A patient with Barrett's esophagus has a 30 to 40 times higher risk of developing EAC [2].

The segment of the Barrett's esophagus length and the degree of dysplasia in Barrett's esophagus are two of the major topics discussed in the literature. Rudolph and colleagues have suggested that no relationship exists between the development of EAC and segment length, whereas Weston and colleagues demonstrated that a length greater than 6 cm of Barrett's esophagus caused the development of EAC or dysplasia [5].

In several studies, low-grade dysplasia has been shown to tend to regress after reaching a rate of 60% and 65%. But over 5 years, high-grade dysplasia has a 59–73% likelihood of causing EAC. The risk of developing EAC with Barrett's esophagus from high-grade dysplasia was 6.5% yearly [25, 26].

The best way to improve esophageal carcinoma survival is to detect esophageal carcinoma at an early stage. Light endoscopy with a biopsy or narrow-band imaging endoscopy without a biopsy is the best recommendation for screening for high-risk patients. If Barrett's esophagus with dysplasia is detected or if EAC is detected at an early stage during surveillance endoscopy, endoscopic ultrasonography is recommended to differentiate between mucosal (T1a) disease and submucosal (T1b) disease. If a patient has Barrett's esophagus with low-grade dysplasia, new guidelines suggest that endoscopic ablation therapy (radiofrequency ablation) or endoscopic surveillance at a 1-year interval could be performed [27, 28].

### 2.2.9 Alcohol

Several studies have suggested that alcohol consumption and tobacco smoking are well-known risk factors for ESCC, and they have synergistic effects. In the United

States, 72.4% of ESCC cases are associated with alcohol consumption. The risk rate of ESCC is related to a person's alcohol consumption amount and to the type of alcohol consumed. High rates of alcohol consumption can increase one's risk rate from 1.8 to 7.4 times. An individual whose alcohol intake is greater than 170 g/week is at a higher risk of developing ESCC. Every 10 g/week of additional alcohol consumption increases one's risk by 3%. The type of alcohol is also important. For example, increasing amounts of beer intake (5% per 10 g/week) have been associated with higher risks of developing ESCC. Even moderate amounts of wine intake (<90 g/week) or liqueur intake (<10 g/week) increase the risk rate of ESCC compared to not drinking. If higher amounts of wine are consumed, the risk rate of developing ESCC also increases [29–31].

Moderate intakes of fermented alcoholic beverages such as wine and beer have been shown to decrease the incidence cardiovascular disease, hypertension, diabetes, and cancers such as colon cancer, basal cell carcinoma, and ovarian and prostate carcinomas. Also, moderate intakes of wine decrease the risk of developing Barrett's esophagus and EAC. The carcinogenic effect of beverages is commonly related to their ethanol content and acetaldehyde content, which have mutagenic metabolites in ethanol. A study by the Department of Pharmacology from Spain demonstrated that exposure to ethanol concentrations between 10% and 15% causes cytotoxic effects on the esophageal epithelium in a dose-dependent manner. To reach the protective effect of alcoholic beverages, only those with noncytotoxic concentrations of ethanol should be consumed [32, 33].

### 2.2.10 Tobacco

Multiple studies have shown that smoking tobacco is a major risk factor of developing ESCC and that the risk rate is increased in a dose-dependent manner. Smoking is also a risk factor for the development of EAC. According to several studies, after 10–30 years of ceasing smoking, the risk of developing esophageal carcinoma decreases for former smoking individuals, but not to the same level as that of non-smoking individuals [34, 35].

Smoking and chewing tobacco have strong relationships with 19 cancers, especially lung cancer, oral cavity cancers, head and neck cancers, esophageal cancer, stomach cancer, breast cancer, bladder cancer, and cervical cancer. Thus, ceasing the smoking and chewing of tobacco is the best recommendation for preventing cancer [36].

### 2.2.11 Diet

A meta-analysis of five cohort studies and 27 case–control studies has suggested that the intake of fruit and vegetables decreases the risk of developing ESCC. An inverse association exists between the development of ESCC and the consumption of fruit and vegetables. It could be explained by the antioxidant and detoxification effects of fruit and vegetables. They could also reduce oxidative stress and inflammation [37].

While the dietary intake levels of folate and serum folate were associated with reduced esophageal cancer risks, no interaction occurred between esophageal cancer and the nutrients vitamin D, vitamin E, selenium, and beta-carotene [2, 38].

Zhao et al. suggested that the dietary intake of vitamin C is associated with a reduced esophageal cancer risk in a dose-dependent manner. They demonstrated a significant inverse association between vitamin C intake and esophageal cancer development. Vitamin C intake is also associated with a reduction in oxidative damage to DNA and free radicals [39].

A meta-analysis of 42,475 participants and 39 case–control studies, especially from South America and Asia, has suggested that individuals who drank hot beverages and foods were at an increased risk of developing esophageal carcinoma. This meta-analysis also showed that the consumption of hot beverages and foods is significantly associated with the development of ESCC rather than EAC. Hot liquids may cause a thermal injury to the esophageal mucosa and thereby cause chronic inflammation [40].

Risch et al. indicated that the consumption of high amounts of red meat and low amounts of vegetables was associated with an increased risk of developing EAC, and the consumption of high-fat poultry meat could cause gastric cardia adenocarcinoma (GCA). Daily multivitamin usage, especially high amounts of vitamin C and folate in one's diet, and consuming high amounts of vegetables may prevent the development of esophageal cancer [41].

### 2.2.12 *Helicobacter pylori*

*Helicobacter pylori* (*H. pylori*), a well-known bacteria, was discovered in 1983. *H. pylori* has been shown to be one of the risk factors of developing gastric cancer [42]. Many studies have shown that *H. pylori* infections decrease the risk of developing EAC because chronic *H. pylori* infections induce atrophic gastritis. Decreased acid secretion due to atrophic gastritis may have a protective effect against the development of EAC [43].

## 2.3 Medications

Many studies have demonstrated that nonsteroidal anti-inflammatory drugs, especially aspirin, reduce the risk of developing esophageal carcinoma, mostly EAC, by inhibiting the cyclooxygenase pathway. A meta-analysis that included two cohort studies, seven case–control studies, and 1813 patients with esophageal carcinoma demonstrated that the use of nonsteroidal anti-inflammatory drugs (NSAIDs) or aspirin decreased the development of esophageal carcinoma by approximately 43% [44].

A study from the Netherlands showed that the synergistic effect of combining the use of NSAIDs and statins decreased the development of EAC. The study included 570 patients with Barrett's esophagus who underwent endoscopy. The rate of the development of high-grade dysplasia and EAC on 4.5-year follow-ups was found to be 1.4 per 100 patient-years. The researchers showed that patients who used statins and NSAIDs had a nearly 50% decreased risk of the progression of Barrett's esophagus [45].

A meta-analysis from China demonstrated that statin usage in patients with esophageal carcinoma reduces the risk of cancer-related mortality. The study consisted of four cohort studies and 20,435 esophageal cancer patients. Of those patients, 5319 used statins after being diagnosed with esophageal carcinoma. They had significantly decreased cancer-specific and all-cause mortality rates than patients who did not use statins after being diagnosed with esophageal carcinoma [46].

## 2.4 Additional Risk Factors

Betel nut/quid chewing, which is common and famous in India and other parts of Asia, is used commonly with tobacco and promotes the development of ESCC. A study from Taiwan that consisted of 513 patients who were newly diagnosed with ESCC and 818 healthy patients were compared for the following behaviors: betel nut/quid chewing, alcohol consumption, and cigarette smoking. They showed that alcohol consumption had the strongest effect on the development of ESCC. The combination of alcohol intake, tobacco smoking, and betel nut/quid chewing can result in a 41.2-fold higher incidence of ESCC, and isolated betel nut/quid chewing increased the risk by 2.9-fold [47].

That antireflux surgery may protect against the progression of Barrett's esophagus to EAC is a misunderstood belief. A study from Sweden and a systematic review by Chang et al. showed no difference in the progression/development of EAC between surgically treated and medically treated groups of patients. In a Swedish population study, 14,102 patients who underwent antireflux surgery were compared with healthy Swedish people over the course of 1965 to 2006. Here, 39 patients had esophageal carcinoma, and the researchers found that patients who underwent antireflux surgery had a 12-fold increased risk of developing EAC [5].

## References

1. Bray F, Ferlay J, Soerjomataram I, Siegel RL, Torre LA, Jemal A. Global cancer statistics 2018: GLOBOCAN estimates of incidence and mortality worldwide for 36 cancers in 185 countries. CA Cancer J Clin. 2018;68:394–424.
2. Uhlenhopp DJ, Then EO, Sunkara T, Gaduputi V. Epidemiology of esophageal cancer: update in global trends, etiology and risk factors. Clin J Gastroenterol. 2020;13:1010–21.
3. Arnold M, Soerjomataram I, Ferlay J, Forman D. Global incidence of oesophageal cancer by histological subtype in 2012. Gut. 2015;64:381–7.

4. Pickens A, Orringer MB. Geographical distribution and racial disparity in esophageal cancer. Ann Thorac Surg. 2003;76(4):S1367–9.
5. Falk GW. Risk factors for esophageal cancer development. Surg Oncol Clin N Am. 2009;18:469–85.
6. Njei B, Mccarty TR, Birk JW. Trends in esophageal cancer survival in United States adults from 1973 to 2009: a SEER database analysis. J Gastroenterol Hepatol. 2016;31:1141–6.
7. SEER cancer statistics review 1975–2016. https://seer.cancer.gov/archive/csr/1975_2016/. Accessed 2 Apr 2023.
8. Van Loon K, Mwachiro MM, Abnet CC, Akoko L, Assefa M, Burgert SL, et al. The African esophageal cancer consortium: a call to action. J Global Oncol. 2018;4:1–9.
9. Guo LW, Huang HY, Shi JF, Lv LH, Bai YN, Mao AY, et al. Medical expenditure for esophageal cancer in China: a 10-year multicenter retrospective survey (2002–2011). Chin J Cancer [Internet]. 2017;36:73. https://cancercommun.biomedcentral.com/articles/10.1186/s40880-017-0242-3.
10. Arnold M, Colquhoun A, Cook MB, Ferlay J, Forman D, Soerjomataram I. Obesity and the incidence of upper gastrointestinal cancers: an ecological approach to examine differences across age and sex. Cancer Epidemiol Biomarkers Prev. 2016;25:90–7.
11. Cronin-Fenton DP, Murray LJ, Whiteman DC, Cardwell C, Webb PM, Jordan SJ, et al. Reproductive and sex hormonal factors and oesophageal and gastric junction adenocarcinoma: a pooled analysis. Eur J Cancer. 2010;46:2067–76.
12. Dhillon PK, Farrow DC, Vaughan TL, Chow W-H, Risch HA, Gammon MD, et al. Family history of cancer and risk of esophageal and gastric cancers in the United States. Int J Cancer. 2001;93(1):148–52.
13. Chen T, Cheng H, Chen X, Yuan Z, Yang X, Zhuang M, et al. Family history of esophageal cancer increases the risk of esophageal squamous cell carcinoma. Sci Rep. 2015;5(1):1–9.
14. Jiang X, Tseng C-C, Bernstein L, Wu AH. Family history of cancer and gastroesophageal disorders and risk of esophageal and gastric adenocarcinomas: a case–control study [Internet]. 2014. http://www.biomedcentral.com/1471-2407/14/60.
15. Rosenberg PS, Greene MH, Alter BP. Cancer incidence in persons with Fanconi anemia. Blood. 2003;101:822–6.
16. Huang FL, Yu SJ. Esophageal cancer: risk factors, genetic association, and treatment. Asian J Surg. 2018;41:210–5.
17. Schulmann K, Sterian A, Berki A, Yin J, Sato F, Xu Y, et al. Inactivation of p16, RUNX3, and HPP1 occurs early in Barrett's-associated neoplastic progression and predicts progression risk. Oncogene. 2005;24:4138–48.
18. Kubo A, Corley DA. Body mass index and adenocarcinomas of the esophagus or gastric cardia: a systematic review and meta-analysis. Cancer Epidemiol Biomarkers Prev. 2006;15:872–8.
19. Whiteman DC, Sadeghi S, Pandeya N, Smithers BM, Gotley DC, Bain CJ, et al. Combined effects of obesity, acid reflux and smoking on the risk of adenocarcinomas of the oesophagus. Gut. 2008;57:173–80.
20. Pandolfino JE, El-Serag HB, Zhang Q, Shah N, Ghosh SK, Kahrilas PJ. Obesity: a challenge to esophagogastric junction integrity. Gastroenterology. 2006;130:639–49.
21. Lassen A, Hallas J, De Muckadell OBS. Esophagitis: incidence and risk of esophageal adenocarcinoma—A population-based cohort study. Am J Gastroenterol. 2006;101:1193–9.
22. Lagergren J, et al. Symptomatic gastroesophageal reflux as a risk factor for esophageal adenocarcinoma. N Engl J Med. 1999;340(11):825–31.
23. Thomas T, Abrams KR, De Caestecker JS, Robinson RJ. Meta analysis: cancer risk in Barrett's oesophagus. Aliment Pharmacol Ther. 2007;26:1465–77.
24. Cameron AJ, Lomboy CT, Pera M, Carpenter HA. Adenocarcinoma of the esophagogastric junction and Barrett's esophagus. Gastroenterology. 1995;109(5):1541–6. https://doi.org/10.1016/0016-5085(95)90642-8. PMID: 7557137.
25. Rastogi A, Puli S, El-Serag HB, Bansal A, Wani S, Sharma P. Incidence of esophageal adenocarcinoma in patients with Barrett's esophagus and high-grade dysplasia: a meta-analysis. Gastrointest Endosc. 2008;67:394–8.

26. Reid BJ, Levine DS, Longton G, Blount PL, Rabinovitch PS. Predictors of progression to cancer in Barrett's esophagus: baseline histology and flow cytometry identify low-and high-risk patient subsets. Am J Gastroenterol. 2000;95(7):1669–76.
27. Qumseya B, Sultan S, Bain P, Jamil L, Jacobson B, Anandasabapathy S, et al. ASGE guideline on screening and surveillance of Barrett's esophagus. Gastrointest Endosc. 2019;90:335–359.e2.
28. Richter JE, Falk GW. Advances in GERD updated guidelines for diagnosing and managing Barrett esophagus. Gastroenterol Hepatol (N Y). 2016;12(7):449.
29. Pandeya N, Williams G, Green AC, Webb PM, Whiteman DC. Alcohol consumption and the risks of adenocarcinoma and squamous cell carcinoma of the esophagus. Gastroenterology. 2009;136:1215–24, e1–2.
30. Choi YJ, Lee DH, Do HK, Kim HS, Yoon H, Shin CM, et al. The relationship between drinking alcohol and esophageal, gastric or colorectal cancer: a nationwide population-based cohort study of South Korea. PLoS One. 2017;12:e0185778.
31. Arnal MJD, Arenas ÁF, Arbeloa ÁL. Esophageal cancer: risk factors, screening and endoscopic treatment in Western and Eastern countries. World J Gastroenterol. 2015;21:7933–43.
32. Arranz S, Chiva-Blanch G, Valderas-Martínez P, Medina-Remón A, Lamuela-Raventós RM, Estruch R. Wine, beer, alcohol and polyphenols on cardiovascular disease and cancer. Nutrients. 2012;4:759–81.
33. Guillén-Mancina E, Calderón-Montaño JM, López-Lázaro M. Avoiding the ingestion of cytotoxic concentrations of ethanol may reduce the risk of cancer associated with alcohol consumption. Drug Alcohol Depend. 2018;183:201–4.
34. Cook MB, Kamangar F, Whiteman DC, Freedman ND, Gammon MD, Bernstein L, et al. Cigarette smoking and adenocarcinomas of the esophagus and esophagogastric junction: a pooled analysis from the International BEACON Consortium. J Natl Cancer Inst. 2010;102:1344–53.
35. Gammon MD, Schoenberg JB, Ahsan H, Risch HA, Vaughan TL, Chow WH, et al. Tobacco, alcohol, and socioeconomic status and adenocarcinomas of the esophagus and gastric cardia [Internet]. J Natl Cancer Inst. 1997. http://jnci.oxfordjournals.org/.
36. Larsson SC, Carter P, Kar S, Vithayathil M, Mason AM, Michaëlsson K, et al. Smoking, alcohol consumption, and cancer: a Mendelian randomisation study in UK biobank and international genetic consortia participants. PLoS Med. 2020;17:e1003178.
37. Liu J, Wang J, Leng Y, Lv C. Intake of fruit and vegetables and risk of esophageal squamous cell carcinoma: a meta-analysis of observational studies. Int J Cancer. 2013;133:473–85.
38. Zhao Y, Guo C, Hu H, Zheng L, Ma J, Jiang L, et al. Folate intake, serum folate levels and esophageal cancer risk: an overall and dose-response meta-analysis [Internet]. www.impactjournals.com/oncotarget.
39. Bo Y, Lu Y, Zhao Y, Zhao E, Yuan L, Lu W, et al. Association between dietary Vitamin C intake and risk of esophageal cancer: a dose-response meta-analysis. Int J Cancer. 2016;138:1843–50.
40. Chen Y, Tong Y, Yang C, Gan Y, Sun H, Bi H, et al. Consumption of hot beverages and foods and the risk of esophageal cancer: a meta-analysis of observational studies. BMC Cancer. 2015;15:449.
41. Navarro Silvera SA, Mayne ST, Risch H, Gammon MD, Vaughan TL, Chow WH, et al. Food group intake and risk of subtypes of esophageal and gastric cancer. Int J Cancer. 2008;123:852–60.
42. Marshall BJ, Warren JR. Unidentified curved bacilli in the stomach of patients with gastritis and peptic ulceration. Lancet. 1984;323(8390):1311–5.
43. Islami F, Kamangar F. Helicobacter pylori and esophageal cancer risk: a meta-analysis. Cancer Prev Res. 2008;1:329–38.
44. Corley DA, Kerlikowse K, Verma R, Buffler P. Protective association of aspirin/NSAIDs and esophageal cancer: a systematic review and meta-analysis. Gastroenterology. 2003;124:47–56.

45. Kastelein F, Spaander MCW, Biermann K, Steyerberg EW, Kuipers EJ, Bruno MJ. Nonsteroidal anti-inflammatory drugs and statins have chemopreventative effects in patients with Barrett's esophagus. Gastroenterology. 2011;141:2000–8.
46. Deng HY, Lan X, Zheng X, Zha P, Zhou J, Wang RL, et al. The association between statin use and survival of esophageal cancer patients a systematic review and meta-analysis. Medicine (Baltimore). 2019;98:e16480.
47. Lee CH, Lee JM, Wu DC, Hsu HK, Kao EL, Huang HL, et al. Independent and combined effects of alcohol intake, tobacco smoking and betel quid chewing on the risk of esophageal cancer in Taiwan. Int J Cancer. 2005;113:475–82.

# Achalasia

# 3

Metin Kement

## 3.1 Background

Achalasia literally means difficulty in relaxation. It is one of the most well-known motor dysfunction diseases of the esophagus. It was first described by Thomas Willis in 1674, who defined the disorder as a lower esophageal sphincter (LES) spasm or lack of relaxation. It is caused by destruction of myenteric neurons, which coordinate LES relaxation with esophageal peristalsis. There are two concomitant disorders in the esophagus of patients with achalasia: impaired relaxation of the LES and the absence of peristalsis in response to swallowing. In at least half of the patients, the resting pressure of the LES is also higher than normal values. As a result, a functional obstruction occurs in the LES [1].

Achalasia is regarded as a rare disease with an annual incidence of about 0.3–1.6 cases per 100,000 individuals and a prevalence of 7–10 cases per 100,000 individuals. The average diagnosis age is more than 50 years in most studies. There is no difference between genders in the incidence [2–6].

Patients with achalasia have an increased risk of esophageal cancer, but the absolute risk is low. In a study in which 448 cases were followed for a median of 9.6 years, esophageal cancer developed in only 15 of them (3.3%) after a mean symptom duration of 13 years. Esophageal cancer secondary to achalasia is typically squamous cell carcinoma (SCC), although some studies have also demonstrated an increased risk of adenocarcinoma. Both the American Society for Gastrointestinal Endoscopy (ASGE) and the American College of Gastroenterology (ACG) do not recommend endoscopic surveillance in patients with achalasia. There are limited data on the risk of developing cancer after Heller myotomy. However,

M. Kement (✉)
General Surgery Department, Bahceşehir University School of Medicine, VM Medical Park Pendik Hospital, Istanbul, Turkey


O. Engin (ed.), *Risk Factors and Therapy of Esophagus Cancer*, https://doi.org/10.1007/978-3-031-47024-0_3

available data suggest that patients remain at an increased risk for esophageal cancer [7–12].

## 3.2 Pathophysiology

Esophageal LES pressure is coordinated with both inhibitory (e.g., vasoactive intestinal peptide, nitric oxide) and excitatory (e.g., substance P, acetylcholine) neurotransmitters. There is progressive degeneration of inhibitory ganglion cells in the myenteric plexus of patients with achalasia. Histopathological examination typically reveals reduced numbers of ganglion cells in the myenteric plexuses, and the remaining ganglion cells are often surrounded by lymphocytes and, less prominently, by eosinophils. This situation leads to an imbalance between inhibitory and excitatory neurotransmitters. The result of this imbalance is a hypertensive LES that cannot relax [13].

## 3.3 Etiology

Although the etiology of primary achalasia is still unclear, it is presumed to result from the inflammation and degeneration of neural cells. Some evidence suggest that the disease may be autoimmune. Some variations in the human leukocyte antigen-DQ (HLA-DQ) region have been shown to be associated with achalasia, wherein circulating antibodies to enteric neurons are frequently detected in the affected patients. Immune-related DNA was compared in patients with achalasia, and 33 single-nucleotide polymorphisms (SNPs) were found to be related to achalasia. All of them were located in the major histocompatibility complex region of chromosome 6, which is a location associated with autoimmune disorders such as type 1 diabetes mellitus (DM), multiple sclerosis (MS), and systemic lupus erythematosus (SLE). A study evaluating T cells in patients with achalasia found reactivity to herpes simplex virus-1 (HSV-1), suggesting that achalasia may be triggered by HSV-1 infection [14–24].

## 3.4 Clinical Presentation

The classic symptom triad of achalasia is dysphagia, regurgitation, and weight loss. Physical examination is usually noncontributory in achalasia. Achalasia should be considered if the following symptoms are present in a patient [25–28]:

- Dysphagia to both solids and liquids
- Heartburn, which is not relieved with acid suppression therapy
- On endoscopy, detecting large amounts of undigested food residues in the esophagus and feeling of resistance during the passage through the esophagogastric junction (EGJ)

## 3.5 Diagnosis

According to the American College of Gastroenterology's guideline, a proper diagnosis of achalasia should include the following [29]:

- Performing an esophageal motility test
- Using an esophagram to support the diagnosis
- Endoscopic evaluation, especially, to rule out pseudoachalasia

The significant findings of the diagnostic tests mainly used in the diagnosis of achalasia are provided in Table 3.1.

## 3.6 Esophageal Manometry

Although it can be diagnosed with a conventional standard manometer, a high-resolution manometer should be preferred. Recent studies have confirmed that high-resolution manometry (HRM) is superior to standard manometry and that it has a higher sensitivity to diagnose achalasia. Today, the gold-standard method for esophageal motility dysfunction diagnosis is HRM.

The classical findings of achalasia on a manometer are as follows:

**Table 3.1** Key findings of the diagnostic methods used in achalasia

| |
|---|
| *Chest X-ray* |
| Mediastinal widening and air liquid level |
| *Barium esophagogram* |
| Delay in the passage of barium into the stomach |
| Esophageal dilatation and air fluid level in the esophagus |
| Falling snow appearance formed by food residues in barium solution |
| Aperistalsis in the esophagus |
| Bird's beak narrowing at the lower end of the esophagus |
| Loss of stomach air pocket |
| Sigmoid esophagus |
| *Manometry* |
| Aperistalsis |
| Incomplete relaxation in the LES |
| Increased resting pressure of the LES |
| *Endoscopy* |
| A dilated esophagus |
| Retained food |
| Nonspecific inflammatory changes |
| Feeling of resistance during the passage through the esophagogastric junction (EGJ) |
| *Endoscopic ultrasonography* |
| A thickened circular muscle layer at the LES and through the smooth muscle layer of esophagus |

- Incomplete relaxation of the LES in response to swallowing (integrated relaxation pressure [IRP] above the upper limit of normal)
- High resting LES pressure
- Absent peristalsis, especially in the distal two-thirds of the esophagus

HRM can be used to classify achalasia into three clinically relevant distinctive subtypes, which can guide prognosis and management. According to the Chicago Classification version 4 (CC-4), three types of achalasia have been defined based on the pattern of contractility in the esophageal body [30–38].

**Type I (classic achalasia)**: No significant change in esophageal pressurization is detected as a response to swallowing. In this type, there is 100% failed peristalsis as indicated by a distal contractile integral (DCI, an index of the strength of distal esophageal contraction) <100 mm Hg·s·cm.

**Type II**: As a response to swallowing, a simultaneous pressurization that extends the entire length of the esophagus is observed. According to CC-4, type II achalasia has 100% unsuccessful peristalsis and only 20% of swallows show pan-esophageal pressurization.

**Type III (spastic achalasia)**: Premature and often lumen-obliterating contractions or spasms are detected as a response to swallowing. According to the CC-4 criteria, type III achalasia has no normal peristalsis and premature (spastic) contractions with distal latency <4.5 s and DCI >450 mm Hg·s·cm are seen in ≥20% of swallows.

## 3.7 Barium Esophagram

Patients drink approximately 100 mL of low-density barium sulfate solution. Oblique films are taken at the first, third, and fifth minutes. Narrow EGJ with a "bird-beak" appearance, dilation of the esophagus, aperistalsis, and delayed emptying of the barium are the suggestive findings of achalasia on a barium esophagogram (Fig. 3.1).

Barium esophagogram is not a sensitive diagnostic method for achalasia, especially in the early stages, as one-third of patients can be interpreted as normal. Barium retention is usually detected in untreated achalasia, and the retention should disappear after appropriate therapy [39, 40].

## 3.8 Endoscopy

Upper gastrointestinal endoscopy should be performed in all patients with dysphagia. This is especially crucial in the differential diagnosis of pseudoachalasia secondary to a malignancy. Endoscopic findings are not evident, especially in the initial stages. As the disease progresses, a dilated esophagus that contains residual material may be revealed. A thickened muscular ring with a rosette configuration can be detected in the LES, which typically does not open spontaneously to allow effortless

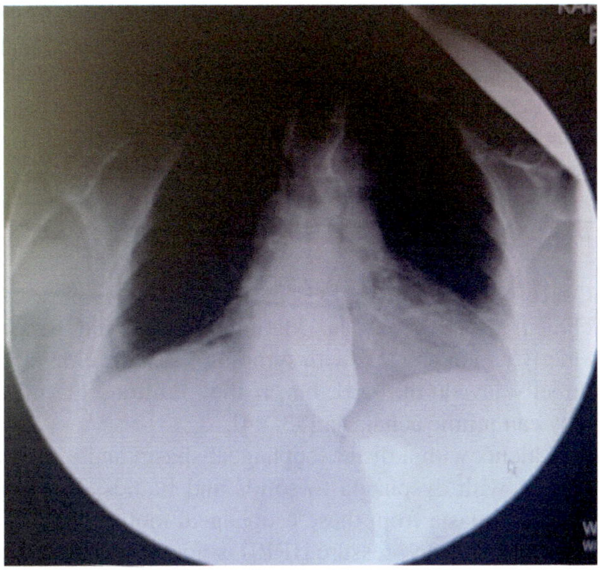

**Fig. 3.1** Bird-beak appearance, dilation of the esophagus, aperistalsis, and delayed emptying of the barium are the suggestive findings of achalasia on a barium esophagogram

passage of the endoscope. Unlike the obstruction caused by fibrotic strictures or malignancies, the LES can usually be passed easily with gentle pressure. Although some nonspecific inflammatory changes including erythema and ulceration may be seen due to retained food and pills, the esophageal mucosa generally appears normal in patients with achalasia on endoscopy [25].

## 3.9 Endoscopic Ultrasonography (EUS)

EUS may reveal a thickened circular muscle layer at the LES and through the smooth muscle layer of the esophagus. Marked (>10 mm) or asymmetric esophageal wall thickening may suggest an underlying malignancy, and this should be confirmed by a biopsy [41].

## 3.10 Functional Lumen Imaging Probe (FLIP)

FLIP is a measurement tool used to measure both diameter and pressure to diagnose and manage various upper gastrointestinal diseases. FLIP was approved by the Food and Drug Administration (FDA). It consists of a catheter (240 mm long with a 3-mm outer diameter) with a balloon mounted on the distal end.

The catheter contains 16 paired impedance planimetry electrodes within the balloon spaced at various intervals ranging from 4 to 10 mm based on bag configuration and length. FLIP can be placed into the esophagus either trans-nasally or trans-orally in an awake or a sedated patient. In achalasia, FLIP reveals a narrowed EGJ segment that has a low distensibility index, and inflation of the FLIP balloon results in abnormal or no esophageal contractions. FLIP may be useful in establishing the diagnosis of achalasia in uncertain cases.

Intraoperative use of FLIP during laparoscopic Heller myotomy or peroral endoscopic myotomy (POEM) also offers the ability to assess the LES myotomy in real time [42].

## 3.11 Differential Diagnosis

Cancers involving the EGJ or tumors that compress from the outside can cause clinical pseudoachalasia. Malignancies should be considered, especially in the elderly and in patients with symptoms that develop in a short time. Tumors may not directly invade the EGJ, but, if they infiltrate the myenteric neural network, then they can mimic achalasia [43, 44].

Patients with a distal esophageal spasm and a jackhammer esophagus may also present with dysphagia to solids and liquids. Esophageal manometry can distinguish achalasia from these esophageal motility disorders, as LES relaxation (integrated relaxation pressure [IRP]) is normal in these disorders [44].

Chagas disease can mimic achalasia. The protozoan *Trypanosoma cruzi* causes Chagas disease that is transmitted to humans by blood-sucking triatomine bugs. It causes chronic destruction in ganglion cells and the myenteric neural network in urinary, gastrointestinal, and respiratory systems. Dilatation in the esophagus, colon, and ureter is detected [44].

Infiltrative diseases such as amyloidosis, sarcoidosis, familial or sporadic visceral neuropathy, diabetes, multiple endocrine neoplasms, and scleroderma also cause pseudoachalasia [44].

## 3.12 Treatment

In achalasia, the primary goal of the current therapies is to eliminate the outflow resistance of the LES. Once the obstruction is relieved, the food bolus can pass through the LES with the contribution of gravity. The advanced technical details of achalasia treatment are beyond the scope of this book. The American College of Gastroenterology guideline recommendations for management of achalasia are as follows [29]:

- When deciding on the initial treatment for achalasia, patient's age, comorbidities, expectations, preferences, and local institutional expertise should be considered.
- It is recommended that the procedures be performed at experienced centers with high volumes.
- Either graded pneumatic dilation (PD) or laparoscopic myotomy is recommended as the initial therapy, if the patient is fit for surgery.
- Botox is recommended for patients who are not suitable for PD or surgery.

- If Botox therapy fails, then pharmacological therapy can be used for patients who are not suitable for PD or surgery.

## 3.13 Pneumatic Dilation (PD)

PD is based on weakening of the LES by rupturing its muscle fibers with the Rigiflex balloon system with an air- or contrast-filled balloon. Pneumatic dilation should be performed by experienced endoscopists. It does not require hospitalization; patients are usually sent home after 2–6 h of observation, and they can return to their normal activities the next day. Multiple procedures are often required for graded dilation. Patients planning PD must have a good status for surgery because perforations related to pneumatic dilation may require emergent surgery.

Pneumatic dilation seems to be a more cost-effective treatment for type II achalasia and has the advantage of being less invasive as compared with POEM or surgery. The initial success rates are high (85% at 1 month) and continue for a while (12–24 months), but effectiveness diminishes over time. Almost one-third of patients have symptom relapse and require retreatment over 4–6 years [45–51].

## 3.14 Peroral Endoscopic Myotomy (POEM)

POEM is an endoscopic method for performing myotomy of the LES, which is a form of natural orifice transluminal endoscopic surgery (NOTES). The usage of POEM is supported by clinical studies and observational data from highly specified centers. POEM is relatively newer than other therapeutic interventions, and long-term data on outcomes are also awaited. Unlike surgical myotomy, POEM does not include any anti-reflux procedures. Therefore, POEM can result in severe gastroesophageal reflux disease (GERD) [52–59].

## 3.15 Surgical Myotomy

Surgical myotomy was first described by Heller in 1913. Today, Heller myotomy is generally performed laparoscopically. Since weakening of the LES can cause GERD and esophagitis, it is frequently combined with an anti-reflux procedure such as a partial fundoplication (Toupet or Dor fundoplication). An significant improvement is achieved in 70–90% of patients with this method. The long-term remission rate is 60–85%.

Surgery poses significant disadvantages, including an extended recovery period and the potential for both early and late complications. These can range from bleeding, perforation, and pneumothorax to vagal nerve injury, infection, and the onset of gastroesophageal reflux disease (GERD). The mortality rate of laparoscopic myotomy is similar to that of pneumatic dilation (about 0.3%).

Laparoscopic Heller myotomy is superior to a single PD in terms of efficacy and permanency. However, the superiority of it over PD is less evident when compared with graded PD, which involves repeated dilations as mandated by the clinical response [60–66].

## 3.16 Botulinum Toxin (BTX) and Medical Treatment

Endoscopic injection of botulinum toxin (BTX) into the LES blocks the excitatory (acetylcholine-releasing) neurons that increase the LES smooth muscle tone. It can be considered in patients who are not good candidates for more definitive therapy with PD, POEM, or surgical myotomy. The initial success rates with BTX are comparable to PD and surgical myotomy. However, relapses are more common and the interval to relapse is shorter in those cases treated with botulinum toxin. With this method, <60% of cases are in remission after 1 year [67].

Medical therapy (e.g., calcium channel blockers and nitrates) is the least effective treatment option in patients with achalasia but should be considered in patients who are unwilling or unable to tolerate invasive therapy for achalasia and for patients who have failed BTX injections.

## 3.17 Prognosis

Without appropriate treatment, achalasia can progress to late- or end-stage disease characterized by angulation, tortuosity, and severe dilatation or megaesophagus (>6 cm).

About 10–15% of cases treated for achalasia will develop end-stage achalasia, and up to 5% of these cases will need esophagectomy according to some series [68, 69].

## References


1. Boeckxstaens GE. The lower oesophagealsphincter. Neurogastroenterol Motil. 2005;17(suppl 1):13–21.
2. Farrukh A, DeCaestecker J, Mayberry JF. An epidemiological study of achalasia among the south Asian population of Leicester, 1986–2005. Dysphagia. 2008;23:161–4.
3. Sadowski DC, Ackah F, Jiang B, et al. Achalasia: incidence, prevalence and survival. A population based study. Neurogastroenterol Motil. 2010;22:e256–61.
4. Birgisson S, Richter JE. Achalasia in Iceland, 1952–2002: an epidemiologic study. Dig Dis Sci. 2007;52:1855–60.
5. Gennaro N, Portale G, Gallo C, et al. Esophageal achalasia in the Veneto region: epidemiology and treatment. Epidemiology and treatment of achalasia. J Gastrointest Surg. 2011;15:423–8.
6. Booy JD, Takata J, Tomlinson G, et al. The prevalence of autoimmune disease in patients with esophageal achalasia. Dis Esophagus. 2012;25:209–13.
7. Sandler RS, Nyrén O, Ekbom A, et al. The risk of esophageal cancer in patients with achalasia. A population-based study. JAMA. 1995;274:1359.

8. Csendes A, Braghetto I, Burdiles P, et al. Very late results of esophagomyotomy for patients with achalasia: clinical, endoscopic, histologic, manometric, and acid reflux studies in 67 patients for a mean follow-up of 190 months. Ann Surg. 2006;243:196.
9. Streitz JM Jr, Ellis FH Jr, Gibb SP, Heatley GM. Achalasia and squamous cell carcinoma of the esophagus: analysis of 241 patients. Ann Thorac Surg. 1995;59:1604.
10. Leeuwenburgh I, Scholten P, Alderliesten J, et al. Long-term esophageal cancer risk in patients with primary achalasia: a prospective study. Am J Gastroenterol. 2010;105:2144.
11. Zendehdel K, Nyrén O, Edberg A, Ye W. Risk of esophageal adenocarcinoma in achalasia patients, a retrospective cohort study in Sweden. Am J Gastroenterol. 2011;106:57.
12. Zaninotto G, Rizzetto C, Zambon P, et al. Long-term outcome and risk of oesophageal cancer after surgery for achalasia. Br J Surg. 2008;95:1488.
13. Reynolds JC, Parkman HP. Achalasia. Gastroenterol Clin North Am. 1989;18:223.
14. Wong RK, Maydonovitch CL, Metz SJ, Baker JR Jr. Significant DQw1 association in achalasia. Dig Dis Sci. 1989;34:349.
15. Verne GN, Sallustio JE, Eaker EY. Anti-myenteric neuronal antibodies in patients with achalasia. A prospective study. Dig Dis Sci. 1997;42:307.
16. Verne GN, Hahn AB, Pineau BC, et al. Association of HLA-DR and -DQ alleles with idiopathic achalasia. Gastroenterology. 1999;117:26.
17. Niwamoto H, Okamoto E, Fujimoto J, et al. Are human herpes viruses or measles virus associated with esophageal achalasia? Dig Dis Sci. 1995;40:859.
18. Birgisson S, Galinski MS, Goldblum JR, et al. Achalasia is not associated with measles or known herpes and human papilloma viruses. Dig Dis Sci. 1997;42:300.
19. Facco M, Brun P, Baesso I, et al. T cells in the myenteric plexus of achalasia patients show a skewed TCR repertoire and react to HSV-1 antigens. Am J Gastroenterol. 2008;103:1598.
20. Spechler SJ, Konda V, Souza R. Can eosinophilic esophagitis cause achalasia and other esophageal motility disorders? Am J Gastroenterol. 2018;113:1594.
21. Goldblum JR, Whyte RI, Orringer MB, Appelman HD. Achalasia. A morphologic study of 42 resected specimens. Am J Surg Pathol. 1994;18:327.
22. Goldblum JR, Rice TW, Richter JE. Histopathologic features in esophagomyotomy specimens from patients with achalasia. Gastroenterology. 1996;111:648.
23. Holloway RH, Dodds WJ, Helm JF, et al. Integrity of cholinergic innervation to the lower esophageal sphincter in achalasia. Gastroenterology. 1986;90:924.
24. Qualman SJ, Haupt HM, Yang P, Hamilton SR. Esophageal Lewy bodies associated with ganglion cell loss in achalasia. Similarity to Parkinson's disease. Gastroenterology. 1984;87:848.
25. Howard PJ, Maher L, Pryde A, et al. Five year prospective study of the incidence, clinical features, and diagnosis of achalasia in Edinburgh. Gut. 1992;33:1011.
26. Eckardt VF, Stauf B, Bernhard G. Chest pain in achalasia: patient characteristics and clinical course. Gastroenterology. 1999;116:1300.
27. Fisichella PM, Raz D, Palazzo F, et al. Clinical, radiological, and manometric profile in 145 patients with untreated achalasia. World J Surg. 2008;32:1974.
28. Spechler SJ, Souza RF, Rosenberg SJ, et al. Heartburn in patients with achalasia. Gut. 1995;37:305.
29. Vaezi MF, Pandolfino JE, Yadlapati RH, et al. ACG clinical guidelines: diagnosis and management of achalasia. Am J Gastroenterol. 2020;115:1393.
30. Pandolfino JE, Ghosh SK, Rice J, et al. Classifying esophageal motility by pressure topography characteristics: a study of 400 patients and 75 controls. Am J Gastroenterol. 2008;103:27.
31. Kahrilas PJ, Ghosh SK, Pandolfino JE. Esophageal motility disorders in terms of pressure topography: the Chicago classification. J Clin Gastroenterol. 2008;42:627.
32. Pandolfino JE, Kwiatek MA, Nealis T, et al. Achalasia: a new clinically relevant classification by high-resolution manometry. Gastroenterology. 2008;135:1526.
33. Roman S, Zerbib F, Quenehervé L, et al. The Chicago classification for achalasia in a French multicentric cohort. Dig Liver Dis. 2012;44:976.
34. Salvador R, Costantini M, Zaninotto G, et al. The preoperative manometric pattern predicts the outcome of surgical treatment for esophageal achalasia. J Gastrointest Surg. 2010;14:1635.

35. Pratap N, Reddy DN. Can achalasia subtyping by high-resolution manometry predict the therapeutic outcome of pneumatic balloon dilatation?: author's reply. J Neurogastroenterol Motil. 2011;17:205.
36. Min M, Peng LH, Yang YS, et al. Characteristics of achalasia subtypes in untreated Chinese patients: a high-resolution manometry study. J Dig Dis. 2012;13:504.
37. Spechler SJ, Castell DO. Classification of oesophageal motility abnormalities. Gut. 2001;49:145.
38. Yadlapati R, Kahrilas PJ, Fox MR, et al. Esophageal motility disorders on high-resolution manometry: Chicago classification version 4.0©. Neurogastroenterol Motil. 2021;33:e14058.
39. Rohof WO, Lei A, Boeckxstaens GE. Esophageal stasis on a timed barium esophagogram predicts recurrent symptoms in patients with long-standing achalasia. Am J Gastroenterol. 2013;108:49.
40. Neyaz Z, Gupta M, Ghoshal UC. How to perform and interpret timed barium esophagogram. J Neurogastroenterol Motil. 2013;19:251.
41. Miller LS, Liu JB, Barbarevech CA, et al. High-resolution endoluminal sonography in achalasia. Gastrointest Endosc. 1995;42:545.
42. Triggs JR, Carlson DA, Beveridge C, et al. Functional luminal imaging probe panometry identifies achalasia-type esophagogastric junction outflow obstruction. Clin Gastroenterol Hepatol. 2020;18:2209.
43. Kahrilas PJ, Kishk SM, Helm JF, et al. Comparison of pseudoachalasia and achalasia. Am J Med. 1987;82:439.
44. Campos CT, Ellis FH Jr, LoCicero J 3rd. Pseudoachalasia: a report of two cases with comments on possible causes and diagnosis. Dis Esophagus. 1997;10:220.
45. Borhan-Manesh F, Kaviani MJ, Taghavi AR. The efficacy of balloon dilation in achalasia is the result of stretching of the lower esophageal sphincter, not muscular disruption. Dis Esophagus. 2016;29:262.
46. Kostic S, Johnsson E, Kjellin A, et al. Health economic evaluation of therapeutic strategies in patients with idiopathic achalasia: results of a randomized trial comparing pneumatic dilatation with laparoscopic cardiomyotomy. Surg Endosc. 2007;21:1184.
47. Hulselmans M, Vanuytsel T, Degreef T, et al. Long-term outcome of pneumatic dilation in the treatment of achalasia. Clin Gastroenterol Hepatol. 2010;8:30.
48. Zerbib F, Thétiot V, Richy F, et al. Repeated pneumatic dilations as long-term maintenance therapy for esophageal achalasia. Am J Gastroenterol. 2006;101:692.
49. Elliott TR, Wu PI, Fuentealba S, et al. Long-term outcome following pneumatic dilatation as initial therapy for idiopathic achalasia: an 18-year single-centre experience. Aliment Pharmacol Ther. 2013;37:1210.
50. Campos GM, Vittinghoff E, Rabl C, et al. Endoscopic and surgical treatments for achalasia: a systematic review and meta-analysis. Ann Surg. 2009;249:45.
51. West RL, Hirsch DP, Bartelsman JF, et al. Long term results of pneumatic dilation in achalasia followed for more than 5 years. Am J Gastroenterol. 2002;97:1346.
52. Pasricha PJ, Hawari R, Ahmed I, et al. Submucosal endoscopic esophageal myotomy: a novel experimental approach for the treatment of achalasia. Endoscopy. 2007;39:761.
53. von Renteln D, Inoue H, Minami H, et al. Peroral endoscopic myotomy for the treatment of achalasia: a prospective single center study. Am J Gastroenterol. 2012;107:411.
54. Inoue H, Minami H, Kobayashi Y, et al. Peroral endoscopic myotomy (POEM) for esophageal achalasia. Endoscopy. 2010;42:265.
55. Swanstrom LL, Kurian A, Dunst CM, et al. Long-term outcomes of an endoscopic myotomy for achalasia: the POEM procedure. Ann Surg. 2012;256:659.
56. Verlaan T, Rohof WO, Bredenoord AJ, et al. Effect of peroral endoscopic myotomy on esophagogastric junction physiology in patients with achalasia. Gastrointest Endosc. 2013;78:39.
57. Inoue H, Ikeda H, Onimaru M, et al. Clinical results in 300 cases of POEM for esophageal achalasia: a single institute registered prospective study (abstract). Gastrointest Endosc. 2013;77:AB121.

58. Von Renteln D, Fuchs KH, Fockens P, et al. Endoscopic versus surgical myotomy for idiopathic achalasia: results of a prospective multicenter study and comparison with laparoscopic surgery (abstract). Gastrointest Endosc. 2013;77:AB122.
59. Li QL, Chen WF, Zhou PH, et al. Peroral endoscopic myotomy for the treatment of achalasia: a clinical comparative study of endoscopic full-thickness and circular muscle myotomy. J Am Coll Surg. 2013;217:442.
60. Hunter JG, Trus TL, Branum GD, Waring JP. Laparoscopic Heller myotomy and fundoplication for achalasia. Ann Surg. 1997;225:655.
61. Vogt D, Curet M, Pitcher D, et al. Successful treatment of esophageal achalasia with laparoscopic Heller myotomy and Toupet fundoplication. Am J Surg. 1997;174:709.
62. Ancona E, Anselmino M, Zaninotto G, et al. Esophageal achalasia: laparoscopic versus conventional open Heller-Dor operation. Am J Surg. 1995;170:265.
63. Holzman MD, Sharp KW, Ladipo JK, et al. Laparoscopic surgical treatment of achalasia. Am J Surg. 1997;173:308.
64. Arreola-Risa C, Sinanan M, Pellegrini CA. Thoracoscopic Heller's myotomy. Treatment of achalasia by the videoendoscopic approach. Chest Surg Clin N Am. 1995;5:459.
65. Luketich JD, Fernando HC, Christie NA, et al. Outcomes after minimally invasive esophagomyotomy. Ann Thorac Surg. 2001;72:1909.
66. Lopushinsky SR, Urbach DR. Pneumatic dilatation and surgical myotomy for achalasia. JAMA. 2006;296:2227.
67. Smith CD, Stival A, Howell DL, Swafford V. Endoscopic therapy for achalasia before Heller myotomy results in worse outcomes than Heller myotomy alone. Ann Surg. 2006;243:579.
68. Eckardt VF, Hoischen T, Bernhard G. Life expectancy, complications, and causes of death in patients with achalasia: results of a 33-year follow-up investigation. Eur J Gastroenterol Hepatol. 2008;20:956.
69. Vela MF, Richter JE, Wachsberger D, et al. Complexities of managing achalasia at a tertiary referral center: use of pneumatic dilatation, Heller myotomy, and botulinum toxin injection. Am J Gastroenterol. 2004;99:1029.

# 4 Risk Factors for Esophageal Carcinoma: Gastroesophageal Reflux Disease and Barrett's Esophagus

Ali Kemal Kayapinar

## 4.1 Introduction

In gastroesophageal reflux (GER), the acid and bile content in the gastric fluid regurgitates into the esophagus in higher amounts than normal due to damage to the anatomic and/or physiological structure of the lower esophageal sphincter (LES) and/or other factors. Furthermore, the regurgitated fluid remains in the esophagus for longer than normal as esophageal clearance is shortened due to esophageal motility disorder and causes macroscopic and/or microscopic injury in the distal segment mucosa of the esophagus. The clinical picture that occurs secondary to this injury is called gastroesophageal reflux disease (GERD), the global prevalence of which has been reported to be in the 8–33% range [1, 2].

Columnar cells take the place of squamous cells in the mucosa of the distal esophagus in response to injuries secondary to chronic GER—a change that was first described by Barrett in 1950 in the literature [3]. The pathophysiology of this conversion has yet to be fully understood [4], although two assumptions related to this change have been put forward: the first is that squamous cells convert into columnar cells (transdifferentiation) and, second, columnar cells develop out of the immature progenitor cells in the esophagus rather than squamous cells (transcommitment) [5]. That said, not all patients with GERD experience this change [5], as Barret's esophagus (BE) develops in 2–20% of all patients with GERD [4].

BE is clinically important as a predisposing factor for adenocarcinoma [5]. Columnar cells undergo a dysplastic change and convert into adenocarcinomas in some patients following the development of BE. BE is believed to develop relatively quickly, and most remain so throughout life. The rate of adenocarcinoma development in patients with non-dysplastic BE is around 0.15% [4].

A. K. Kayapinar (✉)
Department of Gastroenterology Surgery, Izmir City Hospital, Izmir, Turkey



O. Engin (ed.), *Risk Factors and Therapy of Esophagus Cancer*,
https://doi.org/10.1007/978-3-031-47024-0_4

The changes in the distal esophagus are asymptomatic. Adenocarcinoma is generally diagnosed in later stages and has a poor prognosis. GERD and BE are risk factors with the greatest effect on the development of adenocarcinoma. The acknowledgment of the factors that increase GER, the phases of change in the distal esophagus brought on by GER, and the pathogenesis of the development of BE and adenocarcinoma may prevent the development of cancer or increase the chance of an early diagnosis [6, 7].

## 4.2 Gastroesophageal Reflux Disease

GERD is the most common clinical picture encountered in outpatient clinics by gastroenterologists and internal medicine specialists. The prevalence of the reported symptoms was heartburn in 80%, regurgitation in 54%, abdominal pain and cough in 29% each, dysphagia when swallowing solid food in 27%, hoarseness in 21%, hiccup in 15%, and bloating in 15% in a study of 1000 patients with GERD [8]. The prevalence of GERD is around 10–25% in Western populations and <5% in eastern populations [9, 10].

Many factors play a role in the development of GERD, in which the clearance of duodenogastric content is inadequate and slow since the peristaltic movements of the esophageal wall are affected by the condition. The anatomic structure that prevents GER is destroyed in hiatal hernias, in which the supportive tissues of LES are damaged. Therefore, the incidence of GERD in hiatal hernias increases in proportion to the size of the hernia. Obesity causes an increase in intra-abdominal pressure, which, in turn, results in an increase in gastric pressure above the LES. Furthermore, the increased hormone levels associated with the increased adipose tissue (leptin and insulin-like growth factors etc.) lower the LES pressure and facilitate the development of GER. Progesterone and cholecystokinin hormones and calcium channel blocker administrations, treatments including nitrates, consumption of food with a high fat ratio, caffeine intake, consumption of alcohol and spices, and smoking cigarettes all lead to an increase in GER as a result of decreased LES pressure [5, 11, 12].

Recently, the mechanisms behind the histological and immunochemical changes that develop in the esophageal mucosa in patients with GERD have started to be understood. A mucosal defense mechanism starts to work when the distal esophageal mucosa meets the duodenogastric reflux fluid. The first defense mechanism is the prevention of $H^+$ ion passage caused by the tight, adherent, and desmoplastic cellular bonds between the epithelial cells. The mechanism of defense in this process is related to injury-sensitive epithelial cells and the neural plexus in the mucosa [9]. The levels of proteins (disintegrins and metalloproteinases) associated with a weakening of the intercellular bonds have been shown to be increased, and adhesion molecules (cadherin and protein-1) that strengthen the cellular bonds are found to be decreased as a result of the exposition of esophageal squamous cells to acid fluid in experimental studies [13, 14]. Furthermore, proteinase-activated receptor-2 receptors are found to be increased, leading to increased mucosal permeability and the degradation of tight bonds between cells [15]. The mediator release from the mast cells in the esophageal mucosa was found to be increased in proportion to the duration of acid exposure in experimental rat models, and the intercellular permeability ratio was found to be increased in parallel to this increase [16]. The direct damage caused by the acid is made worse by the increased cytokine and other chemoactivator levels. The mediators that are produced as a result of the damage stimulate neural activity and lead to the development of symptoms, which are reported to be increased in proportion to the degree of damage (heartburn etc.) [16, 17].

Gastroscopy will reveal no microscopic pathology in patients with nonerosive GERD, whereas evaluation with electron microscopy can reveal enlarged intercellular spaces in the mucosa. $H^+$ ions passing through the enlarged space into the mucosal cells stimulate the nerve endings and play a role in the pathogenesis of the symptoms [18].

Inflammation in the esophageal mucosa has been shown to be associated with cytokines in patients with GERD in many clinical studies. This process initiates inflammation and results from the stimulation of the immunological pathways rather than the direct effect of acid. Experimental studies have shown that encounters between squamous cells and acid and bile acids result in increased levels of interleukin (IL)-8 and IL-β1, both of which have powerful proinflammatory effects, without initial cell death. Neutrophils and eosinophils are increased by the chemotactic effects of IL-8 and IL-β1, and the degree of esophagitis is found to be proportional to the level of IL-8 in those with erosive and nonerosive GERD. IL-6, monocyte chemoattractant protein-1, IL-33, tumor necrosis factor-α, and prostaglandin E2 have also been found to be increased in these patients [16, 19, 20].

A limited number of Langerhans cells, mast cells, natural killer cells, macrophages, and B lymphocytes are present in the distal esophageal submucosa of normal patients, whereas no neutrophils or eosinophils are present [9].

No erosive lesion is observed in the distal esophageal mucosa in 70% of patients with GERD while the inflammation process is continuing. The neutrophil ratio is <5% in the esophageal mucosa in nonerosive GERD and is 50% in patients with erosive GERD. Granulation tissue and/or fibrin and necrosis are present, in addition to intense neutrophil infiltration in cases of erosive esophagitis [9, 21]. Gastroscopy in GERD revealed erosive esophagitis in 21.7%, in which severe esophagitis (Los Angeles Classification C or D) was present in 9.2% in a national registry study of 543,103 cases. The rate of severe esophagitis has been determined to increase with age (severe esophagitis: 10% in those aged >60 years and 7.7% in those aged <40 years) [22]. Mild or intermediate esophagitis has been shown to develop in 0–30% of patients with GERD in an annual follow-up, and intermediate-level esophagitis was shown to convert into severe esophagitis in 10–22% of the cases during follow-up [1].

As a result of chronic inflammation, basal cells in the mucosa undergo proliferation, papillae elongation, and irregular enlargement in the intercellular space and inflammatory cell depositions are seen. This chronic process sometimes leads to metaplastic changes in patients [9].

## 4.3 Barrett's Esophagus

BE is defined as an acquired condition in which there is displacement of squamous cells in any part of the distal esophagus by mucus-secreting columnar cells; such a change of the columnar mucosa above the esophagogastric junction / Fig. 4.1a for at least 1 cm can be determined by gastroscopy (Fig. 4.1b) [9]. A BE diagnosis is based on the histological confirmation of the biopsy (Fig. 4.2a) results of the four quadrants of visible lesions [tongue-shaped projections/salmon-colored columnar mucosa (Fig. 4.1b)]. When performing the biopsy, two samples should be collected from sites 2 cm above the esophagogastric junction and the remaining two samples should be taken from sites close to the junction. The diagnostic accuracy of more proximal biopsies is decreased [9].

Metaplastic changes in the distal esophagus develop in response to chronic GER. GERD is the main factor in BE development. Inflammation in GERD plays a role in the pathophysiology of carcinogenesis by causing double-strand breaks in the DNA chain [5]. The incidence of GERD has been reported to be 44% in North America, and BE is present in 10–15%. The annual rate of development of adenocarcinoma in individuals with BE has been reported to be 0.3–0.5% [23]. In addition to columnar epithelial changes, the presence of intestinal metaplasia (Fig. 4.2b) increases the rate of cancer development when compared to the cases without metaplasia (annual rate 0.38% vs. 0.22%) [24].

GERD was identified as an independent risk factor in a meta-analysis evaluating GERD, obesity, and alcohol and tobacco consumption in patients with BE [25]. The presence of at least one risk factor, such as male gender (three times the prevalence of females), age >50 years, Caucasian, the presence of hiatal hernia, a high body mass index, and consumption of tobacco, in addition to GERD, increases the possibility of development of adenocarcinoma in patients with BE [4, 5]. No BE was diagnosed in 15% of the patients that developed adenocarcinoma [26].

Abnormalities of esophageal peristalsis, lower esophageal sphincter damage, and excess acid exposure were identified in patients with BE [4, 27]. In esophageal

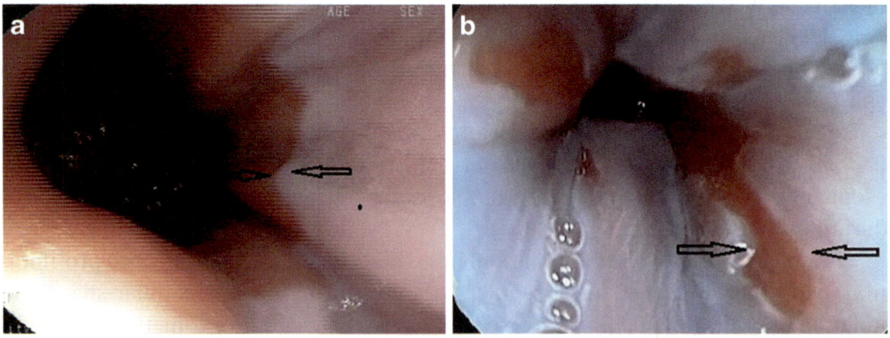


**Fig. 4.1** (**a**) Esophagogastric junction (indicated by the arrow). (**b**) Barrett's esophagus [indicated by the arrow (tongue-shaped projections/salmon-colored columnar mucosa)]

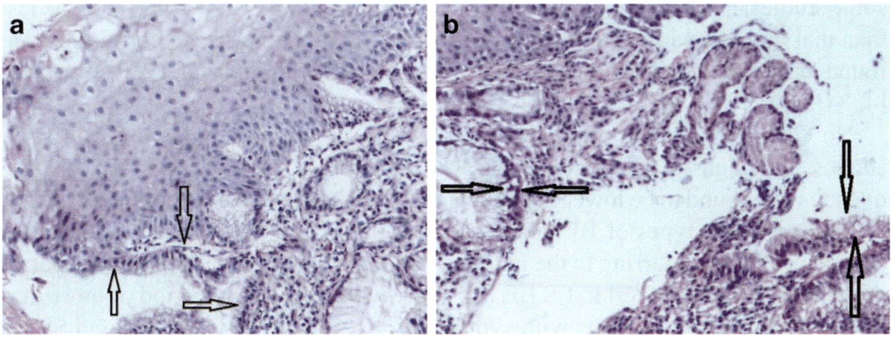


**Fig. 4.2** (**a**) Columnar cells at the esophagogastric junction (cell groups indicated by the arrow) (hematoxylin and eosin (H&E) ×100). (**b**) Presence of focal intestinal metaplasia in Barrett's esophagus (cell groups indicated by the arrow) (H&E ×100)

motility studies, the rate of decrease in distal esophageal peristalsis frequency and amplitude was found to be higher in patients with GERD who developed BE compared to those who did not develop BE., and LES pressure was found to be lower in patients with BE than in those with no BE (45 mmHg vs. 64 mmHg) [28]. It can thus be understood that duodenogastric reflux content stays in the esophagus in larger amounts and for longer durations, thereby increasing the intensity of inflammation, which, in turn, increases the degree of damage. An abnormally high acid level was measured in 93% of the patients with BE using a pH meter, whereas this rate was found to be 75% in erosive esophagitis and 45% in nonerosive esophagitis. The duration of distal esophageal pH <4 measured with a pH meter was found to be longer in patients with GERD and detected BE when compared to other GERD phenotypes [4, 29].

Recent studies have reported a lowered incidence of cancer based on the intense use of proton pump inhibitors (PPIs) [30]. In a study of 540 cases with GERD, intense PPI treatment was shown to decrease the rate of neoplastic change by 75% over 5.2 years [31], although no prevention of bile acid reflux is achieved through PPI use, as it only decreases the acid content of the reflux content. Aspirin or nonsteroidal anti-inflammatory drug use in addition to PPIs have been shown to aid in the regression of BE and prevent the development of adenocarcinoma in many studies [5]. Surgical anti-reflux procedures are effective in BE, although they are not superior to PPI treatment [32]. Despite the fact that no clear-cut results of PPI treatment have been reported in patients with no symptoms of GERD and no esophagitis finding in patients with BE, PPI treatment is still recommended in such patients [5].

PH impedance measures the amount of acid and bile salts in duodenogastroesophageal reflux (DGER) fluid and is reported to be higher in patients with BE than in those without BE. The damage that bile salts inflict on the distal esophageal mucosa is unclear, although PPI treatment has been shown to decrease the severity of the damage by decreasing the amount of acid in the reflux fluid in DGER [1, 33].

The sensitivity of chemoreceptors and mechanoreceptors has been reported to be decreased as a result of the damage caused in patients with BE secondary to GER in some studies, and, so, symptom severity in patients with BE and GERD may be less than that in those with other GERD phenotypes. In other words, no correlation was found between the severity and frequency of the symptoms of GERD and BE [4, 34].

No GERD symptoms were identified in 50% of the patients with BE in some studies, although in patients with GERD symptoms, symptom severity and frequency were found to be lower in patients with BE than in those without BE [35, 36].

There are two types of BE: short-segment (SS) BE (<3 cm) and long-segment (LS) BE (≥3 cm), referring to the length of the metaplastic area [22]. It was reported that SS BE did not convert to LS BE in a study with a follow-up period of more than 5 years [37]. Among patients with symptoms of chronic GERD, LS BE and SS BE have been reported in 3%–8% and 10%–15%, respectively, in the literature [4]. A meta-analysis reported that SS BE was generally not accompanied by GERD symptoms, whereas LS BE was strongly associated with severe symptoms of esophagitis [6]. The rate of development of adenocarcinoma is reported to be higher in cases of LS BE when compared to SS BE [6]. The rate of esophageal motor disorder was found to be higher in LS BE cases when compared to SS BE based on manometric measurements, and esophageal acid exposure was found to be higher in LS BE than in SS BE in pH meter studies. Similarly, pH impedance measurements have revealed a higher rate of esophageal DGER in patients with LS BE than in those with SS BE [4]. Both long- and short-segment BE have been identified in patients with hiatal hernia, although LS BE is more common, which may be attributed to the possibility of SS BE being masked by esophagitis. As such, endoscopy is recommended after the use of PPIs for at least 2 weeks [22].

The development of high-grade dysplasia (HGD) and adenocarcinoma in patients with BE was found to be 0.22% and 0.16%, respectively, in large-series society-based studies [38]. The rate of development of adenocarcinoma in patients with low-grade dysplasia (LGD) has been reported to be 5.7 times that in patients with no dysplasia, the rates of HGD and adenocarcinoma have been reported to be increased by 148% and 112%, respectively, in patients with BE—in other words, the risk of esophageal cancer has been reported to be 30–60 fold higher in patients with BE when compared to the normal population [24, 39].

An increased prevalence of BE was identified in the late twentieth century, continuing into the early twenty-first century. BE was reported in 1.4 of every 1000 gastroscopy applications between 1980 and 1981, whereas this rate was 42.7 between 1992 and 1993 in a study from Scotland, and the rate of adenocarcinoma development was reported to be increased from 1.7/100,000 to 6/100,000 [40]. In another study, the rate of BE in the general population was reported to be 14.3/100,000 and 23.1/100,000 in 1997 and 2002, respectively [41]. The increased prevalence of BE was reversed by the easy access and increased use of PPIs, and a significant decrease has been witnessed in the incidence of BE over the last two decades [10]. In a prospective study of 1109 cases with GERD, the prevalence of BE was found to be 24.3% and 13.5% between 1998 and 2003 and between 2013 and 2015, respectively, and this decrease was found to be statistically significant [10]. That said, no decrease in the incidence of adenocarcinoma has been reported, despite the decreased incidence of BE. Risk factors other than GERD have been suggested to play a role in adenocarcinoma [39]. Some authors have suggested that PPIs would eventually decrease the development of adenocarcinoma in time through the prevention of the development of BE in patients with GERD [42]. The rate of development of cancer in patients with BE is reported to be 05–07% and to be independent of the presence of dysplasia. The prognosis is poor after the development of cancer, and, so, an early diagnosis of cancer is important for a good prognosis [6, 43].

Evidence suggests that screening for BE is not recommended for the general population and only for those who are at risk. An American College of Gastroenterology group suggested cases that should be included in screening programs for BE: patients with at least one symptom of GERD weekly for longer than 5 years, age >50 years, Caucasian, central obesity (waist circumference >102 cm in males and >88 cm in females), cigarette use, and the presence of BE or adenocarcinoma in first-degree relatives [43, 44].

It is recommended that biopsy samples be collected in two sessions. In the first session, the biopsy sample should be collected randomly, as described earlier, and a second biopsy should be performed 2 weeks after the mucosa has healed and should be taken from suspicious areas (nodules, scar tissue, and mucosal irregularities) [9, 43, 45].

Endoscopic imaging methods such as chromoendoscopy or narrow-band imaging rather than classic protocols have been recommended to increase the diagnostic rate of BE and early adenocarcinoma. The reinforcement of the white light used in classic imaging was also found to be effective in early diagnosis [43, 46].

Recently, the improved magnification of imaging optics in addition to advances in technological devices have increased the diagnostic rate of intestinal metaplasia, dysplastic changes, and newly developed adenocarcinomas that previously could not be detected by classical devices and those making use of chromatographic techniques [47].

Endoscopic treatment approaches have been developed for the removal of the BE epithelium making use of such techniques as endoscopic mucosal resection, photodynamic therapy, argon plasma coagulation, and radiofrequency ablation, and complete eradication has been achieved in many patients through these treatment methods [47, 48].

Dysplasia, which is a histological reflection of a DNA abnormality prior to the malignant transformation of cells, may be easily overlooked in biopsies and so is considered a poor marker [5]. The rate of low-grade dysplasia (LGD) was found to be decreased from 100 to 15% based on the evaluation of LGD slides by a field-specific pathologist in a meta-analysis. The authors suggested that HGD is a subjective finding, and, so, slides with dysplasia should be reevaluated by a field-specific pathologist [5, 49].

Gastroenterology societies recommend 6- to 12-month follow-up or endoscopic ablation when an LGD is detected. The rate of development of adenocarcinoma has been reported to be 1.5% in endoscopic ablation and 8.8% in the follow-up group in a randomized controlled study based on the 3-year follow-up of patients with LGD

[50]. Successful results have been achieved recently using ablation techniques, whereas esophagectomy was previously recommended for cases of HGD [5].

## References


1. Chatila AT, Nguyen MTT, Krill T, Roark R, Bilal RG. Natural history, pathophysiology and evaluation of gastroesophageal reflux disease. Dis Mon. 2020;66(1):100848.
2. Gyawali CP, Kahrilas PJ, Savarino E, Zerbib F, Mion F, et al. Modern diagnosis of GERD: the Lyon consensus. Gut. 2018;67(7):1351–62.
3. Barrett NR. Chronic peptic ulcer of the oesophagus and 'oesophagitis'. Br J Surg. 1950;38(150):175–82.
4. Fass R, Teramoto O, Kurin M, Khaless A, Kitayama Y, Shibli F. Esophageal function abnormalities in patients with Barrett's esophagus. J Clin Gastroenterol. 2020;54(6):485–92.
5. Spechler SJ, Souza RF. Barrett's esophagus. N Engl J Med. 2014;371(9):836–45.
6. Eusebi LH, Telese A, Cirota GG, Haidry R, Zagari RM, Bazzoli F, et al. Effect of gastroesophageal reflux symptoms on the risk of Barrett's esophagus: a systematic review and meta-analysis. J Gastroenterol Hepatol. 2022;37(8):1507–16.
7. Hvid-Jensen F, Pedersen L, Drewes AM, Sørensen HT, Funch-Jensen P. Incidence of adenocarcinoma among patients with Barrett's esophagus. N Engl J Med. 2011;365(15):1375–83.
8. Yates RB, Oelschlager BK. Gastroesophageal reflux disease and hiatal hernia. In: Sabiston textbook of surgery. 21st ed. Philadelphia: Elsevier; 2021. p. 1057–78.
9. Mastracci L, Grillo F, Parente P, Unti E, Battista S, Spaggiari P, et al. Gastro-esophageal reflux disease and Barrett's esophagus: an overview with an histologic diagnostic approach. Pathologica. 2020;112(3):117.
10. Hamade N, Weng G, Desai M, Chandrasekar VT, Dasari C, Kennedy K, et al. Significant decline in the prevalence of Barrett's esophagus among patients with gastroesophageal reflux disease. Dis Esophagus. 2021;34(5):doaa131.
11. Fass R, Boeckxstaens GE, El-Serag H, Rosen R, Sifrim D, Vaezi MF. Gastro-oesophageal reflux disease. Nat Rev Dis Primers. 2021;7(1):1–55.
12. Tack J, Pandolfino JE. Pathophysiology of gastroesophageal reflux disease. Gastroenterology. 2018;154(2):277–88.
13. Jovov B, Que J, Tobey NA, Djukic Z, Hogan BL, Orlando RC. Role of E-cadherin in the pathogenesis of gastroesophageal reflux disease. Am J Gastroenterol. 2011;106(6):1039.
14. Okuyama M, Fujiwara Y, Tanigawa T, Watanabe K, Shib M, Tominaga K, et al. Roles of ZO-1 and epidermal growth factor in esophageal epithelial defense against acid. Digestion. 2007;75(2–3):135–41.
15. Kandulski A, Wex T, Mönkemüller K, Kuester D, Fry LC, Roessner A, et al. Proteinase-activated receptor-2 in the pathogenesis of gastroesophageal reflux disease. Am J Gastroenterol. 2010;105(9):1934–43.
16. Ustaoglu A, Nguyen A, Spechler S, Sifrim D, Souza R, Woodland P. Mucosal pathogenesis in gastro-esophageal reflux disease. Neurogastroenterol Motil. 2020;32(12):e14022.
17. Iyengar S, Ossipov MH, Johnson KW. The role of calcitonin gene–related peptide in peripheral and central pain mechanisms including migraine. Pain. 2017;158(4):543.
18. Tobey NA, Hosseini SS, Argote CM, Dobrucali AM, Awayda MS, Orlando RC. Dilated intercellular spaces and shunt permeability in nonerosive acid-damaged esophageal epithelium. Am J Gastroenterol. 2004;99:13–22.
19. Kondo T, Oshima T, Tomita T, Fukui H, Watari J, Okada H, et al. Prostaglandin E2 mediates acid-induced heartburn in healthy volunteers. Am J Physiol Gastrointest Liver Physiol. 2013;304(6):G568–73.

20. Taddei A, Fabbroni V, Pini A, Lucarini L, Ringressi MN, Fantappiè O, et al. Cyclooxygenase-2 and inflammation mediators have a crucial role in reflux-related esophageal histological changes and Barrett's esophagus. Dig Dis Sci. 2014;59:949–57.
21. Souza RF, Huo X, Mittal V, Schuler CM, Carmack SW, Zhang HY, et al. Gastroesophageal reflux might cause esophagitis through a cytokine-mediated mechanism rather than caustic acid injury. Gastroenterology. 2009;137(5):1776–84.
22. Lin EC, Holub J, Lieberman D, Hur C. Low prevalence of suspected Barrett's esophagus in patients with gastroesophageal reflux disease without alarm symptoms. Clin Gastroenterol Hepatol. 2019;17(5):857–63.
23. Siegel RL, Miller KD, Jemal A. Cancer statistics. CA Cancer J Clin. 2019;69(1):7–34.
24. Bhat S, Coleman HG, Yousef F, Johnston BT, McManus DT, Gavin AT, et al. Risk of malignant progression in Barrett's esophagus patients: results from a large population-based study. J Natl Cancer Inst. 2011;103(13):1049–57.
25. Eusebi LH, Telese A, Cirota GG, Haidry R, Zagari RM, Bazzoli F, et al. Systematic review with meta-analysis: risk factors for Barrett's oesophagus in individuals with gastro-oesophageal reflux symptoms. Aliment Pharmacol Ther. 2021;53(9):968–76.
26. Rubenstein JH, Jiang L, Kurlander JE, Chen J, Metko V, Khodadost M, et al. Incomplete response of gastroesophageal reflux symptoms poorly predicts erosive esophagitis or Barrett's esophagus. Clin Gastroenterol Hepatol. 2021;19(11):2284–92.
27. Splittgerber M, Velanovich V. Barrett esophagus. Surg Clin. 2015;95(3):593–604.
28. Campos GM, DeMeester SR, Peters JH, Öberg S, Crookes PF, Hagen JA, et al. Predictive factors of Barrett esophagus: multivariate analysis of 502 patients with gastroesophageal reflux disease. Arch Surg. 2001;136(11):1267–73.
29. Martinez SD, Malagon IB, Garewal HS, Cui H, Fass R. Non-erosive reflux disease (NERD)—acid reflux and symptom patterns. Aliment Pharmacol Ther. 2003;17(4):537–45.
30. Spechler SJ. Barrett's esophagus. In: Principles of deglutition: a multidisciplinary text for swallowing and its disorders; 2013. pp. 723–738.
31. Kastelein F, Spaander MC, Steyerberg EW, Biermann K, Valkhoff VE, Kuipers EJ, et al. Proton pump inhibitors reduce the risk of neoplastic progression in patients with Barrett's esophagus. Clin Gastroenterol Hepatol. 2013;11(4):382–8.
32. Spechler SJ. Does Barrett's esophagus regress after surgery (or proton pump inhibitors). Dig Dis. 2014;32(1–2):156–63.
33. Savarino E, Marabotto E, Zentilin P, Frazzoni M, Sammito G, Bonfanti D, et al. The added value of impedance-pH monitoring to Rome III criteria in distinguishing functional heartburn from non-erosive reflux disease. Dig Liver Dis. 2011;43(7):542–7.
34. Trimble KC, Pryde A, Heading RC. Lowered oesophageal sensory thresholds in patients with symptomatic but not excess gastro-oesophageal reflux: evidence for a spectrum of visceral sensitivity in GORD. Gut. 1995;37(1):7–12.
35. Brandt MG, Darling GE, Miller L. Symptoms, acid exposure and motility in patients with Barrett's esophagus. Can J Surg. 2004;47(1):47.
36. Camilleri M, Dubois D, Coulie B, Jones M, Kahrilas PJ, Rentz AM, et al. Prevalence and socioeconomic impact of upper gastrointestinal disorders in the United States: results of the US upper gastrointestinal study. Clin Gastroenterol Hepatol. 2005;6:543–52.
37. Benipal P, Garewal HS, Sampliner RE, Martinez P, Hayden CW, Fass R. Short segment Barrett's esophagus: relationship of age with extent of intestinal metaplasia. Am J Gastroenterol. 2001;96(11):3084–8.
38. Lagergren J. Adenocarcinoma of oesophagus: what exactly is the size of the problem and who is at risk? Gut. 2005;54(suppl 1):i1–5.
39. Nguyen T, Alsarraj A, El-Serag HB. Brief report: the length of newly diagnosed Barrett's esophagus may be decreasing. Dis Esophagus. 2015;28(5):418–21.
40. Prach AT, MacDonald TA, Hopwood DA, Johnston DA. Increasing incidence of Barrett's oesophagus: education, enthusiasm, or epidemiology? Lancet. 1997;350(9082):933.
41. Van Soest EM, Dieleman JP, Siersema PD, Sturkenboom MC, Kuipers EJ. Increasing incidence of Barrett's oesophagus in the general population. Gut. 2005;54(8):1062–6.

42. He H, Chen N, Hou Y, Wang Z, Zhang Y, Zhang G, Fu J. Trends in the incidence and survival of patients with esophageal cancer: a SEER database analysis. Thorac Cancer. 2020;11(5):1121–8.
43. Elsheaita A, El-Bially MA, Shamseya MM, Ahmed SS, Madkour MA, Shamseya AM, et al. Seattle protocol vs narrow band imaging guided biopsy in screening of Barrett's esophagus in gastroesophageal reflux disease patients. Medicine (Baltimore). 2020;99(8):e19261.
44. Shaheen NJ, Falk GW, Iyer PG, Gerson LB. ACG clinical guideline: diagnosis and management of Barrett's esophagus. Am J Gastroenterol. 2016;111(1):30–50.
45. Kara MA, Peters FP, Ten Kate FJ, Van Deventer SJ, Fockens P, Bergman JJ. Endoscopic video autofluorescence imaging may improve the detection of early neoplasia in patients with Barrett's esophagus. Gastrointest Endosc. 2005;61(6):679–85.
46. Pascarenco OD, Coroş MF, Pascarenco G, Boeriu AM, Draşovean SC, Onişor DM. A preliminary feasibility study: narrow-band imaging targeted versus standard white light endoscopy non-targeted biopsies in a surveillance Barrett's population. Dig Liver Dis. 2016;48(9):1048–53.
47. Kusano C, Singh R, Lee YY, Soh YSA, Sharma P, Ho KY, et al. Global variations in diagnostic guidelines for Barrett's esophagus. Dig Endosc. 2022;34(7):1320–8.
48. Luigiano C, Iabichino G, Eusebi LH, Arena M, Consolo P, Morace C, et al. Outcomes of radiofrequency ablation for dysplastic Barrett's esophagus: a comprehensive review. Gastroenterol Res Pract. 2016;2016:4249510.
49. Wani S, Falk G, Hall M, Gaddam S, Wang A, Gupta N, et al. Patients with nondysplastic Barrett's esophagus have low risks for developing dysplasia or esophageal adenocarcinoma. Clin Gastroenterol Hepatol. 2011;9(3):220–7.
50. Phoa KN, Van Vilsteren FG, Weusten BL, Bisschops R, Schoon E, Ragunath K, et al. Radiofrequency ablation vs endoscopic surveillance for patients with Barrett esophagus and low-grade dysplasia: a randomized clinical trial. JAMA. 2014;311(12):1209–17.

# 5 Esophagus Cancer and Human Papilloma Virus

Şükran Köse, Didem Kıratlı, and Kazım Kıratlı

## 5.1 Introduction

Coronary heart disease is the leading cause of death in the world, followed by malignancies [1]. The two most histopathologically common types of esophageal cancers (ECs) are esophageal squamous cell carcinoma (ESCC) and esophageal adenocarcinoma (EAC). There is a high geographic variation in the incidence and mortality rates of EC types. ESCC is reported at high rates in eastern countries such as Iran, Brazil, India, China, and South Africa, whereas it is observed at lower incidence rates in the United States, Australia, and other Western countries. In Western countries, EAC is seen at higher rates and this type tends to increase in countries where ESCC has been more common in the last 10 years [2–4]. Rare subtypes of ESCCs include basaloid squamous cell carcinoma, undifferentiated carcinoma, spindle cell (squamous) carcinoma (carcinosarcoma), carcinoma cuniculatum, and verrucous (squamous) carcinoma [5–8]. In the report by the International Agency for Research on Cancer (IARC) published in 2012, approximately 456,000 ECs diagnosed in a year are histologically squamous cell cancers [9–11]. The varying incidence rates of ESCC and EAC between countries are related to variable risk factors such as epidemiological and etiological differences, possible dietary habits, and traditional behavioral patterns [12]. ESCC most commonly affects the

S. Köse (✉)
Department of Infectious Diseases and Clinical Microbiology, Dokuz Eylul University Medical Faculty Hospital, Izmir, Turkey

D. Kıratlı
Directorate of Health Care Services, University of Health Sciences Behcet Uz Pediatrics and Surgery Training and Research Hospital, Izmir, Turkey

K. Kıratlı
Department of Infectious Diseases and Clinical Microbiology, Katip Celebi University Ataturk Training and Research Hospital, Izmir, Turkey



O. Engin (ed.), *Risk Factors and Therapy of Esophagus Cancer*,
https://doi.org/10.1007/978-3-031-47024-0_5

squamous cells in the upper two-thirds of the esophagus, whereas EAC associated with Barrett's esophagus (BE) is most common in the lower third of the esophagus, which is close to the stomach, and its incidence increases by 5–10% each year [13, 14]. Considering the survival rates, despite the high technological advances in medicine (both chemotherapy and radiotherapy as well as surgical techniques), the 5-year results are around 20% [15].

## 5.2 Etiology

The etiology of esophageal cancer is not clearly understood. The incidence and diversity of this disease, which varies according to geographical regions and different ethnic groups, indicates that the etiology is multifactorial [16, 17]. Continuous epidemiological and experimental studies are carried out in order to determine the etiology of ESCC, which is a fatal disease with a low cure rate. It is believed that the intake of carcinogens through smoking and alcohol, consumption of hot foods and drinks, various deficiencies of micronutrients such as vitamins and minerals, and the presence of chemicals commonly found in foods, especially nitrosamines, or their precursors may cause ESCC [18–20]. The most important known risk factors for EAC are gastroesophageal reflux (GER) and BE [21, 22]. Although smoking and alcohol consumption are two well-known risk factors for ESCC, it seems that some patients do not have these habits at all. This suggests that some infectious causes, including human papillomavirus (HPV) infection, other than the consumption of carcinogenic foods or hot food, may also be risk factors for the development of ESCC [10]. The low survival rate of EC is actually due to its late detection because it causes dysphagia after the tumor invades the peripheral tissues and shows symptoms at that time. Since an early diagnosis is extremely important in most cancer types and there are no screening methods to detect EC in its early stages, it is important to determine the etiology and take preventive measures to control it [23]. Possible causative agents of EC and infectious agents possibly cooperate in a multistage process to cause this disease [24]. It is well known that some viral infections play a role in various stages of carcinogenesis and cause the formation of malignant tumors. Among these factors, HPV is one of the most important. In fact, 15–20% of all cancers are caused by infectious pathogens. Apart from high-risk human papilloma virus (hrHPV), hepatitis B virus and hepatitis C virus and *Helicobacter pylori*, a bacterial agent, are responsible for almost more than 90% of infectious malignancies. These pathogens are among the preventable risk factors for cancer by preventive public health practices or treatment [25, 26].

## 5.3 HPV

HPV infection is a multifactorial condition that can be transmitted by sexual contact, having multiple sexual partners, indulging in early sexual activity, and coinfection with human immunodeficiency virus (HIV) or other sexually transmitted diseases. HPV is a double-stranded, non-enveloped DNA virus with oncogenic potential that primarily infects basal keratinocytes in the skin or mucous membranes [27–30]. This virus is quite common and highly contagious all over the world. Almost 80% of the population contracts genital HPV infections between the ages of 20 and 30 years [31]. It has been proven by many studies, especially by the IARC, that hrHPV causes anogenital (penis, vulva, vagina), cervical, and some oropharyngeal (including tongue base and tonsils) malignancies. The HPV viral genome has been detected in most of the dysplastic lesions, which are accepted as precursor lesions of cervical malignancies. In recent studies, there is strong evidence that this pathogen, which was previously believed to infect only the squamous epithelium, also shows affinity to the glandular tissue and actually causes adenocarcinoma. In light of this information, it can be said that approximately 85% of cervical malignancies are associated with HPV [25, 26, 32]. Approximately 4.8% of all cancers seen worldwide are due to HPV infection [19]. HPV infection is mostly asymptomatic. Although 90% of the patients clear the virus, in the other 10%, unfortunately, it remains a permanent infection with a high risk of developing cancer [33, 34].

After infection, a five-stage infection cycle begins: 1-infection, 2-protection of the genome, 3-the proliferative phase, 4-genomic amplification, and 5-release of new viral particles. More than 200 HPV subtypes have been detected so far, and they are divided into 2 groups, low-risk and high-risk, according to their capacity to provide cell immortalization. There is also a classification of $\beta$, $\gamma$, $\mu$, and $\nu$ associated with the appearance of papillomas and warts. It was Harald zur Hausen in the 70s who first stated that HPV causes cervical cancer [35, 36]. One of the characteristics of HPV, which is a member of the papilloma virus family, is that it is species-specific and infects only humans. It is known that p16 protein expression is an important marker in the neoplastic process induced by HPV. The replication cascade of the virus is integrally linked to epithelial differentiation, with initial infection of the basal stem cell occurring because of microscopic breaks in the epithelium [2, 18]. Epithelial cell differentiation tightly controls the life cycle of HPV. The natural course of an HPV infection, which is considered high risk, primarily involves the post-replication penetration of the virus into the cells of the basal epithelium, and the persistence of the infection is related to the integration of the virus DNA into the host genome [37–39].

Most cases of cervical cancer are actually due to HPV infection, and HPV-16 is responsible for about 50% and HPV-18 for 20% of the cases [40]. Oropharyngeal cancers due to HPV are primarily detected in the oropharynx, tongue, and tonsil base [41, 42]. Different methods with varying specificities and sensitivities have been used in the temporal process of detecting HPV. Today, in situ hybridization and polymerase chain reaction (PCR) techniques are used reliably. According to the studies, it is seen that types 16 and 18 are the most common oncogenic, followed by types 11, 31, 33, and 52. It is reasonable to assess these types more in studies focusing on malignancies, but, considering that more than 200 types are known, it should not be forgotten that the cancer-forming potential of other untested types may be overlooked [43–47].

## 5.4 Esophagus Cancer and HPV

### 5.4.1 Esophageal Squamous Cell Cancer and HPV

The relationship between HPV infection and EC was explained for the first time in 1982, and many studies on the subject have been published since then [3]. Indeed, the data available for ECs are conflicting, possibly due to incidences that vary between countries. For example, EC is reported to occur 20 times more often in China than in West Africa. In countries with high incidence such as South-Central Asia, southern and eastern Africa, Japan, and Korea, the relationship between HPV and EC appears to be higher than that in Western countries [48]. The existence of a relationship between HPV and ESCC is still unclear. HPV DNA detection rates in the tissue of patients with esophageal cancer vary between 0 and 71%. This wide range of differences may be due to geographical differences and differences in diagnostic techniques as well as their sensitivity and specificity. Two published meta-analyses found a statistically significant association between HPV infection and ESCC with odds ratios of 3.32 and 3.11, respectively [44–47, 49, 50]. In several studies investigating the importance of HPV infection in prognosis, it has been reported that HPV-positive patients with head and neck squamous cell carcinoma have a better prognosis than do HPV-negative patients [51–54]. For example, overexpression of p16 in a cervical malignancy has been accepted as evidence of oncological activity, whereas it has not been confirmed as a safe marker in ESCC [45, 55, 56]. The coexistence of HPV positivity and p16 overexpression was found to be 5% in ESCC [45, 46]. In a study examining 1435 patients in China, it was determined that the presence of the HPV-16 E7 oncoprotein was associated with the risk of developing ESCC [57]. It has also been reported that HPV-16 and HPV-18 are the most common types of genital cancers in HPV-positive patients living in the Kazakh and Xinjiang regions of China and diagnosed with ESCC [58]. In an Australian study conducted by Liyanage et al., with the same number of ESCC and healthy individuals, HPV was evaluated as a risk factor for ESCC [59]. In contrast, a recent study has stated that this pathogen has no place in the etiology due to the scarcity of HPV-related mRNA transcripts detected in ESCCs [60]. In a meta-analysis by Yong et al., a correlation was found between ESCC and HPV in Asians. The same association was not observed in the non-Asian literature [61]. The largest meta-analysis to date (13,401 cases) between the two main subtypes of EC and HPV revealed that hrHPV-16 and hrHPV-18 are potent factors in the etiology and pathogenesis of EC [62]. Another meta-analysis conducted in China concluded that HPV-16 infection may be a risk factor for EC in Chinese patients [63]. In a systematic review and meta-analysis of 3429 EC patients in China, the pooled estimate of HPV-16 positivity was found to be 0.381. The prevalence differed according to the virus detection method, sample type, and geographical regions [64]. In a study involving 8990 patients with ESCC and 174 patients with EA, the prevalence was 22.2% in ESCC cases and 35.0% in EA cases. The most common type was found to be HPV-16 with a rate of 11.4%. As a result of the study, the relationship between HPV infection and EC was found to be significant. However, it was emphasized that more studies are needed, as a strong relationship between cervical and laryngeal cancers could not be detected [65]. In another meta-analysis examining 132 studies in terms of the presence of HPV and ESCC relationship, an increased risk of ESCC was found in patients with HPV. HPV positivity was observed to be 24.8% in ESCC cases [4]. In a meta-analysis of 5755 ESCC cases, the prevalence of HPV-16 was found in 11.67% and HPV-18 in 1.82% of ESCC cases. It was concluded that HPV-16 is a risk factor in ESCC cases, but HPV-18 is not [61]. In another study with 10,234 ESCC cases using different detection techniques for HPV, HPV positivity was found at a rate of 30.6%. A wide variation was found in the rate of cases detected with the virus, which is attributed to geographical differences [66]. In a case–control study of 1223 ESCC cases and 1415 controls, 35% of ESCC cases were positive for HPV. The pooled ratio for HPV and ESCC association was estimated to be 3.04. In this study, the HPV association in countries with a low/moderate incidence of ESCC was more significant than that in countries with a high incidence. It has been emphasized that the doubts about the contribution of HPV to ESCC will decrease with the increase in the number of well-designed studies, that HPV infection increases the risk of ESCC by three times, and that ESCC can be prevented with vaccination, especially in developing countries where a high incidence is observed [44]. In a case–control study, antibodies against HPV E6–E7 proteins (early proteins) and the L1 protein (major capsid protein) were tested in the sera of patients with ESCC. A statistically significant correlation was found between ESCC and HPV-16 ($P = 0.023$) and HPV-6 E6 antibodies ($P < 0.001$). Again, significant correlations were found between ESCC and antibodies against the L1 capsid protein of HPV-33 ($P = 0.047$), HPV-6 ($P = 0.010$), and HPV-11 ($P = 0.0036$). No significant relationship was observed in terms of the E7 antibodies of HPV types [67].

In certain studies, the relationship between HPV and ESCC is not as strong as the relationship observed in cervical and oropharyngeal cancers [45]. This low relationship detected is related to anatomical and environmental factors, for example, high-risk sexual behaviors are less likely to affect the esophageal epithelium than other organs [68]. In developing countries, nutritional deficiencies, low vitamin/mineral intake, and higher hot drink habits are at the forefront, whereas tobacco and alcohol use are more important in Western countries. This may contribute to the differences in the relationship between cancer and HPV [69–72]. In China, HPV positivity was found to be more common in patients with ESCC who smoke and use alcohol [73].

The risk of esophageal papillomas (EPs) transforming into carcinoma is a controversial issue, and there are documented case reports on this. In other words, HPV positivity can be detected in such precursor lesions. In the study by Takeshita et al., HPV positivity was found in 10% of EPs, all of which are in the middle one-third of the esophagus [74, 75].

Some authors think that if HPV is the cause of esophageal papillomas, then it may also be a cause of squamous cell cancer [76]. In an HPV analysis performed on the tissues of 38 patients with EPs in Turkey, HPV positivity was detected in 7 (19%) patients. Three patients were identified as HPV-6, one patient as HPV-81, and the other three patients as HPV-16, HPV-18, and HPV-31, which are known to be oncogenic. No significant correlation was observed between the location of the lesion, reflux esophagitis, age, *H. pylori* positivity, smoking, and HPV positivity. As a result of this study, it was stated that HPV positivity may have a role in the pathogenesis of papilloma [77]. In a cross-sectional study conducted in patients followed between 2000 and 2013 in which Pantham et al. also evaluated EP and HPV positivity, 19 of the 60 patients with papilloma were tested for HPV and 9 were found to be hrHPV-16-positive. There was an approximately fourfold increase between the papilloma patients diagnosed in 2000 and those diagnosed in 2013. With all these findings, it was concluded that HPV infection poses an increasing risk for ESCC in the coming years [78]. Oral HPV positivity was determined as 6.1% (7 people) in HPV tests studied in saliva samples of 114 healthy individuals in Iran. HPV-18 was detected in five people, and HPV-6 and HPV-66 were detected in others. As a result, the relationship of this HPV infection with risk factors and demographic data was not statistically significant [79]. In another case–control study conducted in Iran, HPV DNA L1 gene region analyses were performed in patients with EC and HPV positivity was found in 40% (14 cases) in ESCC and 17.14% (6 cases) in EAC. No positive cases were observed in the control group of this study, which showed 28.57% HPV L1 gene positivity in total [80]. It is known that p16 protein expression is an important marker in the neoplastic process induced by HPV. In the study by Kumar et al., p16 protein expression was observed to be 22% in ESCC and 27.4% in the meta-analysis prepared by Hardefeldt et al. In addition, HPV positivity was found to be 12.2% higher in developing countries than in developed countries [4, 81].

In the study by Antunes et al., it was reported that there was no difference between SCC cases and HPV infection positivity [82].

In another study evaluating 61 patients with ESCC, HPV positivity was found to be 11%. However, the authors stated that it has no prognostic value. In some studies, it was reported that there was no significant relationship between HPV infection and survival [83, 84]. Contrary to these studies, a study published in 2014 showed that HPV-positive ESCC patients had better 5-year survival rates (43.4% versus 65.9%) [85]. Again, Wang et al. found that HPV-16-positive patients with advanced ESCC had significantly better survival than did HPV-negative patients (3-year survival: 55% vs. 21%). In addition, HPV-positive esophageal cancer patients also had a better response to chemotherapy and radiotherapy [86]. Another study similarly found that patients with HPV-positive ESCC had better 5-year survival rates [87]. Kumar et al. found that ESCC patients with p16-positive tumors had better rates of complete remission after chemotherapy than did virus-negative patients [81]. The results are inconsistent between HPV positivity rates in ESCC, possibly due to the differences in testing techniques, sample types, and the sensitivity and specificity of assays [44].

### 5.4.2 Esophageal Adenocarcinoma and HPV

GER disease and BE are among the most important risk factors for EAC, a fast-growing cancer [88]. Studies investigating HPV positivity in EAC yield confusing results. Active HPV infection has been shown to be strongly associated with Barrett's dysplasia (BD) and EAC. There was no relationship found only in those with BE, and these findings suggest that HPV positivity may play a role in EAC [89–91].

For the first time, Rajendra et al. suggested in 2010 that HPV may have a role in the pathogenesis of EAC due to the similar immunogenetic reason in cervical cancer. Three years later, they conducted the first study to prove that hrHPV is strongly associated with EAC and BD [92, 93]. Many studies have been conducted on the active transcriptional activity of hrHPV and its risk of malignant transformation [92, 94–96]. Some systematic reviews and meta-analyses have reported HPV prevalence in EAC ranging from 13 to 35% [65, 97]. Another systematic review reported HPV positivity to be 35% in EAC cases [65]. In a systematic review of 19 studies, the pooled prevalence of HPV in EAC was 13%, suggesting that the relatively low prevalence in this publication may be due to the small sample sizes [97].

In recent years, it has been shown that HPV-positive EAC harbors a different profile of molecular and genetic abnormalities in terms of the biological mechanisms of tumorigenesis compared to HPV-negative EAC. HPV-positive EAC has been found to have somatic mutations. An attempt to prove the interaction between the host and the virus was made with this integration analysis [91]. The high HPV viral load and the integration gradient detected in patients with BD/EAC were found to be significantly associated with disease severity [92]. The majority of BD and EAC patient samples with active hrHPV infection in several studies have found a wild-type TP53 mutation known to be typical for HPV-induced cancers [47, 88, 89]. HPV-positive BD/EAC patients also appear to have a more favorable prognosis than do HPV-negative patients [98].

Despite studies describing a relationship between BD/EAC and HPV, conflicting results have also been reported in some studies. No HPV positivity was detected in 233 EAC tissue samples fixed with formalin [99]. In a case–control study by El-Serag et al., HPV was not found in 127 patients with BE [100]. In a study conducted in the United Kingdom, the presence of HPV infection was not observed in Barrett's metaplasia [101]. In another study, no statistical difference was found between BD/EAC and healthy controls in terms of HPV positivity, and it was suggested that the virus was not involved in the etiology [102].

Detection of HPV in the tissue by PCR is actually a challenging process due to the quality of the tissue sample, storage and storage conditions, inadequacies in the test methodology, the possibility of contamination, and the low viral load in the esophageal tissue. Detecting HPV in fresh frozen tissues is also significantly superior to that in paraffin-embedded samples. The HPV-negative results in EAC may be due to many reasons such as small sample size, geographical and racial differences, and age. Despite all this negativity, HPV positivity rates in EAC patients are reported to be between 13 and 35% [65, 97].

## 5.5 HPV Vaccines

Bivalent (HPV-16/18) and quadrivalent (HPV-6/11/16/18) vaccines produced against common and carcinogenic HPV infections are highly effective in preventing the development of cervical, anogenital and oral cancers [103]. It has been observed that these two vaccines protect individuals against HPV types that are not included in their content but are known to be oncogenic. The vaccine containing nine types (HPV-6/11/16/18/31/33/45/52/58) developed later was also approved in some countries. Currently, studies evaluating the effectiveness of these vaccines in esophageal cancer are not enough. Prophylactic vaccination may have a promising and beneficial effect in reducing HPV-associated ESCC in developing countries, but this requires vaccination of both sexes [104]. In recent years, attempts have been made to develop therapeutic vaccines that aim to induce a T-cell response against tumor-specific antigens. These vaccines are also effective against preexisting lesions. In HPV-infected malignant cells, the oncoproteins E6 and E7 are expressed by the viral genome, and they elicit a strong immunogenic response [104]. Most therapeutic vaccines were developed against the E6 and E7 oncoproteins of HPV-16, and, in a phase II clinical trial involving 20 women with HPV-16-associated grade III vulvar intraepithelial neoplasia, 47% of patients had complete recovery after 1 year [105]. Tipapkinogen Sovacivec HPV vaccine administered to 129 women (diagnosed with cervical intraepithelial neoplasia II/III) provided histological clearance in one-third of the patients, regardless of the HPV type [106].

## 5.6 Conclusions

In conclusion, a growing body of evidence is accumulating as debate continues regarding the role of HPV in ESCC and the correlation between HPV and EAC. Although the picture regarding HPV and BD/EAC appears less blurred, studies should continue for all histopathological types of ECs. Appropriately designed case–control studies with larger sample sizes are needed to detect clear associations in EC, as is the well-known strong association of cervical, anogenital, laryngeal, and oropharyngeal cancers with HPV. It is obvious that ethnic differences, geographical factors, dietary habits, virus detection techniques, and other environmental factors affect the results of the studies, and all these should be taken into consideration. The low viral load in the esophageal epithelium and the high genotype diversity of HPV are other factors that complicate the diagnosis. Studies on vaccination are promising, and the demonstration that therapeutic vaccination can cause reversal even in HPV-related lesions will shed light on personalized therapy based on the virus type in the future.

## References


1. Nagai H, Kim YH. Cancer prevention from the perspective of global cancer burden patterns. J Thorac Dis. 2017;9(3):448–51. https://doi.org/10.21037/jtd.2017.02.75.
2. Agalliu I, Chen Z, Wang T, Hayes RB, Freedman ND, Gapstur SM, Burk RD. Oral alpha, Beta, and gamma HPV types and risk of incident esophageal cancer. Cancer Epidemiol Biomarkers Prev. 2018;27(10):1168–75. https://doi.org/10.1158/1055-9965.EPI-18-0287.
3. Syrjänen KJ. HPV infections and oesophageal cancer. J Clin Pathol. 2002;55(10):721–8. https://doi.org/10.1136/jcp.55.10.721.
4. Hardefeldt HA, Cox MR, Eslick GD. Association between human papillomavirus (HPV) and oesophageal squamous cell carcinoma: a meta-analysis. Epidemiol Infect. 2014;142(6):1119–37. https://doi.org/10.1017/S0950268814000016.
5. Montgomery E, Field JK, Boffetta P, et al. Squamous cell carcinoma of the oesophagus. In: Bosman FT, Carneiro F, Hruban RH, et al., editors. WHO classification of tumours of the digestive system. Lyon: International Agency for Research on Cancer; 2010. p. 18–24.
6. Tripathi M, Swanson PE. Rare tumors of esophageal squamous mucosa. Ann N Y Acad Sci. 2016;1381(1):122–32. https://doi.org/10.1111/nyas.13108.
7. De Petris G, Lewin M, Shoji T. Carcinoma cuniculatum of the esophagus. Ann Diagn Pathol. 2005;9(3):134–8. https://doi.org/10.1016/j.anndiagpath.2005.02.002.
8. Landau M, Goldblum JR, DeRoche T, Dumot J, Downs-Kelly E, Rice TW, Xiao SY, Liu X. Esophageal carcinoma cuniculatum: report of 9 cases. Am J Surg Pathol. 2012;36(1):8–17. https://doi.org/10.1097/PAS.0b013e3182348aa1.
9. Wang Z, Zhang Q, Wu B. Development of an empirically calibrated model of esophageal squamous cell carcinoma in high-risk regions. Biomed Res Int. 2019;2019:2741598. https://doi.org/10.1155/2019/2741598.
10. Abnet CC, Arnold M, Wei WQ. Epidemiology of esophageal squamous cell carcinoma. Gastroenterology. 2018;154(2):360–73. https://doi.org/10.1053/j.gastro.2017.08.023. Epub 2017 Aug 18. Erratum in: Gastroenterology. 2018 Oct;155(4):1281.
11. Goodarzi E. Esophagus cancer geographical distribution, incidence, mortality and their world human development index (HDI) relationship: an ecology study in 2018. World Cancer Res J. 2019;6:8.
12. Recio-Boiles A, Babiker HM. Cancer, esophageal. Treasure Island: StatPearls Publishing; 2018.
13. Arnold M, Soerjomataram I, Ferlay J, Forman D. Global incidence of oesophageal cancer by histological subtype in 2012. Gut. 2015;64(3):381–7. https://doi.org/10.1136/gutjnl-2014-308124.
14. Edgren G, Adami HO, Weiderpass E, Nyrén O. A global assessment of the oesophageal adenocarcinoma epidemic. Gut. 2013;62(10):1406–14. https://doi.org/10.1136/gutjnl-2012-302412.
15. Allemani C, Weir HK, Carreira H, Harewood R, Spika D, Wang XS, Bannon F, Ahn JV, Johnson CJ, Bonaventure A, Marcos-Gragera R, Stiller C, Azevedo e Silva G, Chen WQ, Ogunbiyi OJ, Rachet B, Soeberg MJ, You H, Matsuda T, Bielska-Lasota M, Storm H, Tucker TC, Coleman MP, CONCORD Working Group. Global surveillance of cancer survival 1995-2009: analysis of individual data for 25,676,887 patients from 279 population-based registries in 67 countries (CONCORD-2). Lancet. 2015;385:977–1010.
16. Ferlay J, Shin HR, Bray F, Forman D, Mathers C, Parkin DM. Estimates of worldwide burden of cancer in 2008: GLOBOCAN 2008. Int J Cancer. 2010;127:2893–917.
17. Corley DA, Buffler PA. Oesophageal and gastric cardia adenocarcinomas: analysis of regional variation using the cancer incidence in five continents database. Int J Epidemiol. 2001;30:1415–25.
18. Petrelli F, De Santi G, Rampulla V, Ghidini A, Mercurio P, Mariani M, Manara M, Rausa E, Lonati V, Viti M, Luciani A, Celotti A. Human papillomavirus (HPV) types 16 and 18 infection

and esophageal squamous cell carcinoma: a systematic review and meta-analysis. J Cancer Res Clin Oncol. 2021;147(10):3011–23. https://doi.org/10.1007/s00432-021-03738-9.
19. de Martel C, Ferlay J, Franceschi S, Vignat J, Bray F, Forman D, Plummer M. Global burden of cancers attributable to infections in 2008: a review and synthetic analysis. Lancet Oncol. 2012;13:607–15.
20. Castellsagué X, Muñoz N, De Stefani E, Victora CG, Castelletto R, Rolón PA, Quintana MJ. Independent and joint effects of tobacco smoking and alcohol drinking on the risk of esophageal cancer in men and women. Int J Cancer. 1999;82:657–64.
21. Bhat S, Coleman HG, Yousef F, Johnston BT, McManus DT, Gavin AT, Murray LJ. Risk of malignant progression in Barrett's esophagus patients: results from a large population-based study. J Natl Cancer Inst. 2011;103:1049–57.
22. Hvid-Jensen F, Pedersen L, Drewes AM, Sørensen HT, Funch-Jensen P. Incidence of adenocarcinoma among patients with Barrett's esophagus. N Engl J Med. 2011;365:1375–83.
23. Gholipour M, Islami F, Roshandel G, et al. Esophageal cancer in Golestan Province, Iran: a review of genetic susceptibility and environmental risk factors. Middle East J Dig Dis. 2016;8(4):249–66.
24. Wang J, Zhao L, Yan H, et al. A meta-analysis and systematic review on the association between human papillomavirus (types 16 and 18) infection and esophageal cancer worldwide. PLoS One. 2016;11(7):e0159140.
25. Zeng ZM, Luo FF, Zou LX, He RQ, Pan DH, Chen X, Xie TT, Li YQ, Peng ZG, Chen G. Human papillomavirus as a potential risk factor for gastric cancer: a meta-analysis of 1,917 cases. Onco Targets Ther. 2016;9:7105–14. https://doi.org/10.2147/OTT.S115053.
26. Rajendra S, Sharma P. Causal link of human papillomavirus in Barrett esophagus and adenocarcinoma: are we there yet? Cancers (Basel). 2023;15(3):873. https://doi.org/10.3390/cancers15030873.
27. Hariri S, Unger ER, Sternberg M, Dunne EF, Swan D, Patel S, Markowitz LE. Prevalence of genital human papillomavirus among females in the United States, the National Health and Nutrition Examination Survey, 2003-2006. J Infect Dis. 2011;204:566–73.
28. Chelimo C, Wouldes TA, Cameron LD, Elwood JM. Risk factors for and prevention of human papillomaviruses (HPV), genital warts and cervical cancer. J Infect. 2013;66:207–17.
29. King CC, Jamieson DJ, Wiener J, Cu-Uvin S, Klein RS, Rompalo AM, Shah KV, Sobel JD. Bacterial vaginosis and the natural history of human papillomavirus. Infect Dis Obstet Gynecol. 2011;2011:319460.
30. De Vuyst H, Lillo F, Broutet N, Smith JS. HIV, human papillomavirus, and cervical neoplasia and cancer in the era of highly active antiretroviral therapy. Eur J Cancer Prev. 2008;17:545–54.
31. Chesson HW, Dunne EF, Hariri S, et al. The estimated lifetime probability of acquiring human papillomavirus in the United States. Sex Transm Dis. 2014;41:660–4. https://doi.org/10.1097/OLQ.0000000000000193.
32. IARC Working Group on the Evaluation of Carcinogenic Risks to Humans. Human papillomaviruses. IARC Monogr Eval Carcinog Risks Hum. 2007;90:1–636.
33. Schiffman M, Wentzensen N, Wacholder S, Kinney W, Gage JC, Castle PE. Human papillomavirus testing in the prevention of cervical cancer. J Natl Cancer Inst. 2011;103:368–83.
34. Zandberg DP, Bhargava R, Badin S, Cullen KJ. The role of human papillomavirus in nongenital cancers. CA Cancer J Clin. 2013;63:57–81.
35. Munari FF, Carloni AC, Mariano VS, Syrjanen K, Reis RM, Longatto-Filho A. The relationship between esophageal cancer, chagasic megaesophagus and HPV: myths, tales or reality? Histol Histopathol. 2018;33(11):1135–49. https://doi.org/10.14670/HH-11-993.
36. Nguyen HP, Ramírez-Fort MK, Rady PL. The biology of human papillomaviruses. Curr Probl Dermatol. 2014;45:19–32. https://doi.org/10.1159/000355959.
37. Schiffman M, Castle PE, Jeronimo J, Rodriguez AC, Wacholder S. Human papillomavirus and cervical cancer. Lancet. 2007;370:890–907.
38. Woodman CB, Collins SI, Young LS. The natural history of cervical HPV infection: unresolved issues. Nat Rev Cancer. 2007;7:11–22.

39. Tonon SA, Picconi MA, Bos PD, Zinovich JB, Galuppo J, Alonio LV, Teyssie AR. Physical status of the E2 human papilloma virus 16 viral gene in cervical preneoplastic and neoplastic lesions. J Clin Virol. 2001;21:129–34.
40. De Sanjose S, Quint WGV, Alemany L, et al. Human papillomavirus genotype attribution in invasive cervical cancer: a retrospective cross-sectional worldwide study. Lancet Oncol. 2010;11(11):1048–56.
41. D'Souza G, Kreimer AR, Viscidi R, Pawlita M, Fakhry C, Koch WM, Westra WH, Gillison ML. Case-control study of human papillomavirus and oropharyngeal cancer. N Engl J Med. 2007;356(19):1944–56. https://doi.org/10.1056/NEJMoa065497.
42. Gillison ML, Broutian T, Pickard RK, Tong ZY, Xiao W, Kahle L, Graubard BI, Chaturvedi AK. Prevalence of oral HPV infection in the United States, 2009-2010. JAMA. 2012;307(7):693–703. https://doi.org/10.1001/jama.2012.101.
43. Petrick JL, Wyss AB, Butler AM, Cummings C, Sun X, Poole C, Smith JS, Olshan AF. Prevalence of human papillomavirus among oesophageal squamous cell carcinoma cases: systematic review and meta-analysis. Br J Cancer. 2014;110(9):2369–77. https://doi.org/10.1038/bjc.2014.96.
44. Liyanage SS, Rahman B, Ridda I, Newall AT, Tabrizi SN, Garland SM, Segelov E, Seale H, Crowe PJ, Moa A, Macintyre CR. The aetiological role of human papillomavirus in oesophageal squamous cell carcinoma: a meta-analysis. PLoS One. 2013;8(7):e69238. https://doi.org/10.1371/journal.pone.0069238.
45. Michaelsen SH, Larsen CG, von Buchwald C. Human papillomavirus shows highly variable prevalence in esophageal squamous cell carcinoma and no significant correlation to p16INK4a overexpression: a systematic review. J Thorac Oncol. 2014;9(6):865–71. https://doi.org/10.1097/JTO.0000000000000166.
46. Ludmir EB, Stephens SJ, Palta M, Willett CG, Czito BG. Human papillomavirus tumor infection in esophageal squamous cell carcinoma. J Gastrointest Oncol. 2015;6(3):287–95. https://doi.org/10.3978/j.issn.2078-6891.2015.001.
47. Ojesina AI, Lichtenstein L, Freeman SS, Pedamallu CS, Imaz-Rosshandler I, Pugh TJ, et al. Landscape of genomic alterations in cervical carcinomas. Nature. 2014;506(7488):371–5. https://doi.org/10.1038/nature12881.
48. Koh JS, Lee SS, Baek HJ, Kim YI. No association of high-risk human papillomavirus with esophageal squamous cell carcinomas among Koreans, as determined by polymerase chain reaction. Dis Esophagus. 2008;21(2):114–7. https://doi.org/10.1111/j.1442-2050.2007.00726.x.
49. Matsha T, Erasmus R, Kafuko AB, Mugwanya D, Stepien A, Parker MI, CANSA/MRC Oesophageal Cancer Research Group. Human papillomavirus associated with oesophageal cancer. J Clin Pathol. 2002;55(8):587–90. https://doi.org/10.1136/jcp.55.8.587.
50. Yahyapour Y, Shamsi-Shahrabadi M, Mahmoudi M, Motevallian A, Siadati S, Shefaii S, Shirvani JS, Mollaie HR, Monavari SH, Keyvani H. High-risk and low-risk human papillomavirus in esophageal squamous cell carcinoma at Mazandaran, Northern Iran. Pathol Oncol Res. 2013;19(3):385–91. https://doi.org/10.1007/s12253-012-9590-0.
51. Reimers N, Kasper HU, Weissenborn SJ, Stützer H, Preuss SF, Hoffmann TK, Speel EJ, Dienes HP, Pfister HJ, Guntinas-Lichius O, et al. Combined analysis of HPV-DNA, p16 and EGFR expression to predict prognosis in oropharyngeal cancer. Int J Cancer. 2007;120:1731–8.
52. Syrjänen S. HPV infections and tonsillar carcinoma. J Clin Pathol. 2004;57:449–55.
53. Weinberger PM, Yu Z, Haffty BG, Kowalski D, Harigopal M, Brandsma J, Sasaki C, Joe J, Camp RL, Rimm DL, et al. Molecular classification identifies a subset of human papillomavirus—associated oropharyngeal cancers with favorable prognosis. J Clin Oncol. 2006;24:736–47.
54. Fakhry C, Westra WH, Li S, Cmelak A, Ridge JA, Pinto H, Forastiere A, Gillison ML. Improved survival of patients with human papillomavirus-positive head and neck squamous cell carcinoma in a prospective clinical trial. J Natl Cancer Inst. 2008;100:261–9.
55. Wang L, Li J, Hou J, Li M, Cui X, Li S, Yu X, Zhang Z, Liang W, Jiang J, Pang L, Chen Y, Zhao J, Li F. p53 expression but not p16(INK4A) correlates with human papillomavirus-associated

esophageal squamous cell carcinoma in Kazakh population. Infect Agent Cancer. 2016;11:19. https://doi.org/10.1186/s13027-016-0065-x.
56. Pastrez PRA, Mariano VS, da Costa AM, Silva EM, Scapulatempo-Neto C, Guimarães DP, Fava G, Neto SAZ, Nunes EM, Sichero L, Villa LL, Syrjanen KJ, Longatto-Filho A. The relation of HPV infection and expression of p53 and p16 proteins in esophageal squamous cells carcinoma. J Cancer. 2017;8(6):1062–70. https://doi.org/10.7150/jca.17080.
57. He Z, Xu Z, Hang D, Guo F, Abliz A, Weiss NS, Xi L, Liu F, Ning T, Pan Y, Guo C, Liang Y, Lu C, Zhang L, Cai H, Ke Y. Anti-HPV-E7 seropositivity and risk of esophageal squamous cell carcinoma in a high-risk population in China. Carcinogenesis. 2014;35(4):816–21. https://doi.org/10.1093/carcin/bgt483.
58. Chen WG, Yang CM, Xu LH, Zhang N, Liu XY, Ma YG, Huo XL, Han YS, Tian DA, Zheng Y. Gene chip technology used in the detection of HPV infection in esophageal cancer of Kazakh Chinese in Xinjiang Province. J Huazhong Univ Sci Technolog Med Sci. 2014;34(3):343–7. https://doi.org/10.1007/s11596-014-1280-6.
59. Liyanage SS, Segelov E, Malik A, Garland SM, Tabrizi SN, Cummins E, Seale H, Rahman B, Moa A, Barbour AP, Crowe PJ, MacIntyre CR. A case-control study of the role of human papillomavirus in oesophageal squamous cell carcinoma in Australia. J Oncol. 2014;2014:236482. https://doi.org/10.1155/2014/236482.
60. Cancer Genome Atlas Research Network. Integrated genomic characterization of oesophageal carcinoma. Nature. 2017;541:169–75.
61. Yong F, Xudong N, Lijie T. Human papillomavirus types 16 and 18 in esophagus squamous cell carcinoma: a meta-analysis. Ann Epidemiol. 2013;23(11):726–34. https://doi.org/10.1016/j.annepidem.2013.07.002.
62. Hussain S, Rani J, Tulsyan S, Sisodiya S, Chikara A, Nazir SU, Srivastava A, Khan A, Dash NR, Anoop Saraya A, et al. Influence of HPV infection in esophageal cancer: a systematic review and meta-analysis. Gene Rep. 2022;28:101640.
63. Zhang SK, Guo LW, Chen Q, Zhang M, Liu SZ, Quan PL, Lu JB, Sun XB. The association between human papillomavirus 16 and esophageal cancer in Chinese population: a meta-analysis. BMC Cancer. 2015;15:1096. https://doi.org/10.1186/s12885-015-1096-1.
64. Zhang SK, Guo LW, Chen Q, et al. Prevalence of human papillomavirus 16 in esophageal cancer among the Chinese population: a systematic review and meta-analysis. Asian Pac J Cancer Prev. 2014;15(23):10143–9.
65. Li X, Gao C, Yang Y, et al. Systematic review with meta-analysis: the association between human papillomavirus infection and oesophageal cancer. Aliment Pharmacol Ther. 2014;39(3):270–81.
66. Syrjänen K. Geographic origin is a significant determinant of human papillomavirus prevalence in oesophageal squamous cell carcinoma: systematic review and meta-analysis. Scand J Infect Dis. 2013;45(1):1–18.
67. Sitas F, Egger S, Urban MI, et al. InterSCOPE study: associations between esophageal squamous cell carcinoma and human papillomavirus serological markers. J Natl Cancer Inst. 2012;104(2):147–58.
68. Wong MYW, Wang B, Yang A, Khor A, Xuan W, Rajendra S. Human papillomavirus exposure and sexual behavior are significant risk factors for Barrett's dysplasia/esophageal adenocarcinoma. Dis Esophagus. 2018;31(12):1–7.
69. Tran GD, Sun XD, Abnet CC, Fan JH, Dawsey SM, Dong ZW, Mark SD, Qiao YL, Taylor PR. Prospective study of risk factors for esophageal and gastric cancers in the Linxian general population trial cohort in China. Int J Cancer. 2005;113(3):456–63. https://doi.org/10.1002/ijc.20616.
70. Li Y, Yang H, Cao J. Association between alcohol consumption and cancers in the Chinese population—a systematic review and meta-analysis. PLoS One. 2011;6(4):e18776. https://doi.org/10.1371/journal.pone.0018776.
71. Engel LS, Chow WH, Vaughan TL, Gammon MD, Risch HA, Stanford JL, Schoenberg JB, Mayne ST, Dubrow R, Rotterdam H, West AB, Blaser M, Blot WJ, Gail MH, Fraumeni

JF Jr. Population attributable risks of esophageal and gastric cancers. J Natl Cancer Inst. 2003;95(18):1404–13. https://doi.org/10.1093/jnci/djg047.
72. Freedman ND, Abnet CC, Leitzmann MF, Mouw T, Subar AF, Hollenbeck AR, Schatzkin A. A prospective study of tobacco, alcohol, and the risk of esophageal and gastric cancer subtypes. Am J Epidemiol. 2007;165(12):1424–33. https://doi.org/10.1093/aje/kwm051. Epub 2007 Apr 9.
73. Qi Z, Jiang Q, Yang J, et al. Human papillomavirus (HPV) infection and the risk of esophageal squamous cell carcinoma. Dis Esophagus. 2013;26(1):61–7.
74. Al Juboori AM, Afzal Z, Ahmed N. Esophageal squamous cell papilloma: a not-so-rare cause of dysphagia. Gastroenterol Hepatol (N Y). 2015;11(12):815–6.
75. Takeshita K, Murata S, Mitsufuji S, Wakabayashi N, Kataoka K, Tsuchihashi Y, Okanoue T. Clinicopathological characteristics of esophageal squamous papillomas in Japanese patients—with comparison of findings from Western countries. Acta Histochem Cytochem. 2006;39(1):23–30. https://doi.org/10.1267/ahc.05052.
76. Lavergne D, de Villiers EM. Papillomavirus in esophageal papillomas and carcinomas. Int J Cancer. 1999;80(5):681–4. https://doi.org/10.1002/(sici)1097-0215(19990301)80:5<681::aid-ijc8>3.0.co;2-a.
77. Tiftikçi A, Kutsal E, Altıok E, İnce Ü, Çicek B, Saruç M, Türkel N, Ersoy Ö, Yenmiş G, Tözün N. Analyzing esophageal squamous cell papillomas for the presence of human papilloma virüs. Turk J Gastroenterol. 2017;28(3):176–8. https://doi.org/10.5152/tjg.2017.16636.
78. Pantham G, Ganesan S, Einstadter D, Jin G, Weinberg A, Fass R. Assessment of the incidence of squamous cell papilloma of the esophagus and the presence of high-risk human papilloma virus. Dis Esophagus. 2017;30(1):1–5. https://doi.org/10.1111/dote.12475.
79. Seifi S, Asvadi Kermani I, Dolatkhah R, et al. Prevalence of oral human papilloma virus in healthy individuals in East Azerbaijan province of Iran. Iran J Public Health. 2013;42(1):79–85.
80. Sadeghian Z, Bannazadeh Baghi H, Poortahmasebi V, Sadeghi J, Hasani A, Azadi A, Ahangar OM. Evidence of high-risk human papillomavirus in esophageal cancer in East Azerbaijan Province, northwest of Iran. Can J Infect Dis Med Microbiol. 2022;2022:1099477. https://doi.org/10.1155/2022/1099477.
81. Kumar R, Ghosh SK, Verma AK, Talukdar A, Deka MK, Wagh M, Bahar HM, Tapkire R, Chakraborty KP, Kannan RR. p16 expression as a surrogate marker for HPV infection in esophageal squamous cell carcinoma can predict response to neo-adjuvant chemotherapy. Asian Pacific J Cancer Prev. 2015;16(16):7161–5.
82. Antunes LCM, Prolla JCP, de Barros Lopes A, da Rocha MP, Fagundes RB. No evidence of HPV DNA in esophageal squamous cell carcinoma in a population of southern Brazil. World J Gastroenterol. 2013;19(39):6598.
83. Hippeläinen M, Eskelinen M, Lipponen P, Chang F, Syrjänen K. Mitotic activity index, volume corrected mitotic index and human papilloma-virus suggestive morphology are not prognostic factors in carcinoma of the oesophagus. Antıcancer Res. 1993;13:677–81.
84. Dreilich M, Bergqvist M, Moberg M, Brattström D, Gustavsson I, Bergström S, Wanders A, Hesselius P, Wagenius G, Gyllensten U. High-risk human papilloma virus (HPV) and survival in patients with esophageal carcinoma: a pilot study. BMC Cancer. 2006;6:94.
85. Cao F, Han H, Zhang F, Wang B, Ma W, Wang Y, Sun G, Shi M, Ren Y, Cheng Y. HPV infection in esophageal squamous cell carcinoma and its relationship to the prognosis of patients in northern China. ScientificWorldJournal. 2014;2014:804738.
86. Wang WL, Wang YC, Lee CT, Chang CY, Lo JL, Kuo YH, Hsu YC, Mo LR. The impact of human papillomavirus infection on the survival and treatment response of patients with esophageal cancers. J Dig Dis. 2015;16(5):256–63. https://doi.org/10.1111/1751-2980.12236.
87. Cao F, Zhang W, Zhang F, Han H, Xu J, Cheng Y. Prognostic significance of high-risk human papillomavirus and p16(INK4A) in patients with esophageal squamous cell carcinoma. Int J Clin Exp Med. 2014;7(10):3430–8.
88. Rajendra S. Barrett's oesophagus: can meaningful screening and surveillance guidelines be formulated based on new data and rejigging the old paradigm? Best Pract Res Clin Gastroenterol. 2015;29:65–75.

89. Braakhuis BJM, Snijders PJF, Keune W-JH, et al. Genetic patterns in head and neck cancers that contain or lack transcriptionally active human papillomavirus. J Natl Cancer Inst. 2004;96:998–1006. https://doi.org/10.1093/jnci/djh183.
90. Agrawal N, Frederick MJ, Pickering CR, et al. Exome sequencing of head and neck squamous cell carcinoma reveals inactivating mutations in Notch1. Science. 2011;333:1154–7. https://doi.org/10.1126/science.1206923.
91. Rajendra S, Wang B, Merrett N, et al. Genomic analysis of HPV-positive versus HPV-negative oesophageal adenocarcinoma identifies a differential mutational landscape. J Med Genet. 2016;53:227–31. https://doi.org/10.1136/jmedgenet-2015-103411.
92. Wang B, Rajendra S, Pavey D, Sharma P, Merrett N, Wu X, Snow ET, Kumbhari V, Ball MJ, Robertson IK. Viral load and integration status of high-risk human papillomaviruses in the Barrett's metaplasia-dysplasia-adenocarcinoma sequence. Am J Gastroenterol. 2013;108(11):1814–6. https://doi.org/10.1038/ajg.2013.206. PMID: 24192963.
93. Rajendra S, Wang B, Snow ET, Sharma P, Pavey D, Merrett N, Ball MJ, Brain T, Fernando R, Robertson IK. Transcriptionally active human papillomavirus is strongly associated with Barrett's dysplasia and esophageal adenocarcinoma. Am J Gastroenterol. 2013;108:1082–93.
94. Al-Haddad S, El-Zimaity H, Hafezi-Bakhtiari S, Rajendra S, Streutker CJ, Vajpeyi R, Wang B. Infection and esophageal cancer. Ann N Y Acad Sci. 2014;1325:187–96.
95. Rajendra S, Robertson IK. Barrett's oesophagus; acid and the human papilloma virus? J Clin Virol. 2009;44:176.
96. Nicholson AM, Graham TA, Simpson A, Humphries A, Burch N, Rodriguez-Justo M, Novelli M, Harrison R, Wright NA, McDonald SA, et al. Barrett's metaplasia glands are clonal, contain multiple stem cells and share a common squamous progenitor. Gut. 2012;61:1380–9.
97. Kunzmann AT, Graham S, McShane CM, Doyle J, Tommasino M, Johnston B, Jamison J, James JA, McManus D, Anderson LA. The prevalence of viral agents in esophageal adenocarcinoma and Barrett's esophagus: a systematic review. Eur J Gastroenterol Hepatol. 2017;29(7):817–25. https://doi.org/10.1097/MEG.0000000000000868.
98. Rajendra S, Xuan W, Merrett N, Sharma P, Sharma P, Pavey D, Yang T, Santos LD, Sharaiha O, Pande G, Cosman P, Wu X, Wang B. Survival rates for patients with Barrett high-grade dysplasia and esophageal adenocarcinoma with or without human papillomavirus infection. JAMA Netw Open. 2018;1(4):e181054. https://doi.org/10.1001/jamanetworkopen.2018.1054.
99. Antonsson A, Knight L, Whiteman DC, Australian Cancer Study. Human papillomavirus not detected in esophageal adenocarcinoma tumor specimens. Cancer Epidemiol. 2016;41:96–8. https://doi.org/10.1016/j.canep.2016.01.014.
100. El-Serag HB, Hollier JM, Gravitt P, Alsarraj A, Younes M. Human papillomavirus and the risk of Barrett's esophagus. Dis Esophagus. 2013;26(5):517–21. https://doi.org/10.1111/j.1442-2050.2012.01392.x. Epub 2012 Aug 14.
101. Rai N, Jenkins GJ, McAdam E, Hibbitts SJ, Fiander AN, Powell NG. Human papillomavirus infection in Barrett's oesophagus in the UK: an infrequent event. J Clin Virol. 2008;43(2):250–2. https://doi.org/10.1016/j.jcv.2008.07.004.
102. Iyer A, Rajendran V, Adamson CS, Peng Z, Cooper K, Evans MF. Human papillomavirus is detectable in Barrett's esophagus and esophageal carcinoma but is unlikely to be of any etiologic significance. J Clin Virol. 2011;50(3):205–8. https://doi.org/10.1016/j.jcv.2010.11.015.
103. Skinner SR, Apter D, De Carvalho N, Harper DM, Konno R, Paavonen J, Romanowski B, Roteli-Martins C, Burlet N, Mihalyi A, Struyf F. Human papillomavirus (HPV)-16/18 AS04-adjuvanted vaccine for the prevention of cervical cancer and HPV-related diseases. Expert Rev Vaccines. 2016;15(3):367–87. https://doi.org/10.1586/14760584.2016.1124763.
104. Best SR, Niparko KJ, Pai SI. Biology of human papillomavirus infection and immune therapy for HPV-related head and neck cancers. Otolaryngol Clin North Am. 2012;45(4):807–22. https://doi.org/10.1016/j.otc.2012.04.005.
105. Kenter GG, Welters MJ, Valentijn AR, Lowik MJ, Berends-van der Meer DM, Vloon AP, Essahsah F, Fathers LM, Offringa R, Drijfhout JW, Wafelman AR, Oostendorp J, Fleuren GJ, van der Burg SH, Melief CJ. Vaccination against HPV-16 oncoproteins for vulvar

intraepithelial neoplasia. N Engl J Med. 2009;361(19):1838–47. https://doi.org/10.1056/NEJMoa0810097.

106. Harper DM, Nieminen P, Donders G, Einstein MH, Garcia F, Huh WK, Stoler MH, Glavini K, Attley G, Limacher JM, Bastien B, Calleja E. The efficacy and safety of Tipapkinogen Sovacivec therapeutic HPV vaccine in cervical intraepithelial neoplasia grades 2 and 3: randomized controlled phase II trial with 2.5 years of follow-up. Gynecol Oncol. 2019;153(3):521–9. https://doi.org/10.1016/j.ygyno.2019.03.250.

# Genetic Overview of Esophageal Cancer

# 6

Berk Ozyilmaz and Taha Resid Ozdemir

## 6.1 Esophageal Cancer Epidemiology and Etiology from a Genetic Perspective

Cancer is a polygenic, multifactorial disease. It occurs as a result of the interaction of genetic factors with environmental factors. When evaluated in terms of cancer development risk, while genetic predisposition is more important in some cancer types, environmental factors and lifestyle are more important in some other cancer types. One of the most interesting examples of this situation is esophageal cancer (EC) and colorectal cancer, both of which are gastrointestinal cancers. As will be discussed in more detail in the following sections, esophageal cancer is a type of cancer in which genetic predisposition plays a role in etiology; however, environmental factors and lifestyle play a much more important role. On the other hand, in familial adenomatous polyposis (FAP), which occurs as a result of adenomatous polyposis coli (APC) gene mutations, the risk of developing colorectal cancer throughout life due to these mutations increases up to 95%; thus, this type of colorectal cancer mainly occurs based on genetic predisposition [1].

Cancers are defined according to the cell type they originate from. Carcinomas arise from epithelial cells; however, since epithelial cells are also specialized for different functions, they are classified according to these subtasks. Cancers of epithelial cells with tissue-covering function constitute squamous cell carcinomas, and those with specialized functions such as producing and releasing certain products into body channels and cavities constitute adenocarcinomas [2].

Esophageal cancer (EC) is the seventh most common malignancy worldwide, with more than 500,000 new cases diagnosed each year. The survival rate of EC patients is limited, and it ranks sixth among the causes of death from cancer. The

B. Ozyilmaz (✉) · T. R. Ozdemir
Department of Medical Genetics, University of Health Sciences, Izmir Faculty of Medicine, Izmir City Hospital, Izmir, Turkey



O. Engin (ed.), *Risk Factors and Therapy of Esophagus Cancer*,
https://doi.org/10.1007/978-3-031-47024-0_6

genetic and environmental factors mentioned in the previous section can also determine the histopathological subtype of developing cancers. The majority of esophageal cancers (ECs) are esophageal squamous cell carcinomas (ESCCs) or esophageal adenocarcinomas (EACs). The epidemiological and etiological bases of the histopathological subgroups in EC are different from each other; they have different molecular genetic changes, different risk factors, and even different geographical backgrounds [3].

### 6.1.1 Esophageal Squamous Cell Carcinoma (ESCC)

**ESCC** is the most common type of EC worldwide. It is widely seen in low- and middle-income countries, especially in north-central China, northeastern Iran, South America, Central Asia, and East Africa. Tobacco use, alcohol consumption, a low socioeconomic status, and intake of pickled vegetables and hot foods have been determined as the main factors that increase the frequency of ESCC in South America. N-nitroso compounds, which are especially concentrated in pickled vegetables, are DNA alkylating agents that have shown to be carcinogenic in a mutagenic manner. Apart from that, fungi that produce toxins such as aflatoxin can reduce nitrates to nitroso compounds and show mutagenic and carcinogenic effects by DNA alkylation. Another food-related risk factor is areca nut wrapped in betel leaves, which are common in Asian regions. The high amount of copper ingested as a result of the use of this product plays a role in the development of both esophageal and other gastrointestinal cancers [4].

In East Africa, both high incidence and onset at a young age (one-third of all cases before the age of 45) suggest that it has a specific etiological background. Studies conducted to identify some specific etiologies have added factors such as poor oral hygiene, pest infection in grains and nuts, and exposure to tobacco smoke, in addition to the risk factors in other regions [5].

The fact that ESCC is common in certain geographical regions and that its frequency is more concentrated in some areas within these regions suggests that some genetic factors also play an effective role in the development of ESCC in addition to all these environmental factors. These germline and somatic changes will be discussed in detail in the following sections [6].

### 6.1.2 Esophageal Adenocarcinomas (EAC)

In the last 30 years, the dominant position of ESCC in countries with low socioeconomic conditions has been usurped by EAC, perhaps due to global socioeconomic developments. From another point of view, EAC has shifted its dominance from Western countries to developing eastern countries. In particular, some risk factors brought about by socioeconomic relief have primarily targeted male Caucasian individuals. In fact, socioeconomic improvement alone can be seen as the main risk factor, since most EACs in the United States are caused by Barrett's metaplasia, which is associated with smoking, a high body mass index, gastroesophageal reflux (GER) disease (GERD), and low fruit and vegetable consumption [7].

The majority of EACs arise from Barrett's metaplasia, a pathology mainly associated with smoking; however, genetic factors also play a role in its etiology. Barrett's esophagus (BE) is a condition with an acquired metaplastic epithelial change in the esophagus resulting from gastroesophageal reflux (GER). The transformation of the normal squamous epithelium of the esophagus into a metaplastic columnar epithelium, which can lead to EAC with BE progression, is a complex process involving multiple pathways, including genetic and epigenetic modifications [8].

## 6.2 Genetic Etiology of Esophageal Cancer and Cancer Predisposition by Germline Mutations

**Germline mutations** are inherited. A person with this mutation has a high probability of inheriting this genetic change from one of their parents and carrying it in all their body cells. Since germline mutations are hereditary, there is a 50% probability that they will be passed on to the next generation. The entire genome is copied trillions of times during cell reproduction, which takes place as living organisms transform from a single-cell embryo into a complex organism. However, errors inevitably occur in newly formed DNA sequences. Mutations that occur in the DNA sequence of body cells at a particular moment in the organism's life cycle are defined as **somatic mutations**. Somatic mutations are neither inherited nor passed on to future generations. Using DNA repair mechanisms, attempts have been made to correct these mutations, which inevitably occur continuously. If there is damage that is too severe to be repaired, then that cell is directed to controlled cell death, i.e., "apoptosis." If the DNA repair mechanisms or the apoptosis process do not work and the cell continues to live, then these cells may become cancerous [1].

In this section, germline mutations in the etiology of esophageal cancer, with another definition, and genetic changes that cause esophageal cancer predisposition will be discussed. Somatic mutations used in the diagnosis, prognosis, and treatment planning of this disease will be discussed in the following sections.

Esophageal squamous cell carcinomas (ESCCs) and esophageal adenocarcinomas (ESCs), which are clearly separated epidemiologically and etiologically, are also differentiated in terms of genetic predisposition.

### 6.2.1 Germline Genetic Changes and Hereditary Predisposition to Esophageal Squamous Cell Carcinomas

Despite numerous studies on identifying germline changes that may cause genetic susceptibility to this disease, there is no clear list of the underlying genes. For this reason, it would be a correct approach to use the data obtained from some of these studies as a reference. In this section, data from these studies will be compiled.

In a study conducted in 2021, a mutational signature analysis was performed in 552 ESCC cases. As a result of this study, the 30-kb deletion (rs12628403) detected in the *APOBEC3* gene was associated with both SSCC cancer risk and APOBEC-related mutagenesis. In this study, the 30-kb deletion in the *APOBEC3* gene was detected in 48 (27%) of 552 ESCC patients and 15 of them were even found to be homozygous. This deletion in the *APOBEC3* gene has also been associated with an increased risk for breast and ovarian cancers as well as APOBEC mutagenesis in breast tumors. Second, a single-nucleotide polymorphism (SNP) was found to be associated with ESCC risk. The *ALDH2* gene is involved in alcohol metabolism and catalyzes the conversion of acetaldehyde to acetic acid. Its function in metabolizing acetaldehyde and preventing toxicity-related symptoms is critical, especially following alcohol consumption. The rs671(G>A) SNP, a germline variant in *ALDH2*, restricts the gene's function in alcohol metabolism. Detected almost exclusively in Chinese and Japanese populations, this SNP further increases the risk of alcohol consumption-related ESCC. In addition, it has been shown that germline mutations of the *BRCA2* gene are associated with an increased risk of SSCC [9].

In the study carried out in 2019, whole exome sequencing (WES) was performed to detect germline mutations in 77 patients with SSCC and the results are presented. In this study, 84 different (pathogenic/probably pathogenic) variants were detected in 46 (59.7%) of 77 samples with WES. As a result, it was seen that the p.Gln319* variant in the *CYP21A2* gene was 6.5% (5/77), the c.194+2T>C variant in the *SPINK1* gene was 2.6% (2/77), the p.Glu1048* variant in the *OTOA* gene was 2.6% (2/77), the c.863+1G>T variant in the *PRAMEF7/8* gene was 2.6% (2/77), and the c.866+2T>C variant in the *PRAMEF10/33P* gene was 2.6% (2/77). Apart from these pathogenic/likely pathogenic variants, although it is classified as a variant of uncertain significance (VUS), a rare variant of the *TP53* gene (p.V197E), which is believed to have a clinical effect, has also been detected [10].

In a meta-analysis conducted in 2021, 571 ESCC cases from public databases, the 1000 Genomes Project database from East Asia, and the China Metabolic Analytics Project database were included in the analysis. In this meta-analysis, it was reported that 157 mutations were detected in 75 different cancer susceptibility genes in 25.0% (143/571) of 571 SSCC cases and that more than 5 mutations were detected in each of the 6 genes with the most frequent mutations: *TP53* ($n = 15$), *GJB2* ($n = 8$), *BRCA2* ($n = 6$), *RECQL4* ($n = 6$), *MUTYH* ($n = 6$), and *PMS2* ($n = 5$). Other important data obtained in the study show how the germline mutation carriers transform into cancer in their tissues with the double-hit mechanism. Accordingly, 84 double-hit events (16 germline/somatic double-hit events and 68 somatic/somatic double-hit events) occurred in 18 tumor suppressor genes of 83 patients [11].

Although the examples of these studies in the literature can be multiplied, the data obtained from 1200 patients with ESCC in the 3 studies summarized here show that the diversity of genes that can carry germline mutations and cause a hereditary predisposition to SSCC is quite high (Table 6.1). Despite all this genetic diversity, the *BRCA2* and *TP53* genes seem to have more roles than others [9–11].

**Table 6.1** Most frequently detected germline genetic changes in different publications

| Gene | Variant | Association | Population | Method | Number of detected/ total patients | References |
|---|---|---|---|---|---|---|
| *APOBEC3* | 30-kb deletion (rs12628403) | Increased risk | No data available (NDA) | Mutation signature analysis | 48/552 | Moody [7] |
| *ALDH2* | rs671(G>A) | Increased risk with alcohol consumption | Japan and China | Mutation signature analysis | NDA/552 | Moody [7] |
| *BRCA2* | Deleterious variants | Increased risk | Iran and China | Mutation signature analysis | 16/552 | Moody [7] |
| *CYP21A2* | p.Gln319* | Increased risk | Chinese | Whole exome sequencing | 5/77 | Deng [8] |
| *SPINK1* | c.194+2T>C | Increased risk | Chinese | Whole exome sequencing | 2/77 | Deng [8] |
| *OTOA* | p.Glu1048* | Increased risk | Chinese | Whole exome sequencing | 2/77 | Deng [8] |
| *PRAMEF7/8* | c.863+1G>T | Increased risk | Chinese | Whole exome sequencing | 2/77 | Deng [8] |
| *PRAMEF10/33P* | c.866+2T>C | Increased risk | Chinese | Whole exome sequencing | 2/77 | Deng [8] |
| *TP53* | p.V197E | Increased risk | Chinese | Whole exome sequencing | 1/77 | Deng [8] |
| *TP53* | Different mutations | Increased risk | Mostly Chinese | Meta-analysis | 15/571 | Zeng [9] |
| *GJB2* | Different mutations | Increased risk | Mostly Chinese | Meta-analysis | 8/571 | Zeng [9] |
| *BRCA2* | Different mutations | Increased risk | Mostly Chinese | Meta-analysis | 6/571 | Zeng [9] |
| *RECQL4* | Different mutations | Increased risk | Mostly Chinese | Meta-analysis | 6/571 | Zeng [9] |
| *MUTYH* | Different mutations | Increased risk | Mostly Chinese | Meta-analysis | 6/571 | Zeng [9] |
| *PMS2* | Different mutations | Increased risk | Mostly Chinese | Meta-analysis | 5/571 | Zeng [9] |

### 6.2.2 Germline Genetic Changes and Hereditary Predisposition to Esophageal Adenocarcinomas

It was mentioned in the previous section that EAC often develops based on BE and that some genetic predispositions are associated with BE. Germline genetic changes associated with hereditary susceptibility to both BE and EAC are often considered together.

In a study conducted in 2011, germline mutations in three candidate genes were detected in approximately 11% of the patient series with BE/esophageal adenocarcinoma (AOC). The most frequently affected genes were reported as *MSR1* **(approximately 7%), followed by *ASCC1* and *CTHRC1*** [12]. In a meta-analysis conducted in 2016, null variants **of the *GSTM1* gene, rs4880 SNP of the *SOD2* gene, rs16944 SNP of the *IL1B* gene, rs1052133 SNP of the *OGG1* gene, rs25487 SNP of the *XRCC1* gene, and rs13181 SNP of the *ERCC2*** gene as germline were found to be associated with increased risk [13]. In a study conducted in 2013, it was shown that aberrant **TP53** protein expression determined by immunohistochemistry in biopsy samples is associated with the risk of neoplastic progression in patients with BE and that these data are a much stronger predictor than histological diagnosis [14]. In a genome-wide association study (GWAS) meta-analysis, in which data from 16,790 patients were compiled in 2023, 27 risk loci for BE or EAC were identified, 11 of which were new. All these studies have shown that BE occurs more frequently in individuals carrying certain genetic variants such as *MSR1* mutations and that certain genetic variants such as the *TP53* gene increase the risk of progression from BE to EAC [15].

## 6.3 Somatic Genetic Alterations

The prognosis of esophageal cancer is poor, and perioperative chemotherapy and chemoradiotherapy are used to prolong survival. However, the number of studies on therapeutic targets at the molecular level are less than those for other cancer types. Currently, only trastuzumab (Food and Drug Administration (FDA)-approved) is used in metastatic patients who are ERBB2-positive. In order to overcome this, there are studies performed by many different groups such as The Cancer Genome Atlas (TCGA) and the International Cancer Genome Consortium (ICGC) [16].

Esophagus cancer is histologically classified into two main subtypes: esophageal adenocarcinoma (EAC) and esophageal squamous cell carcinoma (ESCC). There are studies showing that these two subgroups have different molecular genetic characteristics. In this area, whole genome sequencing (WGS), WES, copy number variation (CNV), and gene expression analyses have been performed. Single-nucleotide variants (SNVs), structural rearrangements, and mutation signatures are the prominent genomic biomarkers that have been studied [17].

Point mutations are common in EACs [18]. Genes with the most frequently somatic mutations are *TP53*, *CDKN2A*, *ARID1A*, *SMAD4*, *ERBB2*, *KCNQ3*, *CCDC102B*, and *CYP7B1* [17–21]. These genes play important roles in cell cycle, cell signal transduction, chromatin remodeling, and DNA damage. These findings are consistent with the significance of mutations in the *TP53* and *CDKN2A* genes in dysplastic Barrett's esophagus, which is a precursor of EAC. The *TP53* gene is a tumor suppressor gene (also known as the guardian of the genome). The TP53 protein plays a major role in response to cell damage. Germline mutations in the *TP53* gene lead to Li–Fraumeni syndrome (LFS) that has a predisposition to a wide range of cancers, including breast cancer and childhood cancers (sarcomas, leukemia, brain tumor, adrenocortical carcinoma) [22].

In ESCC, significantly mutated genes were identified as *TP53*, *NFE2L2*, *MLL2*, *ZNF750*, *NOTCH1*, and *TGFBR2* that play a role in cell cycle, chromatin remodeling, and genomic integrity [17, 23–25]. In addition to that, several mutated genes such as *PPFIA2*, *ZBBX*, *ATP13A5*, and IRF2BPL have been newly identified in ESCC through numerous sequencing data. Clinicopathological and epidemiological data of patients provided clinical associations of some mutations. For example, *NOTCH1* mutations are significantly associated with increasing age of diagnosis in ESCC, whereas *NFE2L2* mutations are specifically associated with poor survival in late-stage patients. However, most of the mutations that have prognostic significance have been identified in <5% ESCC patients [26]. While the same pathways are somatically affected in EACs and ESCCs, some genes affected are different from each other. For example, some of the mutations that occurred in both groups are in chromatin regulatory genes. Mutations in genes encoding histone-modifying factors such as KDM6A, KMT2C, and KMT2D are more common in ESCC, whereas genes encoding SWI/SNF family members such as ARID1A, PBRM1, and SMARC4 are more frequently affected in EAC. This likely indicates a different pathophysiology and also suggests different therapeutic modalities [17].

There are differences between EAC and ESCC in terms of genomic alteration patterns. CNVs and structural rearrangements are more prominent among the molecular changes detected in EAC. The CNVs that occur in EAC include amplified loci such as 6p21.1, 17p12, 18q11.2, and 19q12 and a deleted locus such as 18q21.2 (SMAD4). Amplified loci contain genes such as *VEGFA*, *ERBB2* (32%), *GATA6*, and CCNE1. On the other hand, amplified loci are 3q26.33, 5p15.33, 8p11.23, 11q13.3, 12q14.3, and 14q13.2 in ESCC. They include genes such as *SOX2* (48%), *TERT*, *FGFR1*, *CCND1* (57%), *MDM2*, and *NKX2*. The deleted locus is 13q14.2 that contains the *RB1* gene [16].

Mutation and CNV data reveal frequently observed changes in cell cycle regulators. Inactivation of CDKN2A is observed in ~75% of EACs and ESCCs. Inactivation occurs by mutation, epigenetic silencing, or deletion in EAC. Amplification of CCND1 is present in 57% of ESCCs, whereas it is amplified in only 15% of EACs. However, amplification of CCNE1 is observed to be more common than that of CCDN1 in EACs. These data suggest that cell cycle kinase inhibitors may have a potential role in therapy, particularly in ESCCs [23].

Alterations of receptor tyrosine kinases (RTKs) are frequently observed, particularly in EACs. Amplifications of the *ERBB2*, *KRAS*, *EGFR*, *IGF1R*, and *VEGFA* genes are observed in EACs. Therefore, they have therapeutic potential for RTK inhibitors. *ERBB2* gene amplification is the most commonly observed in EACs (32%), whereas it is present in only 3% of ESCCs. Trastuzumab (an anti-ERBB2 antibody) was initially limited to gastric and gastroesophageal junction (GEJ) adenocarcinomas but is now routinely used in many centers for the treatment of ERBB2-positive EACs [27].

A combination of whole genome sequencing (WGS), SNP arrays, and CNV analysis demonstrated that genomic catastrophes frequently occur in EACs. Genomic catastrophes include chromothripsis, kataegis (localized hypermutation), and breakage-fusion-bridge (BFB) events. Chromothripsis comprise tens of hundreds of chromosomal structural rearrangements that occur simultaneously and localize to specific genomic regions. While chromothripsis and kataegis occur in 30–35% and 30–85% of patients with EACs, respectively, they are defined in 55% of ESCCs [19, 20, 23]. These genomic catastrophes may underlie the mechanisms of amplification of oncogenes.

Integrated analyses of somatic copy number alterations (SCNAs), DNA methylation, and mRNA and microRNA expression data revealed the differences between ESCCs and EACs. While E-cadherin-regulating signaling is upregulated in EACs, Wnt, syndecan, and p63 pathways (essential for squamous epithelial cell differentiation) are upregulated in ESCCs. These data suggest that the presence of distinct lineage-specific signaling pathways drives tumorigenesis in both EACs and ESCCs [17].

Three molecular subtypes of ESCC have been identified as ESCC1, ESCC2, and ESCC3 by TCGA based on genetic mutations and gene expression patterns. The majority of cases are in the ESCC1 subtype. It is characterized by three significant events. One of them is NFE2L2 (NRF2) pathway alterations. This pathway is involved in the response to oxidative stress such as carcinogens and chemotherapy agents. In addition to the *NFE2L2* gene, some of the genes in this pathway are *KEAP1*, *CUL3*, *MAFF*, *MAFG*, and *MAFK*. *NFE2L2* mutations are associated with tumor recurrence and poor outcome. Therefore, *NFE2L2* mutations are considered to be applicable as predictive markers of response to chemoradiotherapy [28]. ESCC1 shares similar somatic alterations with head and neck SCCs previously described by TCGA [29, 30]. The other alteration is *TP63*/*SOX2* gene amplifications. They were amplified in 48% of ESCCs. The third event is associated with Hippo pathway activation. It is caused by YAP1 amplification and VGLL4/ATG7 deletion. In ESCC2, *NOTCH1* or *ZNF750* mutations are frequently observed. They are involved in the cell differentiation process. In addition, KDM6A, KMT2D (chromatin remodeling), PTEN, and PIK3R1 (RTK/RAS pathway) inactivating alterations and CDK6 (cell cycle) amplification are also frequently observed. The ESCC3 subtype is a minor group. It has somatic alterations predicted to activate the phosphoinositide 3-kinase (PI3K) pathway. It is also characterized by mutations in the *KMT2D* and *SMARCA4* genes. ESCC subtypes tend to be more common than each other in certain geographical regions. Molecular subtypes appear to be enriched within specific geographic regions: ESCC1 in Asian patients (Vietnamese patients—the only Asian population studied), ESCC2 in Eastern European and South American patients, and ESCC3 in patients from USA and Canada [17].

EAC is more similar to gastric adenocarcinoma (GAC) than is ESCC. GACs are classified into four subtypes based on having:

1. Chromosomal instability (CIN)
2. Microsatellite instability (MSI)
3. Genomic stability (GS)
4. Epstein–Barr virus (EBV) infection [31]

There are similar molecular features between EACs and the CIN subtype of GACs. CIN is highly observed in EACs, extending proximally from the gastro-esophageal junction (71 of 72 EACs classified as CIN) [17]. However, there are somatic alterations that can distinguish EACs from gastric CIN tumors. For example, *SMARCA4* mutations, *RUNX1* deletion, *VEGFA*, and *MYC* amplifications are present at a higher rate in EACs. Additionally, three different molecular subtypes that may have potential therapeutic efficacy were identified [20]:

1. BRCA signature (impaired homologous recombination DNA repair pathway)
2. T>G mutational pattern with a high tumor mutation burden (TMB)
3. C>A/T mutation pattern with signs of aging

The mutagenic subtype may respond better to immunotherapy as it has the highest TMB and neoantigen presentation.

In summary, comprehensive analyses, including SCNAs, gene expression, and unique driver mutations, suggest that the presence of distinct lineage-specific signaling pathways drives tumorigenesis in both EACs and ESCCs. The only targeted therapy is trastuzumab that is routinely used in clinical practice in EACs. However, other RTKs are being evaluated in clinical trials. In ESCC, which is the predominant histological subtype worldwide, therapeutically targetable changes are being investigated in clinical trials. A better understanding of esophageal cancer at the molecular level can provide patient selection for enrollment in clinical trials to determine optimal treatments.

## References

1. Kirbiyik O, Özyilmaz B. Genetic knowledge of colorectal cancer. In: Colon polyps and colorectal cancer; 2021. pp. 481–514.
2. Weinberg RA. The biology of cancer. New York: Garland Science; 2013.
3. Testa U, Castelli G, Pelosi E. The molecular characterization of genetic abnormalities in esophageal squamous cell carcinoma may Foster the development of targeted therapies. Curr Oncol. 2023;30(1):610–40.
4. Liu CQ, Ma YL, Qin Q, Wang PH, Luo Y, Xu PF, et al. Epidemiology of esophageal cancer in 2020 and projections to 2030 and 2040. Thorac Cancer. 2023;14(1):3–11.
5. Buckle GC, Mmbaga EJ, Paciorek A, Akoko L, Deardorff K, Mgisha W, et al. Risk factors associated with early-onset esophageal cancer in Tanzania. JCO Global Oncol. 2022;8:e2100256.
6. Yang CS, Chen XL. Research on esophageal cancer: with personal perspectives from studies in China and Kenya. Int J Cancer. 2021;149(2):264–76.
7. Mukkamalla SKR, Recio-Boiles A, Babiker HM. Esophageal cancer. StatPearls [Internet]: StatPearls Publishing; 2022.
8. Grady WM, Yu M. Molecular evolution of metaplasia to adenocarcinoma in the esophagus. Dig Dis Sci. 2018;63:2059–69.
9. Moody S, Senkin S, Islam SA, Wang J, Nasrollahzadeh D, Cortez Cardoso Penha R, et al. Mutational signatures in esophageal squamous cell carcinoma from eight countries with varying incidence. Nat Genet. 2021;53(11):1553–63.
10. Deng J, Weng X, Ye J, Zhou D, Liu Y, Zhao K. Identification of the germline mutation profile in esophageal squamous cell carcinoma by whole exome sequencing. Front Genet. 2019;10:47.

11. Zeng B, Huang P, Du P, Sun X, Huang X, Fang X, et al. Comprehensive study of germline mutations and double-hit events in esophageal squamous cell cancer. Front Oncol. 2021;11:637431.
12. Orloff M, Peterson C, He X, Ganapathi S, Heald B, Yang Y-r, et al. Germline mutations in MSR1, ASCC1, and CTHRC1 in patients with Barrett esophagus and esophageal adenocarcinoma. JAMA. 2011;306(4):410–9.
13. Findlay JM, Middleton MR, Tomlinson I. Genetic biomarkers of Barrett's esophagus susceptibility and progression to dysplasia and cancer: a systematic review and meta-analysis. Dig Dis Sci. 2016;61:25–38.
14. Kastelein F, Biermann K, Steyerberg EW, Verheij J, Kalisvaart M, Looijenga LH, et al. Aberrant p53 protein expression is associated with an increased risk of neoplastic progression in patients with Barrett's oesophagus. Gut. 2013;62(12):1676–83.
15. Schröder J, Chegwidden L, Maj C, Gehlen J, Speller J, Böhmer AC, et al. GWAS meta-analysis of 16 790 patients with Barrett's oesophagus and oesophageal adenocarcinoma identifies 16 novel genetic risk loci and provides insights into disease aetiology beyond the single marker level. Gut. 2023;72(4):612–23.
16. Jajosky A, Elliott DRF. Esophageal cancer genetics and clinical translation. Thorac Surg Clin. 2022;32(4):425–35.
17. Cancer Genome Atlas Research Network. Integrated genomic characterization of oesophageal carcinoma. Nature. 2017;541(7636):169.
18. Dulak AM, Stojanov P, Peng S, Lawrence MS, Fox C, Stewart C, et al. Exome and whole-genome sequencing of esophageal adenocarcinoma identifies recurrent driver events and mutational complexity. Nat Genet. 2013;45(5):478–86.
19. Nones K, Waddell N, Wayte N, Patch A-M, Bailey P, Newell F, et al. Genomic catastrophes frequently arise in esophageal adenocarcinoma and drive tumorigenesis. Nat Commun. 2014;5(1):5224.
20. Secrier M, Li X, De Silva N, Eldridge MD, Contino G, Bornschein J, et al. Mutational signatures in esophageal adenocarcinoma define etiologically distinct subgroups with therapeutic relevance. Nat Genet. 2016;48(10):1131–41.
21. Weaver JM, Ross-Innes CS, Shannon N, Lynch AG, Forshew T, Barbera M, et al. Ordering of mutations in preinvasive disease stages of esophageal carcinogenesis. Nat Genet. 2014;46(8):837–43.
22. Hampel H, Bennett RL, Buchanan A, Pearlman R, Wiesner GL. A practice guideline from the American College of Medical Genetics and Genomics and the National Society of Genetic Counselors: referral indications for cancer predisposition assessment. Genet Med. 2015;17(1):70–87.
23. Cheng C, Zhou Y, Li H, Xiong T, Li S, Bi Y, et al. Whole-genome sequencing reveals diverse models of structural variations in esophageal squamous cell carcinoma. Am J Hum Genet. 2016;98(2):256–74.
24. Qin H-D, Liao X-Y, Chen Y-B, Huang S-Y, Xue W-Q, Li F-F, et al. Genomic characterization of esophageal squamous cell carcinoma reveals critical genes underlying tumorigenesis and poor prognosis. Am J Hum Genet. 2016;98(4):709–27.
25. Sawada G, Niida A, Uchi R, Hirata H, Shimamura T, Suzuki Y, et al. Genomic landscape of esophageal squamous cell carcinoma in a Japanese population. Gastroenterology. 2016;150(5):1171–82.
26. Lin D-C. Large-scale genomic analyses reveal alterations and mechanisms underlying clonal evolution and immune evasion in esophageal cancer. Nat Commun. 2023;14(1):893.
27. Bang Y-J, Van Cutsem E, Feyereislova A, Chung HC, Shen L, Sawaki A, et al. Trastuzumab in combination with chemotherapy versus chemotherapy alone for treatment of HER2-positive advanced gastric or gastro-oesophageal junction cancer (ToGA): a phase 3, open-label, randomised controlled trial. Lancet. 2010;376(9742):687–97.
28. Shibata T, Kokubu A, Saito S, Narisawa-Saito M, Sasaki H, Aoyagi K, et al. NRF2 mutation confers malignant potential and resistance to chemoradiation therapy in advanced esophageal squamous cancer. Neoplasia. 2011;13(9):864-IN26.

29. Cancer Genome Atlas Research Network. Comprehensive genomic characterization of squamous cell lung cancers. Nature. 2012;489(7417):519.
30. Cancer Genome Atlas Network. Comprehensive genomic characterization of head and neck squamous cell carcinomas. Nature. 2015;517(7536):576.
31. Cancer Genome Atlas Research Network. Comprehensive molecular characterization of gastric adenocarcinoma. Nature. 2014;513(7517):202.

# Anatomy of Important Structures for Esophageal Reconstruction

7

Aydin Ozbek

## 7.1 Esophagus Anatomy

The word esophagus comes from the ancient Greek word ***oisophagos*** **(esophagus, passage for food)**. It is formed by combining the words ***oisein*** **(to carry)** and ***phagos*** **(to eat)** and is used in the sense of **carrying the eaten food**. An adult esophagus is about 23–25 cm long and between 20 and 30 mm in diameter. An esophageal stricture is an abnormal narrowing of the esophagus up to 13 mm or less, causing dysphagia. It has typical narrowness in four places along its entire length. The first narrowing is at the junction of the esophagus and the pharynx, the second is where it crosses the aortic arch, the third is where it crosses the left main bronchus, and the fourth is where it crosses the diaphragm [1, 2].

It is divided into three anatomical parts or segments: cervical, thoracic, and abdominal (Fig. 7.1). The cervical part or segment starts at the level of the cricoid cartilage and ends at the suprasternal notch or jugular notch. This segment lies behind the trachea and is attached to it by loose connective tissue. Posteriorly, the prevertebral fascia connects the esophagus to the bodies of the sixth to eighth cervical vertebrae. The thoracic duct is located on the left side of the sixth cervical vertebra. The lower parts of the carotid sheath and the lateral thyroid gland are located in the lower part of the neck, lateral to the esophagus. Another meaningful relationship between the neck part of the esophagus is the recurrent laryngeal nerves that run along the trachea and lateral surfaces of the esophagus in the tracheoesophageal groove [1, 2] (Fig. 7.1).

A. Ozbek (✉)
Medicine Faculty, Department of Anatomy, Istinye University, Istanbul, Turkey
e-mail: aozbek@istinye.edu.tr


O. Engin (ed.), *Risk Factors and Therapy of Esophagus Cancer*,
https://doi.org/10.1007/978-3-031-47024-0_7

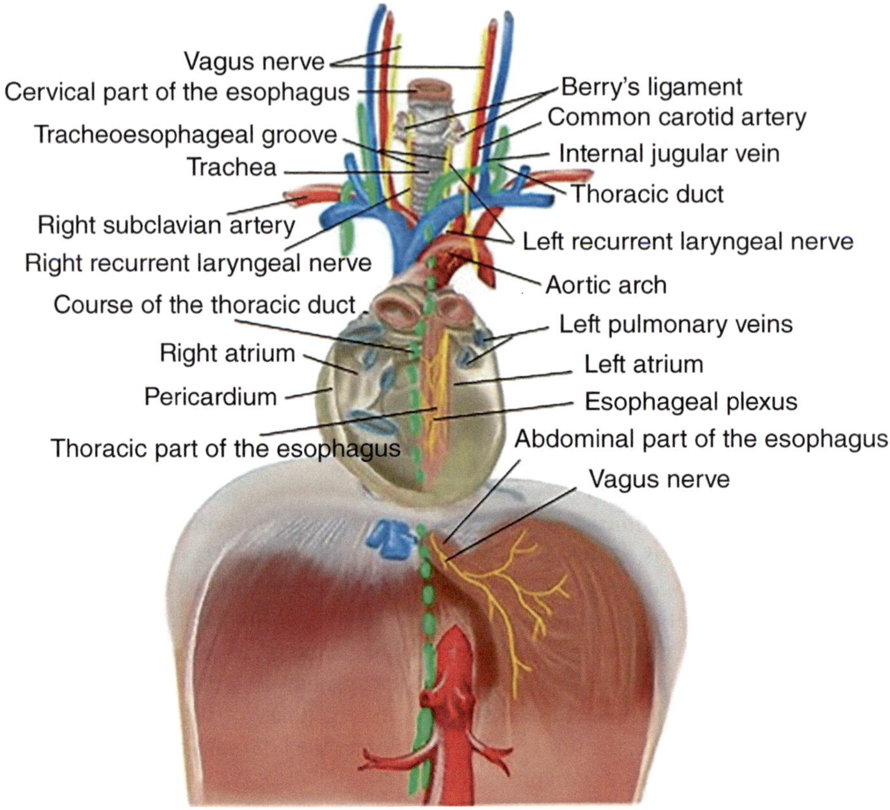


**Fig. 7.1** The position and relations of the esophagus, the thoracic duct, and the recurrent laryngeal nerves in the cervical region and in the posterior mediastinum. The green dotted line is the course of the thoracic duct behind the esophagus. The part of the pericardium in front of the esophagus is removed (illustration by Aydin Ozbek and Mehtap Erdogan)

The thoracal segment is 16–18 cm long and is located in the superior and posterior mediastinum. It lies between the first to the eleventh thoracic vertebrae and does not adapt to the concavity of the vertebral column. The esophagus is located at the level of the first thoracic vertebra to the left of the midline, at the level of the sixth thoracic vertebra to the right of the midline, and at the level of the tenth thoracic vertebra to the left of the midline. Thus, the esophagus makes an inverted "S" just in front of the vertebral column. The parietal pleura is firmly attached to both sides of the vertebral column, thus forming a recessed protruding relationship with the esophagus. This configuration makes it difficult to dissect the esophagus in the thorax. Therefore, pleural rupture is dangerous during surgery [1–3]. In esophageal surgery, one of the most critical structures is the thoracic duct. It is located behind the esophagus along the thoracic cavity. The lower third of the thorax is located slightly apart from the esophagus, whereas the upper part is closer. In front of the thoracic part of the esophagus are the trachea, the aortic arch, the right pulmonary artery, the left main bronchus, the esophageal plexus, the pericardium, the left atrium, and the anterior branch of the vagus nerve. Among its anterior relations, its relationship with the left atrium is clinically significant (Fig. 7.1). The vertebral column, the longus colli muscle, the posterior intercostal arteries, the azygos, the hemiazygos veins, the anterior aortic wall, and the posterior branch of the vagus nerve are found posterior to the esophagus. On the left side of the thoracic part of the esophagus are the aortic arch, the left subclavian artery, the left inferior laryngeal nerve, the left vagus nerve, the thoracic duct, the mediastinal pleura, and the thoracic aorta. On its right side are the azygos vein, the mediastinal pleura, the right main bronchus, and the right vagus nerve [1, 2].

The abdominal part of the esophagus lies between the esophageal hiatus and the cardiac notch of the stomach (incisura cardiaca gastri) and is 2–3 cm long on average (Fig. 7.1). It passes just in front of the left crus of the diaphragm and is located at the level of the eleventh thoracal vertebra. This level corresponds to the front seventh rib. The abdominal part of the esophagus is connected to the spleen, the liver, and the diaphragm by the hepatogastric ligament, the gastrosplenic ligament, and the gastrophrenic ligament [1, 2].

The left and right crus of the diaphragm, the aorta, and the left inferior phrenic artery are posterior to the abdominal part of the esophagus. The left vagus nerve and the esophageal plexus innervating the liver are found anterior to the esophagus. On the right side is the caudate lobe of the liver, and on the left is the stomach's fundus [1, 2].

## 7.2 Weak Points of the Esophagus

There are two weak areas in the esophagus that may be open to mechanical stresses during swallowing and can therefore cause diverticulum formation [1–5]. The weak upper areas are located around the cricopharyngeus muscle. Typically, there are two muscle layers in the esophagus: superficially longitudinal muscle fibers and deep, circular muscle fibers. However, in the posterior part of the esophagus, where it joins the pharynx and just below the cricopharyngeus muscle, there are no longitudinal fibers, only circular fibers. Circular muscle fibers are weaker and thinner than longitudinal muscle fibers. Therefore, this region is less resistant to pressure during swallowing. This region is called "Laimer's triangle," and its borders are formed by the cricopharyngeal muscle at the top and the inner edges of the longitudinal muscles at the lateral margins [1, 2]. Laimer's diverticulum occurs in this region. The regions where "Laimer's triangle" has two upper and lateral angles adjacent to the cricopharyngeal muscle are called the "Killian–Jamieson triangles," and the "Killian–Jamieson diverticulum" is formed in these regions. In this region, there is another triangular area called the "Killian triangle," and the boundaries of this triangle are formed by the parts of the lower constrictor muscle of the pharynx called the cricopharyngeus and thyropharyngeus. These weak areas are also crucial for forming "Zenker's diverticulum" [5].

## 7.3 Blood Supply to the Esophagus

Different arteries supply the three segments of the esophagus. Roughly one-third is supplied by the inferior thyroid artery, one-third by the middle thoracic aorta, and one-third by the inferior left gastric artery [1, 2].

The cervical segment of the esophagus is supplied by the right inferior thyroid arteries originating from the thyrocervical trunk of the right subclavian artery and the left inferior thyroid arteries arising from the left external carotid artery. Branches called tracheoesophageal arteries arise from both inferior thyroid arteries supplying both the cervical esophagus and the trachea [5]. There are branches from the subclavian artery, the superior thyroid artery, the thyroid ima artery, or the common carotid artery to the esophagus, but these variants are rare and insignificant [5–8].

Arteries supplying the lower thoracic segment of the esophagus arise from the thoracic aorta at any level between the fifth and tenth thoracic vertebrae, but usually at the level of the eighth thoracic vertebra. A single arterial branch usually supplies the inferior thoracic segment. Of the 15 cadavers examined in a study, 9 received a single branch, 4 received 2 branches, and 2 received 3 branches [9].

Arteries to the abdominal segment arise from the left gastric artery and the left inferior phrenic artery. Sometimes it receives a branch from the accessory left hepatic artery. Unlike the inferior thoracic segment, the abdominal segment usually receives a double blood supply (10 out of 15 cadavers). These arteries emerge at the level of the twelfth thoracic and first lumbar vertebrae [9].

According to the predominant size of the extramural vessels, the cervical and abdominal arteries provide the main blood supply to the esophagus, whereas the relatively small arteries at the level of the upper thoracic region seem less important [9].

A continuous and regular arterial network connects all the intramural vessels in the submucosa. Therefore, there is no avascular region in the esophagus. Because such anastomoses of vertically extending intramural vessels provide excellent blood supply to the esophagus, this is important for esophageal surgery. As it approaches the periesophageal tissue, the diameter of the extramural vessels narrows and passes vertically into the tunica muscularis layer muscle and proceeds this way. During this progression, they give off horizontal branches in a circular manner and anastomose with the vessels in the opposite region. These circular transverse vessels divide into numerous thin branches along the submucosa. This arterial structure is the same throughout the esophagus [6, 10]. Thus, a continuous, small, dense network is formed in the submucosa to nourish the muscles and mucosa. Therefore, this vascular intramural network provides excellent blood supply to the esophagus.

## 7.4 Venous Drainage of the Esophagus

The veins of the esophagus, like its arteries, vary according to the vessels into which they drain. The venous blood of the cervical part drains into the left brachiocephalic vein through the inferior thyroid vein. The venous blood of the thoracic segment drains into the superior vena cava through the azygos, the hemiazygos, and the accessory hemiazygos veins. The venous drainage of the abdominal part is mainly to the left gastric vein but rarely to the short gastric veins, the splenic vein, the left gastroepiploic vein, and the inferior phrenic veins [1, 2]. The veins from which the abdominal part is drained belong to the portal venous system, and the veins from which the thoracal part is drained belong to the caval venous system. Therefore, there is an anastomosis of these two systems in the lower one-third of the esophagus.

For this reason, in the presence of portal venous hypertension, increased pressure is transmitted to the submucosal plexus of the lower esophagus, forming fragile varices. These esophageal varices are clinically significant as the leading cause of massive upper gastrointestinal bleeding. Direct communication with both the systemic and the portal systems may also be important in the metastatic spread of esophageal carcinoma [11].

## 7.5 Lymphatic Drainage of the Esophagus

Lymphatic drainage of the esophagus is complex, and the presence of lymphatics in its mucosa makes it unique within the gastrointestinal tract [11]. The lymphatics of the cervical part drain into the internal jugular lymph nodes and the superior tracheal lymph nodes. The lymphatics of the thoracic part drain into the posterior parietal lymph nodes, diaphragmatic lymph nodes, tracheobronchial lymph nodes, and infracardiac lymph nodes. The abdominal lymphatics of the esophagus drain into the left gastric lymph nodes and paracardiac lymph nodes, and all these nodes are connected to the celiac lymph nodes. The celiac lymph nodes drain into the cisterna chyli or thoracic duct [1, 11].

## 7.6 Innervation of the Esophagus

Approximately, the proximal third of the esophagus mainly consists of the skeletal muscle, and the distal two-thirds consist of the smooth muscle [1, 12]. However, the esophagus is involuntarily controlled by the autonomic nervous system. The recurrent laryngeal nerve provides parasympathetic innervation of the cervical part, and the cervical sympathetic trunk provides sympathetic innervation. The esophageal plexus innervates the thoracic part of the esophagus. The parasympathetic component of this plexus arises from the vagus nerve and the sympathetic fibers from the sympathetic trunk. Parasympathetic innervation of the abdominal part originates from the thoracic esophageal nerve plexus, and sympathetic innervation originates from the fifth to twelfth thoracic spinal nerves (T5–T12) [1, 12].

## 7.7 Neck Anatomy

The posterior wall of the neck is higher than its anterior wall. Because organs such as the mouth and nose in the anterior are the outward opening regions of organs such as the pharynx and the larynx, which are the continuation of the neck and are located on the face, the pharynx starts at the skull base. The larynx starts at the level of the third cervical vertebra. Therefore, the boundaries of the neck at the top are the lower edge of the mandible, the zygomatic arch, and the upper edge of the first cervical vertebra from anterior to posterior. At the bottom, it is the jugular notch, the clavicle, the acromioclavicular joint, and the seventh cervical vertebra [1, 2]. The neck is subject to various classifications depending on the purpose. Accordingly, the neck is divided into four parts based on its structures: two vascular sections, vertebral sections, and visceral sections [1, 2]. Cervical vertebrae and postural muscles are located in the vertebral section; the common carotid artery, the internal carotid artery, the internal jugular vein, the vagus nerve, and the deep cervical lymph nodes are located in the vascular section; and, finally, the thyroid and parathyroid glands, the thymus, the larynx, the pharynx, and the trachea are located in the visceral section [1, 2].

It is essential to know the anatomy of the neck, as extensive neck dissection is performed during esophagectomy. Although the cervical part of the esophagus is located behind the trachea, it usually protrudes toward the left lateral [13]. Therefore, in esophageal surgery, neck dissection is performed on the left side [13]. Thus, only the thoracic duct, the left thyroid lobe, and the left recurrent nerve located on the left side of the neck become meaningful.

Since the neck is a transition zone between the head and the body, it has a highly complex structure. In particular, the fascia structure is complex and vital both surgically and clinically. In addition, due to the changes in the large vessels and nerve structures in the superior mediastinum on both sides of the body, asymmetrical structuring occurs on the right and left sides of the neck [1, 2, 14].

The fasciae of the neck can also determine the direction in which the infection in the neck can spread. It is defined in two layers: the superficial cervical fascia and the deep cervical fascia. The superficial cervical fascia also forms the subcutaneous part of the neck skin and surrounds the platysma muscle (Fig. 7.2). It attaches posteriorly to the galeal or epicranial aponeurosis and anteriorly to the superficial muscular aponeurotic system (SMAS). Superficial sensory nerves also run in this fascia. Between the platysma muscle and the deep cervical fascia are the external jugular vein and the anterior jugular vein. The external jugular vein crosses the sternocleidomastoid muscle, transverses the cervical nerves, runs toward the middle of the clavicle, pierces the deep fascia in the supraclavicular fossa, and, finally, drains into the subclavian vein or the internal jugular vein. The anterior jugular vein descends bilaterally between the midline and the anterior border of the sternocleidomastoid muscle. It pierces the superficial layer of the deep fascia (investing fascia) and drains directly into the external jugular vein or the subclavian vein [1, 13, 14].

On the other hand, the deep cervical fascia shows different thickenings in many regions of the neck, takes different names, and envelops different structures. These are lamina superficialis (investing fascia), lamina pretrechealis (pretracheal fascia), lamina prevertebralis (prevertebral fascia), carotid sheath, and buccopharyngeal fascia

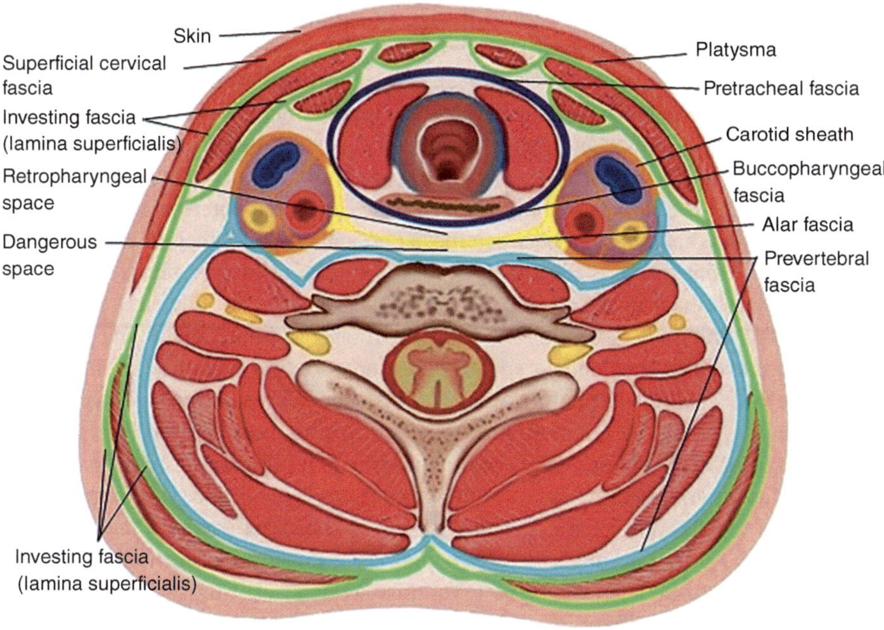


**Fig. 7.2** Transverse section showing the neck fascial layers at the level of the thyroid gland (illustration by Aydin Ozbek and Mehtap Erdogan)

(Fig. 7.2). The deep fascia acts as a canal for nerves and vessels, holding the neck muscles and organs in their compartments. It facilitates the sliding of the compartments on top of each other during the movements of the organs or neck [1, 13, 14].

The investing fascia starts posteriorly from the nuchal ligament, encloses the entire neck, and reattaches to the nuchal ligament (Fig. 7.2). At this time, it splits into two leaves and then rejoins while surrounding the sternocleidomastoid and trapezius muscles. In the upper part of the neck, it attaches to the hyoid bone, the mandible, the mastoid process, and the external occipital protuberance. The lower part of the neck attaches to the acromion, the scapula, the clavicle, and the manubrium of the sternum. It divides into two leaves as it surrounds the submandibular gland and the parotid gland from the upper part of the neck [1, 13, 14].

The pretracheal fascia forms a tube-shaped sheath in the anterior part of the neck and surrounds the structures passing through this tube. These structures are the infrahyoid muscles (sternohyoid, thyrohyoid, omohyoid, sternothyroid), the thyroid and parathyroid glands, the trachea, and the esophagus. For this reason, it is also called the "muscular fascia" (Fig. 7.2). It is also referred to as the middle layer of the deep fascia by some sources [15]. The pretracheal fascia is attached above the hyoid bone and below the cricoid and thyroid cartilages and the fibrous pericardium. It fuses with the carotid sheath on the sides and with the buccopharyngeal fascia of the pharynx posteriorly [1, 13, 14].

The prevertebral fascia forms a tubular sheath around the vertebral column and prevertebral muscles. The muscles that the prevertebral fascia covers anteriorly are the longus colli and the longus capitis, the rectus capitis anterior and the rectus capitis lateralis, and the prevertebral muscles. Laterally, it surrounds the three scalene muscles (anterior, medius, and posterior). It also encircles the sympathetic trunk. The prevertebral fascia attaches superiorly to the occipital bone and inferiorly to the anterior longitudinal ligament and the endothoracic fascia. Laterally, it fuses with the fascia surrounding the axillary vessels and the brachial plexus. This fascia is divided into two layers, the alar leaf and the prevertebral leaf, in the anterior part of the vertebral colon, and there is a gap between these two leaves where there is no formation (Fig. 7.2). The alar fascia is the anteriorly diverging layer of the prevertebral fascia and lies between the transverse processes of the same vertebra. Since this space provides communication between the neck and the thorax and may lead to the spread of infections, it is called the "danger space" or the prevertebral space [1, 13, 14].

The carotid sheath is a tubular passageway for the nerves and vessels formed by the deep neck fascia. The common carotid artery, the internal carotid artery, the internal jugular vein, and the vagus nerve pass through it. In addition, deep cervical lymph nodes, sympathetic fibers, and the carotid sinus nerve are also found in this sheath. The localization of the structures in it is the carotid artery medially, the internal jugular vein laterally, and the vagus nerve posteriorly in the middle. The carotid sheath is fused with the prevertebral fascia posteriorly, the pretracheal fascia medially, and the vestigial fascia anteriorly (Fig. 7.2). The carotid sheath is a tubular fascial tube that starts at the base of the skull above and extends to the root of the neck below. Some authors include the carotid sheath in the pretracheal fascia, whereas *Gray's Anatomy* defines the carotid sheath as the fusion of the pretracheal and other deep fascia leaves together [1, 13–15].

Another fascia originating from the deep fascia is the buccopharyngeal fascia, which is a condensation of the pharyngeal constrictor muscles and the adventitia surrounding the esophagus and separates the visceral compartment from the prevertebral fascia by an open alveolar space in between. After surrounding the buccinator muscle and the pharynx, it fuses with the alar leaf of the prevertebral fascia (Fig. 7.2). The space between the alar leaf of the prevertebral fascia and the buccopharyngeal fascia is called the retropharyngeal space, and this space is filled with loose connective tissue [1, 13, 14].

The retropharyngeal space starts from the skull base and continues until the fusion point of the alar fascia and the buccopharyngeal fascia [1, 16, 17]. This fusion point can be anywhere between the T1 and T6 vertebrae, so the termination of the retropharyngeal space is variable. The retropharyngeal space is anterior to the prevertebral muscles and posterior to the pharynx and the esophagus. It is surrounded anteriorly by the buccopharyngeal fascia, laterally by the carotid sheath, and posteriorly by the prevertebral fascia. Some authors define the retropharyngeal space to include the danger space. Accordingly, the retropharyngeal space is divided into two components by the alar fascia: the "true retropharyngeal space" and the "dangerous area" [16, 17]. The proper retropharyngeal space is located in front of its dangerous area and extends from the base of the skull to the fusion point between T1 and T6 (Fig. 7.3).

On the other hand, the dangerous area runs lower than the proper retropharyngeal space and extends to the diaphragm level [16, 17]. The retropharyngeal space is

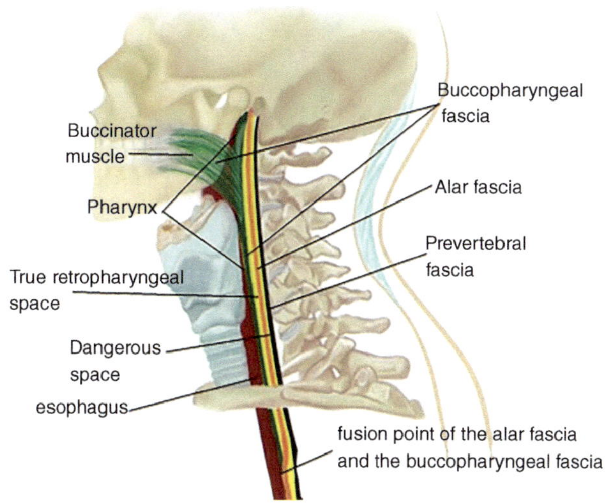


**Fig. 7.3** Sagittal section showing the neck fascial layers (illustration by Aydin Ozbek and Mehtap Erdogan)

divided into suprahyoid and infrahyoid components. The suprahyoid retropharyngeal space consists of adipose tissue and lymph nodes. The infrahyoid retropharyngeal space contains only adipose tissue [16].

While the neck is divided into triangles in classical anatomy, different surgical levels have been determined for clinical applications. The most common of these is the zoning described by Jatin P. Shah et al. in 1981 and has been recommended by the American Head and Neck Society (AHNS) since [18, 19].

In classical triangulation, the sternocleidomastoid and the trapezius muscles are referenced and the neck is first divided into anterior and posterior triangles. The posterior triangle is then divided into two smaller triangular areas and the anterior triangle into four smaller triangular areas. The anterior triangle is located between the anterior margin of the sternocleidomastoid muscle posteriorly, the midline of the neck anteriorly, and the inferior margins of the mandible superiorly and the lines extending from the angulus mandible to the mastoid prominence. The anterior triangle is then divided into four triangles outlined by the superior belly of the omohyoid muscle and the anterior and posterior bellies of the digastric muscle (the submental triangle, the submandibular or digastric triangle, the carotid triangle, and the muscular or visceral triangle) [1, 2].

The posterior triangle is located between the posterior border of the sternocleidomastoid muscle anteriorly, the anterior border of the trapezius muscle posteriorly, and the middle one-third of the clavicle inferiorly. The posterior triangle is divided into two triangles by the posterior belly of the omohyoid muscle. The occipital triangle is located superiorly and the supraclavicular triangle anteriorly [1, 2].

Since a different zoning system is used instead of classical triangles in neck dissection, we will not examine the boundaries and contents of classical triangles here. The leveling recommended by the American Head and Neck Society (AHNS) is as follows. Accordingly, the neck is divided into six surgical levels, and the first, second, and fifth levels are further divided into two subgroups (Figs. 7.4 and 7.5).

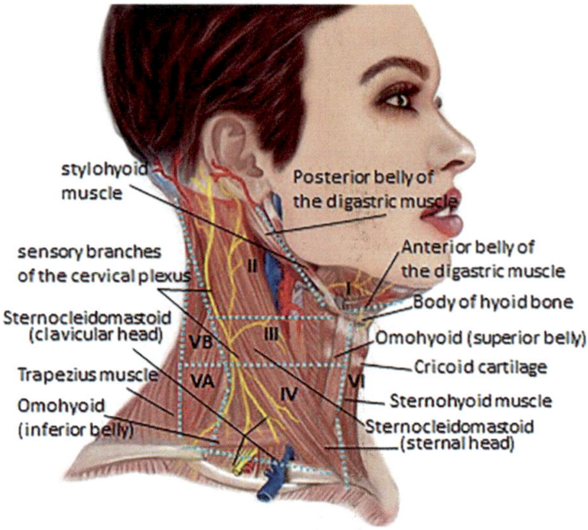


**Fig. 7.4** Regions of the neck divided into surgical levels. Lateral view of the neck (illustration by Aydin Ozbek and Mehtap Erdogan)

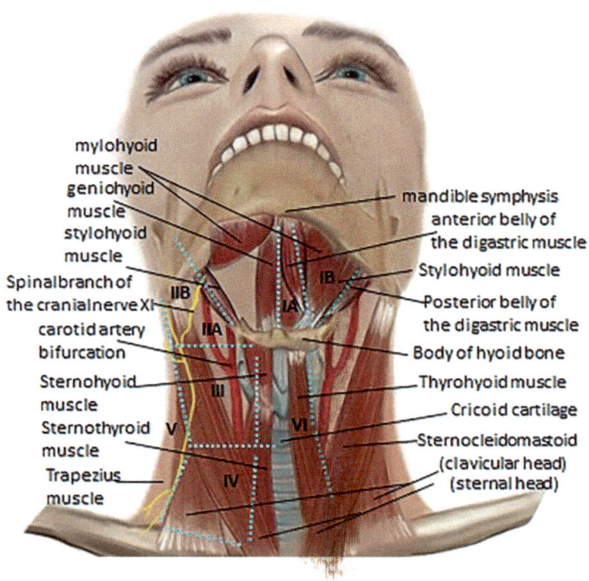


**Fig. 7.5** Regions of the neck divided into surgical levels. Anterior view of the neck with the sternohyoid muscle removed on the right side (illustration by Aydin Ozbek and Mehtap Erdogan)

Level IA is the area between the anterior belly of the digastric muscle and the body of the hyoid bone. Its apex is the mandible symphysis (Fig. 7.5). The superficial or investing layer of the deep fascia makes the roof of this triangle, whereas the muscular fascia or pretracheal fascia surrounding the mylohyoid muscle makes its floor. The significant formations in this region are the submental artery and vein.

Level IB is located between the anterior belly of the digastric muscle anteriorly, the stylohyoid muscle posteriorly, and the base of the mandible above (Fig. 7.5). The floor of this triangle is made of the mylohyoid and hyoglossus muscles, and the roof is made of the deep fascia's superficial (investing) layer. There are many critical anatomical structures at this level. The mandibular and cervical branches of the facial nerve, the facial vein, the artery, the retromandibular vein joining the facial vein, the submandibular gland, the hypoglossal nerve, and the lingual nerve are found at this level.

The second, third, and fourth levels that come after this level are related to the lateral side of the neck. These levels cover the entire neck from the skull base to the clavicle (Fig. 7.4). The superficial leaf or investing leaf of the deep neck fascia forms the roof of these levels. The deep layer, or floor, is the deep leaf of the deep neck fascia, which surrounds the longus coli muscles and the scalene muscles of the neck. These levels' posterior border is the sternocleidomastoid muscle's posterior border. However, some researchers argue that the location of the superficial branches of the cervical plexus is more valuable for the posterior border in neck surgery [19, 20].

Level 2 is the stylohyoid muscle anteriorly and the posterior margin of the sternocleidomastoid muscle posteriorly. It extends from the skull base to the hyoid bone, where the third level starts (Figs. 7.4 and 7.5). However, AHNS has accepted the vertical line passing behind the submandibular gland as the anterior border since 2008 [19, 20]. Level 2 is divided into levels IIA and IIB by the spinal branch of cranial nerve (CN) XI (Fig. 7.5) that runs superficially and obliquely to the levator scapulae muscle in the neck. Therefore, level IIB is located behind and above level IIA. The superficial leaf of the deep neck fascia forms the roof of level 2 in both parts. The floor is made of the deep leaf of the neck fascia surrounding the anterior and middle scalene muscles in the level IIB section, whereas in the level IIA section, it is made of the deep leaf of the neck fascia surrounding the hyoglossus muscle and the buccopharyngeal fascia. In level IIA, there is the external carotid artery, the internal carotid artery, the superior thyroid artery, the lingual artery, the facial artery, the tonsillar artery with branches, the ascending palatine artery, the occipital artery, and the ascending pharyngeal artery. In addition, the internal jugular vein, the facial vein, the retromandibular vein and the lingula vein, the hypoglossal nerve, the accessory nerve, the vagus nerve, and the glossopharyngeal nerves are found at this level. The posterior branch of the spinal portion of the accessory nerve goes to level IIB, whereas the anterior branch goes to level IIA. The superior cervical ganglion, a vital structure, is also at this level [19, 20].

Since the third and fourth levels are located in the lateral region of the neck and below the face region, it is necessary to determine the anterior border of these levels that is formed by the lateral border of the sternohyoid muscle superficially and by the internal carotid artery and the common carotid artery deeply [20]. Since the carotid artery is the most medial structure within the carotid sheath and makes the anterior border of the third to fourth levels, other structures within the sheath (the internal jugular vein and vagus nerve) are considered in the lateral neck area. The area medial to this border is called level VI and represents the anterior-central part of the neck. Since level III represents the lateral part of the upper half of the neck, its anterior border forms the internal carotid artery superiorly and the common carotid artery inferiorly. Because the common carotid artery usually branches at discus levels between C3 and C4, this level corresponds to the upper parts of level III (Fig. 7.5). Therefore, the common carotid artery forms the anterior border of the lower half of level III and all of level IV [1, 21, 22].

The upper limit of level III is the lower edge of the hyoid bone, and the lower border is the lower edge of the cricoid cartilage [19] (Figs. 7.4 and 7.5). Therefore, level 3 lies between levels C3 and C6, and the bifurcation point of the carotid artery coincides with the upper part of level III. For this reason, the lower edge of the hyoid bone uses as the upper border instead of the carotid artery bifurcation, which was previously accepted as the upper border of this level [18]. The superficial layer or roof of the region is made up of the superficial or investing leaf, which also surrounds the sternocleidomastoid muscle of the deep neck fascia. The deep layer or flooring is the deep leaf of the neck fascia. Beneath the floor of this level are the longus colli muscles, which extend to the transverse processes of the cervical spine, and the anterior scalene muscle lateral to them. The structure to be considered surgically here is the phrenic nerve, which runs over the anterior scalene muscle. Level III includes the carotid sheath and the structures within it, the thyroid vessels that cross the carotid sheath anteriorly, the ansa cervicalis, and the juguloomohyoid node. Another important structure, the sympathetic truncus, is located in the posteromedial of the carotid sheath and the deep leaf of the deep fascia surrounding the longus colli muscles [23].

The upper limit of level IV is the lower edge of the cricoid cartilage, and the lower border is the clavicle (Figs. 7.4 and 7.5). The anterior boundary, the floor, and the ceiling of this level are the same as those of level III. The arteries supplying the head and neck enter the neck at level IV. In addition, the lower jugular chain lymph nodes are also located here. Of these level structures, the vertebral artery, the inferior thyroid artery, the truncus sympathicus, and the ductus thoracicus are located at the angle between the longus colli and anterior scalene muscles [1, 2, 14]. The transverse cervical and suprascapular arteries, other branches of the truncus thyrocervicalis, are also located in this region. The central venous structure of this level is the internal jugular vein. The anterior jugular and the external jugular veins join the internal jugular vein or mainly the subclavian vein in this region. The subclavian vein joins with the internal jugular vein behind the medial head of the clavicle to form the brachiocephalic vein. Their junction is called the angulus venosus—the primary lymphatic vessels on the left and right open to these junctions. Level IV also includes the phrenic nerve, the vagus nerve, and the cervical sympathetic truncus. The deep leaf of the deep cervical fascia, the vagus nerve by the carotid sheath, and the cervical sympathetic truncus by the prevertebral fascia and the carotid sheaths surround the phrenic nerve. In addition, the right recurrent laryngeal nerve, which leaves the vagal nerve and curves under the right subclavian artery, returns to the neck, and the left recurrent laryngeal nerve, which curves under the aortic arch and turns into the neck, is also located at this level [19, 20].

Level IV is fundamental in neck anatomy in terms of the structures it contains. The main lymphatic vessels here combine with the venous system, and the distribution of venous vessels has quite a lot of variation. As if that were not enough, there is also mixed neural content, such as the vagus nerve and its descending branches reentering this region [19, 20].

The anterior border of level V is the posterior border of the sternocleidomastoid muscle and the sensory branches of the cervical plexus, and the posterior border is the anterior border of the trapezius muscle. Its upper limit is the junction of the sternocleidomastoid and the trapezius muscles, and its lower limit is the clavicle (Figs. 7.4 and 7.5). This level is divided into two subsections, level VA and level VB, by an imaginary line extending from the lower border of the cricoid cartilage. This level's superficial layer or roof is the investing layer of the deep neck fascia, which surrounds the sternocleidomastoid and trapezius muscles. Its deep layer or floor is the deep leaf of the neck fascia, which also surrounds the splenius capitis, the levator scapula, the middle, and the anterior scalene muscles. The structures at this level are the superficial (transverse) cervical artery, the brachial plexus, part of the subclavian artery and vein, the suprascapular artery, the dorsal scapular artery, and the XI spinal branch of the cranial nerve. Of these structures, the XI spinal branch of the cranial nerve is prone to injury due to its superficial location and is therefore of surgical importance. Another important structure, the brachial plexus, is located between the anterior and middle scalene muscles [19, 20].

Level VI extends from the hyoid bone to the jugular notch of the sternum and represents the anterior and central parts of the neck. The hyoid bone forms the border between levels I and VI. The lateral border of level VI is also the anterior border of levels III and IV. In other words, it is the lateral edge of the sternohyoid muscle superficially, the internal carotid artery at the top, and the common carotid artery at the bottom deeply [20] (Figs. 7.4 and 7.5). The roof of level VI is formed by the pretracheal fascia, which also surrounds the sternohyoid, the thyrohyoid, the omohyoid, and the sternothyroid muscles. In contrast, the deep leaf of the neck fascia forms its floor. At this level, the sternohyoid, the thyrohyoid, the omohyoid, and the sternothyroid muscles, the inferior, the medial, and the superior constrictor muscles of the pharynx, the thyroid and the cricoid cartilages, the cricothyroid membrane, the neck part of the esophagus, the neck part of the trachea, the thyroid gland, the parathyroid gland, the right and the left recurrent laryngeal nerves, the inferior and superior thyroid arteries, rarely the thyroid ima artery, the brachiocephalic artery, the superior thyroid vein, and the venous plexus anterior to the thyroid gland are found. The brachiocephalic artery is sometimes located anterior to the trachea and may extend to the lower edge of the thyroid gland [24]. From a surgical point of view, this should be considered.

## 7.8 Thyroid Gland Anatomy

During esophagectomy, if the thyroid gland is large, then the thyroid lobe on the side of the neck dissection may have to be removed. Therefore, the thyroid gland is a critical structure in esophagus surgery. It is an endocrine gland in the shape of a butterfly or the letter "H," with the right and left lobes corresponding to the butterfly's wings and the isthmus region of its body. The length of the lobes is 4–5 cm, their width is 2–3 cm, and their antero-posterior thickness is 2 cm. The isthmus has a length of 1–2 cm. The gland is located anteriorly and laterally to the trachea and the esophagus below the sternocleidomastoid and infrahyoid muscles. Posterolaterally, it is adjacent to the carotid sheath and the structures it contains. Therefore, it is an organ that needs excellent attention during neck surgery owing to its relations and its variational structure. While the right and left lobes are located at the level of the C5–T1 vertebrae posteriorly, they extend from the upper part of the oblique line of the thyroid cartilage to the fifth tracheal ring anteriorly. The isthmus is at the level of the C7–T1 vertebrae posteriorly and the 2–4 tracheal ring anteriorly [1, 2]. It should also be taken into account that these levels may vary according to some physical characteristics such as age and height. In 50–55% of humans, there is a variational lobe called the pyramidal lobe, which extends from the isthmus or the medial sides of any of the lobes to the prominent laryngeal lobe [25, 26]. This is extremely important for thyroid surgery and cancers. Therefore, in cases where total thyroidectomy is required, the anterior cervical region should be examined and evaluated from an anatomical point of view. Because although total thyroidectomy is required, the disease may recur if the pyramidal lobe is overlooked and not removed. The pyramidal lobe, which is normally inactive, becomes active after thyroidectomy [27]. In addition, the pyramidal lobe must be removed entirely for post-operative radioiodine therapy to be effective in patients with differentiated thyroid carcinoma. Because the pyramidal lobe absorbs most of the radioactive iodine, it reduces the therapeutic benefit of the treatment [26].

The gland tissue is composed of follicles [1, 2, 28], and there are two types of cells in the follicles: central cells (follicular cells) and parafollicular cells (C cells). Follicular cells produce and secrete thyroid hormones, whereas parafollicular cells produce and secrete calcitonin. Calcitonin has the opposite effect of the parathyroid hormone; these two hormones regulate blood calcium levels. The thyroid gland is the only endocrine gland that develops embryologically and can store its secretory product [28]. Thyroid colloids are where the storage takes place.

The thyroid gland has a fibrous capsule, also called the true capsule, which tightly surrounds the organ. Outside this capsule, the pretracheal fascia surrounds the thyroid gland, also called the pseudo-capsule, and is divided into two layers at the posterior border of the gland. One of these layers covers the inner surface of the gland and shows a marked thickening when it reaches the isthmus, connecting the gland to the lower border of the trachea and the cricoid ligament. This ligament is named the lateral ligament of the thyroid gland [1, 2, 29], and it is also called Berry's ligament since Berry first described it in 1888 (Figs. 7.1 and 7.6). It is also called the suspensory ligament of Berry [29, 30]. The other layer extends to the back of the gland and fuses with the prevertebral fascia behind the esophagus and the pharynx. This division of the gland into two fascial sheets creates a fascial compartment on the sides of the esophagus and the trachea, and this space is filled with adipose tissue. The recurrent laryngeal nerve and the inferior thyroid artery lie within this tissue (Fig. 7.6). In this compartment, recurrent laryngeal nerves can travel both medially and laterally to the lateral ligament as well as medially to the ligament, and this variability is significant in terms of surgery. There may also be thin arterial branches of a few millimeters within this ligament, and accidental cutting can cause severe problems because the end of the cut artery is immediately pulled into the gland tissue and disappears [29, 30].

The thyroid gland is supplied by the superior thyroidea artery (a branch of the external carotid artery) and the inferior thyroidea artery (a branch of the thyrocervical truncus). However, the variational thyroidea ima artery, which has been reported at different rates by various researchers, can also supply the thyroid gland. According to many investigators, the thyroidea ima artery can be seen in 1.5–12.2% of cases and may originate from many arteries. Although it most commonly originates from the brachiocephalic trunk (1.9–6%), it can also originate from the right common carotid artery, the aortic arch, the internal thoracic artery, and the subclavian arteries [31, 32]. Therefore, the anterior cervical region should be carefully evaluated in terms of this artery during cricoidectomy, tracheostomy, and neck dissection, and

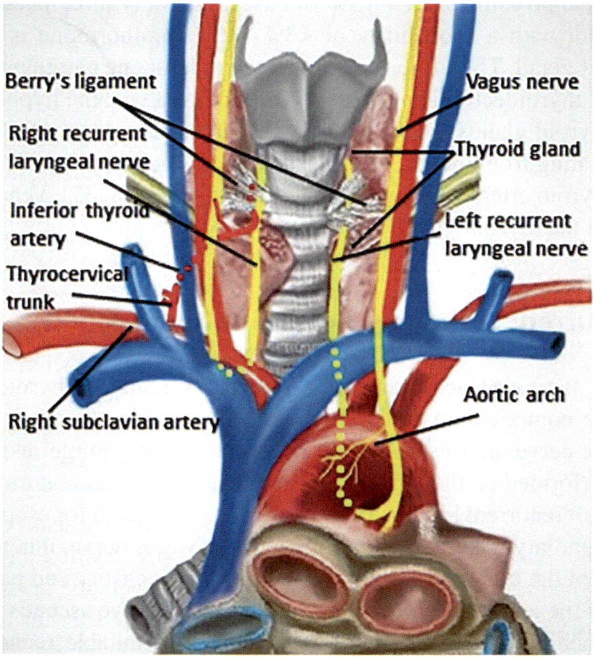


**Fig. 7.6** The recurrent laryngeal nerves and the thyroid gland. The yellow dotted lines are the course of the recurrent laryngeal nerves behind the aortic arch and the right subclavian artery (illustration by Aydin Ozbek and Mehtap Erdogan)

the presence of the artery should be kept in mind. If the thyroidea ima artery originates from a high-pressure artery such as the aortic arch, the brachiocephalic truncus, or the common carotid artery and is injured, it can cause fatal bleeding [33]. Moreover, if this artery is cut, its caudal portion may retract into the upper mediastinum, causing the accumulation of difficult-to-remove blood clots in the chest cavity [34, 35].

The venous drainage of the thyroid gland is through the superior thyroid vein, the middle thyroid vein, and the inferior thyroid vein. The superior thyroid and the middle thyroid veins drain into the internal jugular vein, whereas the inferior thyroid veins drain into the brachiocephalic vein. Parasympathetic innervation is by the vagus nerve, and sympathetic innervation is by the cervical sympathetic ganglia [1, 2].

The parathyroid glands are also located in the fascial compartment on the lateral sides of the thyroid gland and are embedded behind the right and left lobes of the thyroid gland. This situation slightly increases the importance of the fascial compartment in neck and thyroid surgery. It is yellow-brown and has the size of a lentil grain. Since they are located on both the upper and lower sides of the lobes, they are four in number, the upper ones are called the superior parathyroid, and the lower ones are called the inferior parathyroid. While the placement of the upper ones is stable, the placement of the lower ones is extremely variational, and this situation should be considered before surgery. In addition, there may be additional parathyroid glands in approximately 13–15% of cases, and only three parathyroid glands may be present with a probability of <3% [36]. Parathormone is produced and secreted in this gland. Therefore, surgeons leave at least one parathyroid gland, even during radical thyroidectomies, so the patient does not become hypocalcemic [37].

The parathyroid glands are supplied by the superior and the inferior parathyroid arteries originating from the inferior thyroid artery. Therefore, accidental ligation of the inferior thyroid arteries may cause hypoparathyroidism [37]. Venous drainage is the same as in the thyroid gland.

## 7.9 Recurrent Laryngeal Nerve Anatomy

The recurrent laryngeal nerve anatomy is also essential for thyroid surgery. The most common complications after thyroidectomy are due to injury to this nerve; however, these nerve injuries also occur in esophagectomy surgeries. Since esophagectomy is performed on the left side of the neck, anatomical abnormalities or variations of the left recurrent laryngeal nerve are also significant for esophagus surgery.

The recurrent laryngeal nerves, a branch of the vagus nerve, innervate all larynx muscles, except the cricothyroid muscle, and provide sensory and parasympathetic innervation of the larynx. The left recurrent laryngeal nerve ascends below the aortic arch and behind the ligamentum arteriosum. The suitable recurrent laryngeal nerve loops around the right subclavian artery and continues upward in the neck. The recurrent laryngeal nerves then continue bilaterally above and pass medially to the lobes of the thyroid gland as they run along the lateral surfaces of the trachea and the esophagus in the tracheoesophageal groove (Figs. 7.1 and 7.6). As the nerves enter the larynx at this level through the fibers of the inferior constrictor muscles of the pharynx, they pass very close to and behind the cricothyroid joint [1, 2].

The course of the recurrent laryngeal nerve differs on both sides of the neck. The right recurrent laryngeal nerve arises from the vagal nerve in front of the first part of the right subclavian artery and curls under the artery to its posterior surface and ascends obliquely. It is also located behind the right common carotid artery and lateral to the trachea. It then ascends along the right tracheoesophageal groove (Figs. 7.1 and 7.6). At the lower end of the thyroid gland, it crosses the inferior thyroid artery in different positions. The most common condition is that it passes behind the inferior thyroid artery. Less frequently, it passes in front of the inferior thyroid artery and least frequently between its branches [1, 38, 39].

The left recurrent nerve arises from the vagal nerve at the level of the arcus aorta and passes just below the ligamentum arteriosum to the posterior aspect of the arcus and ascends along the left tracheoesophageal groove near the trachea (Figs. 7.1 and 7.6). Its relationship with the inferior thyroid artery is the same as on the right [1, 38–40]. Both nerves enter the larynx at the cricothyroid articulation through the fibers of the inferior constrictor muscles of the pharynx.

The ascent of the recurrent laryngeal nerves in the tracheoesophageal groove is also variational. It rises on both sides, most often in the tracheoesophageal groove. In the second frequency, it rises laterally to the trachea and rarely anterolaterally to the trachea [1, 38, 41, 42].

Recurrent laryngeal nerves show many variations. Many studies report that more than 40% of the nerves split into two or more branches as they approach the inferior constrictor muscle before entering the larynx [38, 40, 42–46]. The branching can occur at any peripheral point where the main trunk of the nerve emerges from the vagus, but, in the inferior thyroid, branching below the arterial level is rare [1, 2, 38]. Recurrent laryngeal nerves sometimes show a fan-shaped branching before entering the larynx [40, 42, 44–46]. They can also enter the larynx by traveling far from the cricothyroid joint, and this distance is more than 5 mm [42]. Sometimes the recurring laryngeal nerves on the left and right do not travel under the arteries and arise directly from the vagus in the neck. In this case, they are referred to as the nonrecurrent inferior laryngeal nerve. In the literature, the left nonrecurrent laryngeal nerve originating directly from the vagus in the neck on the left [42, 46, 47] and the right nonrecurrent laryngeal nerve [42, 47–49] have been reported. In addition, cases of the recurrent laryngeal nerve, which separates directly from the vagal nerve intracranially and follows a convoluted course as it rises in the neck, have also been reported [42].

## 7.10 Thoracic Duct Anatomy

Another vital structure for esophageal surgery is the thoracic duct. An injury to the thoracic duct can cause chylothorax, which is sometimes fatal. In recent years, thoracoscopic esophagectomy applications in the prone position have become widespread due to the precise dissection around the thoracic canal [50, 51]. The neck endings of the thoracic duct show many variations, which makes it vulnerable to injury [52–54]. The thoracic duct is the largest lymphatic vessel in the body and drains 95% of the lymph into the great veins on the left side of the neck [52–54]. It also drains lymph from both the lower extremities, the abdomen (except the diaphragmatic face of the liver), the left hemithorax, the left upper extremity, the left face, and the neck. It starts from the cisterna chyli at the L2 vertebral level, extends to the lower cervical spine, and enters the aortic hiatus of the diaphragm and the thorax behind the aorta as soon as it leaves the cisterna chyli [1, 2, 55]. The thoracic duct continues upward, passing between the aorta and the azygos vein and in front of the vertebral column. It curves to the left at the midthoracic level, runs posterior to the esophagus at the T7 level, and crosses the midline at the T5 vertebral level to the left side of the thorax. At the level of the T1 and T4 vertebrae, the left common carotid artery passes behind the left vagus nerve and the left internal jugular vein and leaves the thorax behind the left subclavian artery and left of the esophagus [1, 2, 55]. It curves laterally behind the common carotid artery and below C6, 3–5 cm above the collarbone. During this course, it is located behind and just lateral to the carotid sheath, where it is most damaged during surgery [55]. It then descends to drain to the junction of the left subclavian and the internal jugular veins (angulus venosus) (Fig. 7.1). During its descent, it is located laterally to the internal jugular vein behind the subclavian artery [1, 2, 55]. At the junction of the lymphatic and venous systems, a bicuspid valve prevents venous backflow into the lymphatic system [56].

The thoracic duct most frequently drains directly into the internal jugular vein, the angulus venosus, and less frequently into the subclavian vein [57, 58]. In <5% of cases, it may drain into other veins, such as the external jugular vein, the vertebral vein, the transverse jugular vein, the brachiocephalic vein, and the suprascapular vein [53, 58]. In addition, the thoracic duct is drained into the right venous system in 2–3% of cases and on both sides in 1.0–1.5% [57].

## 7.11 Gastrointestinal System Anatomy

In esophageal cancers, the organs used for esophageal reconstruction or replacement vary according to the tumor's location. The stomach is used for esophageal reconstruction for tumors in the middle or lower third of the esophagus. In superior mediastinal segment tumors, the use of the stomach is not appropriate, and a flap formed between the terminal ileum and right colon is used for esophageal reconstruction. Due to its vascular structure, the right colon is used more frequently [59, 60]. The last part of the ileum can be mobilized together with the ascending colon and the transverse colon, and the terminal ileum can be anastomosed to the cervical esophagus. Since the left colic artery does not allow, the use of the left colon is not suitable in terms of vascular structure [59, 60]. However, in recent years, suitable parts of the jejunum have started to be preferred more [61, 62]. Compared to the colon or stomach, the jejunum usually does not contain the intrinsic disease, its diameter is very close to that of the esophagus, and it maintains its intrinsic peristalsis after jejunal interposition for esophageal replacement. It also mimics the muscular flexibility of the throat and can thus improve functionality and reduce postoperative reflux. Despite its advantages, the use of the jejunum has been limited for esophageal reconstructions or replacement due to the limitations of the mesenteric blood supply. However, advances in the microsurgical technique now make it possible to replace the entire esophagus with a peduncle jejunal flap [62]. Therefore, it should be expected to be the most outstanding candidate for future esophageal reconstructions. The disadvantages of using the stomach and colon are that previous surgery and the presence of intrinsic diseases such as diverticulosis, polyps, and cancers are at a substantial rate in these organs [62].

As will be understood, the suitability of abdominal structures for esophageal reconstruction or interposition primarily depends on their ability to be mobilized to the extent permitted by their self-supplying vessels. In addition, the lumen diameter and length of the organ to be interposed, whether there are intrinsic diseases, and its ability to maintain aboral peristalsis are also important factors [61, 62]. Therefore, it is necessary to know especially the vascular anatomy and other anatomical features of the stomach, the duodenum, the jejunum, and the colon used in reconstruction after esophagectomy.

## 7.12 General Arterial Supply to the Gastrointestinal Tract

The arterial supply of the intestines is provided by three branches of the abdominal aorta: the celiac trunk, the superior mesenteric artery, and the inferior mesenteric artery. The superior mesenteric artery supplies the small intestines (the jejunum and ileum), whereas branches from the celiac truncus supply the duodenum. The right part of the colon is supplied by the superior mesenteric artery and the left part by the inferior mesenteric artery [1, 2]. The celiac artery or truncus arises from the anterior aspect of the abdominal aorta approximately at the T12 level. Classically, it divides into three arterial branches but shows a significant variation [1, 2, 63]. The most common classical form (trifurcation) has three branches: the left gastric, the splenic, and the common hepatic arteries. True trifurcation occurs in only 25% of cases. In 65–75% of cases, it gives the left gastric artery the first branch and then divides into the splenic and common hepatic arteries. The most common anatomical variant is the origin of the inferior phrenic arteries (35%) or the dorsal pancreatic artery (22%) from the celiac artery [63].

The common hepatic artery first gives the gastroduodenal artery and then divides into the right and left hepatic branches. The most common variation here may also sometimes give off a middle hepatic artery branch to the quadrate lobe [1, 2]. The right gastric artery usually arises from either the common or the left hepatic artery, supplies the pylorus and the lesser gastric curvature, and, eventually, anastomoses with the distal left gastric artery. The gallbladder is supplied by the cystic artery originating from the proper hepatic artery [2, 63].

The gastroduodenal artery courses between the pancreas and the duodenum and gives rise to the superior pancreaticoduodenal arteries as its first branches. It first gives the posterior superior pancreaticoduodenal artery, then the anterior superior pancreaticoduodenal artery, and, finally, the right gastroepiploic (gastro-omental) artery, which supplies the greater curvature of the stomach [1, 63].

The splenic or lienal artery often arises from the celiac truncus distal to the left gastric artery and goes into the upper part of the body and the tail of the pancreas to reach the hilum of the spleen, where it divides into lower and upper branches. With age, the artery lengthens and becomes more tortuous. It goes on along its course, giving off many branches that supply the body and head of the pancreas and giving the more significant pancreatic artery near the tail of the pancreas. The largest branch of the artery is the dorsal pancreatic artery, which gives just after its exit from the celiac truncus. The dorsal pancreatic artery descends behind the pancreas and, after giving a branch supplying the head of the pancreas, runs along the lower border of the body and tail and is called the transverse pancreatic artery. The transverse pancreatic artery (inferior pancreatic artery) anastomoses widely with other pancreatic branches [1, 2, 63].

The superior mesenteric artery arises from the abdominal aorta near the level of L1–2, 1–2 cm below the celiac artery. Where it enters the mesentery, it courses behind the pancreatic body and supplies the distal duodenum, the entire small intestine, and the colon from the cecum to the middle portions of the transverse colon. The first branch of the superior mesenteric artery is the inferior pancreaticoduodenal artery, which sometimes arises as a common trunk with the first jejunal branch. It should be noted that the inferior pancreaticoduodenal artery is part of the arcade that supplies the pancreatic head. The middle colic artery arises proximally from the right side of the superior mesenteric artery as a separate trunk or in common with the right colic artery. Typically, the middle colic artery divides into the right and left branches that supply the ascending colon and the transverse colon, respectively. The right branch of the middle colic artery anastomoses with the ascending branch of the right colic artery, and the left branch joins with the ascending branch of the left colic artery in the splenic flexure (flexura coli sinistra) region to form a vital collateral pathway between the superior and the inferior mesenteric arteries. How the superior mesenteric artery supplies the small intestines is explained in detail in the relevant section [1, 62, 63].

The inferior mesenteric artery originates anterolaterally from the left side of the abdominal aorta around the L3–4 level and supplies the colon from the middle part of the transverse colon to the rectum. Initially, the vessel follows a downward course of several centimeters and then gives off the left colic artery. The ascending branch of the left colic artery anastomoses with the left branch of the middle colic artery at the splenic flexure region. The inferior mesenteric artery and the left colic arteries also give off colic and sigmoid branches descending into the lower descending and sigmoid colon segments. The inferior mesenteric artery then terminates as the superior rectal (hemorrhoidal) artery, which divides into the right and left branches to supply the superior rectum. The middle and lower rectal branches to the rest of the rectum arise from the anterior part of the internal iliac arteries [2, 62, 63].

There are anastomotic connections between the superior mesenteric artery, the inferior mesenteric artery, and the celiac truncus so that the arterial supply of the intestines can be abundant and risk-free. The first of these is between the superior pancreaticoduodenal branches of the celiac truncus and the inferior pancreaticoduodenal of the superior mesenteric artery, known as the Buhler arch. The anterior inferior pancreaticoduodenal and the anterior superior pancreaticoduodenal arteries anastomose between themselves, as do the posterior inferior pancreaticoduodenal and the posterior superior pancreaticoduodenal arteries [1, 2].

There are also two different anastomoses between the superior mesenteric artery and the inferior mesenteric artery. One of these is the structure called "Drummond's marginal artery," "marginal anastomosis," or "paracolic arcade," which is an extensive anastomotic network [1, 61–63]. It is the closest and parallel anastomosis to the intestinal wall. It is an arterial arch that runs along the periphery of the mesentery from the ileocecal junction to the rectosigmoid junction. Even if the celiac truncus and the superior mesenteric artery are occluded, the blood in the inferior mesenteric artery flows in reverse with this arch and continues to supply to the organs supplied by the occluded arteries [63–65].

The anastomosis, called the Riolan arch or a "meandering mesenteric artery," occurs between the middle colic artery of the superior mesenteric artery and the left colic artery of the inferior mesenteric artery and is located at the root of the mesentery [64, 65]. This anastomosis is also essential for the lower extremities. In distal abdominal aortic occlusions, blood flow is provided from the superior mesenteric artery to the inferior mesenteric artery and collateral circulation of the lower extremities is ensured through the superior rectal artery and the iliac vessels from there [63–65].

In addition, we remind here once again of the anastomoses between the right and left gastric arteries and between the right and left gastroepiploic arteries [1, 63].

Despite abundant arterial supply, there are also critical points in the intestines regarding ischemia. One of these is known as the "critical point of the Sudeck" and is a point in the upper part of the rectum [64], where there is no anastomosis between the sigmoid artery, the last branch of the inferior mesenteric artery, and the superior rectal artery, which is a branch of the internal iliac artery. Therefore, this region where the sigmoid artery and the superior rectal artery separate from each other is a critical area for ischemia. Another area is "Griffith's critical point" and is located in the splenic flexura, where a supply deficiency occurs if Drummond's marginal artery is not developed [65].

## 7.13 Stomach Anatomy

The stomach can be used for esophagogastric anastomosis surgically, either by turning it into a tube or as a whole. While some studies say that the whole stomach approach is better because it provides better protection of the submucosal vessels [66, 67], others suggest that the anatomical structure of the gastric tube is more compatible with physiological needs and reduces postoperative complications [68].

Therefore, in our anatomical approach to the stomach, we will pay more attention to the vessels and relations of the stomach. Although the stomach is suitable for esophageal interposition in terms of its mucosa's acid resistance and expansion, it is disadvantaged due to the frequency of intrinsic diseases [62].

The stomach is located in the left upper abdomen in the epigastric, umbilical, and left hypochondriac regions and is like a sac extending between the esophagus and the duodenum. It opens into the esophagus with the gastric cardia and into the duodenum with the pyloric opening and is an intraperitoneal organ. The lesser omentum is connected to the liver, whereas the greater omentum continues down the stomach. The stomach is adjacent to the diaphragm, the left lobe of the liver, and the anterior abdominal wall. It is also adjacent to the base of the left lung and the pericardium of the heart through the diaphragm. In addition, the area directly adjacent to the anterior abdominal wall is called the "Labbe triangle." The base of this triangle is the line connecting the right and left ninth cartilage costae, the left edge is the left arcus costalis, and the right edge is the anterior edge of the liver. The stomach is posteriorly adjacent to the omental bursa, the pancreas, the left kidney and the adrenal gland, the spleen, the third and fourth parts of the duodenum, and the splenic artery. It is adjacent to the esophagus, the diaphragm above, and the transverse mesocolon below and outside [1, 2].

The stomach can be divided into four regions: the cardia, fundus, corpus, and pylorus. The cardia is the point where the esophagus connects to the stomach, and food passes into the stomach. The dome-shaped part located below the diaphragm, above and to the left of the cardia, is called the fundus. The part from the fundus to the pylorus is called the corpus. The pylorus is funnel-shaped and connects the stomach to the duodenum. The broader part of the funnel is called the antrum and is adjacent to the stomach corpus. The narrower end is like a canal and opens into the duodenum and is called the pyloric canal. The junction of the canal with the duodenum is called the pylorus, and the circular smooth muscle fibers here thicken to form the sphincter pyloric muscle. This sphincter controls the emptying of the stomach [1, 2].

The convex edge of the stomach on the left side is called the greater curvature; the concave edge on the right side is called the minor curvature. They have posterior and anterior surfaces extending between these two margins and make the anterior and posterior relations of the stomach. The stomach's blood supply is a complex structure in which many arterial branches participate. The principal arteries of the stomach are the right and left gastric arteries. The left gastric artery is a direct branch of the celiac truncus, whereas the right gastric artery is usually a branch of either the shared or proper hepatic artery. The stomach also receives branches from the splenic artery via the short gastric arteries and the left gastroepiploic arteries. The right gastroepiploic artery, which supplies the right part of the greater curvature of the stomach, arises from the gastroduodenal artery. Both right and left gastroepiploic arteries anastomose at the greater curvature of the stomach and give off branches that supply the mesentery and the greater omentum [1, 63, 69, 70].

The cardia part of the stomach is supplied by anastomoses made by the left gastric artery and the short gastric arteries. Short gastric branches also anastomose with the proper gastric and the left inferior phrenic arteries. These anastomoses also send supplying branches to the fundus of the stomach. Variations in gastric arterial supply are also common. The accessory left gastric artery is relatively common and may originate from the splenic, the main hepatic, celiac, or left hepatic arteries. The left gastric artery may also show frequent variations and give the left hepatic artery a 10–12% probability. Sometimes, 8–13% of the time, the accessory left hepatic branch gives rise [69, 70].

The veins of the stomach also accompany the arteries. Accordingly, the short gastric veins and the left gastroepiploic vein drain into the vena splenica, the left and right gastric veins into the vena porta, and the gastro-epiploic (gastro-omental) vein into the superior vena mesenterica [1, 2].

The nerves of the stomach are the sympathetic nerves from the celiac plexus and the parasympathetic nerves from the vagus nerve (CN X). The sympathetic nerves reach the celiac plexus via nerves from T6 to T10. The left vagus forms the anterior vagal truncus in front of the esophagus and gives off a large branch to the liver and the stomach. The right vagus forms the posterior vagal truncus behind the esophagus and gives off branches to the celiac and mesenteric plexus [1, 2].

## 7.14 Small Intestine Anatomy

The small intestines are divided into the duodenum, the jejunum, and the ileum and vary widely in length and range from 3 to 10 m, with an average length of about 6.5 m or 24 feet. It is the end part of the digestive tract where food digestion, metabolic absorption, and endocrine secretion take place. The jejunum and ileum are the longest, most mobile, and most curved parts of the small intestine and originate from the mesenteron. It starts from the duodenojejunal flexure in the upper left quadrant of the abdominal cavity and ends at the ileocecal junction in the lower right quadrant. These long small intestine sections are suspended on the posterior abdominal wall by the formation of a peritoneum called the mesenterium. It is also referred to by the standard nomenclature of the jejunum and ileum, "mesentery," which can hardly be distinguished by their macroscopic features. There is no clear boundary between the jejunum and the ileum, and an approximate distinction is made according to the differences. The jejunum is usually in the upper left infracolic position, whereas the ileum is in the right and lower abdominal cavity [1, 2]. Since the duodenum is not preferred for esophageal reconstruction, we will not discuss its anatomy here. However, since the jejunum and terminal ileum are frequently used, we will discuss their anatomy.

The jejunum is named after the Latin adjective *jejunus*, meaning "empty or hungry." This is because, at autopsy, this part of the small intestine is empty, often due to terminal peristalsis. That is why this part of the small intestine is called the jejunum, meaning an empty or substance-deprived intestine. In the jejunum, intestinal villi are frequent and high and circular folds (plicae circulares) are numerous and extensive. They decrease as they go down. It is more comprehensive (2–4 cm in diameter), the wall is thicker, the color is redder, and there is a higher degree of vascularization. Peyer's plaques are absent, the mesentery is less fatty, the vasa recta are longer, and the arterial arches have fewer layers (one or two) and wider rings [1, 2].

The ileum is derived from a mixture of the Latin word *ilia* or *ileon* (groin, flank) and the Greek *eileos* (large intestine). The word *eileos* comes from *eilein* (to rotate, to compress by rotation). In this case, there is probably a crossover between the two languages. Its meaning is relatively close to Greek and means "spinning like a spiral," referring to the folds of the large intestines. The ileum is the last part of the small intestine. Circular folds are few and small and absent from the terminal ileum. Its diameter is narrower (2–3 cm), its wall is thinner, and its color is light pink. A large number of lymphoid cells are found in the mucous layer. The mesentery is highly fatty, the vasa recta are short, and the arterial arches have more layers (two or three) with narrower rings [1, 2].

The mesentery of the small intestine is a two-layered peritoneal fold that surrounds the jejunum and ileum and hangs on the posterior abdominal wall. It contains mesenteric vessels, nerves, and mesenteric lymph nodes and lymph vessels. The root of the mesentery (radix mesenterii) averages 15 cm, starts from the flexura duodenojejunalis on the left side of the L2 vertebra, extends obliquely toward the right iliac fossa, and ends at the right sacroiliac joint. Its free edge, about 6 m, attaches to the jejunum and ileum. The radix mesentery crosses from left to right the third part of the duodenum, the aorta, the inferior vena cava, the right ureter, and the right psoas major muscle. The duodenojejunal junction is a landmark easily found during abdominal surgery and is fixed to the posterior abdominal wall by a vertically placed peritoneal fold (Treitz ligament). The inferior mesenteric vein lies retroperitoneally, just lateral to the duodenojejunal junction [1, 2].

The jejunum and ileum are supplied by a single main vessel known as the superior mesenteric artery [1, 2, 71, 72]. The jejunum is supplied by 5–10 jejunal branches arising from the left and anterior aspect of the superior mesenteric artery's superior part. These branches form a single or sometimes double anastomotic arch or arterial arcade before giving off branches to the intestine. The number of these arterial arcades in the ileum is more significant than that in the jejunum. The arterial arcades are parallel and divided into two branches, one ascending and the other descending parallel to the intestine. These branches then fuse with adjacent branches from the nearest jejunal arteries to form the anastomotic arcade. The branches emerging from the most distal of these arterial arcades (the last arch parallel to the intestines) and entering the intestine are called the vasa recta or the arteriae recta and supply the jejunum and ileum. These are terminal vessels about 4–6 cm in size, forming a dense submucosal plexus in the intestinal muscle and mucosa [1, 2, 71, 72].

Our classical knowledge of comparing the anatomy of the jejunum and ileum is that the diameter of the jejunal arteries is larger than that of the ileal arteries and shows a gradual decrease from the jejunum to the ileum. The number of these main branches supplying the jejunum and ileum is between 15 and 18, but the number of ileal branches is more than that of the jejunal branches [1, 2]. In addition, the number of arterial arcade layers in the jejunum (one or two) is less than that of arterial arcade layers in the ileum (two or three). It has also been reported that the length of the vasa recta (arteriae recta) is shorter but more numerous in the ileum [1, 2, 72].

The study by Conley et al. confirmed that the jejunal arteries were slightly larger in diameter than were the ileal arteries and that there were more arterial arcade layers in the ileum compared to the jejunum but showed that, contrary to our classical knowledge, the ileal arteries were not shorter than the jejunal arteries [71]. In addition, this study also confirmed that the length of the vasa recta is shorter and smaller in diameter but more numerous in the ileum [72].

The jejunum is divided into various sections according to the length of its arterial branches to be used for esophageal reconstruction [71]. Accordingly, the first 15 cm of the jejunum is not suitable for isolation for replacement because the first jejunal branch needs to be longer to mobilize this section [71]. The most appropriate section is the loop supplied by the fourth jejunal artery since this branch is the longest and largest jejunal artery [71]. The length of this branch was found to be 45–50 cm in 95% of the cases. Ligation of the first three jejunal arterial branches is not dangerous because it does not cause ischemia. However, the binding of the fourth loop leads to ischemia [70].

The jejunal and ileal veins accompany their arteries and drain into the superior mesenteric vein. The superior mesenteric vein lies to the right of the superior mesenteric artery and crosses the third part of the duodenum and the uncinate process of the pancreas. Then, behind the neck of the pancreas, the superior mesenteric and splenic veins unite and form the portal vein [1, 2, 71, 72].

The nerves of the jejunum and ileum are the sympathetic nerves from the superior mesenteric plexus and the parasympathetic nerves from the vagal nerve. The sympathetic nerves reach the plexus via the lesser splanchnic nerve (ninth to tenth thoracal spinal nerve). The nerves of the duodenum are the sympathetic nerves from the celiac plexus and the parasympathetic nerves from the vagus nerve (CN X). The sympathetic nerves reach the celiac plexus via the greater splanchnic nerves (T5–T9) [1, 2, 71, 72].

## 7.15 Large Intestine Anatomy

The name of the large intestine in medical terminology is "intestinum crassum," which in Latin means an intestine that is twisted or knitted together, often briefly described as the "colon." The large intestine contains the cecum, appendix, entire colon, rectum, and anal canal. The entire colon lies between the cecum and the rectum and is about 1.5 m long. It is divided into ascending colon, descending colon, sigmoid colon, transverse colon sections. The large intestine differs from the small intestine in some features, one of which is the thickened muscle bundles in the form of ribbons called the taeniae coli (also teniae coli or tenia coli). Second, the enlarged parts, such as scoops or pouches between the taenia of the intestine called the haustra coli, and, third, the tiny peritoneal sacs filled with fat called epiploic appendices (appendices omentales) are only specific to the large intestine. In addition, the diameter and lumen of the colon are more significant than those of the small intestines, and they contain mucosal plicas called circular or semicircular folds in their lumens. The large intestine contains three types of taeniae (singular: taenia): liberal or free, mesocolic, and omental taeniae. The taeniae are formed by the condensation of the longitudinal muscle fibers of the large intestine and are not found in the rectum and the appendix vermiformis. The liberal or free taeniae are found on the anterior surface of the cecum, ascending colon, descending colon, and sigmoid colon and on the lower surface of the transverse colon. No structures are attached to the liberal taeniae. The mesocolic taeniae are found on the posterior-interior surface of the cecum, ascending colon, descending colon, sigmoid colon, and the posterior surface of the transverse colon to which the mesocolon transversum is attached. The omental taeniae are located on the posterior outer surface of the cecum, ascending colon, descending colon, sigmoid colon, and the anterior-superior surface of the transverse colon to which the posterior two layers of the greater omentum are attached. The epiploic appendices are tiny peritoneal sacs filled with adipose tissue, primarily lined up along the taenia libera. They are most commonly found in the colon transversum and colon sigmoideum but not in the rectum [1, 2, 73].

The cecum is about 6 cm long and is located intraperitoneally at the ileocecal junction. The appendix is located in different positions and intraperitoneally at the ileocecal junction. The projection of its location is the McBurney point, which corresponds to the one-third outer part of the line extending from the umbilicus to the anterior superior iliac spine. Although the appendix is primarily retrocecal, it can also be found in retrocolic, pelvic, subcecal, pre-ileal, and post-ileal positions. Since they are located intraperitoneally, they also have a mesoappendix. Since the terminal ileum and right colon are the options used together for esophageal reconstruction, this region's folds and blood supply are also necessary [59, 60].

The ascending colon is 15 cm long and extends secondary retroperitoneally from the ileocecal junction to the hepatic flexure. Its anterior surface is adjacent to the anterior abdominal wall when the intestine is entire and to the small intestinal loops when it is empty. Its posterior surface is adjacent to the right subcostal, iliohypogastric, ilioinguinal, femoral, cutaneal, and genitofemoral nerves, the quadratum lumborum and iliacus muscles, the iliac fascia, aponeurosis of the transverse abdominal muscle, and the outer part of the anterior lower surface of the right kidney. It is adjacent to the small intestine loops and major psoas muscle on the inner side and the lateral abdominal wall on the outer side. It is supplied by the ileocolic artery and the right colic artery, whereas its veins drain into the superior mesenteric vein and the lymph into the superior mesenteric lymph nodes [1, 2, 73].

The bend where the ascending colon joins the transverse colon is called the hepatic flexure (the flexura coli dextra or flexura hepatica coli). The hepatic flexura is located intraperitoneally in the right hypochondrium. The transverse colon is 45 cm long and is located intraperitoneally. It is the most mobile and longest part of the large intestine, and the greater omentum adheres to its anterosuperior surface. Since it is located intraperitoneally, it also has a meso. The proximal two-third of the arterial supply is supplied by the middle colic artery, and the distal one-third by the left colic artery. Its venous and lymphatic return is like its arteries, with the proximal two-third part drained by the superior mesenteric vein and the distal one-third part by the inferior mesenteric vein. The proximal two-third part of its lymph is drained into the superior mesenteric lymph nodes, and the distal one-third part is drained into the inferior mesenteric lymph nodes. The bend where the descending colon joins the transverse colon is called the splenic flexura (the flexura coli sinistra or flexura coli splenica). The splenic flexura is intraperitoneally located in the left hypochondrium and is higher than the hepatic flexura. Since the splenic flexura is attached to the diaphragm via the phrenicocolic ligament, it is less mobile than the hepatic flexura [1, 2, 73].

The descending colon is 25 cm long, located secondary retroperitoneally, narrower, and runs more profound than the ascending colon. It joins the sigmoid colon at the entrance to the small pelvis. Its anterior surface is adjacent to the small intestinal loops. Its posterior surface is adjacent to the left subcostal, the left iliohypogastric, the left ilioinguinal, the left femoral cutaneal, and the left genitofemoral nerves, the quadratum lumborum and the iliacus muscles, the iliac fascia, the left testicular (ovarian) vessels, the left ureter, and the outer part of the anterior surface of the left kidney. It is adjacent to the small intestine loops on the inner side and the abdominal side wall on the outer side. The left colic and sigmoid arteries supply it. Its veins drain into the inferior mesenteric vein and its lymph into the inferior mesenteric lymph nodes [1, 2, 73].

The sigmoid colon is 35–40 cm long, located in the small pelvis intraperitoneally, and is highly mobile. It merges with the rectum at the height of S2–S3. Since it is located intraperitoneally, it also has a meso; its position is highly variable because it is extremely mobile. Its position depends on the length of the colon sigmoideum and the mesocolon sigmoideum, the amount of content in it, and the fullness and emptiness of the rectum, bladder, and uterus. While the sigmoid artery supplies it, its veins drain into the inferior mesenteric vein via the sigmoid vein and its lymph into the inferior mesenteric lymph nodes. Arterial anastomoses of the large intestines and poor supplying points will not be mentioned here as they are mentioned in the general information [2, 73].

## References


1. Gray's anatomy: the anatomical basis of medicine and surgery. 38th ed. ELBS; 1995.
2. Moore KL. Clinically oriented anatomy. 3rd ed. Baltimore: Williams & Wilkins; 1992.
3. Minkari T, Ünal G. Surgical anatomy of esophagus. In: Minkari T, editor. Surgery of esophagus. 1st ed. Istanbul: Ceylan Publising; 1980. p. 1–16.
4. Nguyen D, Moslemi M, Rawashdeh B, Meyer M, Garagozlo C, Golestani S, Tempesta B, Maas K, Yousufzai AW, Gharagozlo F. Laimer's diverticulum, a rare true diverticulum inferior to the cricopharyngeus: report of a case and review of the literature. J Clin Case Rep. 2014;4:9.
5. Sato H, Takeuchi M, Hashimoto S, Mizuno K-i, Furukawa K, Sato A, Yokoyama J, Terai S. Esophageal diverticulum: new perspectives in the era of minimally invasive endoscopic treatment. World J Gastroenterol. 2019;25(12):1457–64.
6. Liebermann-Meffert D, Lüscher U, Neff U, Rüedi TP, Allgower M. Esophagectomy without thoracotomy: is there a risk of intramediastinal bleeding? A study on the blood supply of the esophagus. Ann Surg. 1987;206:184–92.

7. Liebermann-Meffert D, Siewert JR. Arterial anatomy of the esophagus. A review of the literature with brief comments on clinical aspects. Gullet. 1992;2:3–10.
8. Vallee B, Hong R, Renelier B, Person H, Huu N. Les artères oesophagiennes d'origine cervicale. Etude anatomique de 23 dissections. Ann Otolaryngol. 1982;99:29–34.
9. Yan Y, Chen C, Chen Y, Wu Y, Shi Z. Arterial patterns in the thoracic and abdominal segments of the esophagus: anatomy and clinical significance. Surg Radiol Anat. 1998;20:399–402.
10. Colas M, Carret JP, Picq P, Le Pivert P, Cuilleret J. Etude de la vascularisation artérielle de l'oesophage par microangiographie. Bull Ass Anat. 1976;60:489–96.
11. Patti MG, Gantert W, Way LW. Surgery of the esophagus. Anatomy and physiology. Surg Clin North Am. 1997;77(5):959–70.
12. Duranceau AC, Liebermann-Meffert D. Embryology, anatomy and physiology of the esophagus. In: Zuidema GD, Orringer MB, editors. Surgery of the alimentary tract. 3rd ed. Philadelphia: W.B. Saunders; 1991. p. 3–49.
13. Lerut T. Technique of cervical approach to the oesophagus. In: Jamieson GG, Debas HT, editors. Surgery of the upper gastrointestinal tract. Boston: Springer. p. 45–51.
14. Morton DA, Bo Foreman K, Kurt H. Albertine the big picture: gross anatomy. 2nd ed. New York: McGraw Hill Professional; 2011.
15. Natale G, Condino S, Stecco A, Soldani P, Belmonte MM, Gesi M. Is the cervical fascia an anatomical proteus. Surg Radiol Anat. 2015;37(9):1119–27.
16. Tomita H, Yamashiro T, Ikeda H, Fujikawa A, Kurihara Y, Nakajima Y. Fluid collection in the retropharyngeal space: a wide spectrum of various emergency diseases. Eur J Radiol. 2016;85(7):1247–56.
17. Debnam JM, Guha-Thakurta N. Retropharyngeal and prevertebral spaces: anatomic imaging and diagnosis. Otolaryngol Clin North Am. 2012;45(6):1293–310.
18. Shah JP, Strong E, Spiro RH, Vikram B. Surgical grand rounds. Neck dissection: current status and future possibilities. Clin Bull. 1981;11(1):25–33.
19. Stack BC, Moreno MA. Chapter 3. Surgical anatomy of the neck. In: Neck dissection. 1st ed. Thieme; 2018.
20. Robbins KT, Shaha AR, Medina JE, et al.; Committee for Neck Dissection Classification, American Head and Neck Society. Consensus statement on the classification and terminology of neck dissection. Arch Otolaryngol Head Neck Surg. 2008; 134(5):536–538.
21. Ozgur Z, Govsa F, Ozgur T. Anatomic evaluation of the carotid artery bifurcation in cadavers; implication for open and endovascular therapy. Surg Radiol Anat. 2008;30:475–80.
22. Ito H, Mataga I, Kageyama I, Kobayashi K. Clinical anatomy in the neck region the position of external and internal carotid arteries may be reversed. Okajimas Folia Anat Jpn. 2006;82:157–67.
23. Civelek E, Karasu A, Cansever T, et al. Surgical anatomy of the cervical sympathetic trunk during the anterolateral approach to the cervical spine. Eur Spine J. 2008;17(8):991–5.
24. Moubayed SP, Ayad T. High-riding innominate artery encountered during neck surgery. Otolaryngol Head Neck Surg. 2014;151(5):888–9.
25. Braun EM, Windisch G, Wolf G, et al. The pyramidal lobe: clinical anatomy and its importance in thyroid surgery. Surg Radiol Anat. 2007;29:21.
26. Geraci G, Pisello F, Li Volsi F, et al. The importance of pyramidal lobe in thyroid surgery. G Chir. 2008;29(11–12):479–82.
27. Mohebati A, Shaha AR. Anatomy of thyroid and parathyroid glands and neurovascular relations. Clin Anat. 2012;25(1):19–31.
28. Nussey S, Whitehead S. Endocrinology. An integrated approach. Oxford: BIOS Scientific Publishers; 2001. isbn-10:1-85996-252-1.
29. Leow CK, Webb AJ. The lateral thyroid ligament of berry. Int Surg. 1998;83(1):75–8.
30. Lekacos NL, Tzardis PJ, Sfikakis PG, Patoulis SD, Restos SD. Course of the recurrent laryngeal nerve relative to the inferior thyroid artery and the suspensory ligament of berry. Int Surg. 1992;77(4):287–8.
31. Moriggl B, Sturm W. Absence of three regular thyroid arteries replaced by an unusual lowest thyroid artery (A. thyroidea ima): a case report. Surg Radiol Anat. 1996;18(2):147–50.

32. Singh R. Study of thyroidea ima artery: narrative review of its prevalence and clinical significance. Basic Sci Med. 2022;11(1):1–4.
33. Simon M, Metschke M, Braune SA, Klaus P, Stefan K. Death after percutaneous dilatational tracheostomy: a systematic review and analysis of risk factors. Crit Care. 2013;17(5):R258.
34. McKenzie GA, Rook W. Is it possible to predict the need for sternotomy in patients undergoing thyroidectomy with retrosternal extension? Interact Cardiovasc Thorac Surg. 2014;19(1):139–43.
35. Shlugman D, Satya-Krishna R, Loh L. Acute fatal haemorrhage during percutaneous dilatational tracheostomy. Br J Anaesth. 2003;90(4):517–20.
36. Wang C. The anatomic basis of parathyroid surgery. Ann Surg. 1976;183:271.
37. Ončar I, Dulfer RR, Massolt ET, Timman R, de Rijke YB, Franssen GJH, Burger PJWA, Smit C, van der Horst FAL, Peeters RP, van Eijck CHJ, van Ginhoven TM. Postoperative parathyroid hormone levels as a predictor for persistent hypoparathyroidism. Eur J Endocrinol. 2020;183(2):149–59.
38. Mishra AK, Amit Agarwal SK, Mishra. Revisited anatomy of the recurrent laryngeal nerves. Am J Surg. 2005;189(5):638.
39. Steinberg JL, Khane GJ, Fernandes CMC, Nel JP. Anatomy of the recurrent laryngeal nerve: a redescription. J Laryngol Otol. 1986;100:919–27.
40. Makay O, Icoz G, Yilmaz M, Akyildiz M, Yetkin E. The recurrent laryngeal nerve and the inferior thyroid artery–anatomical variations during surgery. Langenbecks Arch Surg. 2008;393:681–5.
41. Hunt PS. A reappraisal of the surgical anatomy of thyroid and parathyroid glands. Br J Surg. 1968;55:63.
42. Shao T, Qiu W, Yang W. Anatomical variations of the recurrent laryngeal nerve in Chinese patients: a prospective study of 2,404 patients. Sci Rep. 2016;6:25475. https://doi.org/10.1038/srep25475.
43. Nemiroff PM, Katz AD. Extralaryngeal divisions of the recurrent laryngeal nerve: surgical and clinical significance. Am J Surg. 1982;144:466–9.
44. Ardito G, et al. Revisited anatomy of the recurrent laryngeal nerves. Am J Surg. 2004;187:249–53.
45. Mirilas P, Skandalakis JE. Benign anatomical mistakes: the correct anatomical term for the recurrent laryngeal nerve. Am Surg. 2002;68:95–7.
46. Toniato A, et al. Identification of the non-recurrent laryngeal nerve during thyroid surgery: a 20-year experience. World J Surg. 2004;28:659–61.
47. Henry JF, Audiffret J, Denizot A, Plan M. The non-recurrent inferior laryngeal nerve: a review of 33 cases, including two on the left side. Surgery. 1988;104:977–84.
48. Proye CAG, Carnaille BM, Goropoulos A. Non-recurrent and recurrent inferior laryngeal nerve: a surgical pitfall in cervical exploration. Am J Surg. 1991;162:495–6.
49. Ardito G, Manni R, Vincenzoni C, et al. Il nervo laringeo inferiore non ricorrente: esperienza chirurgica. Ann Ital Chir. 1998;69:21–4.
50. Palanivelu C, Prakash A, Senthilkumar R, Senthilnathan P, Parthasarathi R, Rajan PS, et al. Minimally invasive esophagectomy: thoracoscopic mobilization of the esophagus and mediastinal lymphadenectomy in prone position—the experience of 130 patients. J Am Coll Surg. 2006;203(1):7–16.
51. Fabian T, McKelvey AA, Kent MS, Frederico JA. Prone thoracoscopic esophageal mobilization for minimally invasive esophagectomy. Surg Endosc. 2007;21(9):1667–70.
52. Liu M, Branstetter B, Whetstone J, Escott E. Normal CT appearance of the distal thoracic duct. AJR Am J Roentgenol. 2006;187(6):1615–20.
53. Kinnaert P. Anatomical variations of the cervical portion of the thoracic duct in man. J Anat. 1973;115(Pt 1):45–52.
54. Hematti H, Mehran RJ. Anatomy of the thoracic duct. Thorac Surg Clin. 2011;21(2):229–38.
55. Rosse C, Gaddum-Rosse P. Hollinshead's textbook of anatomy. 5th ed. 1997.
56. Ndiaye A, Di-Marino V, Ba PS, Ndiaye A, Gaye M, Nazarian S. Anatomical variations in lymphatic drainage of the right lung: applications in lung cancer surgery. Surg Radiol Anat. 2016;38(10):1143–51.

57. Skandalakis JE, Skandalakis LJ, Skandalakis PN. Anatomy of the lymphatics. Surg Oncol Clin N Am. 2007;16:1–16.
58. Shimada K, Sato I. Morphological and histological analysis of the thoracic duct at the jugulo-subclavian junction in Japanese cadavers. Clin Anat. 1997;10:163–72.
59. Watanabe M, Mine S, Nishida K, et al. Reconstruction after esophagectomy for esophageal cancer patients with a history of gastrectomy. Gen Thorac Cardiovasc Surg. 2016;64(8):457.
60. Davis PA, Law S. Colonic interposition after esophagectomy for cancer. Arch Surg. 2003;138(3):303–8.
61. Gaur P, Blackmon SH. Jejunal graft conduits after esophagectomy. J Thorac Dis. 2014;6(Suppl 3):S333–40.
62. Ascioti AJ, Hofstetter WL, Miller MJ, Rice DC, Swisher SG, Vaporciyan A, Roth JA, Putnam JB, RoySmythe W, Feig BW, Mansfield PF, Pisters PWT, Torres MT, Walsh GL. Long-segment, supercharged, pedicled jejunal flap for total esophageal reconstruction. J Thorac Cardiovasc Surg. 2005;130(5):1391–8.
63. Gregory Walker T. Mesenteric vasculature and collateral pathways. Semin Intervent Radiol. 2009;26(3):167–74.
64. van Tonder JJ, Boon JM, Becker JH, Van Schoor A. Anatomical considerations on Sudeck's critical point and its relevance to colorectal surgery. Clin Anat. 2007;20(4):424–7.
65. Meyers MA. Griffiths' point: critical anastomosis at the splenic flexure. Significance in ischemia of the colon. AJR Am J Roentgenol. 1976;126(1):77–94.
66. Collard JM, Tinton N, Malaise J, Romagnoli R, Otte JB, Kestens PJ. Esophageal replacement: gastric tube or whole stomach? Ann Thorac Surg. 1995;60(2):261–7.
67. Pierie JP, de Graaf PW, van Vroonhoven TJ. The vascularization of a gastric tube as a substitute for the esophagus is affected by its diameter. Dis Esophagus. 1998;11(4):231–5.
68. Shu YS, Sun C, Shi WP, Shi HC, Lu SC, Wang K. Tubular stomach or whole stomach for esophagectomy through cervico-thoraco-abdominal approach: a comparative clinical study on anastomotic leakage. Ir J Med Sci. 2013;182(3):477–80.
69. Koops A, Wojciechowski B, Broering DC, Adam G, Krupski-Berdien G. Anatomic variations of the hepatic arteries in 604 selective celiac and superior mesenteric angiographies. Surg Radiol Anat. 2004;26(3):239–44.
70. Covey AM, Brody LA, Maluccio MA, Getrajdman GI, Brown KT. Variant hepatic arterial anatomy revisited: digital subtraction angiography performed in 600 patients. Radiology. 2002;224(2):542–7.
71. Van Damme J-P, Bonte J. Vascular anatomy in abdominal surgery. New York: Georg Thieme Verlag; 1990.
72. Conley D, Hurst PR, Stringer MD. An investigation of human jejunal and ileal arteries. Anat Sci Int. 2010;85:23–30.
73. Snell RS. Clinical anatomy for medical students. 4th ed. Boston: Little, Brown, and Company; 1992.

# Histological Features of the Esophagus, Stomach, and Colon

# 8

Feriha Ercan, Dilek Akakın, and Ozlem Tugçe Cilingir-Kaya

## 8.1 General Morphology of the Digestive Tract

The digestive system comprises the digestive tract, also known as the alimentary canal, along with its associated accessory glands. The epithelium of the digestive tract and the glandular structures originate from the endoderm of the primitive gut, whereas the muscular and connective tissue structures arise from the splanchnic mesenchyme. The digestive tract is a hollow tube with varying diameters and includes the oral cavity, esophagus, stomach, small intestine, large intestine, and anus. The digestive system also includes the salivary glands, liver, and pancreas as accessory glands. The wall of the digestive tract is made up of four layers: the mucosa, submucosa, muscularis externa, and adventitia or mesothelium covered by the serosa [1, 2].

The mucosal layer is the innermost layer of the digestive tract and consists of three layers: The epithelial layer surrounds the lumen; the lamina propria layer is composed of loose connective tissue with blood vessels, lymphatics, and glandular structures; and the muscularis mucosae layer consists of smooth muscle cells [2].

The submucosal layer is composed of dense irregular connective tissue with large blood and lymphatic vessels, lymphoid tissue, and submucosal Meissner's plexus of autonomic nerves [2].

The muscularis externa layer consists of smooth muscle cells that are arranged into two or more sublayers. The inner sublayer, located next to the submucosa, is composed of smooth muscle cells organized in a circular pattern. On the other hand, the outer sublayer, which is adjacent to the serosa or adventitia, is arranged longitudinally. Between these two muscular sublayers, there is connective tissue

F. Ercan (✉) · D. Akakın · O. T. Cilingir-Kaya
Department of Histology and Embryology, Marmara University, School of Medicine, Istanbul, Turkey
e-mail: fercan@marmara.edu.tr; dilek.akakin@marmara.edu.tr; tugce.cilingir@marmara.edu.tr


O. Engin (ed.), *Risk Factors and Therapy of Esophagus Cancer*,
https://doi.org/10.1007/978-3-031-47024-0_8

that contains blood and lymphatic vessels as well as Auerbach's (myenteric) nerve plexus [2].

The enteric nervous system (ENS) is the largest portion of the peripheral nervous system, embedded in the wall of the gastrointestinal tract composed of the inner Meissner's plexus, mainly implicated in the regulation of secretion, and the outer Auerbach's plexus involved in the regulation of smooth muscle contractility [3, 4]. The ENS ganglion derives from neural crest cells that originate from the developing dorsal neural tube during development. The enteric ganglion is composed of subtypes of enteric neurons and glial cells, which communicate with each other to modulate intestinal neural reflexes [4].

The outermost layer of the digestive tract is known as the serosa. It is made up of a thin layer of loose connective tissue that contains abundant blood vessels, lymphatics, and adipose tissue. The serosa is surrounded by a simple squamous epithelium or mesothelium. In cases where the serosa is not supported by the mesentery or peritoneal folds, it directly attaches to neighboring structures. This direct attachment can be seen in the esophagus, where the tissue is surrounded by a thick layer called the adventitia. The adventitia is composed of connective tissue that is not surrounded by the mesothelium [2].

## 8.2 Esophagus

The esophagus develops from a small endodermal tube-like structure known as the foregut, which arises during the fourth week of embryonic development. It has two different embryonic origins: the endoderm, which forms the epithelial lining of the esophagus, and the splanchnic mesoderm, which forms the mesenchyme to make up the wall of the esophagus and the outer adventitia [5]. During the fifth week, the middle section of the foregut gives rise to the esophagus. The developmental process includes elongation, crests, thickening, and histological borders [6]. As the heart and lungs descend, the esophagus elongates until the seventh week and becomes lined with specialized cells that secrete mucus. By the end of the eighth week, the esophagus is fully formed and ready to begin its role after birth. Several researchers have suggested that the esophagus can make peristaltic movements during the first trimester. Peristaltic movements may be observed on ultrasound images in the second trimester [5, 7, 8].

The esophagus is a muscular, dynamic, and 25-cm-long tube-like organ that connects the throat (pharynx) to the stomach where digestion and absorption occur. Thus, it plays a crucial role in transporting food and liquids through the alimentary tract, using coordinated muscle contractions known as peristalsis. Its inner lining is made up of a mucous membrane, which secretes mucus to help in clearance and ease food passage and protect the esophagus from damage caused by food or stomach acid [7–10]. The esophagus acts as a conduit for the backward flow of stomach or small intestine contents during episodes of vomiting and reflux [7].

Although the time of existence in various parts of the alimentary canal varies, masticated food is found in the esophagus for about 5 s [10]. The esophagus is

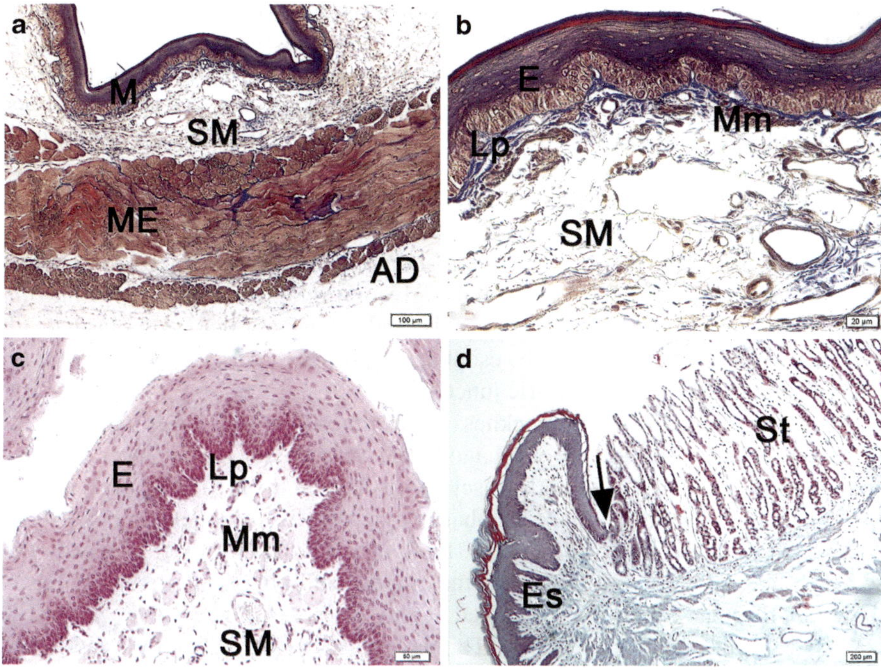


**Fig. 8.1** The esophagus and the esophagogastric junction. (**a**) A cross section of the esophagus showing the mucosa (M), submucosa (SM), muscularis externa (ME), and adventitia (AD) layers. Gomori's one-step staining. Scale bar: 100 μm. (**b**) The stratified squamous epithelium (E), the lamina propria (Lp) in blue color, the muscularis mucosae (Mm) in brown color, and the submucosa (SM) are seen. Gomori's one-step staining. Scale bar: 20 μm. (**c**) The cell layers of the stratified squamous epithelium (E), lamina propria (Lp), muscularis mucosae (Mm), and submucosa (SM) are observed. Hematoxylin and eosin staining. Scale bar: 50 μm. (**d**) The sudden epithelial change from the stratified squamous epithelium to the simple columnar epithelium is seen at the junctional region (arrow) between the esophagus (Es) and cardia (St). Masson's trichrome staining. Scale bar: 200 μm. *As a result of obtaining the samples from the rat esophagus, the epithelium displays a keratin layer, which differs from the human esophagus*

composed of four histological layers: the mucosa, submucosa, muscularis externa, and adventitia (Fig. 8.1) [7–11].

**The mucosal layer** is the innermost layer, which has numerous longitudinal folds with intervening grooves. These folds make the lumen appear obstructed, but, when the esophagus expands, these structures disappear and the lumen becomes patent. The mucosa is composed of three sublayers (Fig. 8.1a) [10].

**Epithelial lining**: The nonkeratinized stratified squamous epithelium surrounding the lumen creates a wet and friction-resistant surface that facilitates the smooth movement of swallowed food masses to the stomach (Fig. 8.1b, c). It makes well-developed interdigitations with the underlying connective tissue. Although it is difficult to measure the thickness of the epithelium due to the interdigitations between the epithelium and lamina propria, it averages 500–800 μm. The glycogen-free basal zone of the epithelium (stratum basale) contains cuboidal/rectangular cells with purple-staining cytoplasm and dark nuclei consisting of several cell layers. There are few melanocytes and neuroendocrine cells scattered in this layer. Epithelial cells increase in size and may accumulate glycogen as they move above the basal zone (stratum intermedium) and eventually flatten out as they approach the lumen (stratum superficiale). Among the keratinocytes of the epithelium, Langerhans cells are found as antigen-presenting cells. The epithelium's renewal rate is slower than those of other parts of the gastrointestinal system. It takes about 3 weeks to reach the surface for newly formed cells in the basal part [8, 9].

**Lamina propria**: This layer is unremarkable and consists of loosely arranged collagen fibers embedded in an acellular glycosaminoglycan matrix. Within this matrix, there are lymphocytes, eosinophils, and occasional mast and plasma cells (Fig. 8.1b, c). This layer houses the esophageal cardiac glands at two sites: near the pharynx and at the esophagogastric junction [8, 9].

**Muscularis mucosae**: The thickness of the smooth muscle layer varies. In the lower part, where it reaches the esophagogastric junction, the muscle layer is thicker and, unusually, consists of smooth muscle fibers located in only one layer (Fig. 8.1b, c). It helps food pass through the esophagus by contracting and relaxing [8, 9].

**The submucosal layer** is a unique, thick layer containing mucous glands that secrete mucus to lubricate and protect the esophageal lining. The secretory units of these tubuloacinar glands are comprised of two distinct cell types, namely, mucous cells and serous cells (Fig. 8.1a–c). This layer also includes the lymphoid tissue, nerves (Meissner's plexus), ganglion cells, and a vascular network (Heller's plexus). Lymphoid cells are concentrated around the glands and their ducts. The presence of a diffuse lymphoid tissue in the esophagus is not as prominent compared to the rest of the gastrointestinal tract, possibly due to the transient exposure to food in this region [7–10].

**The muscularis externa layer** is of varying thickness, consisting of both striated and smooth muscles. Histologically, the muscle layer is organized in two different planes as inner circular and outer longitudinal (Fig. 8.1a). Between the inner and outer smooth muscle layers, a myenteric Auerbach's plexus is found. The upper one-third of the esophagus has the striated muscle that is voluntarily controlled and receives innervation from the somatic nervous system. The smooth muscle makes up the lower two-thirds of the structure and is regulated by the autonomic nervous system, contracting involuntarily. In the middle part of the esophagus, there are both smooth and striated muscles. In the high-pressure zone between the pharynx and the cervical esophagus, a musculocartilaginous structure, the upper esophageal sphincter (UES), is located. The inner circular layer of muscle fibers contracts in a coordinated manner to produce a wave-like motion known as peristalsis. The outer longitudinal layer of muscle fibers helps shorten the esophagus during peristalsis and aids in the relaxation of the lower esophageal sphincter (LES) to allow food to enter the stomach. Any disruption or dysfunction in either of these two sphincters can lead to gastroesophageal reflux, along with its associated symptoms and mucosal alterations [7–10].

**The adventitia layer** is the external covering layer containing fibrous tissue. This loose connective tissue connects the esophagus to the surrounding structures such as the diaphragm and other organs. It covers the esophagus until the diaphragm, and, beneath it, the esophagus is covered by the serosa. In contrast to other regions of the gastrointestinal system, the esophagus lacks a prominent serosal covering, which can facilitate the easier spread of esophageal tumors and pose challenges for surgical treatment. The absence of this serosal layer also makes repairs of luminal disruptions more difficult [7–10].

The esophagus and the stomach are connected by the LES (circular muscle), which helps prevent stomach acid from refluxing back up into the esophagus. The **esophagogastric junction** (squamous/columnar epithelium) is a short area of 1–1.5 cm below the diaphragm and is characterized by a columnar epithelium lining, resembling the stomach (Fig. 8.1d). This junction is a significant site for pathological abnormalities and prevalent diseases, including ulceration, stricture, and cancer [9].

Esophageal cancer, of which the incidence is increasing rapidly worldwide, is a grave malignancy that arises from the cells lining the esophagus. The two predominant forms of esophageal cancer are adenocarcinomas (ACs) and squamous cell carcinoma (SCCs) [12]. For the diagnosis, histological evidence provides the confirmation of a definitive diagnosis [13]. Due to the data suggesting that SCC has a less favorable prognosis compared to AC, a tumor with mixed histopathological characteristics is classified and staged as an SCC [14]. Esophageal AC is the most prevalent type of esophageal cancer and is often detected in the lower segment of the esophagus. The histological features of AC include glandular differentiation, invasion into the lamina propria, muscularis mucosae, submucosa, and beyond [13, 14]. The histological features of SCC include the presence of atypical squamous cells, the invasion of malignant cells into the deeper layers of the esophageal wall, and the presence of keratin pearls, which are clusters of keratinized cells that can be seen under a microscope [13, 14].

## 8.3 Stomach

The surface and glandular epithelium of the stomach is derived from the endoderm of the posterior part of the primordial foregut. The connective and muscular tissues, as well as the peritoneal components, originate from the splanchnic mesenchyme that surrounds the foregut endoderm. During the fifth week of development, the dorsal wall of the stomach grows faster when compared to the ventral wall. This asymmetrical growth results in the formation of a greater curvature on the stomach's dorsal side and a lesser curvature on the ventral side. By the end of the seventh week, continuous dilation of the greater curvature results in the formation of the fundus and the heart incisure. Between the seventh and eighth weeks, the stomach makes a 90° clockwise rotation at the longitudinal axis. As a result, the cranial and caudal ends of the stomach, which were initially positioned in the midline, move to the left and slightly downward, whereas the caudal or pyloric region moves to the right and upward. Thus, the left vagus nerve innervates the anterior wall of the stomach, whereas the right vagus nerve innervates the posterior wall [1, 5, 15].

The stomach is a highly dilated part of the digestive tract. Digestion of carbohydrates continues in the stomach. Acid secretion in the stomach converts the partly digested food into a viscous food material, **chyme**. Production of the pepsin enzyme initiates protein digestion, and lipase production initiates triglyceride digestion. The cardia, fundus, body, and pyloric regions form the stomach. The cardiac region is a narrow transitional zone between the esophagus and the stomach and consists of cardiac glands in the mucosa. The fundus and body regions consist of well-developed gastric tubular glands that secrete acidic gastric juice. The pylorus is a funnel-shaped region of the stomach, consists of pyloric glands in the mucosa, and opens into the duodenum. When the stomach is empty, it consists of numerous, large, longitudinally oriented folds called **rugae** containing the mucosal and submucosal layers, and these folds flatten when filled with food. Like other parts of the digestive tract, the stomach wall consists of four layers: the mucosa, submucosa, muscularis externa, and serosa or the visceral peritoneum (Fig. 8.2) [3, 16].

The mucosa is composed of three sublayers: the epithelial layer, lamina propria, and muscularis mucosae. At the esophagogastric junction, the stratified squamous epithelium transits immediately into the simple columnar epithelium of the stomach. Within the lamina propria, the stomach's epithelium invaginates deeply to form gastric pits, also known as foveola, which open into the stomach's lumen. The gastric glands are connected to these gastric pits and extend throughout the thickness of the lamina propria. These gastric glands consist of various cell types, including

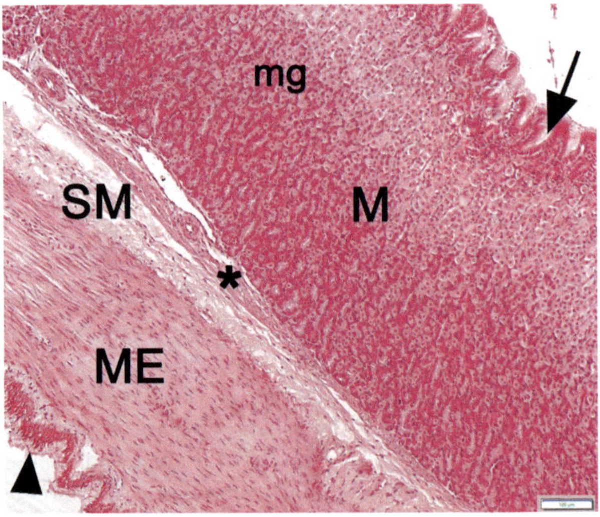


**Fig. 8.2** The stomach. The mucosal (M), submucosal (SM), muscularis externa (ME), and serosa (arrowhead) layers are seen in the fundus region of the stomach. Surface mucous cells cover the luminal surface of the mucosa and gastric pits (arrow). The gastric pits extend into the lamina propria and branch into the tubular mucosal glands (mg). The mucosal glands are located between the gastric pits and the muscularis mucosae (*) along the mucosa's thickness. The muscularis mucosae is seen between the basal ends of the mucosal glands and submucosa. Hematoxylin and eosin staining. Scale bar: 100 μm

mucous neck cells, parietal (or oxyntic) cells, chief (zymogenic) cells, gastroentero-endocrine cells, and stem cells. A gastric gland is divided into three regions: the pit (foveola) is lined by surface mucous cells, the neck contains neck mucous cells, stem cells, and parietal cells, and the body contains the major gastric glands (Figs. 8.2 and 8.3). In the cardiac region of the stomach, the glands are tubular in shape with coiled ends that open into the gastric pits. In the pyloric region, the glands have deeper gastric pits and the mucosa contains highly branched tubular glands. In this region, mostly mucus-secreting cells lining the surface and gastric pits are found, rarely parietal cells are present, and gastrin-secreting G cells are abundant in the glandular epithelium [17, 18].

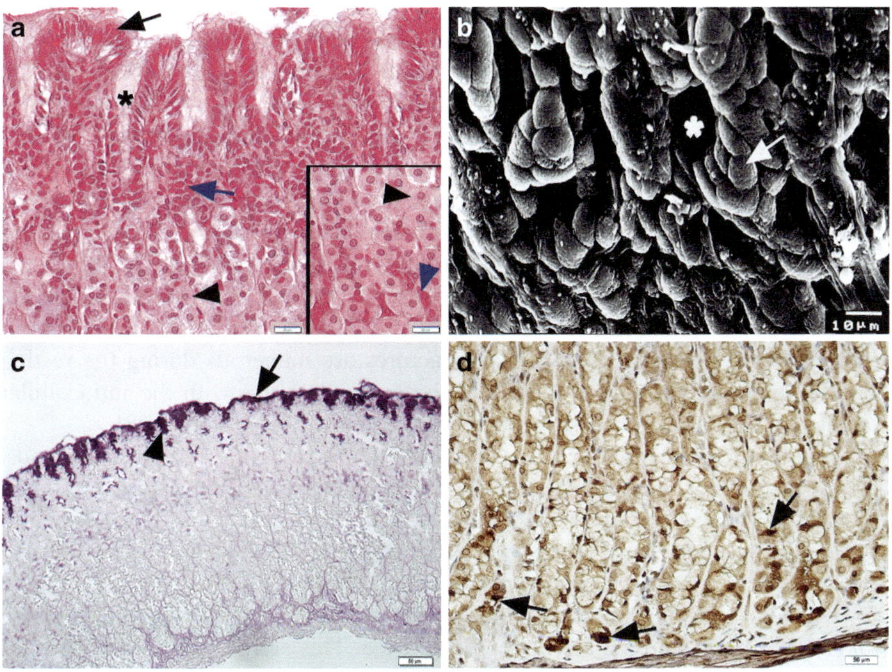


**Fig. 8.3** Gastric pits (foveola) and glandular cells of the stomach. (**a**) Surface mucous cells (black arrow) lie on the apical surface of the mucosa and gastric pits (*). The surface epithelium invaginates toward the lamina propria to form gastric pits. The mucous neck cells (blue arrow) beneath the gastric pits, parietal cells (black arrowheads) with pale pink-stained cytoplasm and a centrally located nucleus, and chief cells (blue arrowhead) pyramidal in shape and a centrally located nucleus are seen. Hematoxylin and eosin staining. Scale bar: 20 µm. (**b**) A scanning electron micrograph showing the apical luminal surface of the stomach with surface mucous cells (white arrow) and gastric pits (*). Scale bar: 10 µm. (**c**) Purple-colored surface mucus as fibrillar morphology (arrow) covers the apical luminal surface of the gastric mucosa and surface mucous cells (arrowhead) lining the apical surface and gastric pits of the mucosa are seen. Periodic acid–Schiff (PAS) staining. Scale bar: 50 µm. (**d**) G cells (arrows) are seen at the lower part of the gastric tubular glands in between the other glandular cells. Gastrin immunohistochemistry. Scale bar: 50 µm

**Surface mucous cells** line the surface of the gastric mucosa and gastric pits. These cells are columnar in shape, and the apical cytoplasm of these cells is filled with mucous granules. **Neck mucous cells** are found as clusters or as a single cell among the other glandular cells of the neck region. The neck mucous cells are less columnar than the surface mucous cells and consist of apical secretory granules. Both mucous cells produce mucins and glycoproteins (Fig. 8.3a–c). The mucus layer consists of mucin and a large amount of water, forming a protective gastric mucosal barrier consisting of an insoluble gel that adheres to the surface of the mucosa. This highly viscous mucus layer is rich in bicarbonate ions that neutralize the microenvironment adjacent to the surface mucus cells and protect the mucosa from the corrosive effects of both partially digested food and stomach acid. Mucus secretion of mucous neck cells is less alkaline than that of the surface mucous cells [2, 18–20].

**Parietal (oxyntic) cells** produce hydrochloric acid and intrinsic factor, a glycoprotein that binds to vitamin B12 in the small intestine. Parietal cells are mostly found among the mucous neck cells in the neck region and upper part of the gastric glands. They are large and morphologically round or pyramidal cells with one centrally located round nucleus. The cytoplasm is eosinophilic due to the presence of numerous mitochondria (Fig. 8.3a). These provide the adenosine triphosphate (ATP) required to pump $H^+$ ions into the **intracellular canaliculus**. The intracellular canaliculus is formed by the invagination of the apical cytoplasm of these cells lined by numerous microvilli and continuous with the lumen of the gastric gland. These cells also contain the $H^+$, $K^+$-dependent ATPase-rich **tubulovesicular membrane system**. These tubulovesicular structures are numerous during the resting phase of these cells. After stimulation, these vesicles fuse with the intracellular canaliculus and release their contents into the lumen of the gland [3, 18].

**Chief (zymogenic) cells** are mostly found in the lower part of the gastric glands. These cells are not found in the glands of the cardiac region but are rarely seen in the pyloric glands. The chief cells have typical characteristics of active protein-secreting cells. These cells have a well-developed rough endoplasmic reticulum and apical secretory granules (**zymogen granules**) containing an inactive **pepsinogen** enzyme (Fig. 8.3a). Pepsinogen is released into the acidic environment of the stomach and converted into the active pepsin enzyme. This active pepsin enzyme initiates the digestion of most proteins. Moreover, chief cells release **gastric lipase**, which initiates lipid digestion [2, 18].

**Gastroenteroendocrine cells** are scattered glandular cells in the gastric mucosa with endocrine and paracrine functions. These cells mostly secrete peptide hormones, and they are dispersed throughout the gastrointestinal tract and regulate the digestive tract function. Transmission electron microscopy or immunohistochemistry techniques using specific antibodies against their products are used to observe these cells (Fig. 8.3d). Some of these cells process amines and were formerly called **amine precursor uptake and decarboxylation (APUD) cells** because of the amine precursor uptake and decarboxylation property of amino acids. Generally, these cells are considered part of the **diffuse neuroendocrine system (DNES)**. There are two types of gastroenteroendocrine cells: The **closed-type cells** lie on the basal lamina and do not reach the gastric lumen and are covered by the neighboring epithelial cells. The **open-type cells** lie on the basal lamina and reach the gastric lumen with their cytoplasmic processes. These cells carry chemoreceptors and sample the contents of the gastric lumen. **Serotonin-secreting enterochromaffin (EC) cells** are located in the fundus region of the gastric mucosa and have a role in the increase of gut motility. **Carcinoid tumors** arising from EC cells are responsible for the overproduction of serotonin. High levels of serotonin cause mucosal vasoconstriction and tissue injury. **Gastrin-secreting G cells** and the other enteroendocrine cells are mostly found in the pyloric region of the gastric mucosa. G cells stimulate the parietal cells for hydrochloric acid secretion. **Gastrinomas (Zollinger–Ellison syndrome**) arising from G cells cause hypertrophy and hyperplasia of the fundic region of the stomach [2, 3, 18, 21].

**Stem cells** are found in the narrow **isthmus** between each gastric pit and gland. These cells divide mitotically to give rise to any type of epithelial cell of the gastric mucosa. Some of these cells move upward to replace surface mucous cells, with a turnover time of 4–7 days. Other progenitor cells move down to give rise to glandular cells of the stomach, which have a much slower turnover time than the surface mucous cells [2, 3, 16].

**The lamina propria** of the mucosa surrounds and supports the gastric pits and gastric glands. This sublayer consists of loose connective tissue containing predominantly reticular and collagen fibers and less elastic fibers, capillaries, lymphatics, fibroblasts, lymphocytes, eosinophils, and mast cells. **The muscularis mucosae**, which is composed of smooth muscle cells, separates the mucosa from the submucosal layer of the stomach [2, 18].

**Other layers**: The **submucosal layer** of the stomach consists of dense irregular connective tissue with adipocytes, capillaries, arterioles, venules, and nerve fibers. The submucosal (Meissner's) plexus consists of ganglionic cells that innervate the blood vessels of the submucosa and smooth muscles of the muscularis mucosae. The **external muscular layer** of the stomach consists of three poorly defined smooth muscle layers: the inner oblique, middle circular, and outer longitudinal. At the pyloric region of the stomach, the middle circular layer becomes thick to form a **pyloric sphincter**. Auerbach's myenteric plexus, located between the muscle layers, regulates the contraction of the muscular layer. The outermost layer of the stomach is the thin **serosa** or visceral peritoneum (Fig. 8.2) [2, 18].

## 8.4 Colon

Three major segments are observed within the large intestine: the **cecum**, **colon**, and **rectum** [3, 18]. The first part of the colon just distal to the ileocecal valve is the cecum, a proximal blind-ended pouch that contains a worm-like extension called the **vermiform appendix**. Lymphatic nodules that extend into the submucosa of the appendix disrupting the continuity of the muscularis mucosae are characteristic for this part of the large intestine. From the ileum, the chyme passes through an anatomical and physiological sphincter (the ileocecal valve) that prevents the reflux of the cecal contents backward. The colon constitutes most of the large intestine and is subclassified into ascending, transverse, descending, and sigmoid colon segments on the basis of its anatomical location. The rectum is the short, dilated, distal portion of the alimentary canal consisting of the upper part, the rectum proper, and the lower part, the anal canal [10]. The mucosa of the rectum is thick with prominent veins and longer crypts of Lieberkühn (fewer numbers per unit area) primarily lined by the goblet cells. It gradually transits from a columnar to a squamous epithelium from the rectum into the anal canal, and the crypts of Lieberkühn gradually disappear at this level. The serosa is replaced by an adventitia in the rectum [2, 3].

The stomach may not be available to use for esophageal reconstruction due to various reasons such as previous gastric resection or tumor involvement. In this condition, using the colon or the jejunum is preferred. The colon offers advantages over the jejunum, particularly in terms of its length, as reconstruction may require the entire length of the esophagus and possibly the stomach as well [22, 23]. Additionally, the colon has a lower potential for reflux and possesses a reservoir-like capacity, making it more suitable for reconstruction. Consequently, the histology of the colon will be discussed in this section of the chapter. Due to its sufficient length and the presence of collateral networks between the middle and left colic arteries, the transverse and left colon segments are commonly utilized as conduits [23, 24].

The epithelium of the large intestine originates from the endoderm of the primitive gut. Muscular and connective tissue, as well as other layers of the alimentary tract wall, are all formed from the splanchnic mesenchyme that surrounds the primitive gut. The cecum, appendix, ascending colon, and the proximal two-thirds of the transverse colon originate from the midgut during development. However, the distal one-third of the transverse colon, descending colon, sigmoid colon, rectum, and the upper two-thirds of the anorectal canal are derived from the hindgut [1]. By the fifth week, the rapid growth of the ileum leads to the formation of the primary intestinal loop of the midgut, which first herniates into the umbilicus by the sixth week and rotates around the axis of the superior mesenteric artery by 90° counterclockwise (from the front view). During the tenth week, by the time the midgut continues to differentiate, the intestinal loop reenters the abdomen and rotates an additional 180° counterclockwise so that the total rotation reaches 270° relative to the posterior abdominal wall. The dorsal mesenteries of the ascending and the descending colon shorten and fold to come in contact with the dorsal body wall; however, the transverse and the sigmoid colon parts remain intraperitoneal [15].

As defined for the typical histological structure of the digestive tube, four layers are observed in the colon: the mucosa, submucosa, muscularis externa, and serosa/adventitia (Fig. 8.4a–d).

The mucosa consists of three components: the epithelium, lamina propria, and muscularis mucosae (Fig. 8.4a, b, and d) [18]. The mucosa has a smooth surface without the plicae circulares or villi and is lined by a simple columnar epithelium. The surface epithelium is made up of absorptive enterocytes and goblet cells. Enterocytes have short apical microvilli, forming a striated apical border, and are responsible for the reabsorption of water and electrolytes (approximately 1400 mL/

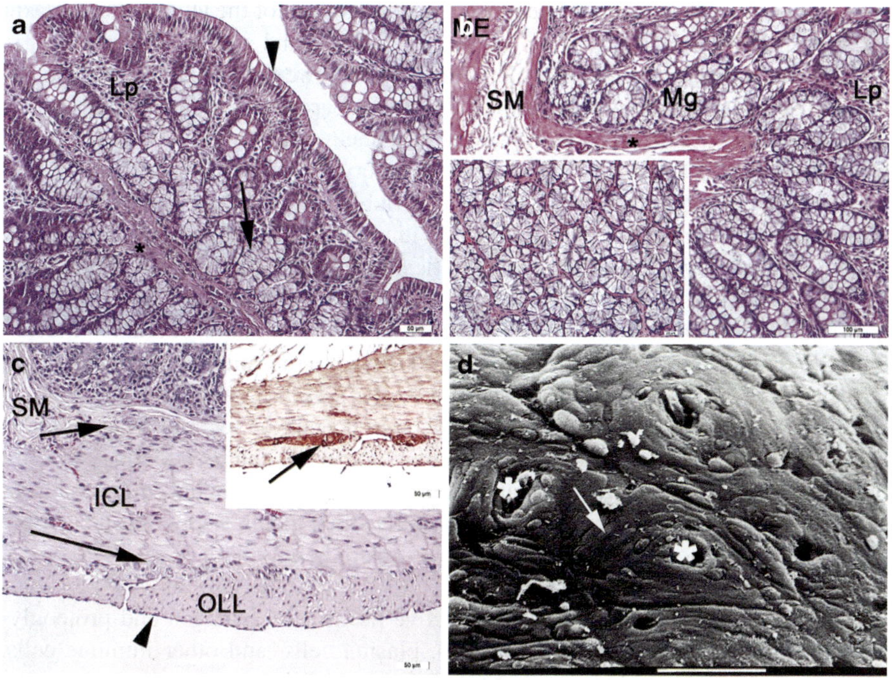


**Fig. 8.4** The colon. (**a** and **b**) Layers of the colon with the crypts of Lieberkühn extending from the lumen. Arrowhead: surface epithelium, arrow: glandular epithelium, *Lp* lamina propria, *Mg* mucosal glands, * muscularis mucosae, *SM* submucosa, *ME* muscularis externa. The inset shows the cross section of crypts with many mucous goblet cells. Hematoxylin and eosin staining. Scale bars: 50 and 100 μm, respectively, and 50 μm for the inset. (**c**) The submucosa (SM), muscularis externa, and serosa (arrowhead) layers of the colon. The submucosal Meissner's plexus (short arrow) and Auerbach's (myenteric) nerve plexus (long arrow) are indicated between the inner circular layer (ICL) and outer longitudinal layer (OLL) of the muscularis externa, respectively. Hematoxylin and eosin staining. The inset shows immunostaining of the neural nitric oxide synthase, and the arrow in the picture indicates the ganglion cell of Auerbach's plexus. Scale bar: 50 μm. (**d**) A scanning electron micrograph of the colon presenting the crypt openings (*) and apical surface of the enterocytes (arrow). Scale bar: 50 μm

day). Reabsorption is achieved by a Na/K-activated ATPase-driven transport system. Na/K-ATPase is abundant and is localized to the lateral plasma membrane. Under the control of mineralocorticoids, $Na^+$ and $Cl^-$ ions are absorbed through the channels of the plasma membrane. The $Na^+$ ions that enter the absorptive enterocytes are expelled by the $Na^+$ pump. The absorptive cells of the colon epithelium secrete glycocalyx that does not contain any digestive enzymes. Goblet cells secrete mucin into the colon that covers the epithelium, lubricates the mucosal surface, and aids in the movement of feces, which facilitates the passage of the increasingly solid contents. The $HCO_3^-$ secreted from the colon adheres to the mucus and acts as a buffer, thus protecting the mucosa from the acidic composition of the feces resulting from acid by-products of bacterial metabolism. Another rare cell type, the caveolated tuft cell, has also been defined in the colonic epithelium and suggested to be a type of goblet cell with fewer mucinogen granules in the central apical cytoplasm [3, 10].

Villi are not seen beyond the ileocecal valve; however, many straight tubular glands (**crypts of Lieberkühn**) are found. These crypts are similar in composition to those of the small intestine; however, no Paneth cells are found in the colon, whereas they may be present in the cecum. The crypts are also longer than those in the small intestine (0.4–0.6 mm) extending through the full thickness of the mucosa. Openings of the glands are examined at the luminal surface of the large intestine at the microscopic level (Fig. 8.4) [25–27]. The **glandular epithelium** lining the tubular glands consists of **stem cells** and **enteroendocrine cells** among the enterocytes and numerous goblet cells. In the colonic epithelium, more abundant mucus-secreting goblet cells are observed compared to that in the small intestine. The goblet cell number increases from the cecum to the sigmoid colon, and the ratio of columnar absorptive cells to goblet cells decreases near the rectum, where there is an abundant number of goblet cells. The few dispersed enteroendocrine cells are located at the base of the tubular glands. Colonic mucosal epithelial cells arise from stem cells located at the lower portion of the intestinal gland. Rapid mitotic activity of these cells replaces the surface and glandular epithelial lining every 6–7 days [3, 10, 18].

The **lamina propria** is a loose connective tissue with collagen and proteoglycans containing fibroblasts, macrophages, plasma cells, and other immune cells. The gut-associated lymphatic tissue in the large intestine is more extensively developed compared to that in the ileum. Lymphatic follicles can be observed under the **muscularis mucosae**, extending into the submucosa. The muscularis mucosae consists of thin strands of smooth muscle fibers that separate the mucosa from the submucosa [3, 10].

The **submucosa** comprises loose connective tissue, thin smooth muscle bundles, and nerve plexus (Meissner's plexus) with ganglion cells, stromal cells, and particularly adipose tissue and blood vessels. Glands are not present in the submucosa (Fig. 8.4c) [3, 10].

The **muscularis externa** consists of inner circular and outer longitudinal layers. Auerbach's nerve plexus is located in between these two muscular layers (Fig. 8.4c) [3, 18]. The inner circular layer of the muscularis is thin and evident, whereas the outer longitudinal layer is practically only found in the taeniae. The longitudinal muscle layer in the colon is not in a continuous pattern. Instead, the smooth muscle tissue is divided into three longitudinally oriented, narrowed, thickened ribbon-like bands (each 1 cm wide) called the **taeniae coli**. The taeniae coli runs the length of the large intestine, primarily visible in the cecum and colon; however, they are absent in the vermiform appendix, rectum, and anal canal. In the rectum, the longitudinal layer has a continuous pattern. As the taeniae coli is shorter than the intestine, contractions of the taeniae coli and circular muscle layer draw the colon into sacculations to form small pouches called **haustra coli** [10].

As the ascending and descending segments of the colon are retroperitoneally located, they are covered by adventitia. The other parts of the colon, however, are invested by the **serosa** and suspended by the mesentery. The serosa (cuboidal mesothelial cells) surrounds the omental **appendices epiploicae**, which are the scattered sacs of adipose tissue, a unique feature of the colon, together with the haustra [3, 12].

## References


1. Moore KL, Persaud TVN, Torchia MG. Chapter 11: Alimentary system. In: The developing human: clinically oriented embryology. 10th ed. Philadelphia: Elsevier; 2016. p. 209–39.
2. Mescher AL. Chapter 15: Digestive tract. In: Junqueira's basic histology. Text and atlas. 13th ed. McGraw-Hill Education; 2018. p. 295–326.
3. Ross MH, Pawlina W. Chapter 17: Digestive system II-esophagus and gastrointestinal tract. In: Histology: a text and Atlas: with correlated cell and molecular biology. 8th ed. New York: Wolters Kluwer Health; 2016. p. 568–600.
4. Furness JB. Types of neurons in the enteric nervous system. J Auton Nerv Syst. 2000;81:87–96.
5. Sadler TW. Chapter 15: Digestive system. In: Langman's medical embryology: Part 2: Systems based embryology. 14th ed. Philadelphia: Wolters Kluwer; 2019. p. 230–55.
6. Carslon BM. Chapter 15: Digestive and respiratory systems and body cavities. In: Human embryology and developmental biology. 4th ed. Missouri: Elsevier; 2009. p. 318–57.
7. Kuo B, Urma D. Reviews part I: oral cavity, pharynx and esophagus. Esophagus—anatomy and development. GI Motility. 2006; https://doi.org/10.1038/gimo6.
8. Lowrie DJ Jr. Chapter 28: Overview of the gastrointestinal system and Chapter 31: pharynx, esophagus, and stomach. In: Histology: an essential textbook. New York: Thieme; 2020. p. 195–205. and 222-231.
9. Stevens A, Lowe JS. Chapter 11: Alimentary tract. In: Stevens & Lowe's human histology. 4th ed. Philadelphia: Elsevier; 2015. p. 186–218.
10. Gartner LP. Chapter 17: Alimentary canal. In: Textbook of histology. 4th ed. Philadelphia: Elsevier; 2017. p. 435–70.
11. Cerit KK, Karakoyun B, Bahadır E, Yüksel M, Bülbül N, Ercan F, et al. Halofuginone improves caustic-induced oxidative injury of esophagus in rats. Esophagus. 2018;15(2):59–68. https://doi.org/10.1007/s10388-017-0594-4.
12. Ovalle WK, Nahirney PC. Chapter 12: Upper digestive tract and Chapter 13: lower digestive tract. In: Netter's essential histology. 2nd ed. Philadelphia: Elsevier; 2013. p. 263–310.
13. Siersema PD. Esophageal cancer. Gastroenterol Clin N Am. 2008;4(37):943–64. https://doi.org/10.1016/j.gtc.2008.09.012.
14. Li Z, Rice TW. Diagnosis and staging of cancer of the esophagus and esophagogastric junction. Surg Clin N Am. 2012;5(92):1105–26.
15. Schoenwolf GC, Bleyl SB, Brauer PR, Francis-West PH. Chapter 14: Development of the gastrointestinal tract. In: Larsen's human embryology. 5th ed. Philadelphia: Elsevier; 2015. p. 341–74.
16. Eroschenko VP. Part II: Organs. Chapter 14: Digestive system Part II: Esophagus and stomach. In: Di Fiore's atlas of histology with functional correlations. 12th ed. Baltimore: Lippincott Williams & Wilkins; 2013. p. 313–37.
17. Atasoy BM, Deniz M, Dane F, Özen Z, Turan P, Ercan F, et al. Prophylactic feeding with immune-enhanced diet ameliorates chemoradiation-induced gastrointestinal injury in rats. Int J Radiat Biol. 2010;86(10):867–79. https://doi.org/10.3109/09553002.2010.487026.
18. Kierszenbaum AL, Tres LL. Part IV: Organ systems: alimentary tract. Chapter 15: Upper digestive segment and Chapter 16: Lower digestive segment. In: Histology and cell biology. An introduction to pathology. 5th ed. Philadelphia: Elsevier Saunders; 2020. p. 511–74.
19. Ercan F, Cetinel S, Contuk G, Cikler E, Sener G. Role of melatonin in reducing water avoidance stress-induced degeneration of the gastrointestinal mucosa. J Pineal Res. 2004;37(2):113–21. https://doi.org/10.1111/j.1600-079X.2004.00143.x.

20. Kumral ZN, Memi G, Ercan F, Yeğen BC. Estrogen alleviates acetic acid-induced gastric or colonic damage via both ERα- and ERβ-mediated and direct antioxidant mechanisms in rats. Inflammation. 2014;37(3):694–705. https://doi.org/10.1007/s10753-013-9786-9.
21. Babayev H, Arabaci-Tamer S, Yildirim A, Kayali D, Ercan F, Yegen C, et al. Sleeve gastrectomy-induced endocrine changes in the remnant stomachs of premenopausal and postmenopausal rats: role of the estrogen receptors. Surg Obes Relat Dis. 2021;17(1):193–207. https://doi.org/10.1016/j.soard.2020.08.011.
22. Watanabe M, Mine S, Nishida K, Kurogochi T, Okamura A, Imamura Y. Reconstruction after esophagectomy for esophageal cancer patients with a history of gastrectomy. Gen Thorac Cardiovasc Surg. 2016;64:457–63.
23. Cha HG, Jeong HH, Kim EK. Microsurgical options after the failure of left colon interposition graft in esophagogastric reconstruction. Arch Craniofac Surg. 2019;20:134–8.
24. Bothereau H, Munoz-Bongrand N, Lambert B, Montemagno S, Cattan P, Sarfati E. Esophageal reconstruction after caustic injury: is there still a place for right coloplasty? Am J Surg. 2007;193:660–4.
25. Karakoyun B, Yüksel M, Ercan F, Salva E, Işik I, Yeğen BC. Halofuginone, a specific inhibitor of collagen type 1 synthesis, ameliorates oxidant colonic damage in rats with experimental colitis. Dig Dis Sci. 2010;55(3):607–16. https://doi.org/10.1007/s10620-009-0798-0.
26. Özbeyli D, Berberoglu AC, Özen A, Erkan O, Başar Y, Şen T, et al. Protective effect of alpha-lipoic acid, aerobic or resistance exercise from colitis in second hand smoke exposed young rats. Clin Exp Pharmacol Physiol. 2017;44(1):62–70. https://doi.org/10.1111/1440-1681.12682.
27. Karakoyun B, Ertaş B, Yüksel M, Akakın D, Çevik Ö, Şener G. Ameliorative effects of riboflavin on acetic acid-induced colonic injury in rats. Clin Exp Pharmacol Physiol. 2018;45(6):563–72. https://doi.org/10.1111/1440-1681.12894.

# Overview of Esophageal Cancer by a Gastroenterologist

9

Gozde Dervis Hakim

## 9.1 Introduction

Esophageal cancer ranks seventh in incidence and sixth in mortality rate among all cancers globally. Regarding the 2020 World data, 604,000 newly diagnosed cases and 544,000 deaths have been observed due to esophageal cancer. The incidence of esophageal cancer ranks in the first place in Asian countries (481,552 cases/year), followed by Europe (52,993 cases/year), Africa (27,546 cases/year), North America (20,806 cases/year), Latin America (19,011 cases/year), and Oceania (2192 cases/year). Mortality and incidence rates were found to differ approximately 2–5 times between both genders. It is seen to be more common in the middle-aged and older population and in the male gender. It is also stated that the frequency is higher in developing countries compared to developed countries [1].

Esophageal cancers occur in various types as: squamous cell cancer (SCC), adenocarcinoma (AC), sarcoma, small cell carcinoma, rarely lymphoma, and melanoma [2, 3]. More than 90% of cases all over the world are in the form of SCC. However, in recent years, the incidence under 50 years of age and the frequency of AC have been increasing gradually, and this increase seems to suppress the incidence of SCC, especially in Europe and North America [2, 3]. While AC is common especially in countries with high socioeconomic status, on the contrary SCC in low socioeconomic status [4].

The anatomical location of esophageal cancer has also changed in recent years. While it used to be located more frequently in the upper 1/3 esophagus part, nowadays, cancer is more common in the lower 1/3 esophagus part with increasing frequency. This difference in esophageal cancer location is due to the increase in the

G. D. Hakim (✉)
Gastroenterology Department, University of Health Sciences, Izmir Medical Faculty Tepecik Training and Research Hospital, İzmir, Turkey





O. Engin (ed.), *Risk Factors and Therapy of Esophagus Cancer*,
https://doi.org/10.1007/978-3-031-47024-0_9

incidence of adeno carcinoma, which is frequently located in the lower esophagus [5].

The incidence of the esophagogastric junction (OGJ) AC appears to have increased moderately in recent years [6]. Like esophageal AC, obesity, gastroesophageal reflux disease, and high fat intake are risk factors for OGJ cancer [7], and Helicobacter pylori infection is inversely related [8].

## 9.2 Risk Factors

### 9.2.1 Esophageal Squamous Cell Carcinoma

SCC is the most common type of esophageal cancer worldwide. Although it is more common in males, gender distribution has been found to differ according to cancer incidence. In countries with lower incidence rates, such as the United States, the female-to-male ratio is 4/1. This rate decreases and even approaches 1/1 in countries with higher incidence, such as China and Iran [2]. SCC etiology and risk factors also differ in high and low-incidence regions, just like gender. Two of the most important risk factors in SCC in industrialized countries are smoking and alcohol consumption. The synergistic effect of these two independent risk factors has also been demonstrated. SCC risk increased 3–9 times in active smokers and 3–5 times in active alcohol consumers [9]. SCC precursor lesions were associated with smoking for more than 20 years (odds ratio: 1.48), alcohol use for more than 30 years (odds ratio: 1.40), and alcohol intake of more than 100 ccs per day (odds ratio: 1.44) [10]. Compared to individuals who never smoked, current or former smokers have a 2–4-fold increased risk. The risk is increased 2–9 times in those who consume alcohol compared to those who do not consume alcohol at all [11, 12].

Hot beverage consumption is also among other factors that increase the risk of SCC. It stimulates the inflammatory cascade, and the resulting endogenous nitrogen species stimulate the TP 53 (tumor protein 53) mutation, which is thought to be effective in the pathogenesis of SCC. In addition, with the thermal damage effect of chronic heat exposure, the barrier effect of the esophageal epithelium disappears, and the passage and interaction of carcinogenic substances become easier. In population-based studies, it has been shown that excessively hot coffee and tea consumption increases the risk of SCC [13].

High rates of nitrosamine formation occur in pickled vegetables due to fermentation. Nitrosamines are associated with SCC formation. Therefore, the risk of SCC is high in societies that consume endemic pickled food. In a meta-analysis including 34 studies involving 225,000 patients, the SCC odds ratio was 2.08 in those who consumed high amounts of pickled food compared to those who did not [14].

Since vitamins A, C, and E prevent the formation of free radicals and nitrosamines, the deficiency of these vitamins is among the risk factors [15]. Low fruit consumption is thought to be associated with SCC [16, 17].

Folic acid, zinc, and selenium deficiencies have also been associated with SCC. Decreased folate intake or impaired metabolism is a risk factor for many gastrointestinal system malignancies such as SCC [18]. In the case-control series, the low folic acid level in serum has been reported to be associated with SCC [16]. Zinc deficiency increases the risk of SCC by potentiating the carcinogenic effect of nitrosamines. A study including a 10-year follow-up period of patients receiving selenium supplementation found that the death rate from esophageal cancer decreased by 17% [19]. In a systemic review reviewing the effect of fresh fruit and vegetable consumption on the reduction of esophageal cancer risk, it was found that daily consumption of fresh, raw vegetables or fruits reduced the cancer rate by 31% and 22%, respectively [20].

Those with a low socioeconomic status have a higher risk of SCC than those with a higher socioeconomic status. Exposure to radiation and agrochemicals, excessive fried food intake, sedentary lifestyle, and low fiber intake are the other risk factors [21, 22] (Table 9.1).

There are controversial results that human papilloma virus (HPV)s serotypes 16–18 are associated with SCC [23]. In studies conducted in regions with a high incidence of SCC, HPV is associated with SCC [24, 25]. However, larger studies are needed. Esophageal lichen planus is associated with the development of SCC in up to 6.1% of patients [26].

Although AC is more common in patients diagnosed with achalasia, SCC can also be observed at a rate of 5% [27]. Approximately 1–24 years after the diagnosis of achalasia, it was found that the risk of SCC increased 16 times, especially in men [28]. Mechanical stenosis occurring in esophageal webs, such as Plummer–Vinson syndrome (iron deficiency anemia, dysphagia, post cricoid webs), increases the risk of SCC with chronic stasis of food and triggering chronic inflammation [29].

Tylosis or hyperkeratosis palmaris et plantaris is a rare but autosomal-dominant genetic disease characterized by abnormalities in the RHBDF2 gene that results in a significant risk of ESCC of at least 80% in a small species [30, 31].

Four genome-wide association studies (GWAS), three conducted in the Chinese population and one in the Japanese population, elaborated on genetic predisposition factors for the development of squamous carcinoma, particularly in heavy alcohol

**Table 9.1** Risk factors of SCC and AC

| Risk factor | Squamous cell cancer | Adeno carcinoma |
|---|---|---|
| Geography | Southeastern Africa, Asia, Iran, South America | Western Europe, North America, Australia |
| Race | Black > white | White > black |
| Gender | Male > female | Male > female |
| Alcohol | ++++ | – |
| Smoking | ++++ | ++++ |
| Obesity | – | ++++ |
| Gastroesophagial reflux | – | ++++ |
| Genetic aspects | ++ | + |
| Socioeconomic Status | ++ | – |

and tobacco users. Two nucleotide polymorphisms (SNPs, single nucleotide polymorphisms) deserve special attention as they encode enzymes that metabolize alcohol: alcohol dehydrogenase 1B (rs1229984, OR = 1.79) and aldehyde dehydrogenase 2 families (rs671, OR = 1.67). The other GWAS found associations at two loci, one in the phospholipase C enzyme and the other in a specific region of chromosome 20 (C20orf54) [32]. A GWAS dataset was reviewed regarding its association with squamous carcinoma, including 453,852 SNPs from 1898 squamous carcinoma patients of the Chinese population and 2100 control subjects. The authors identified candidate causative SNPs and pathways (ICSN Pathway) analysis identified seven candidate SNPs, five genes, and seven pathways, revealing seven hypothetical biological mechanisms together. The three most powerful hypothetical biological mechanisms were rs4135113, rs1800450, and rs3769823 [33].

### 9.2.2 Risk Factors for Adenocarcinoma

AC is the second most common type of esophageal cancer worldwide. It is eight times more common in men than women. In the United States of America (USA), it is five times more common in whites than blacks [34]. Male dominance in SCC and AC derives one to think that female sex hormones may have a protective effect against esophageal cancer. Its incidence is increasing in Western countries, especially in the United Kingdom, Iceland, Australia, and the USA [35–37]. This increase is thought to be due to gastroesophageal reflux, which develops due to increasing obesity in Western countries. Gastroesophageal reflux with acid and bile is the most important risk factor for AC. In population-based case-control studies and meta-analyses, for gastroesophageal reflux, Barrett's esophagus (BE) is associated with AC; an odds ratio of 12.0 (95% Confidence Interval (CI 7.64–18.7) and odds ratio of 4.64 (95% CI 3.28–6.57), respectively [38, 39]. Over the past 30 years, the incidence of BE increased, which is also correlated with the increase in AC. BE develops due to GERD at a rate of 6–14% and causes AC development in 0.5–1% [34]. The largest study on this topic is a nationwide, population-based cohort study using data from all patients with BE from 1992 to 2009 using data from the Danish Pathology Registry and the Danish Cancer Registry. The study included 11,028 patients with BE over a median of 5.2 years. The incidence rate of AC was 1.2 cases per 1000 person-years (95% CI: 0.9–1.5). Compared with the risk in the general population, the risk rate of AC in patients with BE was 11.3 (95% CI: 8.8–14.4). However, the annual risk of esophageal AC was 0.12% (95% CI: 0.09–0.15) [40].

After reflux, obesity, especially central (visceral organ) obesity, is the second strongest risk factor for BE/AC, and these two factors proceed in a synergistic course [41–43]. Obesity may increase reflux through increased intra-abdominal pressure. The obesity-associated metabolic syndrome is also a risk factor for BE, independent of reflux symptoms [44]. In addition, in obese individuals, inflammatory mediators released from adipocytes, insulin-like growth factor, leptin, and adiponectin increase the risk of developing AC from Barret's esophagus by a hormone-dependent mechanism [45]. Although smoking is a moderately strong risk factor for AC, its association with BE is less clear, and alcohol does not appear to increase risk significantly [46].

Other risk factors for BE/AC include high red meat intake (OR 1.91 ranging between 1.07 and 3.38 for highest and lowest ratio), low fruit/vegetable intake and high fat and calorie intake [47].

In contrast, *Helicobacter pylori* infection is inversely associated with BE/AC risk. Decreased population seropositivity for Helicobacter pylori due to improved socioeconomic conditions may also increase AC rates [48].

Various studies have shown that the use of aspirin, nonsteroidal anti-inflammatory, proton pump inhibitor, and statins reduces the risk of AC formation and may have protective effects against AC [49–53] (Table 9.1).

GWAS-type studies have also been conducted to elucidate susceptibility loci. Familial clustering has been observed in Barrett's esophagus and AC. The first genome-wide association study of esophageal AC with BE was recently published. The most significant results were for the combination of cancer and precancerous stages. This suggests that most of the genetic basis for esophageal AC lies in the development of BE rather than esophageal AC. The authors found three novel genome-wide significant loci for esophageal AC and BE and extended existing findings at the FOXF1 and HLA loci. One of the new regions is chromosome 3p13 near FOXP1, a gene that encodes a transcription factor that regulates esophageal development. Interestingly, two other regions (BARX1/9q22.32 and FOXF1/16q24.1) contain risk-associated SNPs that impair FOXP1 binding [54]. Another genome-wide association study identified susceptibility loci for Barrett's esophagus and AC at CRTC1 (encodes a CREB-regulated transcription factor), BARX1 (encodes a protein involved in the esophageal specification), and FOXP1 (located in the esophagus) encodes a protein development [55].

In a genome-wide, confluent association analysis, germline mutations in one of three candidate genes (MSR1, ASCC1, and CTHRC1) were identified in 11% of patients with Barrett's esophagus or AC [55]. Mutant MSR1 is associated with cyclin D1 overexpression resulting in faster cell cycle progression [56]. However, further studies are needed on these issues.

## 9.3 Clinical Features

Despite differences in demographics and risk factors, the clinical presentation is similar between esophageal AC and squamous cell carcinoma. The endoscopic appearance is also similar, although approximately three quarters of all AC lesions are found in the distal esophagus. At the same time, squamous cell carcinoma is more common in the proximal and middle esophagus [57]. Usually, most patients are asymptomatic in the early stages. With the progression of the disease, weight loss, early satiety, and difficulty in swallowing develop. Especially because of difficulty in swallowing, the patient refrains from eating. When the esophageal lumen diameter is 13 mm or less, swallowing difficulty occurs against solid foods. As lumen obstruction increases, difficulty in swallowing becomes more evident; dysphagia develops against liquid foods and is accompanied by weight loss. In the presence of an ulcer lesion, odynophagia develops [57].

Iron deficiency anemia, palpable cervical lymphadenopathy, and chest pain are less common symptoms. Pneumonia or pleural effusion may occur in the development of an esophageal respiratory fistula. Much more rarely, esophageal aortic fistula develops and presents with severe gastrointestinal hemorrhage. Hoarseness is much rarer. Metastases to the lymph node, lung, liver, brain, and bones may occur [5]. Less common symptoms include hoarseness, cough, and laryngeal nerve palsy or pneumonia associated with invasion of the tracheobronchial tree. Patients with head and neck squamous cell carcinoma also have an increased risk of synchronous and metachronous esophageal squamous cell carcinoma [57].

## 9.4 Diagnosis and Screening

Usually, laboratory tests are nonspecific. In advanced stages, anemia (iron deficiency anemia or anemia of chronic disease), hypoalbuminemia, and/or hypercalcemia (mostly due to osteolytic metastasis in bone) develop. Paraneoplastic syndrome is rare, and hypercalcemia due to circulating parathyroid hormone-related protein can be seen in SCC. However, it is quite rare [58]. Squamous dysplasia is the precursor lesion of esophageal squamous cell carcinoma; Barrett's esophagus is the pre-neoplastic lesion before AC [59]. The gold standard for diagnosis is esophagogastroduodenoscopy (EGD) and multiple biopsies taken from suspicious areas during this time (Fig. 9.1). Taking approximately 6–8 biopsies from suspicious areas is

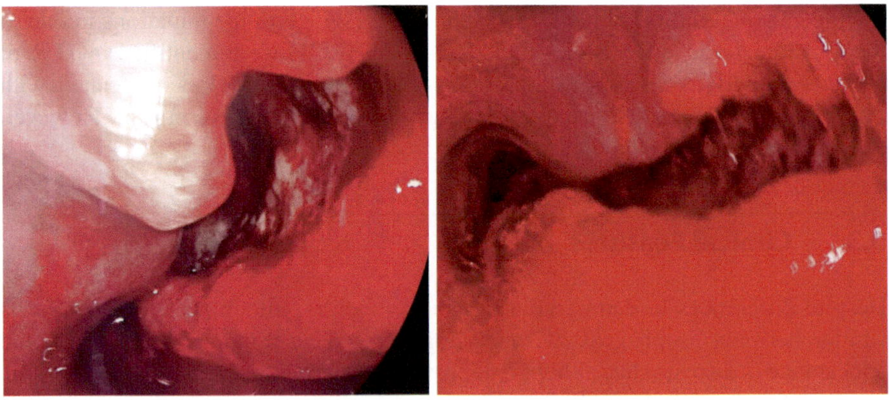

**Fig. 9.1** The appearance of an ulcerovegetative mass with an endoscopic appearance compatible with esophageal cancer, creating narrowing of the esophageal lumen. The biopsy results obtained from the lesion were diagnosed as squamous cell esophageal cancer. This photograph was published with the permission of the patient during the upper gastrointestinal endoscopy performed in the gastroenterology department of Tepecik Training and Research Hospital

recommended to perform pathological and molecular analyses correctly [60]. Histological diagnosis is made according to the World Health Organization (WHO) criteria [61].

Immunohistochemical (IHC) staining is recommended in poorly differentiated and undifferentiated cancers when it is impossible to distinguish between SCC and AC using morphological features [60].

Routine direct chest X-ray may show aspiration pneumonia, air-filled esophagus (pseudo achalasia), metastatic lesion to the lung parenchyma, pleural effusion, and fistula [5].

Barium esophagography may indicate an esophageal mass causing lumen obstruction or stricture. Early stage may indicate abnormal esophageal mucosal streaking, plaque or polypoid lesion, ulceration, or nonspecific focal irregularity. In advanced tumors, the mass may indicate stenosis or luminal narrowing. It can be said that it is superior to endoscopic procedures in esophageal respiratory fistulas. Particular attention should be paid to using barium as a contrast agent instead of hyperosmolar agents (diatrizoate meglumine and diatrizoate sodium), which carry the risk of severe pulmonary edema and pneumothorax [5].

Computerized tomography can denote the presence of focal esophageal stricture or luminal mass with esophageal wall thickening, irregularity, and proximal dilatation and can provide staging information evaluating liver or lung metastases as well as regional lymphadenopathy [5].

Local staging is most accurate with endoscopic ultrasound (EUS), while cross-sectional imaging with CT, PET scan (preferred), or MRI evaluates distant disease [62].

High-resolution endoscopy (>1 million pixels) with magnified endoscopes has been shown in various studies to increase the detection rates of dysplasia and early cancer [63, 64]. Endoscopic findings range from relatively normal-appearing mucosa (submucosal infiltrative pattern) to ulcers, nodules, and prominent masses. It is recommended to take multiple biopsies, including brush cytology. Advances in fluorescence in situ hybridization (FISH) have increased the efficiency of conventional cytology in diagnosing AC and precursors with dysplasia. In the detection of the submucosal infiltrative state of the disease, taking a biopsy with the bite-to-bite technique or biopsy with EUS increases the diagnosis rate. Several other endoscopic techniques may also help identify areas of dysplasia and malignancy, including narrowband imaging (narrow band imagining NBI), chromoendoscopy (conventional or electronic), autofluorescence imaging, and confocal laser endomicroscopy [65].

Conventional chromoendoscopy provides the opportunity for more detailed examination using special dyes. Lugol's iodine, methylene blue, acetic acid, crystal violet, and indigo carmine are the most commonly used dyes. Lugol's iodine solution is the most commonly used dye in cases with suspected SCC, consisting of 0.5–3.0% aqueous potassium iodide solution. Iodine stains glycogen-containing cells of the normal esophageal epithelium and is not uptake by glycogen-depleted dysplastic or malignant cells. Chromoendoscopy with Lugol's has over 90% sensitivity and specificity. Although vital staining with Lugol's solution is straightforward, it is associated with limitations such as cost, possible iodine allergy, and risk of aspiration or esophageal spasm. It can also be associated with heterogeneous coloration, especially in conditions such as inflammation, and the interpretation of this situation is person-based [66]. In diagnosing AC, however, methylene blue, acetic acid, and indigo carmine staining are more useful in detecting glandular abnormalities.

Electronic chromoendoscopy is another method for detecting signs of dysplasia and cancer, using selective light filters to highlight fine details and vascular changes in the mucosa. This method eliminates some of the concerns of traditional chromoendoscopy, such as additional procedure time and potential side effects from the dyes used. Various variations of electronic chromoendoscopy are available from different manufacturers, but most published studies have used narrow band imaging (NBI; Olympus, Tokyo, Japan) in the setting of Barrett's esophagus. NBI selectively filters red light and emits green and blue lights. NBI, electronic chromoendoscopic technique, surveillance shows mucosal histology better throughout and is more successful in diagnosing dysplasia. It has been shown that the diagnosis and classification of BE are better with NBI [67]. In addition, according to the results of systemic review and meta-analysis, conventional or optical chromoendoscopy techniques have been shown to provide a 34% increase in the diagnosis of dysplasia or cancer (95% CI 20–56%) [68]. In a prospective comparative study, the sensitivity and specificity of NBI in the diagnosis of early stage SCC were found to be 88% and 75%, respectively [69].

Autofluorescence imaging (AFI) involves a technique that uses short wavelength blue or ultraviolet light to stimulate biological fluorophores (e.g., collagen, porphyrins, flavins, aromatic amino acids) in the esophagus. It is generally used in the early diagnosis of BE-related cancers. However, this method is not a frequently used method due to the high false positive rate (78%) and low additional diagnostic contribution shown in studies [70].

Confocal laser endomicroscopy provides real-time, in vivo microscopic visualization of the esophageal mucosa. It involves the application of an IV fluorescent dye (most commonly fluorescein sodium) or a topical contrast agent (acriflavine or cresyl violet) taken up by normal mucosal cells. Fluorescent dye uptake is not seen in dysplastic cells, so they appear dark. This method produces approximately 1000x magnification. There are currently two commercially available methods for confocal endomicroscopy. They include an endoscope and a probe-based instrument that can be threaded through an accessory channel on the standard upper endoscope. In the first studies, it was reported that confocal laser endomicroscopy has high accuracy and reliability. Several studies, including a recent prospective randomized double-blind study, reported that confocal laser endomicroscopy significantly improved the diagnostic yield for endoscopically indistinct dysplasia compared with targeted biopsy with high-definition white light endoscopy. It has also been found to reduce the number of biopsies required per patient. However, a subsequent multicenter randomized trial found no increase in efficiency with confocal endomicroscopy compared with high-definition endoscopy for residual metaplasia in patients who had undergone prior ablation [71–74].

Other commercially available technologies include optical coherence tomography, endocytoscopy, and high-resolution microendoscopy. Optical coherence tomography also emits near-infrared light to provide cross-sectional tissue images, which has the potential advantage of identifying submucosal lesions [73]. Endocytoscopy is a fixed-focus, high-power objective lens that projects magnified images of the superficial epithelium.

High-resolution microendoscopy uses light-emitting diodes for illumination and causes fluorescent emission. While these technologies have shown promising initial results, large multicenter studies are warranted for further evaluation. In conclusion, most newer methods have shown high sensitivity in detecting esophageal neoplasia [74]. However, these modalities also showed high false positive rates and limited specificity. With these limitations, new imaging modalities provide only a complementary role to high-definition endoscopy with biopsy.

## 9.5 Screening and Surveying

Screening and surveillance are aimed at increasing survival. Therefore, it is designed to detect the earliest possible histological precursor. While AC screening and surveillance include Barrett's esophagus, since the histological precursors of SCC are dysplasia and carcinoma in situ, screening programs are geared toward their detection [75, 76].

The results of large cohort studies show that the annual cancer risk in patients with non-dysplastic Barrett's esophagus is 0.12–0.40%. Dysplasia in lesions of Barrett's esophagus indicates a marked increase in cancer risk—the annual risk is about 1% for patients with low-grade dysplasia and more than 5% for patients with high-grade dysplasia [40, 77]. However, 80–90% of esophageal AC cases are diagnosed in patients with no known Barrett's esophagus [78]. Endoscopic screening results in detecting Barrett's esophagus in 6–12% of patients with prolonged GERD symptoms, most commonly seen in white men older than 50 [79, 80]. Endoscopic follow-up every 3 years is recommended in patients with known non-dysplastic Barrett's esophagus [79].

The precursor lesion for squamous cell carcinoma is esophageal squamous dysplasia. Patients with mild, moderate, or severe dysplasia have a 3-, 10-, or 30-fold increased risk of squamous cell carcinoma, respectively [81]. In areas with a high incidence of SCC, endoscopic biopsies from unstained areas with Lugol's solution and chromoendoscopic examination are included in SCC screening.

This approach has been associated with an increased five-year survival rate of up to 86% in parts of China with a high incidence of SCC. Chromoendoscopy with Lugol's has a sensitivity and specificity of over 90% [82].

Other previously discussed endoscopy techniques, such as NBI and AFI, have also been evaluated as screening tools. NBI has been shown to detect early esophageal lesions based on superficial vascular pattern and surface structure changes [83, 84]. On the other hand, AFI is not sensitive enough for lesions smaller than 10 mm, so its use for screening is not very common.

## 9.6 Molecular Pathology

For esophageal SCC, expression of death-ligand 1 (PD-L1) programmed by IHC relative to tumor proportion score (TPS) or combined positive score (CPS) is an approved predictive biomarker for treating immune checkpoint inhibitors (ICIs) [60]. Patients with esophageal SCC have been shown to benefit from programmed cell death protein 1 (PD-1) blockade.

## 9.7 Staging and Risk Forecast

After the diagnosis of esophageal cancer, the right treatment can be concluded with clinical staging. Staging should include a complete clinical examination, endoscopic imaging, and computerized tomography (CT) or positron emission tomography (PET) with [18F]2-fluoro-2-deoxy-D-glucose (FDG). Medical risk assessment should complement anatomical staging, particularly in patients scheduled for multimodal therapy and/or surgery. Esophageal cancer should be staged according to the American Joint of Cancer Committee/ International Union for Cancer Control AJCC/UICC TNM (tumor-regional lymph nodes-metastasis) staging system. American joint of Cancer Committee (AJCC) eighth edition of staging epithelial cancers of the esophagogastric junction (EGJ) established separate classifications for clinical (cTNM), pathological (pTNM), and post neoadjuvant (ypTNM) stage groups [85] (Tables 9.2, 9.3, and 9.4).

Histopathological cell type significantly influences the survival of clinically and pathologically staged patients and requires separate grouping for each cell type. Still, the ypTNM groupings are the same for both cell types. Postneoadjuvant staging (ypTNM) was introduced by the AJCC but not accepted by the International Union for Cancer Control (UICC). Therefore, the role of ypTNM classification in adjunctive therapy decision-making is currently limited. In addition, the definition of esophagogastricjunction(EGJ) cancer has changed in the American joint of Cancer Committee (AJCC) eighth edition. According to the new definition, cancers

**Table 9.2** Clinical cTNM stage groups

| C stage group squamous cell carcinoma | cT | cN | cM | C stage group adenocarcinoma | cT | cN | cN |
|---|---|---|---|---|---|---|---|
| 0 | Tis | N0 | M0 | 0 | Tis | N0 | M0 |
| I | T1 | N0–1 | M0 | I | T1 | N0 | M0 |
| II | T2 | N0–1 | M0 | IIA | T1 | N1 | M0 |
| | T3 | N0 | M0 | IIB | T2 | N0 | M0 |
| III | T3 | N1 | M0 | III | T2 | N1 | M0 |
| | T1–3 | N2 | M0 | | T3-4a | N0–1 | M0 |
| IVA | T4 | N0–2 | M0 | IVA | T1–4a | N2 | M0 |
| | T1–4 | N3 | M0 | | T4a | N0–2 | M0 |
| IVB | T1–4 | N0–3 | M1 | | T1–4 | N3 | M0 |
| | | | | IVB | T1–4 | N0–3 | M1 |

**Table 9.3** Patologic pTNM stage groups

| p stage group squamous cell carcinoma | pT | pN | pM | P grade | P location | P stage group adenocarcinoma | cT | cN | cN | P grade |
|---|---|---|---|---|---|---|---|---|---|---|
| 0 | Tis | N0 | M0 | N/A | Any | 0 | Tis | N0 | M0 | N/A |
| IA | T1a | N0 | M0 | G1,x | Any | IA | T1a | N0 | M0 | G1,x |
| IB | T1b | N0 | M0 | G1,x | Any | IB | T1a | N0 | M0 | G2 |
| | T1 | N0 | M0 | G2–3 | Any | | T1b | N0 | M0 | G1–2,x |
| | T2 | N0 | M0 | G1 | Any | IC | T1 | N0 | M0 | G3 |
| IIA | T2 | N0 | M0 | G2–3, x | Any | | T2 | N0 | M0 | G1–2 |
| | T3 | N0 | M0 | Any | Lower | IIA | T2 | N0 | M0 | G3,X |
| | T3 | N0 | M0 | G1 | Upper/middle | IIB | T1 | N1 | M0 | Any |
| IIB | T3 | N0 | M0 | G2–3 | Upper/middle | | T3 | N0 | M0 | Any |
| | T3 | N0 | M0 | X | Any | IIIA | T1 | N2 | M0 | Any |
| | T3 | N0 | M0 | Any | X | | T2 | N1 | M0 | Any |
| | T1 | N1 | M0 | Any | Any | IIIB | T4a | N0–1 | M0 | Any |
| IIIA | T1 | N2 | M0 | Any | Any | | T3 | N1 | M0 | Any |
| | T2 | N1 | M0 | Any | Any | | T2–3 | N2 | M0 | Any |
| IIIB | T4a | N0–1 | M0 | Any | Any | IVA | T4a | N2 | M0 | Any |
| | T3 | N1 | M0 | Any | Any | | T4b | N0–2-3 | M0 | Any |
| | T2–3 | N2 | M0 | Any | Any | IVB | T1–4 | N3 | M0 | Any |
| IVA | T4a | N2 | M0 | Any | Any | | T1–4 | N0–3 | M1 | Any |
| | T4b | N0–2 | M0 | Any | Any | N/A: not applicable | | | | |
| | T1–4 | N3 | M0 | Any | Any | | | | | |
| IVB | T1–4 | N0–3 | M1 | Any | Any | X: not defined | | | | |

**Table 9.4** Postneoadjuvant (ypTNM) theraphy stage groups

| ypStage group | ypT | ypN | ypM |
|---|---|---|---|
| I | T0–2 | N0 | M0 |
| II | T3 | N0 | M0 |
| IIIA | T0–2 | N1 | M0 |
| IIIB | T4a | N0 | M0 |
| | T3 | N1–2 | M0 |
| | T0–3 | N2 | M0 |
| IVA | T4a | N1–2, X | M0 |
| | T4b | N0–2 | M0 |
| | T1–4 | N3 | M0 |
| IVB | T1–4 | N0–3 | M1 |
| X, NOT DEFİNED | | | |

that extend <2 cm into the gastric cardia will be classified as EGJ cancer, and cancers that extend 2 cm or more will be classified as gastric cancer [85].

Tumor invasion depth (T stage) is important in predicting lymph node metastasis and distant metastasis. Carcinoma in situ Tis and T1 tumors are classified as superficial cancers. T1 tumor is divided into T1a and T1b according to the depth of submucosal invasion. While lymph node metastasis is 8% in Tis and T1a tumors, this rate rises to 56% when it rises to T1b level [86–88].

Tx: Tumor cannot be assessed.
T0: No evidence of primary tumor.
Tis: High-grade dysplasia, defined as malignant cells confined by the basement membrane.
T1: Invades the lamina propria, muscularis mucosae, or submucosa.
T1a: M1: Intraepithelial Ca.
T1a: M2: Invades the lamina propria.
T1a: M3: Invades the muscularis mucosa.
T1b: SM1: Invades to the upper 1/3 of the submucosa.
T1b: SM2: Invades to the middle 1/3 of the submucosa.
T1b: SM3: Invades to the lower 1/3 of the submucosa.
T2: Invades the muscularis propria.
T3: Invades adventitia.
T4: Invades adjacent structures.
T4a: Invades the pleura, pericardium, azygos vein, diaphragm, or peritoneum.
T4b: Invades other adjacent structures, such as aorta, vertebral body, or trachea.

NX: Regional lymph nodes cannot be assessed.
N0: No regional lymph node metastasis.
N1: Metastasis in 1–2 regional lymph nodes.
N2: Metastasis in 3–6 regional lymph nodes.
N3: Metastasis in 7 or more regional lymph nodes.

M0: No distant metastasis.
M1: Distant metastasis.

Grade III histology of the tumor, SM3 invasion depth, lymphatic or vascular invasion, and SM2 or SM1 invasion were associated with lymph node involvement. The presence of vascular invasion and SM3 invasion depth are predictors of lymph node metastasis in SCC. In contrast, the presence of lymphatic invasion in AC is the best predictor of lymph node metastasis [89].

### 9.7.1 Adenocarcinoma G (Grade) Category According to Histopathological Findings [85]

Gx: Differentation cannot be assessed.
G1: Well differentiated. >95% of tumor is composed of well-formed glands.
G2: Moderately differentiated. 50–95% of tumor shows gland formation.
G3: Poorly differentiated. Tumor is composed of nest and sheets of cells with <50% of tumor demonstrating glandular formation.

### 9.7.2 Squamous Cell Carcinoma G (Grade) Category (Histological Grade) [85]

Gx: Differentation cannot be assessed.
G1: Well differentiated. Prominent keratinization with pearl formation and a minor component of nonkeratinizing basal like cells. Tumor cells are arranged in sheets and mitotic counts are low.
G2: Moderately differentiated. Variable histologic features, ranging from parakeratotic to poorly g category keratinizing lesions. Generally, pearl formation is absent.
G3: Poorly differentiated. Consists predominantly of basal-like cells forming large and small nests with frequent central necrosis. The nests consist of sheets or pavement like arrangements of tumor cells, and occasionally are punctuated by small numbers of parakeratotic or keratinizing cells.
Squamous cell carcinoma L category (location category; classify according to the cancer location) [85].
Lx: Location unknown.
Upper: cervical esophagus to lower border of azygos vein.
Middle: Lower border of azygos vein to lower border of inferior pulmonary vein.
Lower: Lower border of inferior pulmonary vein to stomach, including esophagogastric junction.

Biopsies taken during endoscopy, endoscopic resection material, endoscopic ultrasound, and multidetector tomography with $1^8$ f–fluoro-2 deoxy-D glucose PET, CT, are methods that help in the staging of esophageal cancer [90].

Endoscopic ultrasound (EUS) can be used for tumor (T) and lymph node (N) staging but has low accuracy for T1 tumors; in these cases, endoscopic resection offers more precise staging in addition to the therapeutic benefit [91, 92]. EUS is particularly useful in determining the therapeutic strategy in two ways:

(i) for assessment of T4b status by invasion into the airways, pericardium, or aorta, and,
(ii) for identification and biopsy of suspected lymph node metastases outside the normal radiation area or beyond the planned resection margins. In advanced T stages, tumor stenosis may preclude the use of EUS [91, 92].

In assessing tumor growth into the central airways, bronchoscopy with endobronchial ultrasonography is a useful complement to EUS, especially when tumor stenosis precludes using EUS. Endoscopic ultrasound of the esophagus provides a detailed examination of the esophageal wall and is currently the procedure of choice for determining cT. The esophageal wall is displayed as alternating hyperechoic (white) and hypoechoic (black) layers in EUS. The muscularis propria, displayed as the fourth layer (hypoechoic), is vital in distinguishing between T1, T2, and T3 cancers. Hypoechoic cancers are cT1 if there is no invasion into the fourth layer, cT2 if there is an invasion into the fourth layer, or cT3 if there is an invasion beyond the fourth layer [93].

In addition, EUS is used to assess the interface between the primary cancer and adjacent structures (between layers 4 and 5). If the invasion of the fifth layer is detected, the cancer is cT4. The performance index for distinguishing T1 or T2 cancers from T3 or T4 cancers with EUS is 0.89 for esophageal cancers and 0.91 for EGJ cancers [93]. This distinction is important for decision-making: typically, T3–4 cancers have a high probability of N+ and require neoadjuvant therapy, while T1–2 cancers are likely N0 and require resection alone [94]. Clinical categorization of cT1–2 cancer guides future therapy. EUS is used to evaluate regional lymph nodes' size, shape, margin, and internal echocardiographic features. Larger, rounder, well-defined hypoechoic lymph nodes are more likely to contain metastases.

However, reliance on the EUS imaging evaluation of the cN is problematic.

In patients with a 60% prevalence of pN+, EUS criteria were 5 mm, using rounded edges, smooth shape, and a hypoechoic center for cN+, whereas EUS was only 20% specific for N+ and resulted in overstating in 80% of pN0 cancers [95]. An enlarged lymph node on CT suggests nodal metastasis. In a recent review, CT was 50% sensitive (range 41–60%) and 83% specific (range 77–89%) in cN assessment [62].

FDGePET (typically performed as PETeCT) helps identify undetected distant metastases. FDGe PET should be performed in patients who are candidates for esophagectomy, as it may help to avoid unnecessary surgery; however, the availability of PETeCT differs between countries and centers [62, 96–98].

Esophageal SCCs are often accompanied by second primary tumors of the head and neck (HNSPTs).

Patients with an additional HNSPT have a worse prognosis than patients with only esophageal SCC. The combined prevalence of HNSPT in patients with esophageal SCC is 6.7%. Therefore, early detection of HNSPTs may improve the overall outcome of patients with esophageal SCC [99]. Patients with esophageal SCC should undergo a qualified head and neck clinical examination to exclude HNSPTs. Laparoscopy should be performed to exclude peritoneal metastases found in locally advanced (T3/T4) ACs of OGJ infiltrating the anatomical cardia [100].

The presence of unknown peritoneal metastases may prevent them from undergoing unnecessary surgery.

Medical risk assessment should include differential blood count and liver, pulmonary, cardiac and renal function tests.

Nutritional status and weight loss history should be evaluated according to European Society for Clinical Nutrition and Metabolism (ESPEN) guidelines [101]. More than half of patients lose >5% of their body weight before admission for esophagectomy, and 40% lose >10%.

Regardless of body mass index, weight loss increases the risk of surgery, worsens the patient's quality of life (QoL), and is associated with poor survival in advanced diseases. Therefore, according to the ESPEN guidelines, nutritional support is integral to medical care for patients with esophageal cancer in both curative and palliative settings [102].

Decreased physical activity is associated with worse outcomes following perioperative treatment.

In addition, low physical fitness is a negative predictor of long-term survival in esophagogastric cancer [103].

## 9.8 Treatment

The histological subtype, clinical TNM stage, location of the tumor, and the patient's performance status, comorbidities, and estimated treatment tolerance should be determined multidisciplinary based on. This team should include a gastroenterologist, surgeon, radiation oncologist, medical oncologist, dietitian, and palliative support physicians. Nutritional support should be provided to the patient during and after treatment. If necessary, enteral nutrition is performed through a feeding jejunostomy or nasogastric tube.

### 9.8.1 Early Stage Disease cT1 N0 M0

In lesions with high-grade intraepithelial dysplasia and mostly T1 tumors, after correct staging, endoscopic treatments should be preferred if there is no risk of deep resection margin or lymph node metastasis. T1a tumors, formerly called mucosal tumors, consist of mucosa (M1 or intraepithelial), lamina propria (M2), or muscularis mucosa (M3). These tumors have a very low risk of lymph node metastasis. However, T1b, formerly known as submucosal tumors, was classified as SM1 (superficial submucosal invasion, SM1, invasion depth < 500 mm, no ulceration), SM2 (invasion into the submucosa), or SM3 (deep submucosal invasion) and have a lymph node metastasis rate that ranges from 21% in SM1 to up to 56% in SM3 [87, 88]. Other risk factors for lymph node metastasis include invasion depth, lymphovascular invasion, low degree of differentiation, ulceration, and large tumor size [104, 105]. Endoscopic treatments are applicable for T1a tumors, but caution should be exercised for T1b tumors due to the risk of lymph node metastasis.

Endoscopic mucosal resection (EMR) or endoscopic submucosal dissection (ESD) are the preferred endoscopic treatment methods [106, 107]. ESD or EMR are endoscopic methods used for the removal of target tissue with intact margins in nodular or flat high-grade dysplasia-containing Barrett's esophagus epithelium or T1a cancers. ESD should be preferred for T1b and lesions >20 mm in size [108]. Endoscopic resection is generally considered curative for T1a cancers and the most superficially submucosal involved T1b cancers, in the absence of other risk factors for lymph node metastasis, in the context of esophageal intestinal metaplasia [107, 108] (Fig. 9.2).

The EMR method should be preferred for ulcer-free or nodular, well, or moderately differentiated, intra-mucosal, and lymphovascular invasion-free lesions with a diameter of <20 mm. It is known that the best results and curative disease can be achieved when used for these lesions. EMR should not be preferred for multifocal or known lymph node metastases. The success rate for T1a cancers is between 91 and 98% [109, 110].

Complications of EMR procedure include bleeding up to 10%, perforation <3%, and stricture development. Post-EMR strictures are generally related to the length and circumference of mucosal resection and respond well to endoscopic balloon dilation [111, 112].

The risk of lymph node metastasis is generally higher in esophageal SCC than in AC, and even deep intramucosal T1a cancers (m3) require additional treatment if other risk factors are present [105]. Studies from Asia show that ESD results in a higher rate of complete resection and lower risk of local recurrence compared to EMR [113].

In studies conducted in Japan with extensive experience in ESD, it has been reported that the ESD with en bloc resection rate for SCC is 100% and the curative

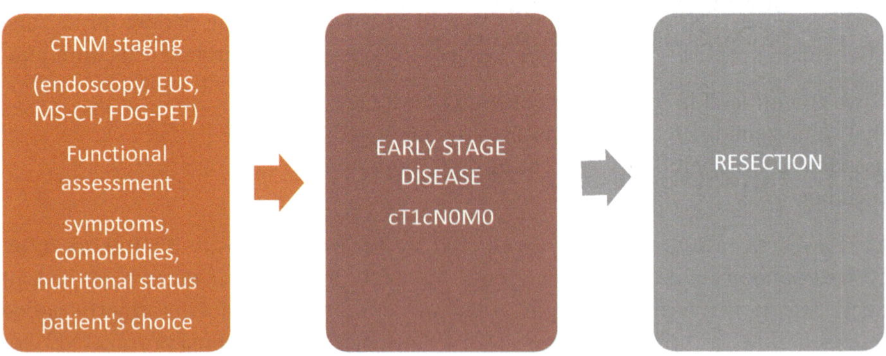


**Fig. 9.2** Treatment algorithm for local/locoregional resectable esophageal; early stage disease*MS-CT* multislice-computed tomography, *EUS* endoscopic ultrasound, *FDGePET* [18F]2-fluoro-2-deoxy-D-glucose positron emission tomography, *cTNM* clinical tumourenodeemetastasis

resection rate is 80% [114, 115]. The complication rates for ESD procedures are 2–5% for perforation and 5–17% for stricture formation [114, 110]. For both histological subtypes, patients with deep endoscopic resection margins or lymph node metastases and significant risk factors should be recommended for further resective surgery with appropriate lymphadenectomy; however, chemoradiotherapy (CRT) can be considered as a treatment option for organ-preserving stage IA SCC [116]. In a meta-analysis of five case-control studies, which included 319 lesions treated with ESD and 476 lesions treated with EMR, ESD was found to have lower recurrence rates than EMR, with better en bloc and histologically superior resection rates without increasing procedural incidence, but with higher procedure-related complications, longer processes, and higher costs [117].

Indeed, in a similar meta-analysis of 21 studies with 1152 patients and 1240 lesions treated with ESD, with an average follow-up period ranging from 12–53 months, the overall resection rate was found to be 99% (95% CI: 99–100%), with a 90% R0 resection rate. A higher R0 resection rate was obtained in lesions smaller than 25 mm (92% vs. 85%, $P < 0.001$). The complication rate was very low, with the most important being stenosis with an incidence of 5% (95% CI: 3–8%). Therefore, it was concluded that this method is a safe and effective technique [118].

Ablation can be performed as photodynamic therapy (PDT), radiofrequency ablation (RFA), or cryotherapy, either alone or more commonly in conjunction with resection techniques. PDT can eliminate T1a lesions despite having high recurrence and complication rates (strictures and photosensitivity) [119]. RFA is increasingly used in patients with high-grade dysplasia of Barrett's and in situ AC. Unlike PDT, RFA is associated with fewer complications and greater preservation of esophageal function [120, 121]. Although there is less evidence, cryotherapy is also effective in early esophageal cancer [122]. Ablation therapy should be applied in combination with a resection technique in patients who are not candidates for surgery. The main limitations of ablation therapy are that it does not provide solid tissue for advanced pathological evaluation and staging, and recurrence is common.

#### 9.8.1.1 Local Advanced Resectable Disease (CT2-T4 OR CN1–3 M0)

For locally advanced resectable esophageal cancer (cT2-T4a or cN1–3), surgery remains the first choice for curative treatment for both histological subtypes. However, in cases of previously resectable esophageal SCC, surveillance and salvage esophagectomy with definitive chemoradiotherapy (CRT) are also recommended when necessary for local tumor control. The preferred procedure is radical transthoracic esophagectomy with en bloc two-field lymphadenectomy in appropriate patients. However, the success of esophagectomy depends on the patient's overall condition, comorbidities, performance status, and disease stage, as well as the experience of the performing team and the volume of the center. Mortality rates can rise up to 20% in low-volume centers (<5 esophagectomies per year) [123–126]. Generally, esophagectomy has a significant perioperative morbidity rate of 40–50% and a mortality rate of 3–13% [127–130]. However, it is known that these rates are lower than 2% in high-volume centers (>20 per year) [131, 132].

There are many surgical techniques available for esophagectomy in esophageal cancer. Factors such as lymph node size, anastomosis type, the characteristics of the replaced part of the esophagus, and pyloric drainage are influential in determining the surgical technique. Generally, two techniques are adopted such as transthoracic or transhiatal methods. The transthoracic method is divided into two: (1) Ivor-Lewis esophagectomy (right thoracotomy and laparotomy), (2) McKeown-type esophagogastrectomy (thoracotomy, laparotomy, and cervical anastomosis). Transhiatal methods involve laparotomy and cervical anastomosis [133, 134].

For distal tumors, abdominal and right chest incisions are used, and reconstruction is performed with a gastric tube conduit with an esophagogastric anastomosis in the upper mediastinum (Ivor Lewis procedure). While the Ivor Lewis procedure enables radical resection and provides a wide radial resection margin, there is a risk of intrathoracic anastomotic leakage, and the primary tumor may become unresectable after complete abdominal mobilization [135].

For middle and upper esophageal tumors, a combination of abdominal, right thoracic, and cervical access is used with a reconstruction similar to that of the cervical esophagus (McKeown procedure). The McKeown procedure provides a wide axial and radial resection margin, allowing for radical resection and the opportunity for a cervical anastomosis. However, it has the disadvantage of requiring three separate incisions and being a long surgical procedure [135].

In weak patients with distal tumors, transhiatal esophagectomy can be performed without thoracotomy, with less extensive lymphadenectomy and lower morbidity [108]. Advantages of this technique include providing a wide axial margin, not requiring thoracotomy, being a one-stage procedure, and enabling a cervical anastomosis. However, its disadvantages include providing a limited radial resection margin and causing more significant blood loss. Additionally, this technique is not suitable for patients with limited cardiac reserve [135].

Minimal invasive esophagectomy (MIE) techniques, including robotic procedures, have become increasingly common in clinical practice in recent years. With this method, radical resection is possible without thoracotomy. Furthermore, the anastomosis can be placed in the neck or chest, and it entails a much faster recovery period, shorter hospital stay, and lower cost. However, it is an equipment-dependent technique [135]. Three randomized controlled trials comparing MIE with open esophagectomy reported lower postoperative morbidity, faster functional recovery, and better quality of life (QoL) with MIE up to 1 year after surgery [136–139]. A recent population-based cohort study from Sweden and Finland reported better long-term overall survival (OS) after MIE than after open esophagectomy [140]. Experienced centers recommend MIE as the surgical approach.

### Lymph Node Dissection

Lymphatic spread is commonly observed in early and advanced stages of esophageal cancer. When the tumor reaches the muscularis mucosae, there is a probability of 8–30% for lymph node metastasis, and when it reaches the submucosa, this probability increases to 30–58%. Lymph node status is an independent predictor factor in esophageal cancer survival [141]. NCCN guidelines recommend the removal of

15 or more lymph nodes in patients who will undergo esophagectomy without neoadjuvant chemoradiation [142]. However, the number of lymph nodes has not been found to be associated with increased survival in patients who will receive neoadjuvant chemoradiation [143].

## Pre- and Perioperative Chemotherapy or CRT

Should be considered for all patients with locally advanced resectable disease.

There are two options for locally advanced esophageal SCC: either it should be treated with CRT followed by surgery, or close monitoring and salvage surgery should be performed to prevent local tumor persistence and progression (Fig. 9.3).

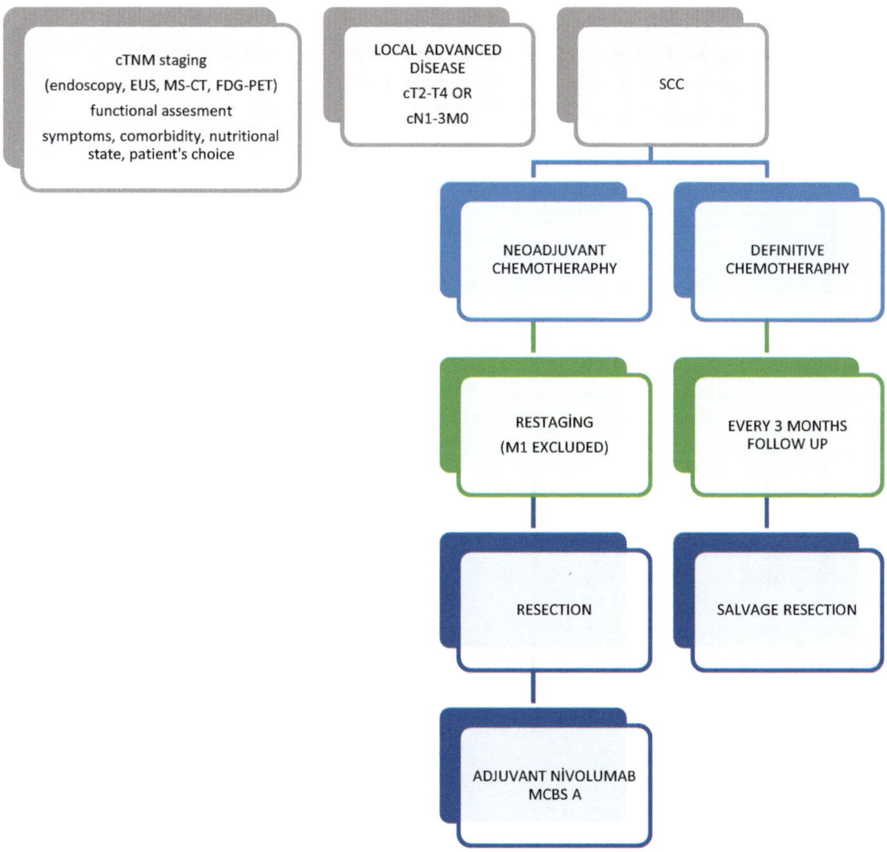


**Fig. 9.3** Treatment algorithm for local advanced squamous cell esophageal cancer *AC* adenocarcinoma, *ChT* chemotherapy, *CRT* chemoradiotherapy, *cTNM* clinical tumourenodeemetastasis, *EMA* European Medicines Agency, *EUS* endoscopic ultrasound, *FDA* Food and Drug Administration, *FDGePET* [18F]2-fluoro-2-deoxy-D-glucose positron emission tomography, *FLOT* 5-fluorouracileleucovorineoxaliplatinedocetaxel, *GoR* grade of recommendation, *MCBS* magnitude of clinical benefit score, *MS-CT* multislice-computed tomography, *OGJ esophagogastric* junction, *SCC* squamous-cell carcinoma

A comprehensive meta-analysis has shown that neoadjuvant chemotherapy increases survival and increases the rate of complete resection (R0) [144].

Based on numerous meta-analyses and prospective studies, neoadjuvant chemoradiotherapy has become the standard treatment for locally advanced esophageal cancer [145, 146].

Definitive CRT is recommended for tumors with cervical involvement requiring laryngectomy.

Preoperative CRT or pre- and perioperative chemotherapy (ChT) is recommended as standard regimens for locally advanced AC of the esophagus and OGJ cancer.

Resectable, locally advanced esophageal AC or OGJ cancer patients should be treated with neoadjuvant CRT based on the CROSS regimen or perioperative ChT (FLOT) and then undergo surgery (Fig. 9.4). Even after a complete clinical tumor

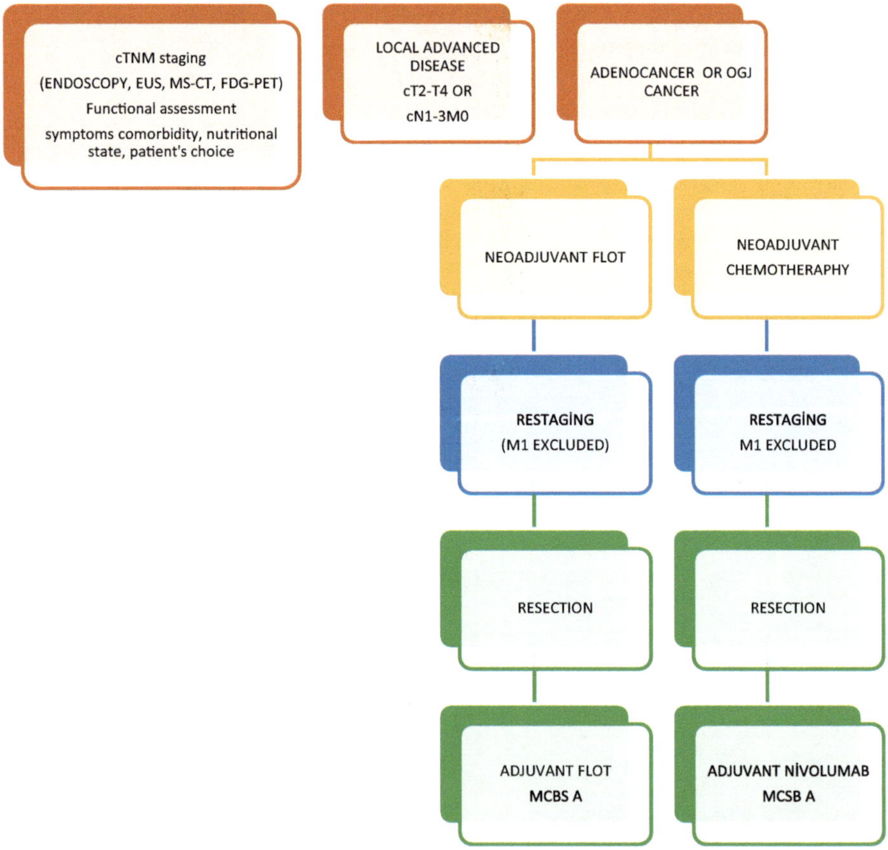


**Fig. 9.4** Treatment algorithm for local advanced adenocancer or sephagogastric junction cance-r*AC* adenocarcinoma, *ChT* chemotherapy, *CRT* chemoradiotherapy, *cTNM* clinical tumoureno-deemetastasis, *EMA* European Medicines Agency, *EUS* endoscopic ultrasound, *FDA* Food and Drug Administration, *FDGePET* [18F]2-fluoro-2-deoxy-D-glucose positron emission tomography, *FLOT* 5-fluorouracileleucovorineoxaliplatinedocetaxel, *GoR* grade of recommendation, *MCBS* magnitude of clinical benefit score, *MS-CT* multislice-computed tomography, *OGJ* esophagogastric junction, *SCC* squamous-cell carcinoma

response to preoperative CRT or ChT, patients with resectable esophageal or OGJ cancer should continue with surgery as data on watch and wait strategy is limited. Patients with esophageal SCC or AC, including OGJ cancer with residual pathological disease (ypT1 and/or ypN1) after neoadjuvant CRT and resection, should be treated with adjuvant nivolumab. Definitive CRT is recommended for patients with unresectable and locally advanced esophageal SCC or AC or those who are not surgical candidates or do not wish to undergo surgery [60].

### 9.8.2 Advanced Stage and Metastatic Disease

Prognosis of patients with metastatic or unresectable esophageal cancer who cannot be treated with curative intent CRT is poor. Treatment for advanced SCC, AC, or OGJ is shaped according to PD-L1 expression (Fig. 9.5). Pembrolizumab is an FDA-approved antibody to programmed death ligand-1 (PD-L1). It is recommended in the treatment of refractory cancers with PDL1 positivity or tumors with microinstability or DNA mismatch gene defects [147].

Advanced stage AC or OGJ cancers receive chemotherapy or CRT according to the guidelines for advanced gastric cancer (Fig. 9.6). Esophageal AC tumor biopsy

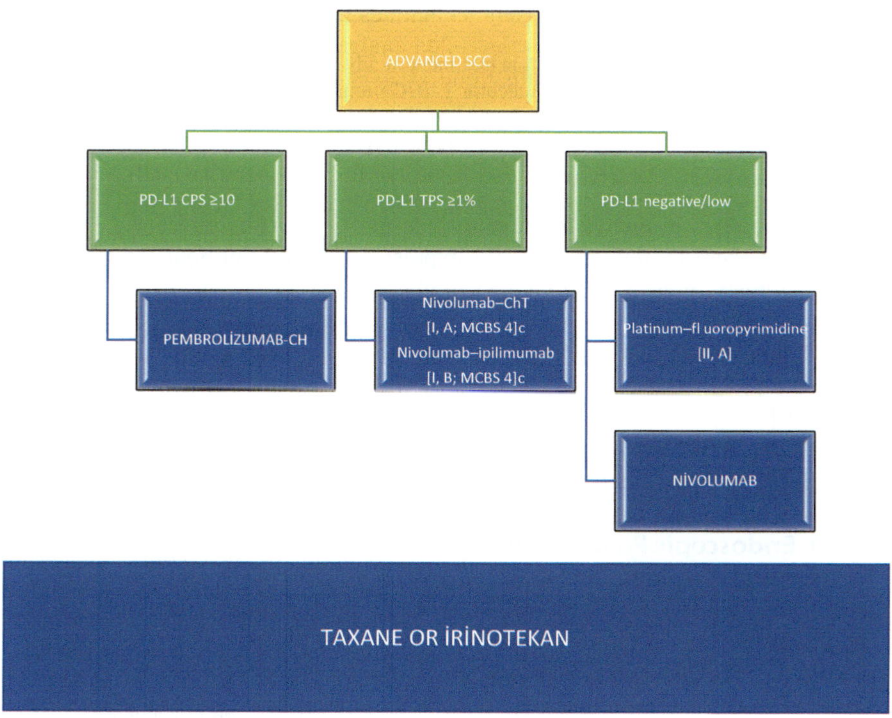


**Fig. 9.5** Treatment algorithm for advanced esophageal SCC*MCBS* magnitude of clinical benefit score, *OGJ* esophagogastric junction, *PDL1* programmed death-ligand 1, *SCC* squamous-cell carcinoma, *TPS* tumor proportion score

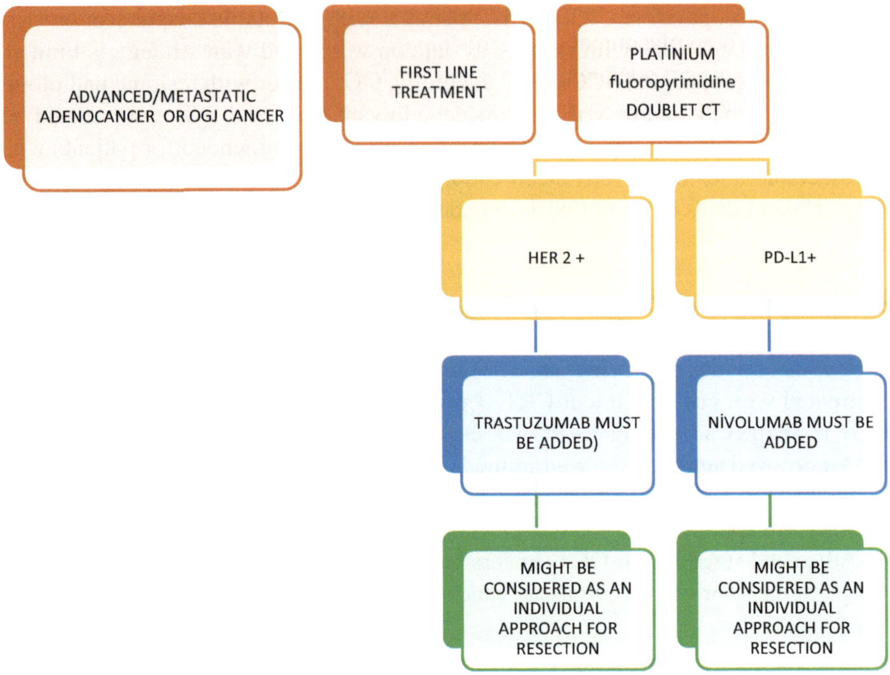


**Fig. 9.6** Treatment algorithm for first-line treatment of advanced/metastatic unresectable gastric. *HER2* human epidermal growth factor receptor 2, *IHC* immunohistochemistry, *MCBS* magnitude of clinical benefit scale, *ESMO* European Society for Medical Oncology, *PD-L1* programmed death-ligand 1

materials should be evaluated for human epidermal growth factor receptor 2 (HER2) positivity. If there is high-level HER2 expression, HER2 antibodies trastuzumab and pertuzumab can be added to the chemotherapy regimen in metastatic adenocarcinomas or locally advanced carcinomas that are not suitable for local treatment [148]. Ramucirumab, a VEGF receptor 2 antibody, has been approved by the FDA for refractory advanced OGJ adenocarcinomas in standard chemotherapy regimens [149].

NCCN has indicated that radiation therapy can be performed in patients who are not eligible for chemotherapy and are planned for palliative treatment [142].

#### 9.8.2.1 Endoscopic Palliative Treatment

In patients with dysphagia, endoscopic dilatation or stent placement can be applied. Stents applied by endoscopic methods, especially self-expanded and metallic stents, will reduce the risk of tumor occlusion. It has been observed that small diameter (18 mm) or large diameter (23 mm) stents have the same effect [150, 151]. In addition to chemotherapy, radiotherapy, or brachytherapy, endoscopic stent placement is recommended as palliative treatment [152]. Also, covered self-expanded stents are effective in closing fistulas in tracheoesophageal fistulas by 86% [153].

In patients with severe weight loss and swallowing difficulties, if not used as a gastric conduit, the placement of gastrostomy or jejunostomy feeding tubes is recommended to support adequate calorie intake [154].

#### 9.8.2.2 Prognosis

Esophageal cancer has a poor prognosis due to late diagnosis. In the United States, 40% of esophageal cancers are found after spreading to distant organs or lymph nodes, while 32% are detected after regional spread to nearby organs and lymph nodes. The best predictors of survival in esophageal cancer are the depth of invasion (T stage) and lymph node involvement (N stage) [155, 156]. Histological type, degree of differentiation, and tumor location also affect survival [157].

In patients undergoing surgical resection, there has been a significant improvement in overall and progression-free survival. Although survival based on cancer stage follows a predictable model, survival in localized disease is still <50% (expected five-year survival rate of 46.7%). Regional and distant metastatic esophageal cancer show five-year survival rates of 25.1% and 4.8%, respectively [158].

In the United States, the average five-year survival rate for esophageal cancer is 19.9%. Caucasians have a 21% five-year survival rate, while Blacks have a 13% rate. The overall five-year survival rate for esophageal AC patients in the United States is about 17%, slightly higher than the rate for squamous cell carcinoma patients [159]. Although incidence rates differ significantly between genders, five-year survival is similar in men (19.4%) and women (21.5%) [158].

While early stage esophageal AC can be detected through screening and follow-up, most tumors are found when regional metastasis (in 30% of cases) or distant metastasis (in 40% of cases) has occurred, the five-year survival rate drops from 39% in localized disease to 4% in cases with distant metastasis [159].

The median survival time for all esophageal cancers in the United States is 9 months. Localized, regional, and distant metastatic disease show median survival times of 30, 13, and 6 months, respectively. For EAC patients in the United States, median survival is 11 months, while for ESCC patients it is 8 months [160]. China has shown 20.9% five-year survival rates for esophageal cancer, similar to those in the United States [161]. European survival rates are lower, with 1- and 5-year survival rates of 33.4% and 9.8%, respectively.

## 9.9 Other Esophageal Tumors

### 9.9.1 Malignant Epithelial Tumors

*Squamous cell carcinoma variants*:

Verrucous carcinoma and carcinosarcoma, both variants are rare and have a poor prognosis [162].

*Small cell carcinoma*:

Occurs at a rate of 0.8–3.1%. It is highly aggressive and has a very poor prognosis [163].

*Malignant melanoma*:

A rare tumor that occurs at a rate of 0.1–0.5%. Esophageal malignant melanoma is often located in the middle or lower esophagus. It appears as a blackish polypoid lesion on endoscopy due to pigmentation. Diagnosis is made by imaging methods and histopathologically [164].

### 9.9.2 Benign Epithelial Tumors

*Squamous papilloma*:

An asymptomatic, endoscopically visible, white-pinkish, solitary, exophytic lesion generally located in the lower 1/3 of the esophagus [165].

*Adenoma*:

Rare polypoid lesions that are believed to be associated with Barrett's metaplasia [166].

*Inflammatory fibroid polyp*:

Also known as inflammatory pseudopolyp or eosinophilic granuloma. These polypoid lesions show increased eosinophil cells, perivascular, concentric fibroblastic proliferation [167].

### 9.9.3 Malignant Non-Epithelial Tumors

*Lymphoma*:

Can be primary or secondary. Endoscopically, they can present as submucosal nodules, masses, ulcers, or polypoid lesions. Diffuse large B-cell lymphoma is the most common type of non-Hodgkin lymphoma [168].

*Sarcoma*:

These are rare mesenchymal tumors of the esophagus. They can present as leiomyosarcoma, gastrointestinal stromal tumors, rhabdomyosarcoma, fibrosarcoma, liposarcoma, fibrous histiocytoma, Kaposi sarcoma, or choriocarcinoma [169].

*Metastases*:

Melanoma and breast cancer can metastasize to the esophagus [5].

### 9.9.4 Benign Non-Epithelial Tumors

*Leiomyoma*:

They are seen endoscopically as submucosal masses. EUS is important for differential diagnosis. Large leiomyomas (>5 cm) should be removed using the ESD method [170].

*Granular cell tumor*:

These are mostly asymptomatic tumors detected incidentally. They should be removed endoscopically [171].

*Fibrovascular polyps*:

They are mostly seen in the cervical esophagus. They are incidental pedunculated polyps consisting of blood vessels, adipose cells, and stroma covered with normal epithelium [172].

*Hamartoma*:

These are rare tumors that can contain multiple tissue types, such as cartilage, bone, adipose tissue, smooth muscle, and skeletal muscle. They should be removed endoscopically [173].

*Hemangioma*:

Endoscopically, they appear as submucosal nodules that are bluish or reddish and can be either cavernous or capillary. They can cause bleeding or dysphagia [174].

*Lipoma*:

These are rare tumors that are usually located in the proximal esophagus and appear as yellowish nodules. If symptomatic (causing dysphagia or aspiration), they should be removed endoscopically or surgically [175].

## References

1. Sung H, Ferlay J, Siegel RL, et al. Global Cancer Statistics 2020: GLOBOCAN estimates of incidence and mortality worldwide for 36 cancers in 185 countries. CA Cancer J Clin. 2021;71(3):209–49.
2. Arnold M, Abnet CC, Neale RE, et al. Global burden of 5 major types of gastrointestinal cancer. Gastroenterology. 2020;159(1):335–49.
3. Codipilly DC, Sawas T, Dhaliwal L, et al. Epidemiology and outcomes of young-onset esophageal adenocarcinoma: an analysis from a population-based database. Cancer Epidemiol Biomarkers Prev. 2021;30(1):142–9.
4. Hongo M, Nagasaki Y, Shoji T. Epidemiology of esophageal cancer: orient to occident. Effects of chronology, geography and ethnicity. J Gastroenterol Hepatol. 2009;24:729–35.
5. Feldman M, Friedman LS, Brandt LJ. Sleisenger and Fordtran's gastrointestinal and liver disease-2 volume set: pathophysiology, diagnosis, management. 11th ed. Elsevier; 2010.
6. Parfitt JR, Miladinovic Z, Driman DK. Increasing incidence of adenocarcinoma of the gastroesophageal junction and distal stomach in Canada—an epidemiological study from 1964–2002. Can J Gastroenterol. 2006;20(4):271–6.
7. O'Doherty MG, Freedman ND, Hollenbeck AR, et al. A prospective cohort study of obesity and risk of oesophageal and gastric adenocarcinoma in the NIH-AARP Diet and Health Study. Gut. 2012;61(9):1261–8.
8. Parsonnet J, Friedman GD, Vandersteen DP, et al. Helicobacter pylori infection and the risk of gastric carcinoma. N Engl J Med. 1991;325(16):1127–31.
9. Freedman ND, Abnet CC, Leitzman MF, et al. a prospective study of tobacco, alcohol, and the risk of esophagial and gastric cancer subtypes. Am J Epidemiol. 2007;165:1424–33.
10. Lu P, Gu J, Zhang N, et al. Risk factors for precancerous lesions of esophageal squamous cell carcinoma in high-risk areas of rural China: a population-based screening study. Medicine. 2020;99(31):e21426.
11. Wang QL, Xie SH, Li WT, et al. Smoking cessation and risk of esophageal cancer by histological type: systematic review and meta-analysis. J Natl Cancer Inst. 2017;109(12):djx115.

12. Engel LS, Chow WH, Vaughan TL, et al. Population attributable risks of esophagealand gastric cancers. J Natl Cancer Inst. 2003;95:1404–13.
13. Islami F, Boffetta P, Ren J, et al. High-temperature beverages and foods and esophageal cancer risk—a systematic review. Int J Cancer. 2009;125:491–524.
14. Islami F, Ren JS, Taylor PR, et al. Pickled vegetables and the risk of oesophageal cancer: a meta-analysis. Br J Cancer. 2009;101:1641–7.
15. Rogers MA, Thomas DB, Davis S, et al. A case-control study of element levels and cancer of the upper aerodigestive tract. Cancer Epidemiol Biomarkers Prev. 1993;2(4):305–12.
16. Liu J, Wang J, Leng Y, et al. Intake of fruit and vegetables and risk of esophageal squamous cell carcinoma: a meta-analysis of observational studies. Int J Cancer. 2013;133:473–85.
17. Liu X, Wang X, Lin S, et al. Dietary patterns and oesophageal squamous cell carcinoma: a systematic review and meta-analysis. Br J Cancer. 2014;110:2785–95.
18. Blot WJ, Li JY, Taylor PR, et al. Nutrition intervention trials in Linxian, China: supplementation with specific vitamin/mineral combinations, cancer incidence, and disease-specific mortality in the general population. J Natl Cancer Inst. 1993;85:1483–92.
19. Mark SD, Qiao YL, Dawsey SM, et al. Prospective study of serum selenium levels and incident esophageal and gastric cancers? J Natl Cancer Inst. 2000;92:1753–63.
20. Engel LS, et al. Population attributable risks of esophageal and gastric cancers. J Natl Cancer Inst. 2003;95(18):1404–13.
21. Jansson C, Johansson ALV, Nyrén O, et al. Socioeconomic factors and risk of esophageal adenocarcinoma: a nationwide Swedish case-control study. Cancer Epidemiol Biomarkers Prev. 2005;14:1754.
22. Talagala IA, Nawarathne M, Arambepola C. Novel risk factors for primary prevention of oesophageal carcinoma: a case-control study from Sri Lanka. BMC Cancer. 2018;18:1135.
23. Farhadi M, Tahmasebi Z, Merat S, et al. Human papillomavirus in squamous cell carcinoma of esophagus in a high-risk population. World J Gastroenterol. 2005;11:1200–3.
24. Guo F, Liu Y, Wang X, et al. Human papillomavirus infection and esophageal squamous cell carcinoma: a case-control study. Cancer Epidemiol Biomarkers Prev. 2012;21:780–5.
25. Sitas F, et al. InterSCOPE study: associations between esophageal squamous cell carcinoma and human papillomavirus serological markers. J Natl Cancer Inst. 2012;104(2):147–58.
26. Ravi K, Codipilly DC, Sunjaya D, et al. Esophageal lichen planus is associated with a significant increase in risk of squamous cell carcinoma. Clin Gastroenterol Hepatol. 2019;17:1902–3.
27. Chuong JJ, DuBovik S, McCallum RW. Achalasia as a risk factor for esophageal carcinoma. A reappraisal. Dig Dis Sci. 1984;29:1105–8.
28. Sandler RS, Nyren O, Ekbom A, et al. The risk of esophageal cancer in patients with achalasia. A population-based study. J Am Med Assoc. 1995;274:1359–62.
29. Bakari G, et al. Endoscopic treatment of 135 cases of Plummer-Vinson web: a pilot experience. Gastrointest Endosc. 2014;80(4):738–41.
30. Ellis A, Risk JM, Maruthappu T, et al. Tylosis with oesophageal cancer: diagnosis, management and molecular mechanisms. Orphanet J Rare Dis. 2015;10:126.
31. Ellis A, Field JK, Field EA, et al. Tylosis associated with carcinoma of the oesophagus and oral leukoplakia in a large Liverpool family–a review of six generations. Eur J Cancer B Oral Oncol. 1994;30b:102–12.
32. Zhang HZ, Jin GF, Shen HB. Epidemiologic differences in esophageal cancer between Asian and Western populations. Chin J Cancer. 2012;31:281–6. https://doi.org/10.5732/cjc.011.10390.
33. Yang X, Zhu H, Qin Q, Yang Y, Yang Y, Cheng H, Sun X. Genetic variants and risk of esophageal squamous cell carcinoma: a GWAS-based pathway analysis. Gene. 2015;556:149–52. https://doi.org/10.1016/j.gene.2014.11.049.
34. Wheeler JB, Reed CE. Epidemiology of esophageal cancer. Surg Clin North Am. 2012;92:1077–87. https://doi.org/10.1016/j.suc.2012.07.008.
35. Lepage C, Rachet B, Jooste V, et al. Continuing rapid increase in esophageal adenocarcinoma in England and Wales. Am J Gastroenterol. 2008;103:2694–9.

36. Lord RV, Law MG, Ward RL, et al. Rising incidence of oesophageal adenocarcinoma in men in Australia. J Gastroenterol Hepatol. 1998;13:356–62.
37. Bollschweiler E, Wolfgarten E, Gutschow C, et al. Demographic variations in the rising incidence of esophageal adenocarcinoma in white males. Cancer. 2001;92:549–55.
38. Anderson LA, et al. Risk factors for Barrett's oesophagus and oesophageal adenocarcinoma: results from the FINBAR study. World J Gastroenterol. 2007;13:1585–94.
39. Cook MB, et al. Gastroesophageal reflux in relation to adenocarcinomas of the esophagus: a pooled analysis from the Barrett's and Esophageal Adenocarcinoma Consortium (BEACON). PLoS One. 2014;9:e103508.
40. Hvid-Jensen F, Pedersen L, Drewes AM, Sørensen HT, Funch-Jensen P. Incidence of adenocarcinoma among patients with Barrett's esophagus. N Engl J Med. 2011;365:1375–83. https://doi.org/10.1056/NEJMoa1103042.
41. Stein DJ, El-Serag HB, Kuczynski J, Kramer JR, Sampliner RE. The association of body mass index with Barrett's oesophagus. Aliment Pharmacol Ther. 2005;22:1005–10.
42. Smith KJ, et al. Interactions among smoking, obesity, and symptoms of acid reflux in Barrett's esophagus. Cancer Epidemiol Biomarkers Prev. 2005;14:2481–6.
43. Akiyama T, et al. Visceral obesity and the risk of Barrett's esophagus in Japanese patients with non-alcoholic fatty liver disease. BMC Gastroenterol. 2009;9:56.
44. Leggett CL, et al. Metabolic syndrome as a risk factor for Barrett esophagus: a population-based case-control study. Mayo Clin Proc. 2013;88:157–65.
45. Garcia JM, et al. Circulating inflammatory cytokines and adipokines are associated with increased risk of Barrett's esophagus: a case-control study. Clin Gastroenterol Hepatol. 2014;12(2):229–38.
46. Oze I, Matsuo K, Ito H, Wakai K, Nagata C, Mizoue T, Tanaka K, Tsuji I, Tamakoshi A, Sasazuki S, Inoue M, Tsugane S. Cigarette smoking and esophageal cancer risk: an evaluation based on a systematic review of epidemiologic evidence among the Japanese population. Jpn J Clin Oncol. 2012;42:63–73. https://doi.org/10.1093/jjco/hyr170.
47. Zhang ZF, Kurtz RC, Yu GP, et al. Adenocarcinomas of the esophagus and gastric cardia: the role of diet. Nutr Cancer. 1997;27:298–309.
48. Zhuo X, Zhang Y, Wang Y, et al. Helicobacter pylori infection and oesophageal cancer risk: association studies via evidence-based meta-analyses. Clin Oncol. 2008;20:757–62.
49. Anderson LA, Johnston BT, Watson RG, et al. Nonsteroidal anti-inflammatory drugs and the esophageal inflammation-metaplasia-adenocarcinoma sequence. Cancer Res. 2006;66:4975–82.
50. Fortuny J, Johnson CC, Bohlke K, et al. Use of anti-inflammatory drugs and lower esophageal sphincter-relaxing drugs and risk of esophageal and gastric cancers. Clin Gastroenterol Hepatol. 2007;5:1154–9.
51. Nguyen DM, Richardson P, El-Serag HB. Medications (NSAIDs, statins, proton pump inhibitors) and the risk of esophageal adenocarcinoma in patients with Barrett's esophagus. Gastroenterology. 2010;138(7):2260–6.
52. Singh S, et al. Acid-suppressive medications and risk of oesophageal adenocarcinoma in patients with Barrett's oesophagus: a systematic review and meta-analysis. Gut. 2014;63(8):1229–37.
53. Singh S, et al. Statins are associated with reduced risk of esophageal cancer, particularly in patients with Barrett's esophagus: a systematic review and meta-analysis. Clin Gastroenterol Hepatol. 2013;11(6):620–9.
54. Levine DM, Ek WE, Zhang R, Liu X, Onstad L, Sather C, Lao- Sirieix P, Gammon MD, Corley DA, Shaheen NJ, Bird NC, Hardie LJ, Murray LJ, Reid BJ, Chow WH, Risch HA, Nyrén O, Ye W, Liu G, Romero Y, Bernstein L, Wu AH, Casson AG, Chanock SJ, Harrington P, Caldas I, Debiram-Beecham I, Caldas C, Hayward NK, Pharoah PD, Fitzgerald RC, Macgregor S, Whiteman DC, Vaughan TL. A genome-wide association study identifies new susceptibility loci for esophageal adenocarcinoma and Barrett's esophagus. Nat Genet. 2013;45:1487–93. https://doi.org/10.1038/ng.2796.

55. Orloff M, Peterson C, He X, et al. Germline mutations in MSR1, ASCC1, and CTHRC1 in patients with Barrett esophagus and esophageal adenocarcinoma. JAMA. 2011;306:410–9.
56. Shan J, Zhao W, Gu W. Suppression of cancer cell growth by promoting cyclin D1 degradation. Mol Cell. 2009;36:469–76.
57. Rustgi AK, El-Serag HB. Esophageal carcinoma. N Engl J Med. 2014;371(26):2499–509. https://doi.org/10.1056/NEJMra1314530.
58. Watanabe HA, et al. Esophageal carcinoma with high serum parathyroid hormone-related protein (PTHrP) level. J Gastroenterol. 1999;34(4):510–5.
59. Lao-Sirieix P, Fitzgerald RC. Screening for oesophageal cancer. Nat Rev Clin Oncol. 2012;9:278–87.
60. Obermannová R, Alsina M, Cervantes A, Leong T, Lordick F, Nilsson M, van Grieken NCT, Vogel A, Smyth EC, ESMO Guidelines Committee. Oesophageal cancer: ESMO Clinical Practice Guideline for diagnosis, treatment and follow-up. Ann Oncol. 2022;33(10):992–1004. https://doi.org/10.1016/j.annonc.2022.07.003.
61. Nagtegaal ID, Odze RD, Klimstra D, et al. The 2019 WHO classification of tumours of the digestive system. Histopathology. 2020;76(2):182–8.
62. van Vliet EPM, Heijenbrok-Kal MH, Hunink MGM, Kuipers EJ, Siersema PD. Staging investigations for oesophageal cancer: a meta-analysis. Br J Cancer. 2008;98(3):547–57. https://doi.org/10.1038/sj.bjc.6604200.
63. Guelrud M, Ehrlich EE. Enhanced magnification endoscopy in the upper gastrointestinal tract. Gastrointest Endosc Clin N Am. 2004;14:461–73.
64. Kumagai Y, Inoue H, Nagai K, et al. Magnifying endoscopy, stereoscopic microscopy, and the microvascular architecture of superficial esophageal carcinoma. Endoscopy. 2002;34:369–75.
65. Kara MA, et al. High-resolution endoscopy plus chromoendoscopy or narrow-band imaging in Barrett's esophagus: a prospective randomized crossover study? Endoscopy. 2005;37(10):929–36.
66. Shimizu Y, et al. Endoscopic diagnosis of early squamous neoplasia of the esophagus with iodine staining: high-grade intra-epithelial neoplasia turns pink within a few minutes. J Gastroenterol Hepatol. 2008;23(4):546–50.
67. Sharma P, et al. Development and validation of a classification system to identify high-grade dysplasia and esophageal adenocarcinoma in Barrett's esophagus using narrow-band imaging. Gastroenterology. 2016;150(3):591–8.
68. Qumseya BJ, et al. Advanced imaging technologies increase detection of dysplasia and neoplasia in patients with Barrett's esophagus: a meta-analysis and systematic review. Clin Gastroenterol Hepatol. 2013;11(12):1562–70.
69. Nagami Y, et al. Usefulness of non-magnifying narrow-band imaging in screening of early esophageal squamous cell carcinoma: a prospective comparative study using propensity score matching. Am J Gastroenterol. 2014;109(6):845–54.
70. Boerwinkel DF, et al. Effects of autofluorescence imaging on detection and treatment of early neoplasia in patients with Barrett?s esophagus? Clin Gastroenterol Hepatol. 2014;12(5):774–81.
71. Dunbar KB, Okolo P 3rd., Montgomery E, et al. Confocal laser endomicroscopy in Barrett's esophagus and endoscopically inapparent Barrett's neoplasia: a prospective, randomized, double-blind, controlled, crossover trial. Gastrointest Endosc. 2009;70:645–54.
72. Sharma P, Meining AR, Coron E, et al. Real-time increased detection of neoplastic tissue in Barrett' s esophagus with probe-based confocal laser endomicroscopy: final results of an international multicenter, prospective, randomized, controlled trial. Gastrointest Endosc. 2011;74:465–72.
73. Isenberg G, Sivak MV Jr, Chak A, et al. Accuracy of endoscopic optical coherence tomography in the detection of dysplasia in Barrett's esophagus: a prospective, double-blinded study. Gastrointest Endosc. 2005;62:825–31.

74. Leggett CL, et al. Comparative diagnostic performance of volumetric laser endomicroscopy and confocal laser endomicroscopy in the detection of dysplasia associated with Barrett's esophagus. Gastrointest Endosc. 2016;83(5):880–8.
75. Wang JW, et al. Natural history analysis of 101 severe dysplasia and esophageal carcinoma cases by endoscopy. Gastroenterol Res Pract. 2017;2017:9612854.
76. Wang GQ, Jiao GG, Chang FB, et al. Long-term results of operation for 420 patients with early squamous cell esophageal carcinoma discovered by screening.? Ann Thorac Surg. 2004;77:1740–4.
77. de Jonge PJ, van Blankenstein M, Looman CW, Casparie MK, Meijer GA, Kuipers EJ. Risk of malignant progression in patients with Barrett's oesophagus: a Dutch nationwide cohort study. Gut. 2010;59:1030–6.
78. Dulai GS, Guha S, Kahn KL, Gornbein J, Weinstein WM. Preoperative prevalence of Barrett's esophagus in esophageal adenocarcinoma: a systematic review. Gastroenterology. 2002;122:26–33.
79. Spechler SJ, Sharma P, Souza RF, Inadomi JM, Shaheen NJ. American Gastroenterological Association technical review on the management of Barrett's esophagus. Gastroenterology. 2011;140(3):e18–52.
80. Sharma P. Barrett's esophagus. N Engl J Med. 2009;361:2548–56. [Erratum, N Engl J Med 2010;362:1450.]
81. Wang GQ, Abnet CC, Shen Q, et al. Histological precursors of oesophageal squamous cell carcinoma: results from a 13 year prospective follow up study in a high risk population. Gut. 2005;54:187–92.
82. Shahid MW, Wallace MB. Endoscopic imaging for the detection of esophageal dysplasia and carcinoma. Gastrointest Endosc Clin N Am. 2010;20:11–24.
83. Morita FH, et al. Narrow band imaging versus lugol chromoendoscopy to diagnose squamous cell carcinoma of the esophagus: a systematic review and meta-analysis? BMC Cancer. 2017;17(1):54.
84. Inoue H, et al. Magnification endoscopy in esophageal squamous cell carcinoma: a review of the intrapapillary capillary loop classification. Ann Gastroenterol. 2015;28(1):41–8.
85. Rice TW, Ishwaran H, Blackstone EH, et al. Recommendations for clinical staging (cTNM) of cancer of the esophagus and esophagogastric junction for the 8th edition AJCC/UICC staging manuals. Dis Esophagus. 2016;29(8):913–9.
86. Takubo K, et al. Early squamous cell carcinoma of the oesophagus: the Japanese viewpoint. Histopathology. 2007;51(6):733–42.
87. Sepesi B, Watson TJ, Zhou D, et al. Are endoscopic therapies appropriate for superficial submucosal esophageal adenocarcinoma. An analysis of esophagectomy specimens. J Am Coll Surg. 2010;210:418–27.
88. Holscher AH, Bollschweiler E, Schroder W, et al. Prognostic impact of upper, middle, and lower third mucosal or submucosal infiltration in early esophageal cancer. Ann Surg. 2011;254:802–7.
89. Sgourakis G, Gockel I, Lyros O, et al. The use of neural networks in identifying risk factors for lymph node metastasis and recommending management of t1b esophageal cancer. Am Surg. 2012;78:195–206.
90. Low DE. Update on staging and surgical treatment options for esophageal cancer. J Gastrointest Surg. 2011;15:719–29.
91. Catalano MF, Van Dam J, Sivak MV. Malignant esophageal strictures: staging accuracy of endoscopic ultrasonography. Gastrointest Endosc. 1995;41(6):535–9.
92. Krill T, Baliss M, Roark R, et al. Accuracy of endoscopic ultrasound in esophageal cancer staging. J Thorac Dis. 2019;11(Suppl. 12):s1602–9.
93. Kelly S, Harris KM, Berry E, et al. A systematic review of the staging performance of endoscopic ultrasound in gastro-oesophageal carcinoma. Gut. 2001;49:534–9.
94. Rice TW, Ishwaran H, Hofstetter WL, et al. Esophageal cancer: associations with (pN+) lymph node metastases. Ann Surg. 2017;265:122–9.

95. Kutup A, Link BC, Schurr PG, et al. Quality control of endoscopic ultrasound in preoperative staging of esophageal cancer. Endoscopy. 2007;39:715–9.
96. Flamen P, Lerut A, Van Cutsem E, et al. Utility of positron emission tomography for the staging of patients with potentially operable esophageal carcinoma. J Clin Oncol. 2000;18(18):3202–10.
97. Heeren PAM, Jager PL, Bongaerts F, et al. Detection of distant metastases in esophageal cancer with 18F-FDG PET. J Nucl Med. 2004;45(6):980–7.
98. Findlay JM, Bradley KM, Maile EJ, et al. Pragmatic staging of oesophageal cancer using decision theory involving selective endoscopic ultrasonography, PET and laparoscopy. Br J Surg. 2015;102(12):1488–99.
99. van de Ven S, Bugter O, Hardillo JA, et al. Screening for head and neck second primary tumors in patients with esophageal squamous cell cancer: a systematic review and meta-analysis. United Eur Gastroenterol J. 2019;7(10):1304–11.
100. Gertsen EC, Brenkman HJF, van Hillegersberg R, et al. 18F-fludeoxyglucose- positron emission tomography/computed tomography and laparoscopy for staging of locally advanced gastric cancer: a multicenter prospective Dutch cohort study (PLASTIC). JAMA Surg. 2021;156(12):e215340.
101. Cederholm T, Barazzoni R, Austin P, et al. ESPEN guidelines on definitions and terminology of clinical nutrition. Clin Nutr. 2017;36(1):49–64.
102. Bischoff SC, Austin P, Boeykens K, et al. ESPEN guideline on home enteral nutrition. Clin Nutr. 2020;39(1):5–22.
103. Whibley J, Peters CJ, Halliday LJ, et al. Poor performance in incremental shuttle walk and cardiopulmonary exercise testing predicts poor overall survival for patients undergoing esophago-gastric resection. Eur J Surg Oncol. 2018;44(5):594–9.
104. Pimentel-Nunes P, Dinis-Ribeiro M, Ponchon T, et al. Endoscopic submucosal dissection: European Society of Gastrointestinal Endoscopy (ESGE) Guideline. Endoscopy. 2015;47(9):829–54.
105. Yamashina T, Ishihara R, Nagai K, et al. Long-term outcome and metastatic risk after endoscopic resection of superficial esophageal squamous cell carcinoma. Am J Gastroenterol. 2013;108(4):544–51.
106. di Pietro M, Canto MI, Fitzgerald RC. Endoscopic management of early adenocarcinoma and squamous cell carcinoma of the esophagus: screening, diagnosis, and therapy. Gastroenterology. 2018;154(2):421–36.
107. Weusten B, Bisschops R, Coron E, et al. Endoscopic management of Barrett's esophagus: European Society of Gastrointestinal Endoscopy (ESGE) position statement. Endoscopy. 2017;49(2):191–8.
108. Hulscher JBF, van Sandick JW, de Boer AGEM, et al. Extended transthoracic resection compared with limited transhiatal resection for adenocarcinoma of the esophagus. N Engl J Med. 2002;347(21):1662–9.
109. Ell C, May A, Pech O, et al. Curative endoscopic resection of early esophageal adenocarcinomas (Barrett's cancer). Gastrointest Endosc. 2007;65:3–10.
110. Ishihara R, Tanaka H, Iishi H, et al. Long-term outcome of esophageal mucosal squamous cell carcinoma without lymphovascular involvement after endoscopic resection. Cancer. 2008;112:2166–72.
111. Pouw RE, van Vilsteren FG, Peters FP, et al. Randomized trial on endoscopic resection-cap versus multiband mucosectomy for piecemeal endoscopic resection of early Barrett's neoplasia. Gastrointest Endosc. 2011;74:35–43.
112. Chennat J, Konda VJ, Ross AS, et al. Complete Barrett's eradication endoscopic mucosal resection: an effective treatment modality for high-grade dysplasia and intramucosal carcinoma, an American single-center experience. Am J Gastroenterol. 2009;104:2684–92.
113. Cao Y, Liao C, Tan A, et al. Meta-analysis of endoscopic submucosal dissection versus endoscopic mucosal resection for tumors of the gastrointestinal tract. Endoscopy. 2009;41(9):751–7.

114. Ono S, Fujishiro M, Niimi K, et al. Long-term outcomes of endoscopic submucosal dissection for superficial esophageal squamous cell neoplasms. Gastrointest Endosc. 2009;70:860–6.
115. Takahashi H, Arimura Y, Masao H, et al. Endoscopic submucosal dissection is superior to conventional endoscopic resection as a curative treatment for early squamous cell carcinoma of the esophagus. Gastrointest Endosc. 2010;72:255–64.
116. Kato K, Ito Y, Nozaki I, et al. Parallel-group controlled trial of surgery versus chemoradiotherapy in patients with stage I esophageal squamous cell carcinoma. Gastroenterology. 2021;161(6):1878–86.
117. Wang J, Ge J, Zhang XH, Liu JY, Yang CM, Zhao SL. Endoscopic submucosal dissection versus endoscopic mucosal resection for the treatment of early esophageal carcinoma: a meta-analysis. Asian Pac J Cancer Prev. 2014;15:1803–6. https://doi.org/10.7314/APJCP.2014.15.4.1803.
118. Sun F, Yuan P, Chen T, Hu J. Efficacy and complication of endoscopic submucosal dissection for superficial esophageal carcinoma: a systematic review and meta-analysis. J Cardiothorac Surg. 2014;9:78. https://doi.org/10.1186/1749-8090-9-78.
119. Gray J, Fullarton GM. Long term efficacy of Photodynamic Therapy (PDT) as an ablative therapy of high grade dysplasia in Barrett's oesophagus. Photodiagn Photodyn Ther. 2013;10(4):561–5.
120. Shaheen NJ, Sharma P, Overholt BF, et al. Radiofrequency ablation in Barrett's esophagus with dysplasia. N Engl J Med. 2009;360:2277–88.
121. Beaumont H, Gondrie JJ, McMahon BP, et al. Stepwise radiofrequency ablation of Barrett's esophagus preserves esophageal inner diameter, compliance, and motility. Endoscopy. 2009;41:2–8.
122. Dumot JA, Vargo JJ 2nd, Falk GW, et al. An open-label, prospective trial of cryospray ablation for Barrett's esophagus high-grade dysplasia and early esophageal cancer in high-risk patients. Gastrointest Endosc. 2009;70:635–44.
123. Swisher SG, Deford L, Merriman KW, et al. Effect of operative volume on morbidity, mortality, and hospital use after esophagectomy for cancer. J Thorac Cardiovasc Surg. 2000;119:1126–32.
124. Miller JD, Jain MK, de Gara CJ, et al. Effect of surgical experience on results of esophagectomy for esophageal carcinoma. J Surg Oncol. 1997;65:20–1.
125. Wouters MW, Wijnhoven BP, Karim-Kos HE, et al. High-volume versus low-volume for esophageal resections for cancer: the essential role of case-mix adjustments based on clinical data. Ann Surg Oncol. 2008;15:80–7.
126. Millikan KW, Silverstein J, Hart V, et al. A 15-year review of esophagectomy for carcinoma of the esophagus and cardia. Arch Surg. 1995;130:617–24.
127. Svanes K, Stangeland L, Viste A, et al. Morbidity, ability to swallow, and survival, after oesophagectomy for cancer of the oesophagus and cardia. Eur J Surg. 1995;161:669–75.
128. Birkmeyer JD, Siewers AE, Finlayson EV, et al. Hospital volume and surgical mortality in the United States. N Engl J Med. 2002;346:1128–37.
129. Chang AC, Ji H, Birkmeyer NJ, et al. Outcomes after transhiatal and transthoracic esophagectomy for cancer. Ann Thorac Surg. 2008;85:424–9.
130. Reames BN, et al. Hospital volume and operative mortality in the modern era. Ann Surg. 2014;260(2):244–51.
131. Meguid RA, Weiss ES, Chang DC, et al. The effect of volume on esophageal cancer resections: what constitutes acceptable resection volumes for centers of excellence? J Thorac Cardiovasc Surg. 2009;137:23–9.
132. Dimick JB, Pronovost PJ, Cowan JA, et al. Surgical volume and quality of care for esophageal resection: do high-volume hospitals have fewer complications? Ann Thorac Surg. 2003;75:337–41.
133. Hagen JA, DeMeester SR, Peters JH, et al. Curative resection for esophageal adenocarcinoma: analysis of 100 en bloc esophagectomies. Ann Surg. 2001;234:520–30.

134. Orringer MB, Marshall B, Iannettoni MD. Transhiatal esophagectomy: clinical experience and refinements. Ann Surg. 1999;230:392–400. discussion 400–393
135. Mwachiro M, White R. Management of esophageal cancer treatment in resource-limited settings. Thorac Surg Clin. 2022;32(3):397–404. https://doi.org/10.1016/j.thorsurg.2022.04.007.
136. Biere SSAY, van Berge Henegouwen MI, Maas KW, et al. Minimally invasive versus open oesophagectomy for patients with oesophageal cancer: a multicentre, open-label, randomised controlled trial. Lancet. 2012;379(9829):1887–92.
137. Maas KW, Cuesta MA, van Berge Henegouwen MI, et al. Quality of life and late complications after minimally invasive compared to open esophagectomy: results of a randomized trial. World J Surg. 2015;39(8):1986–93.
138. Mariette C, Markar SR, Dabakuyo-Yonli TS, et al. Hybrid minimally invasive esophagectomy for esophageal cancer. N Engl J Med. 2019;380(2):152–62.
139. van der Sluis PC, van der Horst S, May AM, et al. Robot-assisted minimally invasive thoracolaparoscopic esophagectomy versus open transthoracic esophagectomy for resectable esophageal cancer: a randomized controlled trial. Ann Surg. 2019;269(4):621–30.
140. Gottlieb-Vedi E, Kauppila JH, Mattsson F, et al. Long-term survival in esophageal cancer after minimally invasive esophagectomy compared to open esophagectomy. Ann Surg. 2021; https://doi.org/10.1097/SLA.0000000000004645.
141. Mariette C, et al. The number of metastatic lymph nodes and the ratio between metastatic and examined lymph nodes are independent prognostic factors in esophageal cancer regardless of neoadjuvant chemoradiation or lymphadenectomy extent. Ann Surg. 2008;247(2):365–71.
142. NCCN Guidelines Version 2. 2018, Esophageal and esophagogastric junction cancers 2018.
143. Noordman BJ, et al. Impact of surgical approach on long-term survival in esophageal adenocarcinoma patients with or without neoadjuvant chemoradiotherapy. Ann Surg. 2018;267(5):892–7.
144. Kidane B, et al. Preoperative chemotherapy for resectable thoracic esophageal cancer. Cochrane Database Syst Rev. 2015;(5):CD001556.
145. Sjoquist KM, et al. Survival after neoadjuvant chemotherapy or chemoradiotherapy for resectable oesophageal carcinoma: an updated meta-analysis. Lancet Oncol. 2011;12(7):681–92.
146. Pasquali S, et al. Survival after neoadjuvant and adjuvant treatments compared to surgery alone for resectable esophageal carcinoma: a network meta-analysis. Ann Surg. 2017;265(3):481–91.
147. Doi T, et al. Safety and antitumor activity of the anti-programmed death-1 antibody pembrolizumab in patients with advanced esophageal carcinoma. J Clin Oncol. 2018;36(1):61–7.
148. Bang YJ, et al. Trastuzumab in combination with chemotherapy versus chemotherapy alone for treatment of HER2-positive advanced gastric or gastro-oesophageal junction cancer (ToGA): a phase 3, open-label, randomised controlled trial. Lancet. 2010;376(9742):687–97.
149. Wilke H, et al. Ramucirumab plus paclitaxel versus placebo plus paclitaxel in patients with previously treated advanced gastric or gastro-oesophageal junction adenocarcinoma (RAINBOW): a double-blind, randomised phase 3 trial? Lancet Oncol. 2014;15(11):1224–35.
150. Vakil N, et al. A prospective, randomized, controlled trial of covered expandable metal stents in the palliation of malignant esophageal obstruction at the gastroesophageal junction. Am J Gastroenterol. 2001;96(6):1791–6.
151. White RE, et al. Randomized trial of small-diameter versus large-diameter esophageal stents for palliation of malignant esophageal obstruction. J Clin Gastroenterol. 2015;49(8):660–5.
152. Lai A, et al. Role of esophageal metal stents placement and combination therapy in inoperable esophageal carcinoma: a systematic review and meta-analysis. Dig Dis Sci. 2018;63(4):1025–34.
153. Kim KR, Shin JH, Song HY, et al. Palliative treatment of malignant esophagopulmonary fistulas with covered expandable metallic stents. AJR Am J Roentgenol. 2009;193:W278–82.
154. Ellrichmann M, et al. Prospective evaluation of malignant cell seeding after percutaneous endoscopic gastrostomy in patients with oropharyngeal/esophageal cancers. Endoscopy. 2013;45(7):526–31.

155. Rice TW, Zuccaro G Jr, Adelstein DJ, et al. Esophageal carcinoma: depth of tumor invasion is predictive of regional lymph node status. Ann Thorac Surg. 1998;65:787–92.
156. Daly JM, Karnell LH, Menck HR. National cancer data base report on esophageal carcinoma. Cancer. 1996;78:1820–8.
157. Altorki NK, Zhou XK, Stiles B, et al. Total number of resected lymph nodes predicts survival in esophageal cancer. Ann Surg. 2008;248:221–6.
158. Howlader N, Noone AM, Krapcho M, et al. SEER Cancer Statistics Review, 1975–2016, National Cancer Institute. Bethesda, MD, https://seer.cancer.gov/csr/1975_2016/, based on November 2018 SEER data submission, posted to the SEER web site, April 2019. Accessed 23 February 2020.
159. Rustgi AK, El-Serag HB. Esophageal carcinoman. N Engl J Med. 2014;371:26.
160. Njei B, McCarty TR, Birk JW. Trends in esophageal cancer survival in United States adults from 1973 to 2009: a SEER database analysis. J Gastroenterol Hepatol. 2016;31:1141–6.
161. Zeng H, Zheng R, Guo Y, et al. Cancer survival in China, 2003–2005: a population-based study. Int J Cancer. 2015;136:1921–30.
162. Lam AK. Histopathological assessment for esophageal squamous cell carcinoma. Methods Mol Biol. 2020;2129:7–18. https://doi.org/10.1007/978-1-0716-0377-2_2.
163. Li J, Zhang X, Xu X, Zhao Q, Yang Q, He M, Chen X, Zhao J. The survival and prognosis characteristics of primary esophageal small-cell carcinoma. Dis Markers. 2022;2022:5615009. https://doi.org/10.1155/2022/5615009.
164. Zheng J, Mo H, Ma S, Wang Z. Clinicopathological findings of primary esophageal malignant melanoma: report of six cases and review of literature. Int J Clin Exp Pathol. 2014;7(10):7230–5.
165. Mavilia MG, Wu GY. Esophageal squamous papilloma: a case series and literature review. J Dig Dis. 2018;19(4):254–6. https://doi.org/10.1111/1751-2980.12535.
166. Keeffe EB, Hisken EC, Schubert F. Adenomatous polyp arising in Barrett's esophagus. J Clin Gastroenterol. 1986;8(3 Pt 1):271–4. https://doi.org/10.1097/00004836-198606000-00014.
167. Garmpis N, Damaskos C, Garmpi A, Georgakopoulou VE. Inflammatory fibroid polyp of the gastrointestinal tract: a systematic review for a benign tumor. In Vivo. 2021;35(1):81–93. https://doi.org/10.21873/invivo.12235.
168. Quiroga-Centeno AC, Bautista-Parada IR, Tapias LF, Gómez-Ochoa SA. Primary esophageal non-Hodgkin's lymphoma: demographics, clinical characteristics, histopathologic types, and survival in 179 patients from the SEER program and systematic review of the literature. Esophagus. 2021;18(4):734–42. https://doi.org/10.1007/s10388-021-00842-0.
169. Ishida H, Fujishima F, Onodera Y. Esophageal carcinosarcoma with basaloid squamous cell carcinoma: a case report and review of the literature. Tohoku J Exp Med. 2019;249(4):255–63. https://doi.org/10.1620/tjem.249.255.
170. Karagülle E, Akkaya D, Türk E, Göktürk HS, Yildirim E, Moray G. Giant leiomyoma of the esophagus: a case report and review of the literature. Turk J Gastroenterol. 2008;19(3):180–3.
171. Chen WS, Zheng XL, Jin L, Pan XJ, Ye MF. Novel diagnosis and treatment of esophageal granular cell tumor: report of 14 cases and review of the literature. Ann Thorac Surg. 2014;97(1):296–302. https://doi.org/10.1016/j.athoracsur.2013.08.042.
172. Nie D, Zong Y, Li J. Difficult endoscopic resection of a giant esophageal fibrovascular polyp: case report and literature review. J Int Med Res. 2021;49(8):3000605211039801. https://doi.org/10.1177/03000605211039801.
173. Trindade AJ, Fan C, Bienstock B. Endoscopic resection of a rare subepithelial esophageal hamartoma. Dig Liver Dis. 2018;50(6):617. https://doi.org/10.1016/j.dld.2017.12.019.
174. Araki K, Ohno S, Egashira A, Saeki H, Kawaguchi H, Ikeda Y, Kitamura K, Sugimachi K. Esophageal hemangioma: a case report and review of the literature. Hepato-Gastroenterology. 1999;46(30):3148–54.
175. Cuttitta A, Annese V, Tancredi A, Clemente C, Scaramuzzi R. Giant esophageal lipoma. Updates Surg. 2011;63:125–7.

# 10 Thoracic Imaging During Diagnosis, Treatment, and Follow-Up in Esophageal

Hilal Şahin

## 10.1 Imaging Techniques

### 10.1.1 Barium Esophagography

Fluoroscopic studies with swallowing of Barium are used as initial imaging modality to evaluate structural and functional abnormalities of the esophagus [1]. Dysphagia, odynophagia, the sensation of "*a lump in the throat*" (globus sensation), and aspiration are all symptoms of swallowing disorders. Since the swallowing starts in the mouth and finishes in the stomach, the upper GI tract should be assessed as a whole mechanism [2].

For the opacification of the esophagus, thick and thin barium preparations are used as positive contrast agents. However, in case of suspicion of perforation, a diluted water-soluble contrast agent is typically used, followed by diluted barium solution if no perforation is seen [3]. In elderly patients or in those with neurological problems, barium studies should be done cautiously due to risk of aspiration. A deep aspiration of barium into the lungs may cause barium plugs in the bronchi and predisposes to pneumonia. Therefore, the risk of aspiration should be assessed before the barium swallow. A history of coughing after swallowing suggests aspiration, but in patients with an absent cough reflex, history may not be reliable. In those patients, upper GI study should start with the imaging of pharynx after the patient swallows a teaspoonful of a water-soluble nonionic contrast agent with low osmolarity such as iohexol or iopamidol. Those agents are readily absorbed if they enter the bronchi.

H. Şahin (✉)
Radiology Department, University of Health Sciences, Tepecik Training and Research Hospital, Izmir, Türkiye

Radiology Department, University of Health Sciences, Izmir Faculty of Medicine, Izmir, Türkiye
e-mail: hilal.sahin1@sbu.edu.tr



O. Engin (ed.), *Risk Factors and Therapy of Esophagus Cancer*,
https://doi.org/10.1007/978-3-031-47024-0_10

If the risk of aspiration is considered small, then a thin barium solution may be used, similar to the steps in suspicion of perforation [1, 3].

The barium study techniques include upright double-contrast fluoroscopy images with a high-density (200 w/v) barium suspension, single-contrast images with a low-density (60 w/v) barium suspension [2]. The double-contrast technique requires ingestion of effervescent agent first, followed by rapid gulp of high-density barium [4]. It is particularly useful for demonstration of reflux disease, infectious esophagitis, esophageal carcinoma, and other structural lesions [1]. The single-contrast views include images of the esophagus distended with barium, allowing for identification of esophageal cancers, esophageal rings and webs, hiatal hernias [2]. Additional views such as mucosal relief views are beneficial in suspected tumors, esophagitis, or varices.

In general, barium esophagography allows to determine changes in the contours of esophagus (e.g., irregular contours, filling defects), mucosal deformities, changes in peristalsis (i.e., motility disorders), extraluminal pathologies, and expulsion difficulties. Most of the esophageal pathologies present as intra- or extra-luminal changes, with interruption of the normal featureless intraluminal appearance of the esophagus with smooth, thin walls. Intraluminal or intrinsic lesions usually cause symmetrical shouldering of the esophageal contours, so called the "*shoulder sign*". Mucosal lesions such as esophageal neoplasia often cause concentric narrowing in the esophageal lumen whereas submucosal or extramural lesions present as eccentric narrowing (Fig. 10.1) [2].

Malignancy criteria in barium esophagography can be summarized as luminal narrowing, thickening of the wall, irregular contours, mucosal destruction, loss of peristalsis (rigidity), short segment involvement, and sharp transition zone (Fig. 10.2). Early esophageal lesions may appear as plaque like lesions, small polypoid lesion with narrow or wide base, or just focal wall irregularity on double-contrast studies. Poorly defined nodules in a merging fashion may point to superficial spreading carcinoma. On the other hand, advanced esophageal cancers may manifest as infiltrative, ulcerative, polypoidal, or varicoid type on double-contrast views [4]. Among those types, infiltrative lesions are the most common with variable

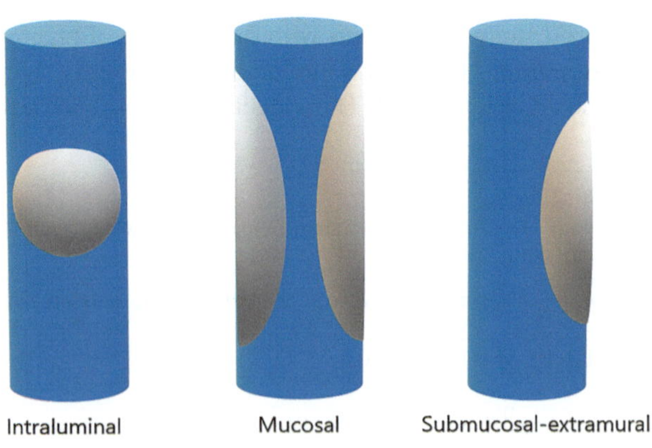


**Fig. 10.1** Schematic drawing of esophageal contour abnormalities according to the localization of the lesions in the esophageal wall

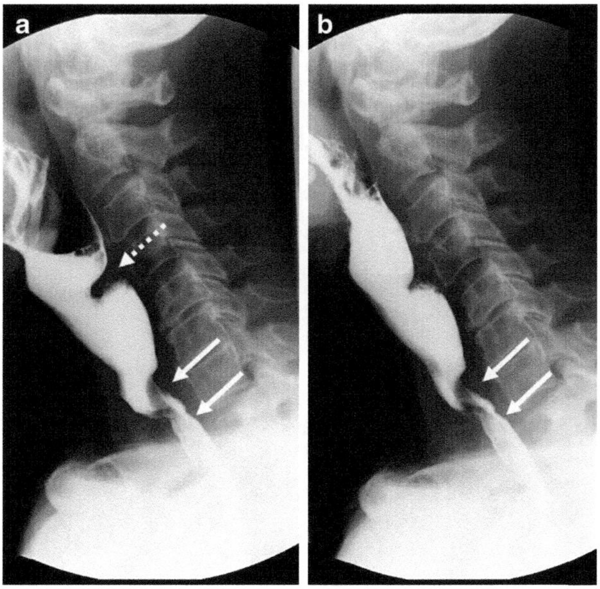


**Fig. 10.2** Esophageal carcinoma (**a**, **b**). Distal cervical esophagus presents luminal narrowing and mucosal irregularity (solid arrows). Note that cricopharyngeal bar/muscle spasm (dashed arrow) is demonstrated as a smooth well-defined impression on the posterior esophageal wall at the C4 level in (**a**) and it is relaxed in (**b**)

appearances of luminal narrowing, mucosal irregularity or nodularity, ulceration, and shouldering of margins. Giant ulcers surrounded by tumor rind are seen occasionally in ulcerative carcinomas. Polypoid lesions are classically seen as lobulated intraluminal masses with or without ulceration. In varicoid type lesions, thickened fixed longitudinal filling defects are seen due to submucosal infiltration of the tumor. In patients with motility disorders, multiple non-peristaltic tertiary contractions may be seen producing a wall irregularity [4]. In those cases, to avoid from a misdiagnosis of esophageal cancer, fluoroscopic images should be carefully watched to demonstrate the resolution of contractions and change in shape in time (Fig. 10.3).

Apart from great value in primary diagnostic procedures of esophageal pathologies, barium studies still remain valuable in assessment of complications after treatment. Double or single contrast views may be used to show esophageal stricture and dysmotility after definitive radiotherapy for unresectable locally advanced esophageal tumors. In addition, fluoroscopic studies are often used to demonstrate possible complications such as anastomotic leaks after esophagectomy and gastric pull-through procedures in adjunct with the other imaging modalities (e.g., chest X-ray and CT) [5]. Anastomotic leaks may manifest either in the early postoperative period (2–3 days) as a result of technical failure, or later in the following days (3–7 days) due to ischemic changes usually at or below the anastomosis site, often as a consequence of necrosis of the proximal end of the pulled-through stomach [6]. A single contrast esophagogram is recommended between postoperative days 6 and 10 depending on the perioperative findings and postoperative general status of the patient. However, it must be kept in mind that after esophagectomy, the risk of aspiration increases because of possible recurrent laryngeal nerve injury. In those group of patients, using a low-osmolar, nonionic, water-soluble contrast agent, positioning

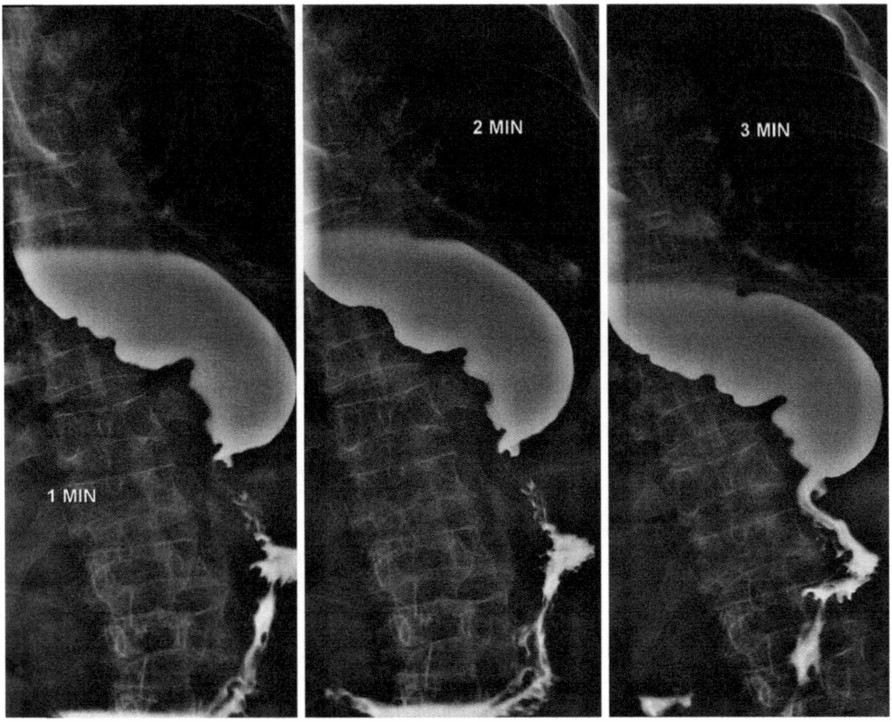


**Fig. 10.3** Motility disorder and multiple tertiary contractions in a patient with dysphagia. Marked narrowing of the distal esophagus, dilation, and contrast stasis in upper esophageal segments, which may mimic esophageal carcinoma. Multiple non-peristaltic tertiary contractions are seen in the anterior wall, which change shape in following fluoroscopic images

the head of the fluoroscopy table high enough and cautiously watching for aspiration throughout the study are mandatory to avoid the risk of pulmonary complications from aspiration. An esophagographic technique including hand injection of the contrast via a nasogastric tube above the anastomosis is recommended by Flanagan et al. to evaluate the conduit under pressure and detect anastomotic leaks, which may otherwise be missed at a passive swallow test [5].

### 10.1.2 Chest X-ray

Chest X-ray (radiography) is the most frequently requested radiologic modality in the preoperative and postoperative period. It employs ionizing radiation (X-rays) to generate the images of the chest. The routine posterior–anterior (PA) view allows the evaluation of lungs, heart, large arteries, ribs, and diaphragm. Lesions obscured on the PA view, such as lesions superimposed on the heart shadow, are often clearly demonstrated on the lateral view. Other views in different positions (e.g., apical or decubitus) may be useful for certain diagnostic difficulties before proceeding to the more complex or expensive techniques [7].

The common symptoms that give rise to a chest X-ray order are persistent or bloody cough, chest pain, difficulty in breathing, and fever. X-rays are used to diagnose many conditions such as pneumonia, pneumothorax, lung diseases, heart failure, bone fractures, and diaphragmatic or hiatal hernia. Esophagus itself cannot be differentiated in any of the views unless it contains contrast. Air in the esophagus can be a frequent finding on normal PA views. However, a large air column in the esophagus may refer to distal involvement or narrowing due to tumor, achalasia, or systemic sclerosis (Fig. 10.4) [8]. Therefore, further evaluation is warranted in those cases.

In patients with esophageal cancer, barium studies are frequently used either in the primary diagnosis or early after the operation. In case of aspiration of barium during the study, the radiopaque barium spreads to the bronchi and bronchioles. Involved lung segments could be easily defined either in fluoroscopy images or chest X-rays (Fig. 10.5) [5].

Surgical treatment of esophageal cancer requires resection of the esophagus with variations of techniques according to different choices of conduit (i.e., stomach, colon, or jejunum) [5]. Chest X-rays, esophagograms, and CT scans play an important role in the early identification of complications. Accurate interpretation of postoperative images is vital in those patients and when interpreting the images, radiologist should be familiar with different surgical techniques used and their potential complications. After esophagectomy and gastric pull-through or bowel interposition procedures, the air column of the conduit can be seen on mediastinum or right paravertebral space as an expected finding on PA chest-X rays (Fig. 10.6). For the assessment of complications after the surgery, particularly the pulmonary

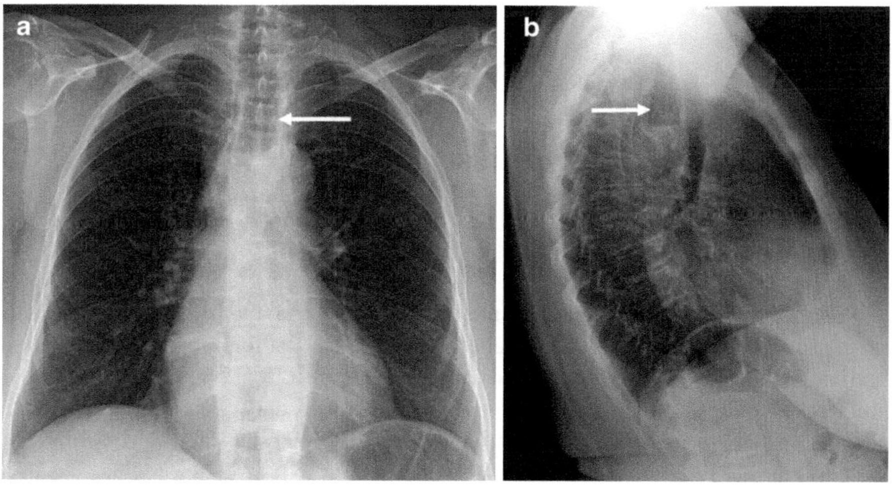


**Fig. 10.4** Large air column in the proximal esophagus. Posterior–anterior (**a**) and lateral (**b**) chest X-rays show dilation in the esophagus with an air-fluid level (arrows). On lateral radiography, esophagus is seen posterior to the tracheal air column. Patient was diagnosed as achalasia after further evaluation

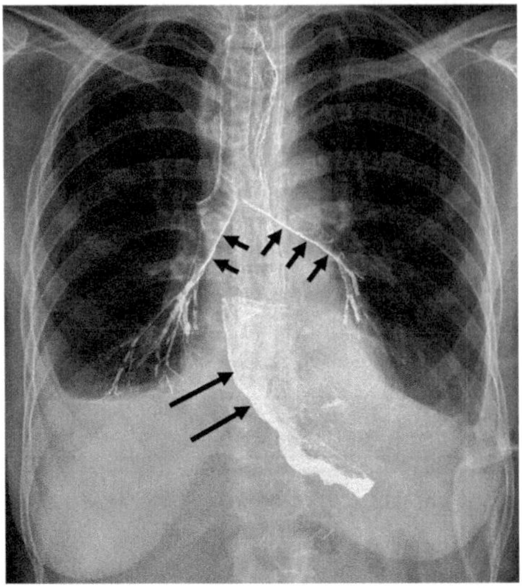

**Fig. 10.5** Barium aspiration in the postoperative period. PA chest X-ray shows barium lining the walls of the trachea and lower lobe bronchi (short arrows) due to deep aspiration during fluoroscopy scan. Contrast retention is seen in the pulled-through stomach (long arrows)

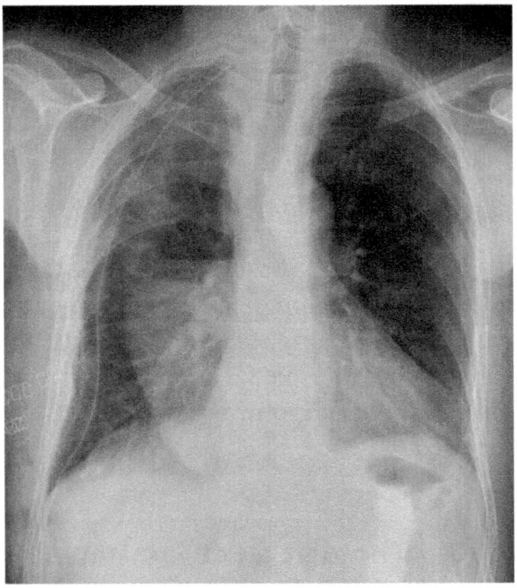

**Fig. 10.6** PA chest X-ray after esophagectomy and gastric pull-through operation. The dilated "gastric conduit" is located posteriorly in the right paravertebral space. Air-fluid level is seen in the lumen. Additional findings include right pleural catheter

and pleural complications including atelectasis, pneumonia, liquid aspiration, pleural effusion, and respiratory failure, chest X-ray is the first imaging modality due to high availability even in the intensive care units. Therefore, it has become a routine practice to obtain an immediate post-esophagectomy chest X-ray to ensure the absence of pneumothorax, significant atelectasis or collapsed lung, or distention of the conduit that requires immediate intervention [9].

### 10.1.3 Computed Tomography

Thoracic CT scanning is a cross-sectional diagnostic modality, which is a relatively high radiation dose technique, capable of exposing an effective dose 50–500 times higher than a conventional chest radiogram. Therefore, appropriate patient selection and correct choice of the scan parameters are important. With the improvements in CT technologies, multidetector or multislice CT machines have been developed allowing larger volumes to be scanned with thinner sections up to 0.625 mm for thoracic imaging, and yet shorter scan times. As a result, the demonstration of thoracic vasculature, including pulmonary arteries and thoracic aorta, has become possible with shorter contrast agent administration thus reducing contrast usage. Thoracic CT is performed to improve visualization of a lesion, which is not clearly demonstrated on chest X-ray, to localize a lesion, to evaluate the hilum and proximal airways, to search for a suspected lesion, and to evaluate the mediastinum and chest wall. Esophagus is normally seen as a collapsed tubular structure in the posterior mediastinum on CT scans. Normal esophageal wall thickness is expected to be less than 3 mm for a distended esophagus and 5 mm for a collapsed lumen. Any wall thickness greater than 5 mm on CT is considered abnormal [10]. Esophageal tumors usually appear as eccentric or concentric mural thickening (Fig. 10.7).

In patients with esophageal cancer, preoperative staging is of paramount importance due to stage specific treatment options. Endoscopic ultrasonography (EUS) and CT have complementary roles in preoperative staging of esophageal carcinomas. EUS can show the layers of the esophageal wall, therefore have a place in local tumor staging with a sensitivity of 81–92% and specificity of 94–97% for correct evaluation of T category [11]. The accuracy of CT in the initial staging of esophageal tumors increases in cases with more advanced disease. CT has a value particularly in assessing locally advanced tumors, distant lymphadenopathies, and other

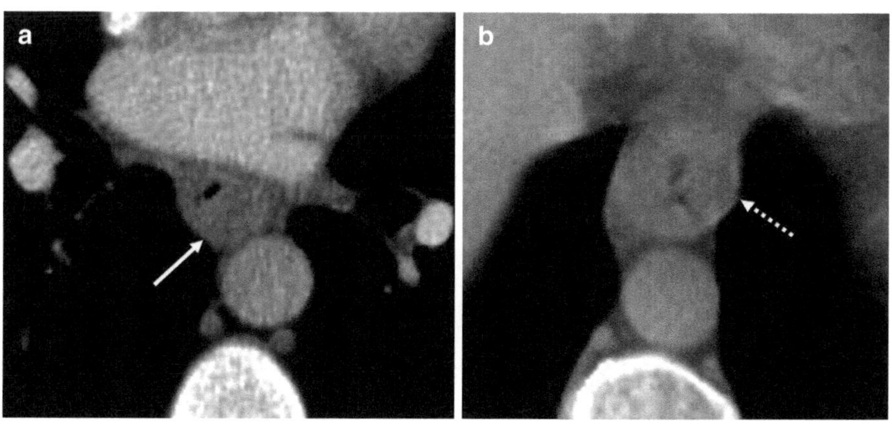


**Fig. 10.7** Esophageal carcinoma. CT images show eccentric (solid arrow in **a**) and concentric (dashed arrow in **b**) mural thickening in two different patients with the diagnosis of esophageal carcinoma

distant metastatic sites. According to the recent American College of Radiology (ACR) appropriateness criteria, CT of the chest and abdomen with intravenous contrast media or FDG-PET/CT is appropriate for use at initial staging of newly diagnosed esophageal cancer as they provide additional information about distant nodal and metastatic disease [12]. Similarly, according to the European Society for Medical Oncology (ESMO) guidelines, staging of esophageal cancer should include a complete clinical examination and a CT scan of the neck, chest, and abdomen. FDG-PET should be carried out in patients who are candidates for esophagectomy [13].

With the eight-edition staging of cancer of the esophagus and esophagogastric junction by AJCC/UICC, clinical stage grouping (cTNM) before treatment decision is newly introduced, in which TNM categories are typically defined by imaging [14]. Separate clinical groupings were implicated for adenocarcinoma and squamous cell carcinoma (SCC). For SCC, localization of primary site (L category; upper, middle, and lower) is defined by epicenter of esophageal tumor. The definition of the esophagogastric junction tumors was revised. Cancers involving the esophagogastric junction (EGJ) that have their epicenter within the 2 cm of the cardia (Siewert I/II) are now staged as esophageal cancers, whereas cancers whose epicenter is more than 2 cm distal from the EGJ (Siewert III), even if the EJG is involved, are staged according to stomach cancer TNM and stage groups (Fig. 10.8) [15].

According to TNM categories, T1 cancers invade the lamina propria, muscularis mucosa, or submucosa, T2 cancers invade the muscularis propria, and T3 cancers invade the adventitia [14]. EUS is capable of differentiating T1, T2, and T3 tumors due to better delineation of esophageal wall layers. Although the accuracy of EUS

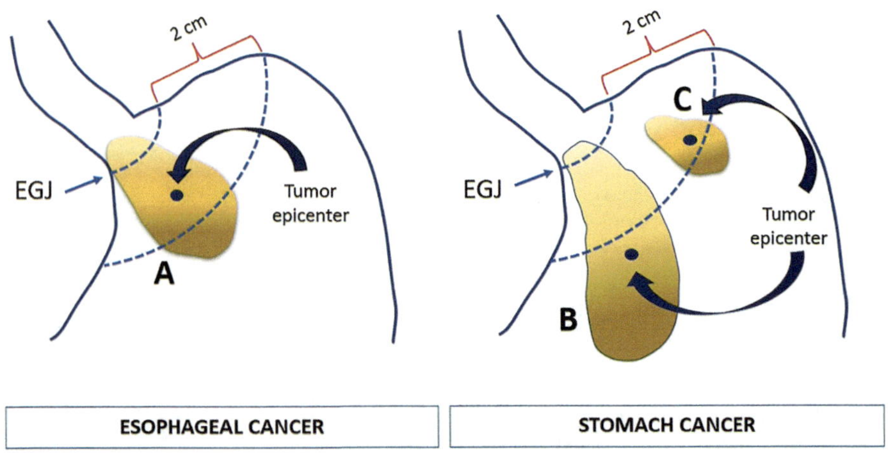


**Fig. 10.8** Schematic drawing of definition of the esophagogastric junction tumors. A tumor with its epicenter located within 2 cm of esophagogastric junction (EGJ) and involves the EGJ (shown as **A**) is classified as esophageal cancer. A tumor with its epicenter located >2 cm from the EGJ and involves EGJ (shown as **B**) or a tumor located within 2 cm of EGJ but do not involve the EJG (shown as **C**) is classified as stomach cancer

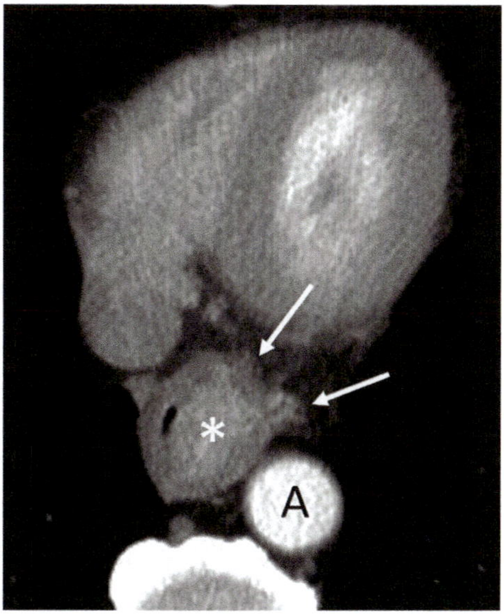


**Fig. 10.9** Esophageal carcinoma with T3 category. CT image shows luminal narrowing and eccentric mural thickening of the inferior third of thoracic esophagus regarding the esophageal tumor (star). Arrows point to ill-defined soft tissue around the lesion in consistent with adventitial invasion (T3 category). Note that, fat planes are preserved between the tumor and the aorta (A)

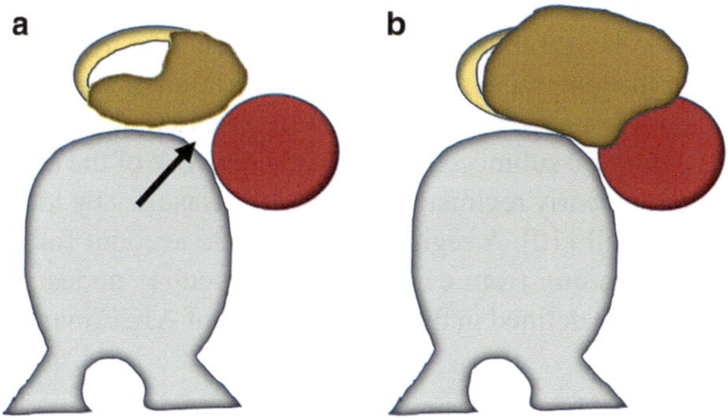


**Fig. 10.10** Schematic drawing of invasion of aorta in esophageal tumor. Picture (**a**) shows normal anatomical triangular fat plane (arrow) between esophagus, vertebral body, and the aorta (red circle). Picture (**b**) shows obliteration of the triangular fat between the esophageal tumor, the spine, and the aorta, which increases the suspicion of aortic invasion by the tumor

for T staging is high, it is an operator-dependent procedure and interobserver variation may occur due to different experience levels. On the other hand, CT is considered as the most accurate imaging modality for ruling out local invasion to adjacent structures (i.e., T4 tumor) which defines the appropriateness for surgical resectability. T3 tumors demonstrate definite wall thickening or an esophageal mass causing luminal obstruction on CT scans. Invasion of adventitia regarding the T3 category may appear as ill-defined soft tissue density around the tumor (Fig. 10.9). Nonetheless, the triangular fat space between the esophageal tumor, aorta, and spine should be preserved to exclude T4 tumor (Fig. 10.10) [10].

The loss of intervening fat planes between the tumor and the adjacent organs, or displacement or indentation of adjacent mediastinal structures by the tumor are criteria for local tumoral invasion on CT. However, in the posterior mediastinum, fat is usually absent between the esophagus and neighborhood structures, especially in severely underweight patients or patients with previous radiotherapy. Therefore, absence of fat planes should be used as an adjunct to the other criteria for deciding local invasion [10].

According to eighth edition of AJCC/UICC esophageal cancer staging manual, T4a category refers to the invasion of pleura, pericardium, azygos vein, diaphragm, and peritoneum, which is also accepted as resectable disease [14]. The obliteration of fat plane between the tumor and the pericardium, the presence of pericardial thickening, pericardial effusion, or indentation of the left atrium creating a concave deformity of the heart contour suggest pericardial invasion. More than 1 cm direct contact of the tumor with the diaphragmatic crus suggests invasion [10].

T4b tumors show invasion to the aorta, carotid vessels, trachea, bronchi, or vertebral body, which precludes resection. Direct extension of the esophageal tumor to the lumen of trachea or the presence of a tracheobronchial fistula are obvious findings of airway invasion. In addition, posterior wall indentation of the trachea or bronchus with a concave contour or displacement of them increase the suspicion of tumoral invasion and should be confirmed with bronchoscopy and biopsy (Fig. 10.11). For the invasion of the aorta, the presence of a circumferential interface >90° between the tumor and the aorta, or obliteration of the triangle fat between the spine, aorta, and esophageal tumor should be assessed on axial CT images [10].

Owing to the extensive submucosal lymphatic network of the esophagus, it is not surprising to encounter early regional lymph node metastases by longitudinal spread along the muscular wall [10]. A regional lymph node account for any paraesophageal lymph node extending from cervical nodes to celiac nodes. Twenty regional lymph node stations are defined in the eighth edition of AJCC manual including left

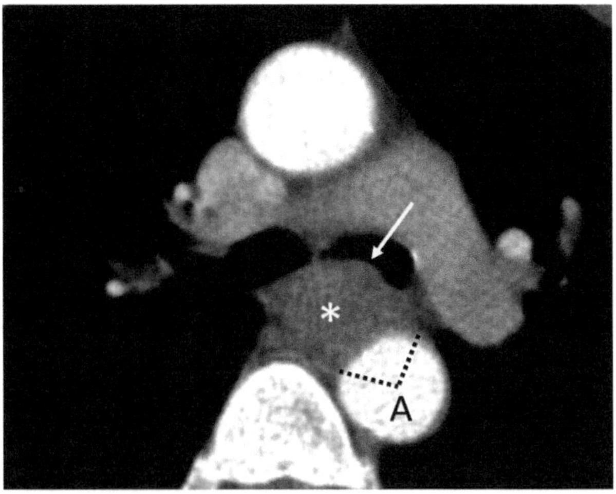


**Fig. 10.11** Esophageal carcinoma with T4 category. The posterior wall indentation of the left main bronchus with a concave contour (arrow) is suspicious for airway invasion by the esophageal tumor (star). In addition to obliteration of the triangular fat plane between the tumor and the aorta (**A**), the circumferential interface between them is >90° (dashed lines) is consistent with T4 tumor category

gastric, common hepatic, splenic, and celiac nodes [14]. Lymph node status is one of the most prognostic factors in the prognosis of esophageal cancer. However, CT is a poor predictor of tumoral metastasis in especially small regional lymph nodes. According to a meta-analysis, the pooled sensitivity and specificity of CT for regional lymph node metastases in esophageal cancer were 51.7% and 80.3%, while for abdominal lymph node metastases were 41.5% and 91.2%, respectively [16]. On CT imaging, lymphadenopathy is diagnosed according to the short axis criterion in which 10 mm is usually taken as the threshold for mediastinal and upper abdominal lymph nodes, whereas 6 mm is the cut off for retrocrural lymph nodes and 5 mm for supraclavicular nodes [17]. Apart from size criterion, clusters of smaller nodes, ill-defined mass in a lymph node area, nodal mass with central low density indicating necrosis and loss of smooth well-defined borders with heterogeneous internal density are all ancillary features to decide the lymph node metastasis (Fig. 10.12) [16]. The eighth edition of AJCC manual classifies 1–2 suspicious regional lymph nodes as N1, 3–6 as N2, and 7 or more as N3 category. Nevertheless, it may be difficult to give the exact number of positive lymph nodes on CT and even PET/CT since peri-esophageal lymph node involvement may be indistinguishable from the tumoral mass leading to underestimation of the N stage. On the other hand, EUS can accurately determine the number of positive regional lymph nodes with capability of adding tissue sampling to EUS findings improving the pooled sensitivity to 96.7% and 95.5%, respectively [18]. Histologic confirmation of nodal status is critical for the accurate clinical staging; therefore, EUS-directed fine needle aspiration biopsy is strongly suggested by the AJCC [15].

The fundamental use of CT in the initial evaluation of patients with esophageal cancer is in detection of distant metastasis (M category). Intravenous contrast administration is recommended by the American College of Radiology for optimal performance when chest and abdominal-pelvic CT are used in the initial staging

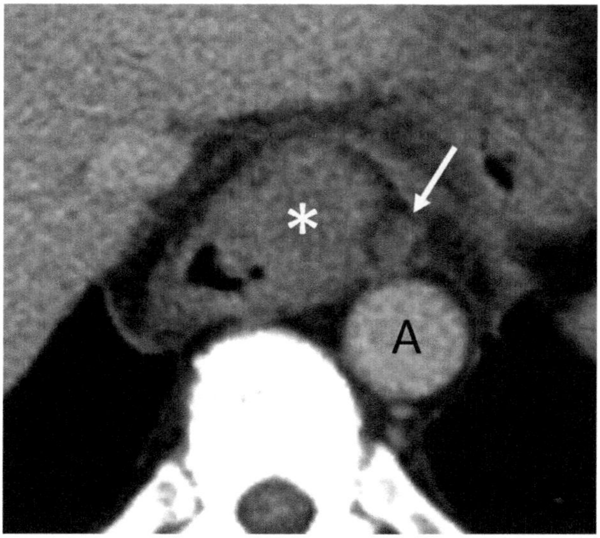


**Fig. 10.12** Esophageal carcinoma with regional lymph node metastasis. CT image shows an eccentric esophageal tumor (star) invading the adventitia. An ill-defined soft tissue mass (arrow) separate from the tumor is seen in the peri-esophageal area regarding the regional lymph node metastases. *A* aorta

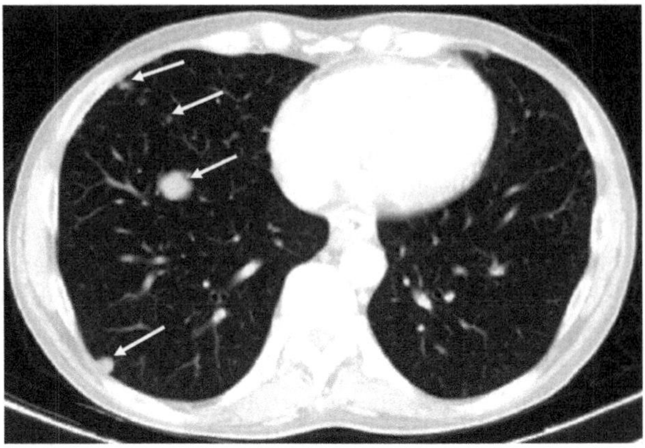

**Fig. 10.13** Lung metastases. CT image in lung window shows multiple round metastases (arrows) in a patient with diagnosis of distal esophageal carcinoma

[12]. The most common sites for distant metastatic involvement are non-regional lymph nodes, liver, lung, and adrenal gland (Fig. 10.13) [19]. Brain CT is not regularly performed in routine clinical practice due to low rate of brain metastasis (<1%). However, routine chest and abdominopelvic CT covers majority of the possible metastatic sites.

Response to neoadjuvant treatment is routinely assessed by evaluation of tumor-related symptoms such as dysphagia, endoscopy, and CT examination [13]. On CT, response prediction could be difficult due to therapy-related changes. Especially, an increase in the density of paraoesophageal fat planes due to treatment creates an important limitation [20]. Indeed, the main role of CT or PET/CT in staging after neoadjuvant treatment is to rule out development of interval metastases between therapy and surgery, where resection is performed unless there is radiologically demonstrated metastasis [13, 18].

Various surgical techniques are used in esophageal cancer surgery. Those techniques include transthoracic esophagectomy procedures (Ivor Lewis, McKeown procedures, left thoracoabdominal technique) and different forms of bypass surgeries. When the stomach is not available to use due to previous or synchronous partial or total gastrectomy, colon or jejunum is used as an esophageal substitute for reconstruction [5]. The conduit may be placed in a substernal, posterior mediastinal, or rarely intrapleural position. Those sophisticated procedures can alter the normal anatomy; hence image interpretation becomes difficult. Therefore, radiologists should be aware of the details of the surgical procedure and should have the knowledge of how these procedures affect images (e.g., postoperative anatomic changes) and possible postoperative complications. Complications of esophagectomy could be intraoperative or postoperative. CT has a major role in both early and late postoperative complications. Pulmonary complications, anastomotic leaks, strictures of the anastomosis site, chylothorax, redundancy and delayed emptying, diaphragmatic hernia, and reflux esophagitis constitute a broad spectrum of complications after the surgery [6]. Pulmonary and pleural complications, which include atelectasis, pneumonia, respiratory failure, pulmonary embolism, pleural effusion, pneumothorax, are the most important causes of early postoperative mortality. Anastomotic leaks occasionally occur within the first 10 days after surgery due to inappropriate tension [5]. Although esophagogram is part of routine postoperative assessment at most centers, the role of chest CT should not be overlooked particularly in unstable patients or critically ill patients who cannot stand in upright position. CT may be performed without or with intravenous contrast or with oral contrast as CT esophagography according to the suspected complication. In the literature, the sensitivity and specificity of CT esophagography for are reported as 59–100% and 80–100%, respectively. In this technique, after a precontrast CT scan from the angle of the mandible to iliac crests, low-osmolar oral contrast material is given either by active drinking of the patient or by nasogastric tube, which is placed above the level of cricopharyngeal sphincter [21]. When compared with fluoroscopy, CT esophagography may identify small leaks that can be extremely difficult with fluoroscopy. In addition, fluoroscopy is an operator-dependent technique and requires sufficient experience to perform and interpret the study, whereas CT esophagography is more consistent in terms of performance, scan protocol, and interpretation. CT may show direct leakage of contrast material from the esophagectomy site, visible discontinuity of the conduit wall, or esophagopleural fistula (Fig. 10.14) [22]. In addition, extraesophageal findings such as mediastinal fluid collection or abscess, mediastinal gas, small bowel obstruction, or more distal small bowel injuries or leaks can be demonstrated by CT.

After the definitive treatment by esophagectomy or multimodality treatment options, tumor recurrence may occur in the follow-up. Distant metastases are much more common than local recurrence and may occur in the non-regional lymph nodes or distant organs [17]. Development of a new soft tissue thickening or a mass at the surgical anastomosis site or new regional lymphadenopathy should rise the suspicion of local recurrence on CT (Fig. 10.15). PET/CT may provide additional information in suspicion of recurrence compared to conventional CT imaging;

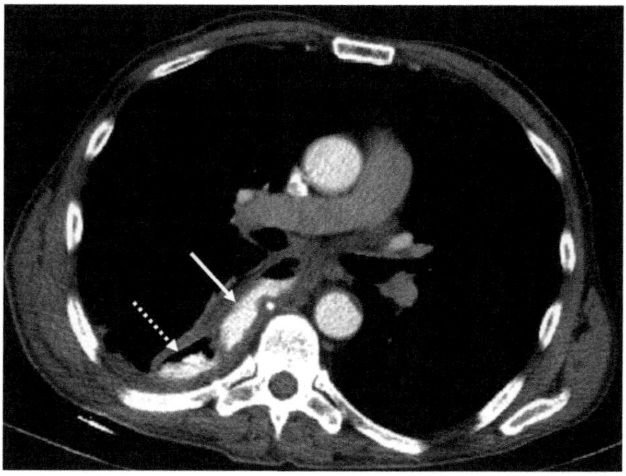

**Fig. 10.14** Esophagopleural fistula. CT esophagography image with oral contrast shows gastric conduit (solid arrow) in the right paravertebral space after Ivor Lewis procedure. Filling of contrast material into the right pleural space (dashed arrow) is consistent with esophagopleural fistula

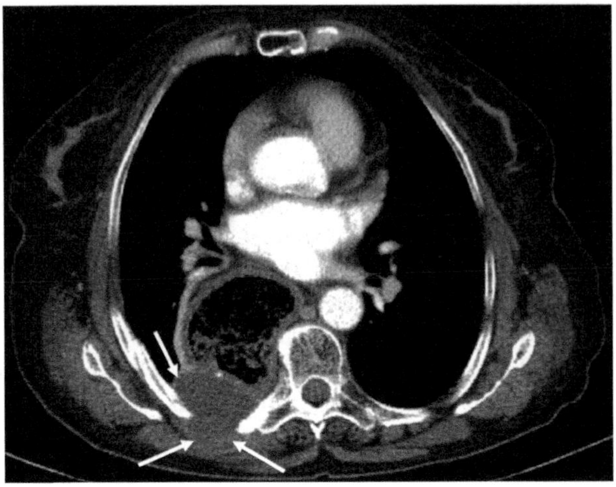

**Fig. 10.15** Regional recurrence after esophagectomy. CT image shows a lobulated low density soft tissue mass (arrows) posterior to the gastric conduit, destructing the ribs. It was a new finding in the follow-up and was proved to be metastasis of esophageal carcinoma pathologically

however, confounding factors that cause increased FDG uptake such as inflammation and ulceration should be kept in mind [17].

### 10.1.4 Ultrasonography

Ultrasonography is an easily applied imaging technique in the emergency and critical care setting. It is particularly beneficial in critically ill unstable patients who could not be transported to CT room safely. In contrast to imaging techniques acknowledged up to now, it does to expose ionizing radiation and hence, repeatable as much as required. For thorax imaging, is it useful in assessing superficial pulmonary, pleural-based and chest wall lesions. In fact, the acoustic beam almost totally reflects from the aerated lungs due to acoustic mismatch between the lungs and the chest wall. Nonetheless, it is extraordinarily sensitive for pleural effusion and collections as low as 5–20 mL [23]. Moreover, it may characterize the pleural fluid with demonstration of septations, loculations, and complexity (whether simple or loculated).

Thorax ultrasonography is mostly used in esophageal cancer patients after the surgery to determine the early pleural and pulmonary complications on bedside. Pleural fluid appears as an echo-free area delineating the pleural space. Internal echoes may be seen in the pleural fluid regarding blood or pus. A thick wall suggests empyema, in which accompanying gas may be identified. A consolidation makes the tissues denser and less well aerated which results in a hyperechoic appearance as a solid organ on ultrasonography, which is also termed as hepatization [23, 24].

In Mc Keown procedure or trans-hiatal esophagectomy, a left neck incision is performed to create a cervical anastomosis particularly for more proximal esophageal tumors [5]. Early complications around the cervical anastomosis site after surgery, such as hematoma or collections due to anastomotic leaks, abscess, or thoracic duct injury, are easily assessed by ultrasonography.

Ultrasonography is also beneficial as a guide in percutaneous drainage of fluid collections either in the pleural space, intraperitoneal space, or in the neck [25]. It ensures the appropriate position of the drainage catheter in the collection and demonstrates the possible complications such as malpositioning or kinking of the catheter.

### 10.1.5 Magnetic Resonance Imaging (MRI)

MRI is a cross-sectional imaging method with multiplanar facility and high soft tissue contrast discrimination. This allows mediastinal lesions to be differentiated from normal tissues without contrast media administration. Respiratory and cardiac motion artifacts, and flow artifacts from aorta and pulmonary vessels are the main disadvantages that cause technical challenges particularly in MRI of the esophagus [26]. Nonetheless, faster MRI sequences with single breath-hold or the use of cardiac or respiratory-gated techniques may overcome those artefacts [27]. Moreover, for the best MRI performance for assessment of mediastinal structures, a 3.0-T scanner with a 32-channel phased-array body coil is recommended with high-resolution image protocols including motion compensation methods [28].

Unlike CT imaging, evaluation of lung parenchyma is very limited on MRI owing to low signal intensity from aerated lung spaces and motion artefacts. However, cystic lesions of the lung such as bronchogenic cysts and mucoceles can be clearly demonstrated with very high T2 signal intensity [29].

MRI can delineate the borders of normal anatomic structures in the mediastinum due to excellent soft tissue contrast. With the identification of normal layers of the esophageal wall, MRI has a potential to improve stratification of patients toward endoscopic resection, upfront surgery, or neoadjuvant therapy [27]. Especially, high-resolution T2-weighted sequences enables the detailed imaging of the anatomical layers of the esophagus and preserved surrounding peri-esophageal tissues [26]. According to a meta-analysis, MRI appears to differentiate organ confined disease (T1–T2 stage) from advanced disease (T3–T4 stage) with a high diagnostic performance (pooled sensitivity and specificity of 86%) [28]. However, in differentiating positive nodes, depending on the size threshold, reported sensitivity and specificity of MRI vary between 59–100% and 57–92%, respectively [27].

Besides, current role in staging of the esophageal cancer, MRI may also be beneficial for delineation of tumor borders and radiation treatment planning (Fig. 10.16) [30]. The delineation of the gross tumor volume is particularly important for cone-down boost techniques of radiotherapy, which aims to ensure adequate target volume coverage and limit the dose to surrounding organs at risk. MR-guided radiotherapy for esophageal cancer is an emerging technique that may find a place for possible applications in clinical practice in the future [31].

With the improvement of functional MRI techniques such as diffusion-weighted imaging (DWI) and dynamic contrast-enhanced (DCE) MRI sequences, response assessment after neoadjuvant chemoradiotherapy (NACT) or re-staging via MRI has been studied in different tumors such as rectal cancer, and promising results

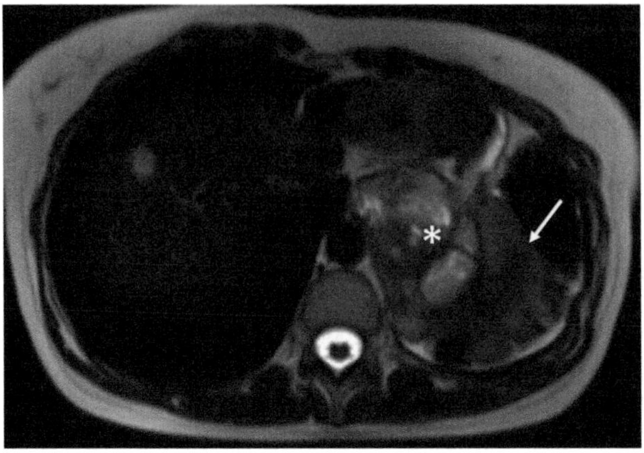


**Fig. 10.16** Esophageal tumor. Axial plane T2-weighted MR image shows gross mass (star) originating from distal esophagus. The tumor is well defined with a T2 hypointense capsule and contains cystic areas. The atelectasis of the left lower lung lobe (arrow) can be differentiated from the tumor by differences in signal intensity. The pathology of the tumor was gastrointestinal stromal tumor of the esophagus

have been achieved. Although there are limited studies in the current literature on response assessment of esophageal cancer with MRI, results show that change in ADC values derived from DWI images can be used for detection of residual disease after NACT with high sensitivity and specificity over 92% [28]. However, further research investigating the role of MRI in esophageal cancer staging, re-staging, and treatment planning including more validation studies is required [32].

## References

1. Levine MS, Rubesin SE. Diseases of the esophagus: diagnosis with esophagography. Radiology. 2005;237(2):414–27. https://doi.org/10.1148/radiol.2372050199.
2. Keshav N, Khalid S, Parasher G, Cassidy F, Thompson W, Shiehmorteza M. Dots, lines, contours, and ends: an image-based review of esophageal pathology. Eur J Radiol Open. 2021;8:100361. https://doi.org/10.1016/j.ejro.2021.100361.
3. Marini T, Desai A, Kaproth-Joslin K, Wandtke J, Hobbs SK. Imaging of the oesophagus: beyond cancer. Insights Imaging. 2017;8(3):365–76. https://doi.org/10.1007/s13244-017-0548-3.
4. Debi U, Sharma M, Singh L, Sinha A. Barium esophagogram in various esophageal diseases: a pictorial essay. Indian J Radiol Imaging. 2019;29(2):141–54. https://doi.org/10.4103/ijri.IJRI_465_18.
5. Flanagan JC, Batz R, Saboo SS, Nordeck SM, Abbara S, Kernstine K, et al. Esophagectomy and gastric pull-through procedures: surgical techniques, imaging features, and potential complications. Radiographics. 2016;36(1):107–21. https://doi.org/10.1148/rg.2016150126.
6. Kim TJ, Lee KH, Kim YH, Sung SW, Jheon S, Cho SK, Lee KW. Postoperative imaging of esophageal cancer: what chest radiologists need to know. Radiographics. 2007;27(2):409–29. https://doi.org/10.1148/rg.272065034.
7. Ho ML, Gutierrez FR. Chest radiography in thoracic polytrauma. AJR Am J Roentgenol. 2009;192(3):599–612. https://doi.org/10.2214/AJR.07.3324.

8. Olivé A, Juncosa S, Evison G, Maddison PJ. Air in the oesophagus: a sign of oesophageal involvement in systemic sclerosis. Clin Rheumatol. 1995;14(3):319–21. https://doi.org/10.1007/BF02208346.
9. Gabriel E, Shah R, Attwood K, Kukar M, Hochwald S. The first postesophagectomy chest X-ray predicts respiratory failure and the need for tracheostomy. J Surg Res. 2018;224:89–96. https://doi.org/10.1016/j.jss.2017.11.057.
10. Hong SJ, Kim TJ, Nam KB, Lee IS, Yang HC, Cho S, et al. New TNM staging system for esophageal cancer: what chest radiologists need to know. Radiographics. 2014;34(6):1722–40. https://doi.org/10.1148/rg.346130079.
11. Puli SR, Reddy JB, Bechtold ML, Antillon D, Ibdah JA, Antillon MR. Staging accuracy of esophageal cancer by endoscopic ultrasound: a meta-analysis and systematic review. World J Gastroenterol. 2008;14(10):1479–90. https://doi.org/10.3748/wjg.14.1479.
12. Expert Panels on Thoracic and Gastrointestinal Imaging; Raptis CA, Goldstein A, Henry TS, Porter KK, Catenacci D, Kelly AM, et al. ACR appropriateness criteria® staging and follow-up of esophageal cancer. J Am Coll Radiol. 2022;19(11S):S462–72. https://doi.org/10.1016/j.jacr.2022.09.008.
13. Lordick F, Mariette C, Haustermans K, Obermannová R, Arnold D, Guidelines ESMO, Committee. Oesophageal cancer: ESMO Clinical Practice Guidelines for diagnosis, treatment and follow-up. Ann Oncol. 2016;27(Suppl. 5):v50–7. https://doi.org/10.1093/annonc/mdw329.
14. Rice TW, Ishwaran H, Ferguson MK, Blackstone EH, Goldstraw P. Cancer of the esophagus and esophagogastric junction: an eighth edition staging primer. J Thorac Oncol. 2017;12(1):36–42. https://doi.org/10.1016/j.jtho.2016.10.016.
15. Rice TW, Patil DT, Blackstone EH. 8th edition AJCC/UICC staging of cancers of the esophagus and esophagogastric junction: application to clinical practice. Ann Cardiothorac Surg. 2017;6(2):119–30. https://doi.org/10.21037/acs.2017.03.14.
16. Sgourakis G, Gockel I, Lyros O, Hansen T, Mildenberger P, Lang H. Detection of lymph node metastases in esophageal cancer. Expert Rev Anticancer Ther. 2011;11(4):601–12. https://doi.org/10.1586/era.10.150.
17. Godoy MC, Bruzzi JF, Viswanathan C, Truong MT, Guimarães MD, Hofstetter WL, Erasmus JJ, Marom EM. Multimodality imaging evaluation of esophageal cancer: staging, therapy assessment, and complications. Abdom Imaging. 2013;38(5):974–93. https://doi.org/10.1007/s00261-013-9986-7.
18. Li Z, Rice TW. Diagnosis and staging of cancer of the esophagus and esophagogastric junction. Surg Clin North Am. 2012;92(5):1105–26. https://doi.org/10.1016/j.suc.2012.07.010.
19. D'Journo XB. Clinical implication of the innovations of the 8th edition of the TNM classification for esophageal and esophago-gastric cancer. J Thorac Dis. 2018;10(Suppl. 22):S2671–81. https://doi.org/10.21037/jtd.2018.03.182.
20. Encinas de la Iglesia J, Corral de la Calle MA, Fernández Pérez GC, Ruano Pérez R, Álvarez DA. Esophageal cancer: anatomic particularities, staging, and imaging techniques. Radiologia. 2016;58(5):352–65. https://doi.org/10.1016/j.rx.2016.06.004.
21. Norton-Gregory AA, Kulkarni NM, O'Connor SD, Budovec JJ, Zorn AP, Desouches SL. CT esophagography for evaluation of esophageal perforation. Radiographics. 2021;41(2):447–61. https://doi.org/10.1148/rg.2021200132.
22. Veziant J, Gaillard M, Barat M, Dohan A, Barret M, Manceau G, Karoui M, Bonnet S, Fuks D, Soyer P. Imaging of postoperative complications following Ivor-Lewis esophagectomy. Diagn Interv Imaging. 2022;103(2):67–78. https://doi.org/10.1016/j.diii.2021.09.003.
23. Hendin A, Koenig S, Millington SJ. Better with ultrasound: thoracic ultrasound. Chest. 2020;158(5):2082–9. https://doi.org/10.1016/j.chest.2020.04.052.
24. Joshi P, Vasishta A, Gupta M. Ultrasound of the pediatric chest. Br J Radiol. 2019;92(1100):20190058. https://doi.org/10.1259/bjr.20190058.
25. Ghaye B, Dondelinger RF. Imaging guided thoracic interventions. Eur Respir J. 2001;17(3):507–28. https://doi.org/10.1183/09031936.01.17305070.

26. van Rossum PSN, van Lier ALHMW, Lips IM, Meijer GJ, Reerink O, van Vulpen M, Lam MGEH, van Hillegersberg R, Ruurda JP. Imaging of oesophageal cancer with FDG-PET/CT and MRI. Clin Radiol. 2015;70(1):81–95. https://doi.org/10.1016/j.crad.2014.07.017.
27. Withey SJ, Goh V, Foley KG. State-of-the-art imaging in oesophago-gastric cancer. Br J Radiol. 2022;95(1137):20220410. https://doi.org/10.1259/bjr.20220410.
28. Lee SL, Yadav P, Starekova J, Christensen L, Chandereng T, Chappell R, Reeder SB, Bassetti MF. Diagnostic performance of MRI for esophageal carcinoma: a systematic review and meta-analysis. Radiology. 2021;299(3):583–94. https://doi.org/10.1148/radiol.2021202857.
29. Geiger J, Zeimpekis KG, Jung A, Moeller A, Kellenberger CJ. Clinical application of ultra-short echo-time MRI for lung pathologies in children. Clin Radiol. 2021;76(9):708.e9–708.e17. https://doi.org/10.1016/j.crad.2021.05.015.
30. van Rossum PSN, van Hillegersberg R, Lever FM, Lips IM, van Lier AL, Meijer GJ, van Leeuwen MS, van Vulpen M, Ruurda JP. Imaging strategies in the management of oesophageal cancer: what's the role of MRI? Eur Radiol. 2013;23(7):1753–65. https://doi.org/10.1007/s00330-013-2773-6.
31. Lee SL, Bassetti M, Meijer GJ, Mook S. Review of MR-guided radiotherapy for esophageal cancer. Front Oncol. 2021;11:628009. https://doi.org/10.3389/fonc.2021.628009.
32. Foley K, Findlay J, Goh V. Novel imaging techniques in staging oesophageal cancer. Best Pract Res Clin Gastroenterol. 2018;36-37:17–25. https://doi.org/10.1016/j.bpg.2018.11.009.

# Radiologic Evaluation: Diagnosis of Postoperative Complications and Evaluation of Intraabdominal Metastases in Esophageal Cancer

# 11

Serap Bas and Fatma Busra Ulas

In 2020, 604,100 people have been diagnosed with cancer of the esophagus, which constituted 3.3% of all cancer diagnoses according to World Cancer Research Fund International statistics. Esophagus cancer (EC) has the eighth highest incidence and sixth most deadly type of cancer worldwide [1–3]. Esophagus cancer has a higher incidence in men than women for 70% of all esophageal cancers worldwide and affects the elderly predominantly, and 60% of cases are >65 years old [1].

Esophageal squamous cell carcinoma (ESCC) is the most prevalent histological type worldwide, while the United States (US) and other Western countries have predominantly esophageal adenocarcinoma (EAC) [2–4]. Globally, 87% of all esophageal cancers are ESCC with 11% constituting EAC. ESCC is typically found in the proximal two-thirds of the esophagus [1]. Squamous dysplasia known as precursor lesion of squamous carcinoma is hardly detectable and there is no standardized screening program. Chemo endoscopic techniques such as Lugol staining have been suggested for the diagnosis of precancerous squamous lesions [2]. EAC typically occurs in the distal third of the esophagus and at the gastroesophageal junction (GEJ) and it is related to Barret's esophagus (BE), which increases a patient's risk of EAC 30-to 40-fold the most important factor in EAC. Dysplasia within BE lesions signals a marked increase in cancer risk, but screening of BE-associated adenocarcinoma by endoscopy has not been proven cost effective [4].

Malignancy of the esophagus has a particularly poor prognosis because they typically cause no symptoms, so they are diagnosed late in their course [1]. Most often preceded symptoms are progressive dysphagia, odynophagia, and weight loss [3]. Asymptomatic patients may present with anemia, mediastinal lymphadenopathy, and hoarseness due to recurrent laryngeal nerve encasement [3]. Upper endoscopy is the gold standard for the evaluation of esophageal symptoms, which not only visualizes the tumor but also does the tissue sampling for pathological

S. Bas (✉) · F. B. Ulas
Radiology Department, Basaksehir Cam ve Sakura City Hospital, Istanbul, Turkey





O. Engin (ed.), *Risk Factors and Therapy of Esophagus Cancer*,
https://doi.org/10.1007/978-3-031-47024-0_11

confirmation. Esophageal cancer can present as a luminal obscuring mass, flat lesion, or subtle area [5].

## 11.1 Staging of EC

The outcome for patients with EC is strongly associated with the stage at initial diagnosis. Appropriate staging of the patient before curative surgery and evaluation of the response to neoadjuvant therapy are very important in determining the most appropriate treatment for the patient and performing the appropriate operation in curative surgery [6]. The American Cancer Committee (AJCC) has created separate classifications for clinical, pathological, and post-neoadjuvant stage groups in the final staging (TNM) published for esophageal and esophagogastric junction cancers (eighth edition of AJCC) [6].

**TMN stage of esophageal cancer [6]**

| Category | Criteria |
|---|---|
| *T category* | |
| TX | Tumor cannot be assessed |
| T0 | No evidence of primary tumor |
| Tis | High-grade dysplasia, defined as malignant cells confined by the basement membrane<br>T1 Tumor invades the lamina propria, muscularis mucosae, or submucosa |
| T1a | Tumor invades the lamina propria or muscularis mucosae |
| T1b | Tumor invades the submucosa |
| T2 | Tumor invades the muscularis propria |
| T3 | Tumor invades the adventitia |
| T4 | Tumor invades adjacent structures |
| T4aa | Tumor invades the pleura, pericardium, azygos vein, diaphragm, or peritoneum |
| T4ba | Tumor invades other adjacent structures, such as the aorta, vertebral body, or trachea |
| *N category* | |
| NX | Regional lymph nodes cannot be assessed |
| N0 | No regional lymph node metastasis |
| N1 | Metastasis in 1–2 regional lymph nodes |
| N2 | Metastasis in 3–6 regional lymph nodes |
| N3 | Metastasis in ≥7 regional lymph nodes |
| *M category* | |
| M0 | No distant metastasis |
| M1 | Distant metastasis |

## 11.2 Imaging Modalities of EC for Clinical Staging

Clinical staging is based on imaging modalities with minimal histologic information and is also limited by the resolution of imaging methods. The assessment of cancer location is crucial, which is made during esophagoscopy alternatively location may be determined from chest CT [7].

Esophageal ultrasound (EUS) provides a detailed examination of the esophageal wall and the current procedure of choice determining clinical T. The muscularis propria is vital for the differentiation of T1, T2, and T3 cancers. In T1 cancers, there is no invasion of muscularis propria. In T2 cancers, there is muscularis propria invasion, if the invasion is beyond the muscularis propria, the cancer is T3. The clinical catheterization of T1–T2 cancer directs future therapy [6].

EUS, CT, and FDG-PET are the principal non-invasive modalities for clinical lymph node determination [7–10]. EUS is used to evaluate the size, shape, border, and internal echogenic characteristics of regional lymph nodes [11]. Larger, more rounded, well-demarcated hypoechoic lymph nodes are most likely to metastasize. Round-shaped and enlarged short-axis lymph node on CT suggests nodal metastasis. Intrathoracic and abdominal lymph nodes >1 cm are considered enlarged [11]. In a recent review, CT was 50% sensitive (41–60%) and 83% specific (77–89%) in lymph node assessment [11, 12]. FDG-PET relies on metabolic evaluation and intensity of FDG uptake and decay. Adding CT to FDG-PET increases accuracy, sensitivity, specificity, and negative predictive value minimally, it has the biggest impact on positive predictive value that increase 82% from 69% [13].

EUS, CT, and FDG-PET have very similar rates in terms of accuracy, sensitivity and specificity in lymph node evaluation. (Accuracy 66% for EUS, 63% for CT and 68% for PET; sensitivity 42% for EUS, 35% for CT, and 35% for PET; specificity 91% for EUS, 93% for CT, and 87% for PET) [7, 9, 13].

Endosonographic-directed fine needle aspiration (EUS-FNA) provides histologic confirmation which is critical for accurate clinical staging and strongly recommended by the AJCC [11]. In a multicenter study, sensitivity, specificity, positive predictive value, and negative predictive value for lymph node assessment were 92%, 93%, 100%, and 86% respectively [11].

For the assessment of distant metastases, the value of EUS is extremely limited. Visualization of ascites with EUS may raise suspicion of intraperitoneal metastases. Thoracic and abdominal CT with intravenous and oral contrast has been reported to be 37–66% sensitive to detect distant metastases [9]. MRI staging has been shown to have an accuracy of 40% with very low sensitivity and specificity [14]. FDG-PET/CT imaging increases the detection of distant metastases [15].

## 11.3 Treatment Strategies of EC According to Staging

The treatment of EC is directed by the stage of the tumor. For intramucosal tumors, endoscopic resection is diagnostic and curative. The role of surgical therapy for early EC continues to be debated. For tumors that involve the deeper layers of the esophagus (T2 and beyond) and/or with nodal involvement, neoadjuvant therapy is recommended [16]. When distant metastases have been identified, treatment options are severely limited, and the focus shifts to palliation [17]. Median survival can only be 9–10 months despite treatment with chemotherapy [17, 18].

## 11.4 Surgical Treatment

Curative treatment for EC is primarily surgery, and about 20% of those who receive the diagnosis undergo surgery [11]. Supplementary neoadjuvant chemotherapy or radio chemotherapy increases survival. A variety of surgical procedures are used in the treatment of esophageal cancer. These procedures include transthoracic esophagectomy, trans hiatal esophagectomy, and various forms of bypass surgery [10, 19, 20].

Esophagectomy for EC is a highly complex and demanding two-cavity (abdominothoracic) procedure [21]. Recent studies conducted at large surgical centers have reported an associated high morbidity rate ranging from 30% to 50% [22].

Postoperative tumor recurrence is not uncommon in patients undergoing curative resection for esophageal cancer and can be categorized as either locoregional lymph node metastases, anastomotic recurrence) or distant (hematogenous metastases, pleural or peritoneal seeding) [23]. Hematogenous metastases most commonly involve the liver, lungs, and bones, followed by the adrenal glands, brain, and kidneys [24].

## 11.5 Complications After Surgery

The spectrum of potential surgical complications following esophagectomy includes necrosis, anastomotic leak (with mediastinitis, pleural empyema/abscess, tracheobronchial lesion, bleeding, etc.), aspiration pneumonia (Fig. 11.1), dense pleural effusion, and abscess formation (Fig. 11.1), recurrent laryngeal nerve palsy, chylothorax, intrathoracic herniation, and functional gastric tube outflow obstruction [24]. Pleural effusion, atelectasis, and pneumonia may also develop in the lung in the postoperative period, and CT imaging can be used in suspected patients (Fig. 11.2). Metastasectomy can be performed in some EC patients with liver

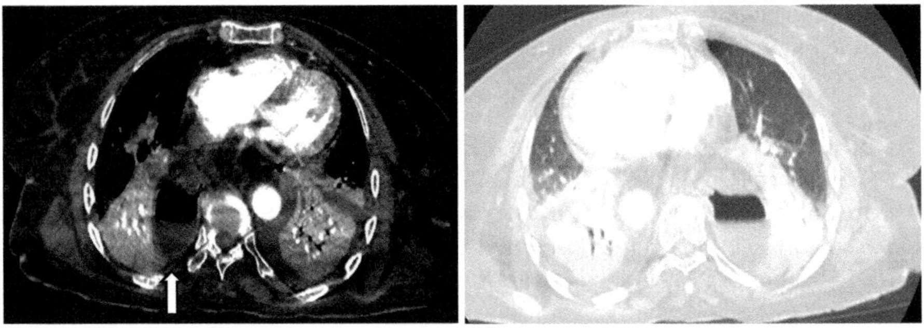

**Fig. 11.1** A 72-year-old female patient who was operated on for esophageal cancer developed postoperative aspiration pneumonia, dense pleural effusion, and abscess formation. In thoracic CT, there are infiltrative areas of aspiration pneumonia in the bilateral lung parenchyma, a dense collection area with air-fluid leveling in the right lung (white arrow), atelectatic areas, and bilateral pleural effusion

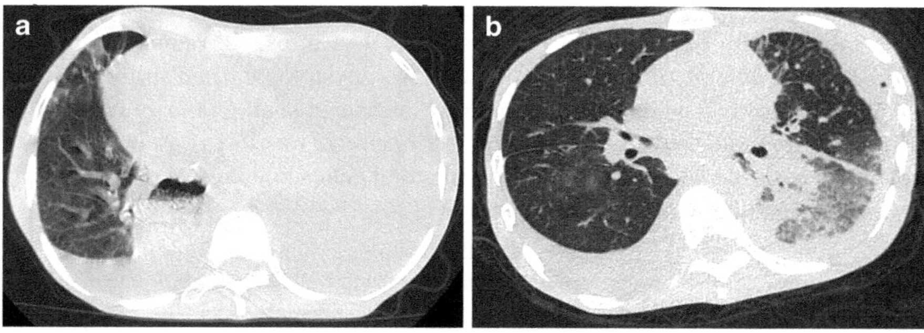


**Fig. 11.2** A 60-year-old female patient who had been operated on for esophageal cancer. Postoperative complications are seen in thorax CT. There are bilateral pleural effusion and areas of atelectasis and pneumonic infiltration, especially in the lower lobes

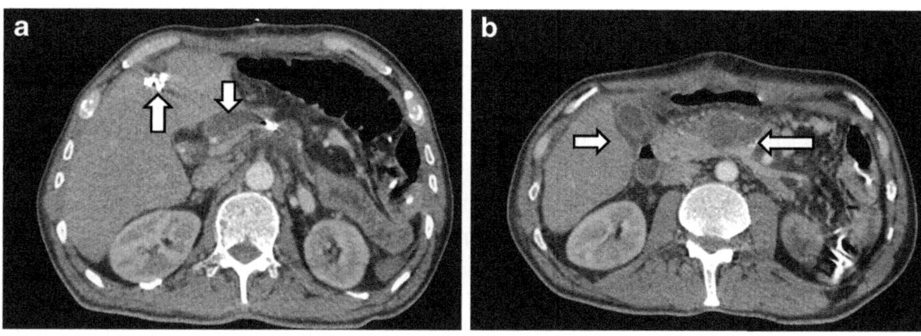


**Fig. 11.3** In a 49-year-old patient who underwent esophagectomy due to malignant mesenchymal tumor of the distal esophagus and metastasectomy for liver metastasis, postoperative fluid collection extending to the peripancreatic, pericholecystic, and periportal areas is observed. (**a**) Fluid collection in the periportal area and the metastasectomy area (white arrow). (**b**) Pericholecystic and peripancreatic fluid collections (white arrows)

metastases. In these patients, fluid collection may develop in the abdomen (for example, perihepatic, pericholecystic, peripancreatic) as a postoperative complication after metastasectomy (Fig. 11.3). Conduit necrosis and anastomotic insufficiency continue to be a source of considerable morbidity and mortality after esophageal resection [21].

Whereas esophageal conduit necrosis is somewhat rare, with average rates of ischemic complications for stomach, colon, and jejunum of 3.2%, 5.1%, and 4.2% respectively, anastomotic leaks up to 30% may occur, depending on their intrathoracic or cervical localization [21]. Endoscopy and computed tomography (CT) scan (thorax/abdomen) are the current diagnostic means of choice with a view to the consequences of decision-making regarding further therapeutic-surgical or conservative/interventional options. The false-negative rate for the detection of anastomotic insufficiencies in esophagogram is 30–50% in the current literature [25]. In recent clinical studies, a concept called Fast-track recovery surgery (FTS) has also been used in patients with esophageal cancer, and this system is mainly used for preoperative health education for patients, control of infusion volume during surgery, advanced enteral nutrition after surgery, and physiological and surgical effects caused by surgery. It includes peri-operative measures such as rehabilitation that can reduce psychological stress reactions. Perioperative measures based on the FTS concept have shown that patients undergoing total endoscopic resection for EC can significantly facilitate postoperative recovery [26].

## 11.6 Recurrence of EC After Surgery

The recurrence of esophageal cancer after curative surgery can be classified as locoregional or distant. Local recurrence is defined as a recurrent disease at the site of anastomosis, esophageal resections, and lymph node dissection. Distant recurrence is defined as hematogenous if the disease develops within a solid organ or the pleura and as trans celomic if metastatic lesions develop within the peritoneal cavity. The reported rate of locoregional recurrence (21–68% of cases) is slightly higher than that of distant recurrence (18–68%) [22]. Distant recurrence has been shown to occur more frequently than locoregional recurrence with lower third tumors, whereas the opposite is true for upper- or middle-third lesions. Other factors affecting locoregional recurrence include depth of tumor invasion, number of metastatic lymph nodes, and radicality of surgical procedures. Factors affecting distant recurrence include tumor staging, vascular invasion, and the oncologic behavior of the tumor [22, 27, 28].

It is generally agreed that the presence of lymph node metastasis associated with resectable esophageal cancer is the strongest known predictor of post-esophageal resection recurrence and mortality [29]. Lymph node metastasis at the time of surgery was most frequently found in the right recurrent laryngeal nerve nodes, right pericardiac nodes, peri-esophageal nodes, and lesser curvature nodes [12]. In contrast, postoperative lymph node recurrence was more frequently found in the left upper recurrent laryngeal nerve nodes and the right supraclavicular, celiac, and abdominal paraaortic nodes [12, 22, 30].

Anastomotic recurrence occurs infrequently (3–9% of cases). CT is a useful tool for detecting local recurrence at anastomosis sites. Tumor recurrence manifests at CT as soft-tissue masses or as intra-mural nodular wall thickening of the stomach or esophagus at the anastomosis site [12, 25].

## 11.7 Locally Advanced and Metastatic EC

EC is notorious for its aggressive behavior; it may invade local, regional, or distant structures by various pathways, including direct extension, lymphatic spread, and hematogenous metastasis [17]. Age, lower third location, high grade and large tumors, poor performance status, multiple metastasis sites, and presence of bone secondary metastatic EC are associated with poor prognosis [23, 31–33].

### 11.7.1 Direct Extension

The spread of esophageal cancers to the mediastinum is rapid and easy since there is no serosa in the esophageal wall and it is attached to neighboring structures only by a loose adventitia [9, 34]. Therefore, esophageal cancer can easily spread to adjacent structures in the neck or thorax (e.g., the trachea, thyroid gland, larynx, bronchi, aorta, lung, pericardium, and even diaphragm) [34, 35]. Tracheobronchial invasion may result in tracheoesophageal or broncho esophageal fistula [36].

### 11.7.2 Lymphatic Spread

The flow of lymph in the upper two-thirds of the esophagus tends to be upward, whereas that in the distal third tends to be downward; however, all lymphatic channels intercommunicate, and there is bidirectional flow in the tracheal bifurcation [27, 37]. Thus, lymphatic fluid from any portion of the esophagus may move to any other portion and may spread to any region of the thorax or drain the nodal bed. Therefore, although tumors in the distal esophagus are more likely to metastasize to the abdomen, the lymphatic spread of cancer in the upper or mid esophagus can also result in metastasis to celiac or other intraabdominal lymph nodes [37].

### 11.7.3 Hematogenous Metastasis

Hematogenous metastases are often found in patients with advanced esophageal cancer [9]. The most common sites include the liver, lungs, bones, adrenal glands, kidneys, and brain in a descending order of frequency of occurrence [38].

## 11.8 Metastases of EC

In a novel study, 54.5% had multiple (three or more) metastases, 23.9% had two metastases, and 21.6% had only one metastasis, among 268 esophageal cancer patients [27]. Overall, esophageal cancer patients presented most frequently with liver, distant lymph node, and lung metastases (56.0%, 52.6%, and 50.0% respectively). Metastases to the liver were most common in AC (59.9%), whereas metastases to the lungs were most frequently seen in SCC (57.4%). There were three major differences in metastatic patterns between histological subtypes [27].

Peritoneal and bone metastases were detected more frequently in AC compared to SCC, 34.7% versus 15.8% ($P < 0.01$) and 29.9% versus 17.8% ($P < 0.01$), respectively. 0.05. In contrast, lung metastases were observed more frequently in AC (45.5%, $P = 0.059$) than in SCC (57.4%) [27, 39]. Patients with only one metastatic location mostly seem to have liver metastasis in AC and liver or lung metastasis in SCC esophageal cancer.

Proximal and middle esophageal carcinomas and distal esophageal and GEJ carcinomas: A sub analysis for the metastatic site of proximal and middle to distal esophageal cancer (including GEJ carcinoma) was inadequate due to the small number of upper esophageal carcinomas ($n = 25$). Upper esophageal carcinomas tended to metastasize to the spleen more frequently [3 of 25 (12%) and 2 of 174 (1.1%, $P < 0.01$)], while distal esophageal carcinomas more frequently metastasized to the peritoneum [3 of 25 patients (12%), 57 vs. 174 patients (32.8%), $P < 0.05$] [27]. Distal esophagus, GEJ, and cardia carcinomas: Comparison of distal esophagus, GEJ, and cardia adenocarcinomas (bowel and diffuse type), and non-cardia gastric adenocarcinomas showed differences in the metastatic pattern.

Non-cardia gastric cancer frequently metastasizes to the peritoneum and female reproductive organs (56.3% vs. 37.6%, $P < 0.001$ and 12.2% vs. 2.1%, $P < 0.001$, respectively). Distal esophageal, GEJ, and cardia carcinomas more often showed metastases to the liver (61.5 vs. 47.2%, $P < 0.05$), pleura (27.8% vs. 17.9%, $P < 0.05$), and heart (12.0% vs. 6.1%, $P < 0.05$) compared with non-cardia gastric carcinomas. Lung metastases were more frequently found when comparing only distal esophageal and GEJ carcinomas with cardia adenocarcinomas (49.2% vs. 36.2%, $P < 0.05$) [27].

The venous drainage of the distal esophagus is partly provided by the left gastric vein and by the gastroepiploic veins for the stomach which both drain directly into the portal vein. This may explain the high frequency of liver metastases in both groups. The other part of the venous drainage of the distal esophagus, as well as the mid and proximal part of the esophagus, is provided by the azygos vein which directly drains to the superior vena cava which probably explains the high frequency of lung metastases [17, 40]. In addition to anatomical factors that promote specific spreading, the organ-specific tropism of circulating tumor cells as suggested by the seed and soil hypothesis may also account for frequent metastases to the liver and lung [27]. In esophageal and gastric cancer patients with metastatic disease, we unusually also observed numerous metastases in the adrenal gland (27% and 23%), heart (13% and 7%), and kidney (10% and 7%) [27]. Curiously, it is shown that peritoneal metastases are also generally observed in patients with metastatic distal esophageal and GEJ AC (38%). Few clinical studies do show the added value of diagnostic laparoscopy for occult metastatic disease in distal esophageal and GEJ adenocarcinoma patients, while other studies report a relatively low rate of positive findings for routine laparoscopy in these patients [27, 41]. Further clinical studies are needed to investigate whether pretreatment diagnostic laparoscopy may be beneficial in this patient group. Furthermore, knowledge of the preferred location of metastases may help to develop individualized treatment strategies in case of metastatic disease such as Selective Liver Internal Radiation therapy (SIRT) for liver metastases or adjuvant pressurized intraperitoneal aerosol chemotherapy or hyperthermic intraperitoneal chemotherapy for peritoneal metastases [27].

### 11.8.1 Imaging Techniques

The liver is the organ in which intra-abdominal metastases are most common in primary esophageal cancers [23]. After the diagnosis of esophageal primary cancer, intra-abdominal metastasis scanning and whole-body metastasis scanning are performed with the help of US, CT, MRI, and PET-CT. The patient is followed up with imaging methods in terms of possible metastases after neoadjuvant chemoradiotherapy and/or the operation [42–44].

Detection and characterization of liver metastases depend on the optimization of imaging methods. MRI images taken using hepatocyte-specific contrast media are more sensitive than CT and PET-CT in detecting liver metastases. The fact that MRI includes diffusion-weighted imaging in detecting malignant cells also provides an advantage over other imaging methods [7]. MRI is, therefore, more sensitive in detecting liver metastases smaller than 1 cm in the early stages [45]. Imaging of other T1- and T2-weighted MRI sequences with or without fat suppression and CT are required to characterize liver lesions.

### 11.8.2 Ultrasonography

Ultrasound images of hepatic metastases may have different echogenicity and characteristics according to the metastasis origin. The presence of hepatic steatosis may affect the sonographic appearance of liver lesions. With the ultrasound appearance pattern of hepatic metastases, the primary, malignant-benign distinction of some cancers can be predicted. Hepatic metastases can appear hypoechoic, hyperechoic, cystic, or calcific and may contain peripheral halo signs [46]. Doppler ultrasound may be useful to assess the vascularity of lesions and/or to guide biopsy. We can evaluate the vascularity of metastatic liver lesions with Doppler ultrasonography and have an idea about their origin and type according to whether they are hypo/hyper vascular. For example, neuroendocrine cancer metastases appear hyper vascular, while squamous cell carcinoma and adenocarcinoma appear more hypo vascular [47].

### 11.8.3 Endoscopic Ultrasonography

Endoscopic ultrasonography is also used to determine the T stage of the primary tumor [6]. The sensitivity and specificity of endoscopic ultrasonography were found to be higher than CT. In addition, endoscopic ultrasonography allows the sampling of suspicious lymph nodes to assess the N stage [11]. Visualization of ascites with EUS may raise suspicion of intraperitoneal metastases.

### 11.8.4 Computed Tomography

Detection of distant metastases on CT guides patients for systemic therapy or other multimodality treatments [9, 45]. Contrast-enhanced CT is the first step and mainstay in evaluating patients with esophageal cancer and whether they have distant metastases [46], CT has an established role in the detection of liver metastases of many primary tumoral lesions [7]. Contrast-enhanced spiral(multi-detector) CT is one of the most preferred methods for liver imaging today [7, 45]. Spiral CT has a very high sensitivity in detecting lesions of 10 mm and above. Liver metastases are usually seen as hypodense lesions on CT (Figs. 11.4 and 11.5). Most liver metastases are best seen in the portal venous phase in contrast-enhanced series.

### 11.8.5 Magnetic Resonance

MRI is a very sensitive method for detecting liver metastases [7]. Due to its superior sensitivity, MRI is an imaging modality that has the potential to provide accurate staging and active surveillance of advanced invasive metastatic disease in patients with biopsy-proven esophageal carcinoma [48]. With an increase in the number of new studies with high diagnostic performance, MRI is an imaging method that has

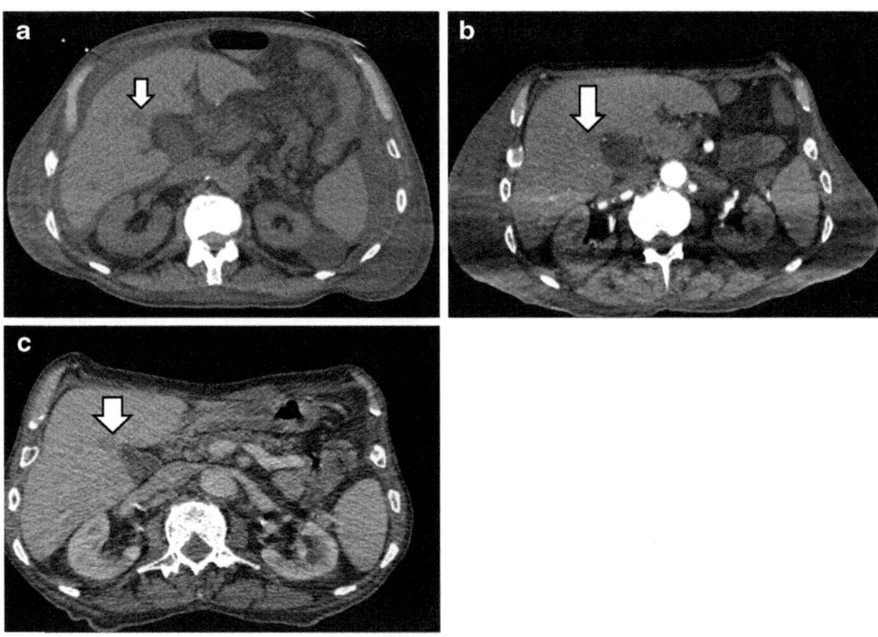


**Fig. 11.4** A 72-year-old male patient with a diagnosis of distal esophageal adenocarcinoma and liver metastasis. Esophageal adenocarcinoma metastasis observed as hypodense lesion in non-contrast (**a**), as hypovascular lesion in intravenous contrast-enhanced arterial phase (**b**) and venous-phase (**c**) abdominal CT images in hepatic segment 5 indicated by arrow

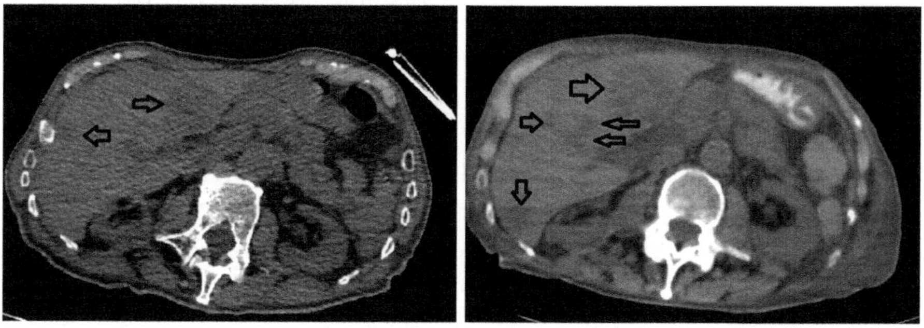

**Fig. 11.5** A 72-year-old male patient with a diagnosis of distal esophageal adenocarcinoma and multiple liver metastases. There are multiple hypodense lesions of different sizes and heterogeneous appearance, indicated by arrows on CT images of the abdomen without contrast

the potential to play a routine role in the detection of metastases of esophageal cancer and in determining the appropriate treatment [49]. The advantage of MR imaging over CT is the detection of non-hepatocyte cells using liver-specific contrast material and the ability to distinguish malignant cells and their density in apparent diffusion coefficient (ADC) and diffusion arrays. Metastases are hypointense on hepatobiliary phase images because they lack normal hepatocytes on imaging using hepatocyte-specific contrast media [50]. Diffusion can be measured using the ADC with low ADC corresponding to limited diffusion. Other T1- and T2-weighted MRI sequences with or without fat suppression are also required to characterize focal liver lesions [45]. Metastasis appearances may differ according to the type of cancer cell.

Metastatic adenocarcinomas show varying degrees of fibrosis, liquefied necrosis, and degeneration, mostly in central areas [45]. On MRI, fibrous change or old bleeding is shown as hypo intensity on T1- and T2-weighted images, while liquefaction necrosis or degeneration is shown as areas of clear hyperintensity on T2-weighted images, and mild hyperintensity may be seen on T1-weighted images [45]. Mucinous adenocarcinomas may appear hyperintense on T2 series (Fig. 11.6a, b) due to dense extracellular mucin density and may contain punctate calcifications [45]. In addition, diffusion-weighted and ADC sequences show significant diffusion restriction in esophageal adenocarcinomas (Fig. 11.6c, d). If peripherally dominant viable tumor cells are present, they appear as moderate-hyperintense lesions on T2-weighted images and as hypointense lesions on T1-weighted images [51]. The contrast difference between the central and peripheral areas can be seen as a target mark on T2-weighted images [51]. In metastases of esophageal squamous cell carcinomas, hemorrhage may be seen in the central part of the lesion. The bleeding area appears centrally more hyperintense than the lesion on T2-weighted sequences (Fig. 11.7a–d). If the bleeding becomes chronic, hypointensity is seen on the diffusion weighted sequence and hyperintensity is seen on the ADC (Fig. 11.7e, f). MR imaging is the preferred method for the suspicion of hepatic metastasis in

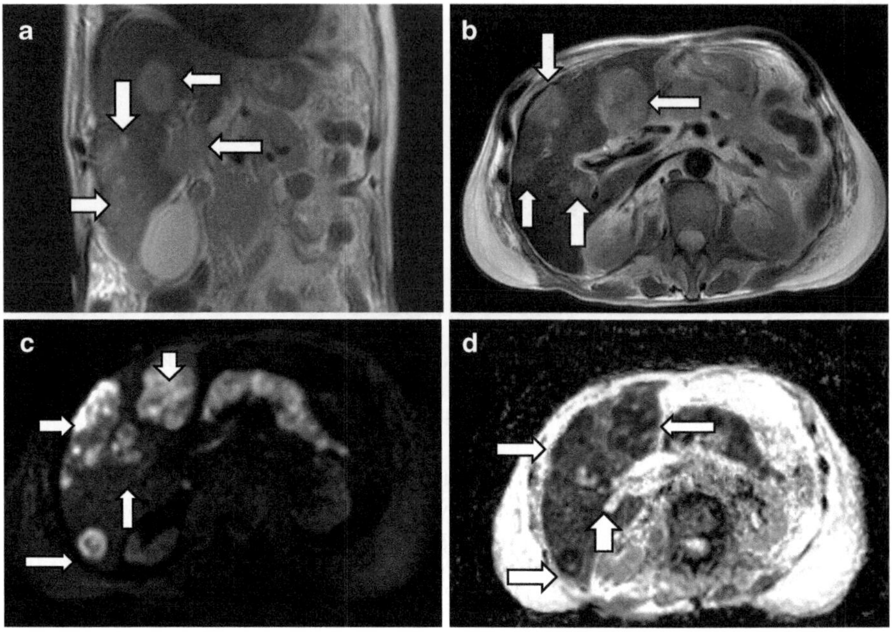


**Fig. 11.6** MRI images of a 72-year-old male patient (in Fig. 11.5) diagnosed with distal esophageal adenocarcinoma and multiple liver metastases (white arrows). (**a**) T2-weighted coronal section and (**b**). T2-weighted axial section images show multiple metastatic lesions with hyperintense heterogeneous appearance. The metastatic lesions are hyperintense in the DWI (diffusion-weighted) sequence axial section (**c**) and are hypointense in the ADC sequence axial section (**d**) and shows significant diffusion restriction (white arrows)

esophageal cancers and its sensitivity is high when evaluated in correlation with PET-CT [50, 52].

### 11.8.6 PET CT

PET-CT helps to detect malignant cells with F-18 fluoro-2-deoxy-glucose (FDG) uptake in any tissue in the body in oncological patients. PET CT is one of the most sensitive noninvasive imaging methods for detecting liver metastases in esophageal cancers [7, 45]. It is useful in detecting the presence of liver metastases in esophageal cancers and detecting areas with focal increased FDG uptake in the liver (Figs. 11.8 and 11.9). The disadvantage of PET is the lack of detailed anatomical information [9]. It is important to visualize the intrahepatic location of the metastasis, the relevant hepatic segment, and the relationship between the lesion and the surrounding vessels in the patient's treatment decision. It was observed that high sensitivity values were obtained when PET CT results were interpreted together with MR and/or CT [45]. FDG PET/CT is sensitive to detect early changes in glucose metabolism that accompany response to therapy and is used to monitor

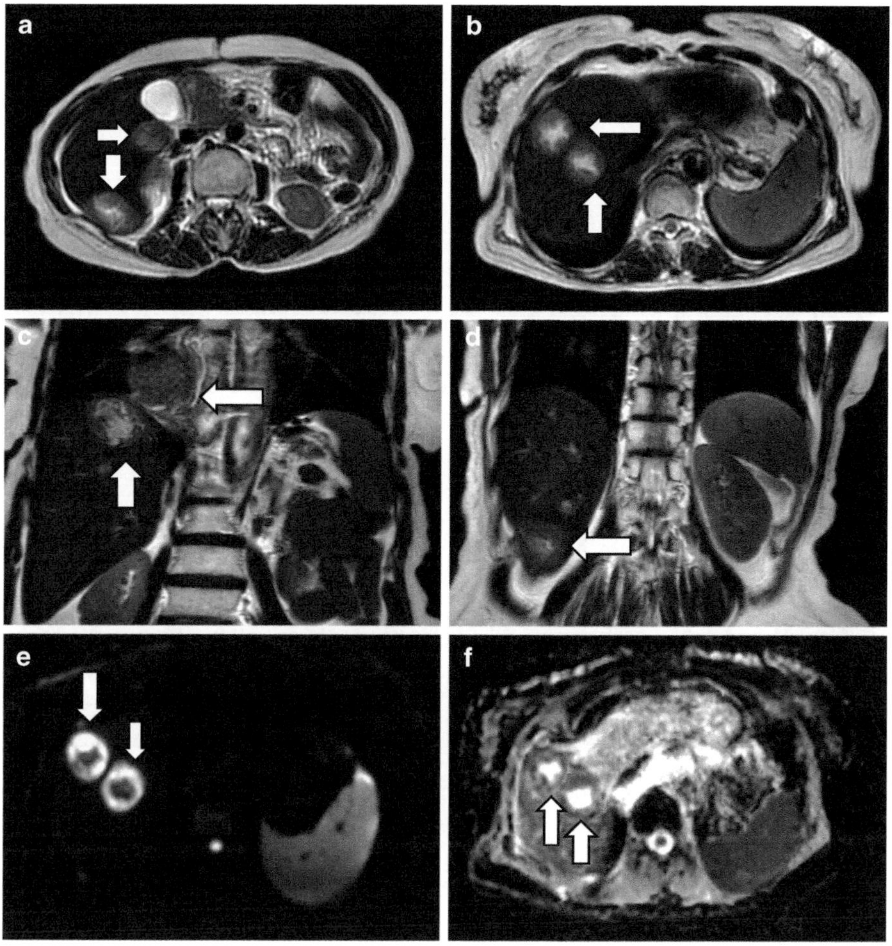


**Fig. 11.7** Primary lesion (**c**. black arrow) and multiple liver metastases in a 49-year-old female patient with distal esophageal squamous cell carcinoma. In T2-weighted axial (**a**, **b**) and coronal (**c**, **d**) sections, there are multiple metastatic lesions that are hyperintense and centrally more hyperintense in heterogeneous appearance indicated by white arrows. On diffusion-weighted images (DWI), metastatic lesions appear hyperintense and centrally hypointense (**e**). In ADC sequence, metastatic lesions appear hypointense and centrally hyperintense (**f**). Findings show diffusion restriction in the metastatic lesion and chronic hemorrhage in the central of the lesions

response to therapy [42]. These metabolic changes can often be used to assess early response to therapy in malignancies [42]. Response evaluation criteria help to gain insight into disease survival.

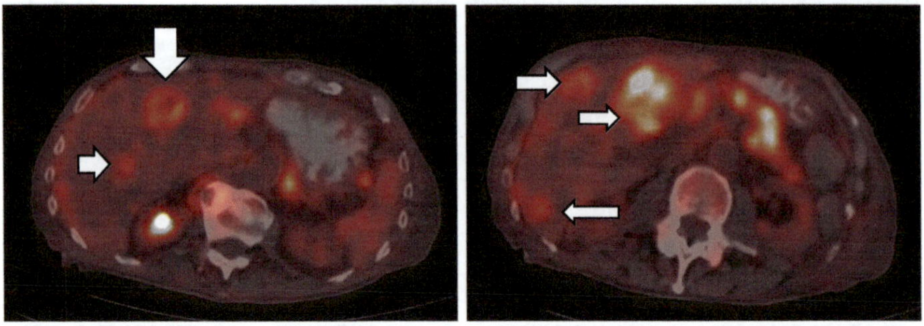

**Fig. 11.8** Hypermetabolic multiple metastatic liver lesions (arrows) showing FDG uptake on PET CT in a 72-year-old male patient with diagnosis of distal esophageal adenocarcinoma

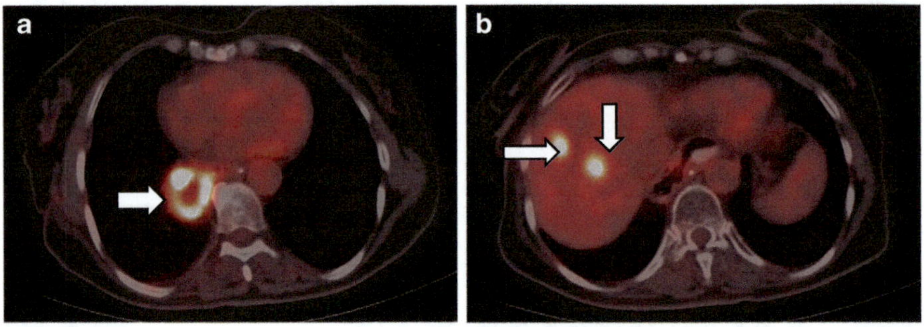


**Fig. 11.9** Primary lesion (**a**, arrow) and hypermetabolic liver metastases (**b**, arrows) of esophageal carcinoma showing FDG uptake in PET CT examination in a 49-year-old female patient with distal esophageal squamous cell carcinoma

## 11.9 Conclusion

Esophageal cancer is a rare cancer with high mortality worldwide. There are two different types of esophageal cancer, esophageal squamous cell carcinoma (ESCC), and adenocarcinoma (EAC). Although it is mostly seen in the elderly, its symptoms start nonspecifically and therefore early detection can be difficult. Intra-abdominal metastases of esophageal cancer are rare and the liver is the most common solid organ of intra-abdominal metastases. US, endoscopic US, CT, MRI, and PET are imaging modalities that play an important role in the diagnosis, staging, detection of regional and distant metastases, and evaluation of postoperative complications in patients with esophageal cancer. US can be used as the first examination, especially in the evaluation of the liver metastasis, in estimating the type and origin of liver metastases according to the pattern. CT is a useful initial screening method for detecting the operability of the patient's primary esophageal mass and whether there is distant metastasis. CT is also helpful in the detection of metastatic lymph nodes in the mediastinum and abdomen, and complications such as postoperative necrosis, anastomotic leak (with mediastinitis, pleural empyema/abscess, tracheobronchial lesion, bleeding, etc.), chylothorax, intrathoracic herniation, and functional gastric tube outflow obstruction. Endoscopic US is one of the best methods to determine the depth of tumor invasion and the presence of regional lymph node involvement. MRI is more sensitive than other imaging modalities in detecting hepatic metastases, especially thanks to the use of liver-specific contrast media, ADC, and diffusion-weighted sequences. PET is used to detect distant metastases, segment localization of liver metastases, and is useful in restaging after neoadjuvant therapy. However, detailed anatomical information cannot be obtained in PET CT. Each method has advantages and disadvantages; therefore, US, endoscopic US, CT, MRI, and PET should be considered as complementary modalities in the staging of esophageal cancer and in the evaluation of metastases.

## References


1. Uhlenhopp DJ, Then EO, Sunkara T, Gaduputi V. Epidemiology of esophageal cancer: update in global trends, etiology and risk factors. Clin J Gastroenterol. 2020;13(6):1010–21. https://doi.org/10.1007/s12328-020-01237-x.
2. Smyth EC, Lagergren J, Fitzgerald RC, Lordick F, Shah MA, Lagergren P, Cunningham D. Oesophageal cancer. Nat Rev Dis Primers. 2017;3:17048. https://doi.org/10.1038/nrdp.2017.48.
3. Alsop BR, Sharma P. Esophageal cancer. Gastroenterol Clin N Am. 2016;45(3):399–412. https://doi.org/10.1016/j.gtc.2016.04.001.
4. Domper Arnal MJ, Ferrández Arenas Á, Arbeloa ÁL. Esophageal cancer: risk factors, screening and endoscopic treatment in Western and Eastern countries. World J Gastroenterol. 2015;21(26):7933–43. https://doi.org/10.3748/wjg.v21.i26.7933.
5. Lewis RB, Mehrotra AK, Rodriguez P, Levine MS. From the radiologic pathology archives: esophageal neoplasms: radiologic-pathologic correlation. Radiographics. 2013;33(4):1083–108. https://doi.org/10.1148/rg.334135027.
6. D'Journo XB. Clinical implication of the innovations of the 8th edition of the TNM classification for esophageal and esophago-gastric cancer. J Thorac Dis. 2018;10(Suppl. 22):S2671–81. https://doi.org/10.21037/jtd.2018.03.182.
7. Kinkel K, Lu Y, Both M, Warren RS, Thoeni RF. Detection of hepatic metastases from cancers of the gastrointestinal tract by using noninvasive imaging methods (US, CT, MR imaging, PET): a meta-analysis. Radiology. 2002;224(3):748–56. https://doi.org/10.1148/radiol.2243011362.
8. Beukinga RJ, Hulshoff JB, Mul VEM, Noordzij W, Kats-Ugurlu G, Slart RHJA, Plukker JTM. Prediction of response to neoadjuvant chemotherapy and radiation therapy with baseline and restaging 18F-FDG PET imaging biomarkers in patients with esophageal cancer. Radiology. 2018;287(3):983–92.
9. Kim TJ, Kim HY, Lee KW, Kim MS. Multimodality assessment of esophageal cancer: preoperative staging and monitoring of response to therapy. Radiographics. 2009;29(2):403–21. https://doi.org/10.1148/rg.292085106.
10. Borggreve AS, Kingma BF, Domrachev SA, Koshkin MA, Ruurda JP, van Hillegersberg R, Takeda FR, Goense L. Surgical treatment of esophageal cancer in the era of multimodality management. Ann N Y Acad Sci. 2018;1434(1):192–209. https://doi.org/10.1111/nyas.13677.
11. Puli SR, Reddy JB, Bechtold ML, Antillon MR, Ibdah JA. Accuracy of endoscopic ultrasound in the diagnosis of distal and celiac axis lymph node metastasis in esophageal cancer: a meta-analysis and systematic review. Dig Dis Sci. 2008;53(9):2405–14.
12. Kim TJ, Lee KH, Kim YH, Sung SW, Jheon S, Cho SK, Lee KW. Postoperative imaging of esophageal cancer: what chest radiologists need to know. Radiographics. 2007;27(2):409–29. https://doi.org/10.1148/rg.272065034.

13. Parihar AS, Dehdashti F, Wahl RL. FDG PET/CT-based response assessment in malignancies. Radiographics. 2023;43(4):e220122. https://doi.org/10.1148/rg.220122.
14. Lee SL, Yadav P, Starekova J, Christensen L, Chandereng T, Chappell R, Reeder SB, Bassetti MF. Diagnostic performance of MRI for esophageal carcinoma: a systematic review and meta-analysis. Radiology. 2021;299(3):583–94. https://doi.org/10.1148/radiol.2021202857.
15. Block MI, Patterson GA, Sundaresan RS, Bailey MS, Flanagan FL, Dehdashti F, Siegel BA, Cooper JD. Improvement in staging of esophageal cancer with the addition of positron emission tomography. Ann Thorac Surg. 1997;64(3):770–6.; discussion 776–7. https://doi.org/10.1016/s0003-4975(97)00619-x.
16. di Pietro M, Canto MI, Fitzgerald RC. Endoscopic management of early adenocarcinoma and squamous cell carcinoma of the esophagus: screening, diagnosis, and therapy. Gastroenterology. 2018;154(2):421–36. https://doi.org/10.1053/j.gastro.2017.07.041.
17. Iitaka D, Shiozaki A, Fujiwara H, Ichikawa D, Okamoto K, Komatsu S, Murayama Y, Ikoma H, Kuriu Y, Nakanishi M, Ochiai T, Kokuba Y, Sonoyama T, Otsuji E. Case involving long-term survival after esophageal cancer with liver and lung metastases treated by multidisciplinary therapy: report of a case. Surg Today. 2013;43(5):556–61. https://doi.org/10.1007/s00595-012-0240-7.
18. Noordman BJ, Wijnhoven BP, van Lanschot JJ. Optimal surgical approach for esophageal cancer in the era of minimally invasive esophagectomy and neoadjuvant therapy. Dis Esophagus. 2016;29(7):773–9. https://doi.org/10.1111/dote.12407.
19. Flanagan JC, Batz R, Saboo SS, Nordeck SM, Abbara S, Kernstine K, Vasan V. Esophagectomy and gastric pull-through procedures: surgical techniques, imaging features, and potential complications. Radiographics. 2016;36(1):107–21. https://doi.org/10.1148/rg.2016150126.
20. Grøtting MS, Løberg EM, Johannessen HO, Johnson E. Resection for oesophageal cancer—complications and survival. Tidsskr Nor Laegeforen. 2016;136(9):809–13. https://doi.org/10.4045/tidsskr.15.1136.
21. Gockel I, Niebisch S, Ahlbrand CJ, Hoffmann C, Möhler M, Düber C, Lang H, Heid F. Risk and complication management in esophageal cancer surgery: a review of the literature. Thorac Cardiovasc Surg. 2016;64(7):596–605. https://doi.org/10.1055/s-0034-1399763.
22. Miyawaki Y, Sato H, Oya S, Sugita H, Hirano Y, Sakuramoto S, Okamotom K, Yamaguchim S, Koyama I. Clinical impact of abdominal versus mediastinal metastases as a prognostic factor for poor outcomes following esophageal cancer surgery: a retrospective study. BMC Cancer. 2021;21(1):725. https://doi.org/10.1186/s12885-021-08484-2.
23. Ghazy HF, El-Hadaad HA, Wahba HA, Abbas R, Abbas OA. Metastatic esophageal carcinoma: prognostic factors and survival. J Gastrointest Cancer. 2022;53(2):446–50. https://doi.org/10.1007/s12029-021-00610-4.
24. Booka E, Takeuchi H, Nishi T, Matsuda S, Kaburagi T, Fukuda K, Nakamura R, Takahashi T, Wada N, Kawakubo H, Omori T, Kitagawa Y. The impact of postoperative complications on survivals after esophagectomy for esophageal cancer. Medicine (Baltimore). 2015;94(33):e1369. https://doi.org/10.1097/MD.0000000000001369. Erratum in: Medicine (Baltimore) 2015;94(39):1. PMID: 26287423; PMCID: PMC4616453
25. Fabbi M, Hagens ERC, van Berge Henegouwen MI, Gisbertz SS. Anastomotic leakage after esophagectomy for esophageal cancer: definitions, diagnostics, and treatment. Dis Esophagus. 2021;34(1):doaa039. https://doi.org/10.1093/dote/doaa039.
26. Jia Y, Xing J, Li Y, Du J, Li L. A systematic review and meta-analysis of nursing effect of fast-track recovery surgery on patients undergoing total endoscopic resection of esophageal cancer: fast-track recovery surgery *vs.* nursing care as usual. J Gastrointest Oncol. 2023;14(2):572–84. https://doi.org/10.21037/jgo-23-101.
27. Verstegen MH, Harker M, van de Water C, van Dieren J, Hugen N, Nagtegaal ID, Rosman C, van der Post RS. Metastatic pattern in esophageal and gastric cancer: Influenced by site and histology. World J Gastroenterol. 2020;26(39):6037–46. https://doi.org/10.3748/wjg.v26.i39.6037.

28. Kauppila JH, Johar A, Lagergren P. Postoperative complications and health-related quality of life 10 years after esophageal cancer surgery. Ann Surg. 2020;271(2):311–6. https://doi.org/10.1097/SLA.0000000000002972.
29. Liu S, Bai Y, Zhao B, Ren H, Qin X, Qi B. Analysis of prognostic factors in patients with recurrent and metastatic esophageal carcinoma. Zhonghua Zhong Liu Za Zhi. 2015;37(2):143–7.
30. Ninomiya I, Osugi H, Fujimura T, Fushida S, Okamoto K, Maruzen S, Oyama K, Kinoshita J, Tsukada T, Kitagawa H, Takamura H, Nakagawara H, Tajima H, Hayashi H, Makino I, Ohta T. Thoracoscopic esophagectomy with extended lymph node dissection in the left lateral position: technical feasibility and oncologic outcomes. Dis Esophagus. 2014;27(2):159–67. https://doi.org/10.1111/dote.12071.
31. Lindner K, Fritz M, Haane C, Senninger N, Palmes D, Hummel R. Postoperative complications do not affect long-term outcome in esophageal cancer patients. World J Surg. 2014;38(10):2652–61. https://doi.org/10.1007/s00268-014-2590-3.
32. Kauppila JH, Johar A, Lagergren P. Medical and surgical complications and health-related quality of life after esophageal cancer surgery. Ann Surg. 2020;271(3):502–8. https://doi.org/10.1097/SLA.0000000000003097.
33. Li KK, Wang YJ, Liu XH, Tan QY, Jiang YG, Guo W. The effect of postoperative complications on survival of patients after minimally invasive esophagectomy for esophageal cancer. Surg Endosc. 2017;31(9):3475–82. https://doi.org/10.1007/s00464-016-5372-1.
34. Durmaz F, Özgökçe M, Toprak N, Oğuzlar FÇ, Göya C. The comparison of wall thickness of esophagus and gastroesophageal junction using computed tomography with endoscopy and biopsy results. Turk Gogus Kalp Damar Cerrahisi Derg. 2020;28(3):488–95. https://doi.org/10.5606/tgkdc.dergisi.2020.19072.
35. Li ZX, Li XD, Liu XB, Xing WQ, Sun HB, Wang ZF, Zhang RX, Li Y. Clinical evaluation of right recurrent laryngeal nerve nodes in thoracic esophageal squamous cell carcinoma. J Thorac Dis. 2020;12(7):3622–30. https://doi.org/10.21037/jtd-20-774.
36. Karande M, Kang M, Lazarow F. Bronchoesophageal fistula diagnosed on modified barium swallow, a unique presentation. Radiol Case Rep. 2022;17(12):4855–8. https://doi.org/10.1016/j.radcr.2022.09.057.
37. Gotohda N, Nishimura M, Yoshida J, Nagai K, Tanaka N. The pattern of lymphatic metastases in superficial squamous cell carcinoma of the esophagus. Hepato-Gastroenterology. 2005;52(61):105–7.
38. Huddy JR, Thomas RL, Worthington TR, Karanjia ND. Liver metastases from esophageal carcinoma: is there a role for surgical resection? Dis Esophagus. 2015;28(5):483–7. https://doi.org/10.1111/dote.12233.
39. Quint LE, Hepburn LM, Francis IR, Whyte RI, Orringer MB. Incidence and distribution of distant metastases from newly diagnosed esophageal carcinoma. Cancer. 1995;76(7):1120–5. https://doi.org/10.1002/1097-0142(19951001)76:7<1120::aid-cncr2820760704>3.0.co;2-w.
40. Ai D, Chen Y, Liu Q, Deng J, Zhao K. The effect of tumor locations of esophageal cancer on the metastasis to liver or lung. J Thorac Dis. 2019;11(10):4205–10. https://doi.org/10.21037/jtd.2019.09.67.
41. Yoon HH, Lowe VJ, Cassivi SD, Romero Y. The role of FDG-PET and staging laparoscopy in the management of patients with cancer of the esophagus or gastroesophageal junction. Gastroenterol Clin N Am. 2009;38(1):105–20., ix. https://doi.org/10.1016/j.gtc.2009.01.007.
42. Erasmus JJ, Munden RF. The role of integrated computed tomography positron-emission tomography in esophageal cancer: staging and assessment of therapeutic response. Semin Radiat Oncol. 2007;17(1):29–37. https://doi.org/10.1016/j.semradonc.2006.09.005.
43. Rai V, Abdo J, Agrawal DK. Biomarkers for early detection, prognosis, and therapeutics of esophageal cancers. Int J Mol Sci. 2023;24(4):3316. https://doi.org/10.3390/ijms24043316.
44. Cerfolio RJ, Bryant AS, Ohja B, Bartolucci AA, Eloubeidi MA. The accuracy of endoscopic ultrasonography with fine-needle aspiration, integrated positron emission tomography with computed tomography, and computed tomography in restaging patients with esophageal cancer after neoadjuvant chemoradiotherapy. J Thorac Cardiovasc Surg. 2005;129(6):1232–41. https://doi.org/10.1016/j.jtcvs.2004.12.042.

45. Ozaki K, Higuchi S, Kimura H, Gabata T. Liver metastases: correlation between imaging features and pathomolecular environments. Radiographics. 2022;42(7):1994–2013. https://doi.org/10.1148/rg.220056.
46. Watt I, Stewart I, Anderson D, Bell G, Anderson JR. Laparoscopy, ultrasound and computed tomography in cancer of the oesophagus and gastric cardia: a prospective comparison for detecting intra-abdominal metastases. Br J Surg. 1989;76(10):1036–9. https://doi.org/10.1002/bjs.1800761017.
47. Segura Grau A, Valero López I, Díaz Rodríguez N, Segura Cabral JM. Ecografía hepática: lesiones focales y enfermedades difusas [Liver ultrasound: focal lesions and diffuse diseases]. Semergen. 2016;42(5):307–14. https://doi.org/10.1016/j.semerg.2014.10.012.
48. Guo J, Wang Z, Qin J, Zhang H, Liu W, Zhao Y, Lu Y, Yan X, Zhang Z, Zhang T, Zhang S, Dominik NM, Kamel IR, Li H, Qu J. A prospective analysis of the diagnostic accuracy of 3 T MRI, CT and endoscopic ultrasound for preoperative T staging of potentially resectable esophageal cancer. Cancer Imaging. 2020;20(1):64. https://doi.org/10.1186/s40644-020-00343-w.
49. Pellat A, Dohan A, Soyer P, Veziant J, Coriat R, Barret M. The role of magnetic resonance imaging in the management of esophageal cancer. Cancers (Basel). 2022;14(5):1141. https://doi.org/10.3390/cancers14051141.
50. Choi SH, Kim SY, Park SH, Kim KW, Lee JY, Lee SS, Lee MG. Diagnostic performance of CT, gadoxetate disodium-enhanced MRI, and PET/CT for the diagnosis of colorectal liver metastasis: systematic review and meta-analysis. J Magn Reson Imaging. 2018;47(5):1237–50. https://doi.org/10.1002/jmri.25852.
51. Sica GT, Ji H, Ros PR. Computed tomography and magnetic resonance imaging of hepatic metastases. Clin Liver Dis. 2002;6(1):165–79. https://doi.org/10.1016/s1089-3261(03)00071-0.
52. Schulz A, Viktil E, Godt JC, Johansen CK, Dormagen JB, Holtedahl JE, Labori KJ, Bach-Gansmo T, Kløw NE. Diagnostic performance of CT, MRI and PET/CT in patients with suspected colorectal liver metastases: the superiority of MRI. Acta Radiol. 2016;57(9):1040–8. https://doi.org/10.1177/0284185115617349.

# Nuclear Medicine in Esophageal Cancer

# 12

Emel Ceylan Gunay

## 12.1 Introduction

Esophageal cancer is a significant public health concern and is among the 10 most common malignancies in the World. It is a complex disease with multiple genetic and environmental factors involved in its pathogenesis. Because of the late onset of symptoms, diagnosis has usually been made in an advanced stage which results in a poor prognosis [1–3].

Due to the difficulty in diagnosis and severity of the disease, esophageal cancer represents a clinical challenge that requires a multidisciplinary approach, coordinating specialist research teams, and optimizing knowledge and technology developments ranging from primary healthcare to digestive and nuclear medicine departments.

The treatment of esophageal cancer depends on the stage of the disease and the patient's overall health. Surgery is the primary treatment for early stage esophageal cancer, while chemotherapy and radiation therapy are used for locally advanced or metastatic disease. Early detection and accurate staging of esophageal cancer are crucial for optimal management and improved survival outcomes. Since local and systemic recurrences are common even after a proper surgical approach, the use of careful follow-up in these patients also improves patient outcomes after recurrence [4, 5].

Nuclear medicine imaging techniques have been increasingly utilized for the diagnosis, staging, and treatment response of esophageal cancer. Detection of molecular and metabolic changes in cancer cells enables the assessment of primary tumor extent, lymph node involvement, and distant metastases [6].

PET imaging has been used in the detection and staging of esophageal cancer and can provide additional information to conventional imaging techniques [7].

E. Ceylan Gunay (✉)
Faculty of Medicine, Department of Nuclear Medicine, Istinye University, Istanbul, Turkey



O. Engin (ed.), *Risk Factors and Therapy of Esophagus Cancer*,
https://doi.org/10.1007/978-3-031-47024-0_12

PET imaging can also be used to assess treatment response and guide decisions on subsequent treatment strategies.

## 12.2 Diagnostic Imaging in Staging

Determining optimal management of the disease and prediction of outcome in esophageal cancer are based on accurate staging [8]. The American Joint Committee on Cancer (AJCC) staging system, which is based on the extent of tumor invasion, lymph node involvement, and distant metastasis, is commonly used for staging [9].

Conventional diagnostic imaging techniques such as computed tomography (CT) and magnetic resonance imaging (MRI) provide valuable information about the size and location of the tumor and the presence of lymph node involvement as well as distant metastases. When tracheobronchial invasion is suspected, endoscopic ultrasonography may have additional value, especially for evaluating the depth of tumor invasion. On the other hand, these techniques have limitations for the detection of small lesions and in differentiating between tumor and inflammation or fibrosis [10, 11]. Additionally, the evaluation of response to neo-adjuvant therapy or definitive CRT is inadequate.

The main nuclear medicine imaging technique that has been utilized for the staging of esophageal cancer is positron emission tomography (PET) [12, 13]. Flourodeoxyglucose (FDG) PET imaging is a highly accurate method for the staging of esophageal cancer, with sensitivity and specificity ranging from 77–93% to 75–91%, respectively. FDG PET/CT plays an important role especially in detecting distant metastases besides loco-regional spread but is inferior in assessing local tumor status. PET/CT imaging—followed by endoscopic ultrasonography (EUS)—has been proposed as the most cost-effective strategy for initial staging [10–14].

## 12.3 PET Imaging

PET is a tomographic imaging method that shows the three-dimensional distribution of positron emitter radiopharmaceuticals.

The most widely used PET radiopharmaceutical is F-18 labeled FDG. $^{18}F$ is a cyclotron-produced radioisotope of fluorine that emits positrons and has a half-life of 109.7 min and allows labeling of molecular tracers that can be imaged within a few hours after injection. FDG is a glucose analog trapped by viable cells through glucose transporters of cell membrane. Therefore, 18F-FDG uptake is proportional to glucose consumption of the tissue. Because of the increased glucose consumption, increased GLUT expression, and hexokinase activity in cancer tissues, 18F-FDG uptake increases [15].

Ga-68-labeled fibroblast activation protein inhibitor is one of the recently developed PET radiopharmaceuticals ([68Ga]-FAPI), which targets the tumor microenvironment. 68Ga-FAPI has been shown to demonstrate increased uptake in a wide range of cancer types. On 68Ga-FAPI-PET/CT, high uptake values have been observed in esophageal cancers [16]. 68Ga-FAPI may be of value in better differentiating viable esophageal malignancy from adjacent esophagitis. Based on the developments in the field of radiopharmacy, different radionuclide agents may come to the fore in the future.

PET scanning is performed on an integrated hybrid system combining PET with either multi-detector CT components or MR system. In routine practice, PET-CT has been widely used. CT component is mainly used for attenuation correction and anatomical correlation. Combined or integrated PET and MR systems (PET/MR) have also come onto the market. Although this technology is not yet widely available, the use of PET-MR systems and the number of research articles are increasing steadily in the literature. PET/MR imaging demonstrated acceptable accuracy for T staging compared with EUS, and accuracy is also high for prediction of N staging. With adjustments in protocols, PET/MR imaging may play an important role in preoperative esophageal cancer staging in the future [17, 18].

## 12.4 Procedure in FDG PET

Patient preparation includes fasting and not consuming beverages, except for water for at least 4–6 h before FDG injection. Intravenous fluids containing dextrose or parenteral feedings also should be withheld for 4–6 h. Oral hydration with water is encouraged. Tumor uptake of 18F-FDG is reduced in hyperglycemic states. The preferred serum glucose level is <160 mg/dL. The blood glucose level should be checked before FDG administration. If the blood glucose level is >200 mg/dL, rescheduling the patient or administering insulin can be considered, but the administration of 18F-FDG should be delayed after insulin administration.

At least 45 min, approximately 60–90 min after administration of 18F-FDG, PET images are acquired. CT images are usually reconstructed with slice thicknesses of 3–5 mm. Skull base-to-proximal thigh imaging generally is recommended to scan for most tumor types. A low milliampere-seconds setting is recommended to decrease the radiation dose to the patient. A second late imaging for suspicious areas might be considered to assess the change of FDG uptake over time. If there is no contraindication or unnecessity, administration of oral and intravenous contrast agents improves the ability to identify the anatomical location and lesion boundaries [15].

In addition to visual evaluation, quantitative parameters such standardized uptake value (SUV), total lesion glycolysis (TLG), and metabolic tumor volume (MTV) are derived from the activity within the region of interest, estimating the tumor glucose metabolism [19–24]. Semiquantitative estimation of tumor metabolism can be based on the ratio of 18F-FDG uptake in a lesion compared to the uptake in reference regions, such as the blood pool, mediastinum, or normal liver parenchyma.

## 12.5 Primary Tumor Staging (T Stage)

The T-stage is determined by the depth of tumor infiltration through the esophageal wall. EUS is the preferred method for primary tumor staging with a pooled sensitivity for T-stages between 81% and 92% [25].

18F-FDG PET-CT has a limited role for evaluating the depth of invasion. Besides, visualization of early stage carcinomas with small volumes is not easy because of the spatial resolution. On the other hand, it is possible to exclude irresectable T4b disease by demonstrating preserved fat planes between the esophagus and surrounding structures [26].

False-positive results may result from benign lesions and inflammation; however, nonmalignant 18F-FDG PET hypermetabolism is often linear, involving a long craniocaudal segment with relatively low intensity, whereas malignant lesions are more focal and have more intensive uptake allowing to distinguish from benign lesions [27, 28].

## 12.6 Lymph Node Metastases (N Stage)

The status of regional lymph nodes is among the most important prognostic factors in esophageal cancer. Patients with lymph node metastases have a higher likelihood of systemic spread. The high prevalence of lymph node involvement is due to the rich lymphatic network along the entire esophagus. Accurate preoperative assessment of the lymph node metastases is crucial for the prediction of prognosis and for treatment planning either with surgery or radiotherapy. Regional lymph node involvement is currently evaluated by EUS, CT, and/or 18F-FDG PET [29].

FDG PET-CT can improve preoperative nodal staging; on the other hand, the sensitivity of PET-CT is not enough to use in clinical decision-making. In a meta-analysis, the reported pooled sensitivity is 51% (34–69%) and specificity is 84% (76–91%) [30]. FDG PET/CT is a complementary study for regional lymph node evaluation for assessment of loco-regional lymph node involvement in esophageal cancer.

Lymph nodes with microscopic involvement may not show sufficient 18F-FDG uptake. On the other hand, there may be false-positive results because of the inflammatory disease. Small lymph nodes (especially smaller than 1 cm) that are very close to the primary tumor may not be detected separately by PET scan. 18F-FDG uptake of the primary tumor may obscure uptake in peri-tumoral lymph nodes. However, these lesions are removed surgically with the primary tumor and do not alter management [31].

## 12.7 Distant Metastatic Disease (M Staging)

Identifying patients with distant metastases is essential for proper management of esophageal cancer. The prognosis is very poor when there are distant metastases. Major surgery and ineffective and debilitating treatments are not justified in this group of patients. The use of PET-CT for staging esophageal cancer provides reduction of both cost and morbidity.

Expected sites of metastases are distant lymph nodes, liver, and lung before other organs. 18F-FDG PET/CT is more sensitive than conventional imaging for the demonstration of the extent of metastatic disease. Metabolic imaging is superior to conventional strategies, especially when there is a radiologically occult disease. The value of 18F-FDG PET/CT in the management of esophageal cancer depends on its ability to detect unexpected distant metastases at initial presentation [26]. Detecting unusual or unexpected metastatic sites using whole-body 18F-FDG PET/CT decreases the number of inappropriate surgical attempts. Therefore, 18F-FDG PET/CT should be a routine part of initial staging (Fig. 12.1).

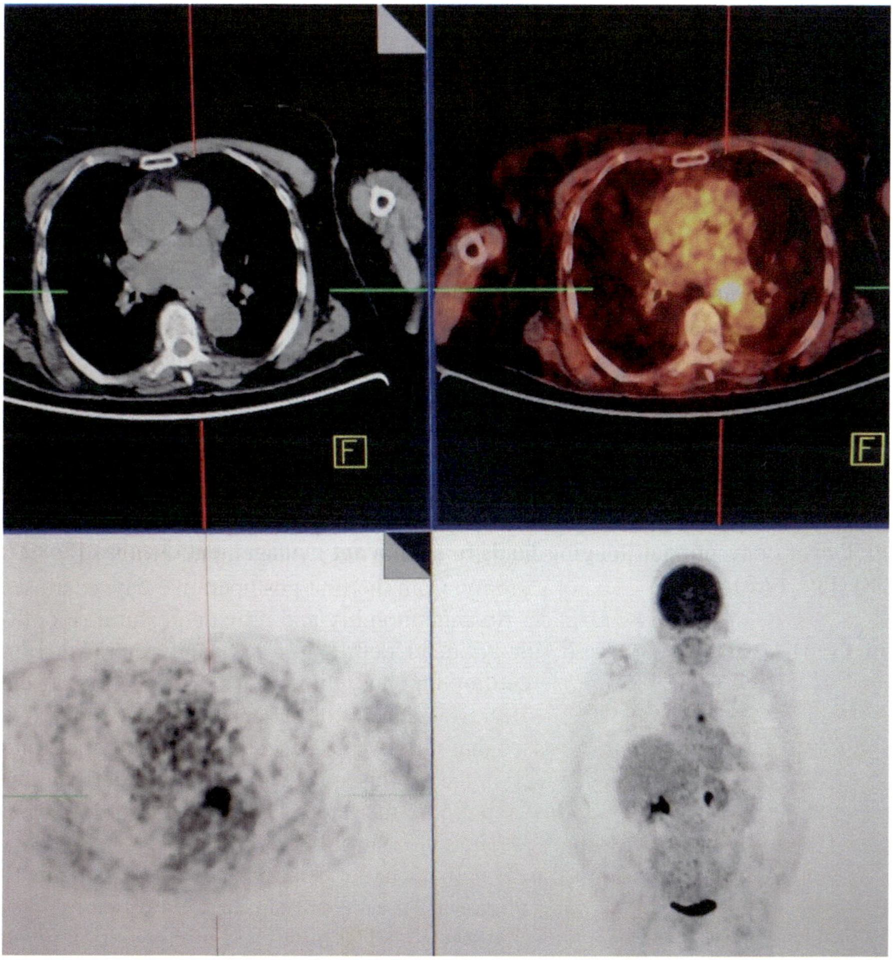

**Fig. 12.1** 18F-FDG PET-CT images including CT, PET, fusion, and whole-body MIP images. Lower esophageal malignancy with high FDG uptake has been observed, but there was no other pathological uptake suggestive of metastases

## 12.8 Radiation Treatment Planning

Chemoradiotherapy is the standard treatment of locally advanced or inoperable squamous cell carcinoma of esophagus [14]. Accurate delineation of tumor volume is very important to optimize the delivered target dose for loco-regional tumor control by radiotherapy. Besides, minimizing the volume of irradiated surrounding tissues is crucial to avoid excessive toxicity [32].

FDG PET/CT may provide valuable information for radiation treatment planning. Definitive demonstration of the esophageal tumor length and the proximal and distal margins of tumors may not be possible with CT. Adapting the target volumes and boundaries on the basis of FDG-PET/CT images enables characterization of the biologically active tumor volume and better reflection of histopathologic tumor extent [33]. Better sparing of the adjacent organs, spinal cord, lugs, and normal surrounding tissues might be possible. The use of FDG PET/CT changes the target volume in 10–63% of patients when compared to other methods such as CT and EUS [34].

## 12.9 Re-staging/Recurrence

After surgical resection, it is often difficult to differentiate scar tissue and recurrent or residual tumor tissue where FDG PET/CT may change clinical decision-making. For the detection of local recurrence, the sensitivity of FDG PET is more valuable than its specificity because of the physiological or inflammatory FDG accumulation. Being aware of the inflammatory conditions and physiological uptakes would result in a more accurate evaluation. For the detection of nodal recurrence and distant metastases, FDG PET/CT was found to be more accurate than CT alone [35, 36]. FDG PET/CT has been found useful for the detection of new interval metastases after neoadjuvant therapy too [37]. Diagnostic information provided by FDG PET over conventional imaging leads to significant management changes [26, 27, 38] (Fig. 12.2).

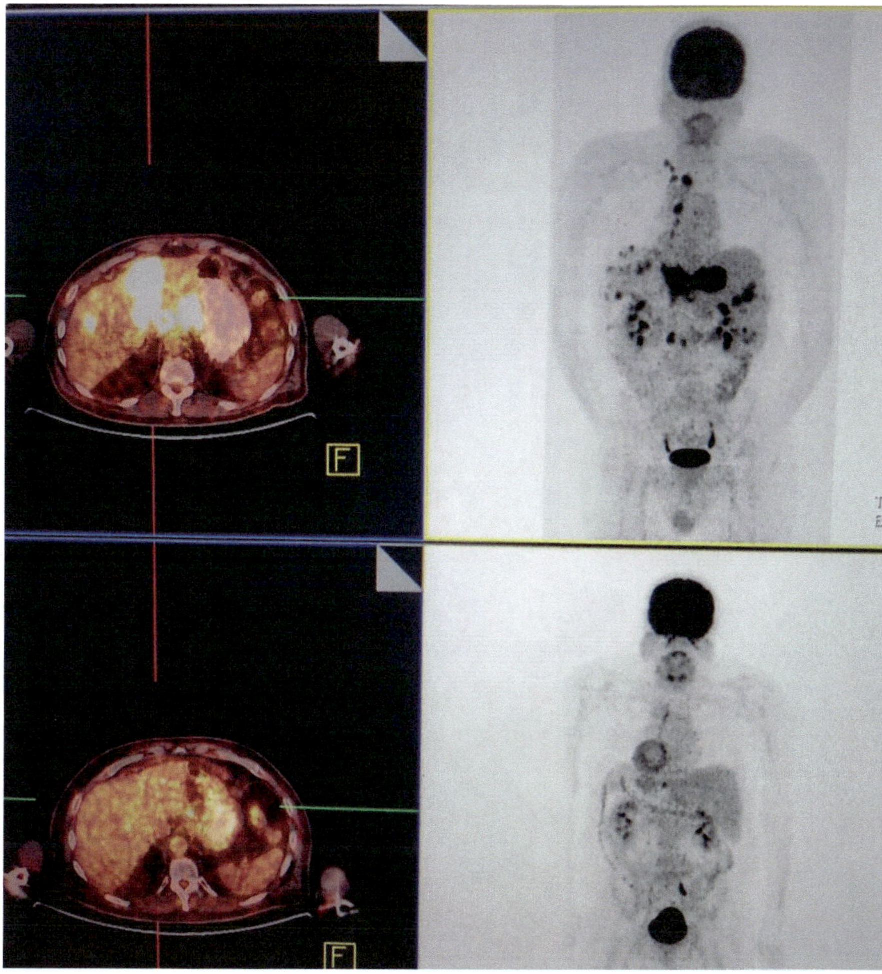

**Fig. 12.2** After completion of the first-line therapy for esophageal cancer, partial response to treatment (lower line) was observed in a patient with lymph node metastasis. Recurrence with multiple distant metastases is observed on F-18FDG- PET scan (upper line) within a year after chemoradiotherapy

## 12.10 Assessing Treatment Response, Prediction of Survival, and Prognosis

Not only staging or restaging but also treatment response is an important parameter in oncology practice for several disease (Fig. 12.3). Esophageal tumors such as adenocarcinomas or squamous cell carcinomas tend to respond differently to neoadjuvant chemotherapy or definitive CRT. If complete response is achieved disease-free, overall survival rates increase. In those cases, with a complete

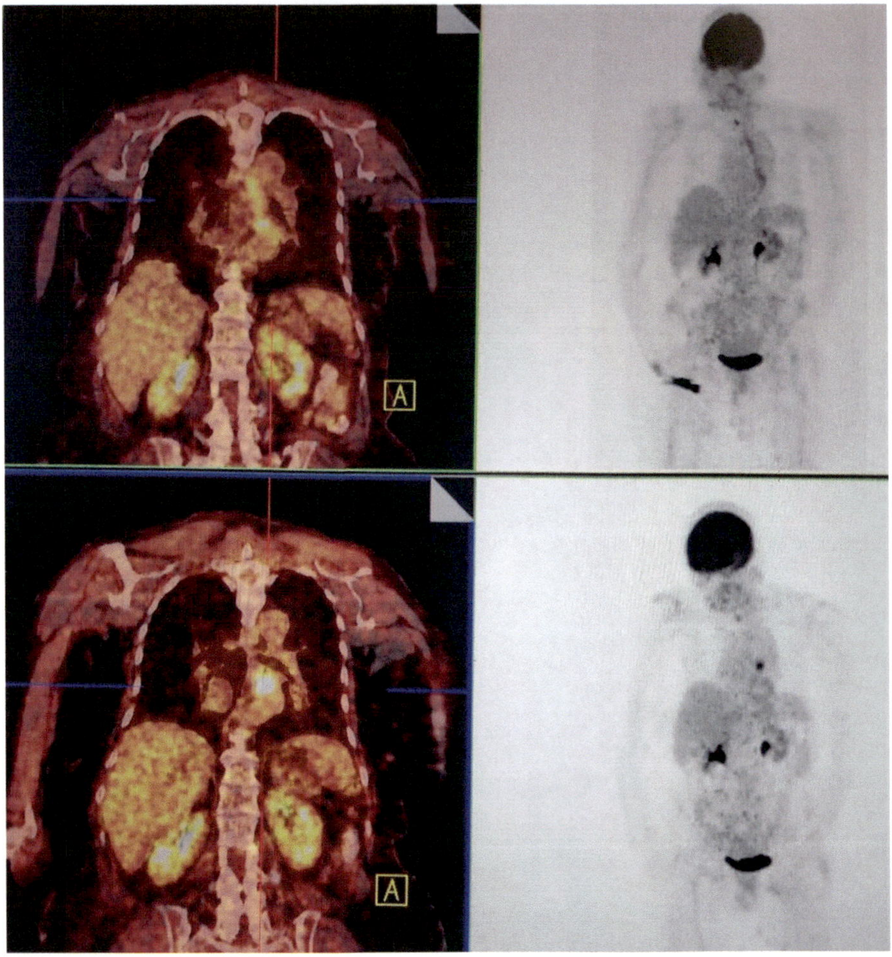


**Fig. 12.3** T3 esophageal squamous cell cancer showing high uptake on PET scan with no lymph node or distant metastasis (lower line) revealed a good response to chemoradiotherapy (upper line). But there was a diffuse uptake along the line of esophagus probably because of the inflammation related to radiotherapy

response, surgery with an organ-preserving approach and avoiding unnecessary surgical morbidity might be possible. Early identification of nonresponders to chemoradiotherapy is also critical to avoid ineffective therapy, lower the toxicity of therapies, and discontinue or modify the treatment not providing prognostic benefit. The Response Evaluation Criteria in Solid Tumors (RECIST) is usually used when CT is the choice for treatment evaluation [39]. However, it has a poor sensitivity and moderate specificity for pathologic response in esophageal cancer [40]. Besides, a correlation between treatment response and prognosis could not be demonstrated.

For detecting residual tumors, EUS after treatment has a high sensitivity (96%) but very low specificity (11%). Inversely posttreatment endoscopic biopsy has a high specificity (91%) but poor sensitivity (35%) [41].

The advantages of FDG PET/CT are rapid evaluation of all body parts and lesions in a single session, assessing viable tissue in residual masses, metabolic information besides size measurements, and low inter-observer variability. Many evaluation criteria have been proposed for standardization and interpretation of PET/CT. PET-based standardized uptake values (SUV) are used to evaluate and predict treatment response [42].

The clinical TNM-stage is the most important prognostic factor before treatment. Other factors such as, the initial SUVmax value and SUVmax after chemoradiotherapy, response to neoadjuvant therapy, TNM-staging after surgery, resection status, extracapsular lymph node involvement have prognostic impact, too [26, 43].

The FDG uptake of the primary tumor was found to be an independent prognostic factor along with pathological stage based on both seventh and eighth AJCC/UICC staging systems in patients with esophageal squamous cell carcinoma. The suggested staging system, including SUVmax, was better for predicting prognoses than the conventional staging system [44].

Management of treatment strategy, selecting the proper treatment option for the patients depends on the stratification according to the expected prognosis. After treatment with curative intent, the number of patients with early progression within 1 year has been reported between 24% and 41% [45]. Adding to routine clinical parameters, the need for sufficient predictive ability for pathologic response is still on the table. There is a need of an approach which may guide decision-making and contribute to more individualized treatment strategies in clinical practice.

SUV has been widely used parameter for evaluation of FDG uptake degree of several tumor types to quantify metabolic tumor activity including FDG PET studies in esophageal cancer. Changes in the rate of SUV can be used reliably to differentiate histological responders from non-responders after neoadjuvant treatment with either chemoradiotherapy or chemotherapy [46].

Since most of the tumors have nonhomogeneous 18F-FDG uptake pattern, SUV could be a rough parameter in the evaluation of total lesion glucose metabolism. SUVmax does not characterize the total activity nor heterogeneity of the FDG uptake for the entire tumor. Metabolic tumor volume (MTV) and total lesion glycolysis may provide additional and more useful information [22–24].

The field of radiomics focuses on improvement of image analysis using quantitative features of medical images, including shape, intensity, filter-based, or textural features. When radiomics was firstly introduced, the scope was limited to radiological images, more specifically to computed tomography. The aim was to provide a macroscopic phenotyping of tumors that could reflect the underlying pathophysiological processes. PET radiomics is a promising field for better understanding, depending on the recent reviews in the literature [47].

Since radiomics involves post-processing techniques on standard CT and PET images, there is no need for an additional imaging. The information taken from routine imaging has been used for quantitative analysis. It has been hypothesized that quantification of tumor heterogeneity may provide important information for staging, predicting response to treatment, chemoradiation-resistance, and predicting prognosis in cancer patients. Higher clinical stage and node-positive tumors were associated with increased tumor heterogeneity that generally decreases following treatment probably due to a reduction in cellular density and normalization of the vasculature [48, 49].

Overall, all the information obtained from imaging can be used to adjust treatment plans and optimize treatment outcomes. PET-CT is an important tool in the management of esophageal cancer and can provide valuable information for guiding treatment decisions and improving patient outcomes. Further studies would help to validate the utility and determine the optimal use of nuclear medicine for esophageal cancer in the clinical setting.

## References


1. Napier KJ, Scheerer M, Misra S. Esophageal cancer: a review of epidemiology, pathogenesis, staging workup and treatment modalities. World J Gastrointest Oncol. 2014;6(5):112–20.
2. World Health Organization International Agency for Research on Cancer (IARC). Globocan 2020; Cancer Fact Sheets, Esophageal Cancer [homepage on the internet]; Available from: https://gco.iarc.fr/today/data/factsheets/cancers/15-Esophagus-fact-sheet.pdf.
3. Liu WJ, Zhao Y, Chen X, Miao ML, Zhang RQ. Epigenetic modifications in esophageal cancer: an evolving biomarker. Front Genet. 2023;13:1087479.
4. Shridhar R, Park KU, Schefter TE, Karam SD. Local and systemic recurrences after definitive chemoradiation for esophageal cancer: a systematic review and meta-analysis. Radiother Oncol. 2014;111(2):175–81.
5. Berry MF. Esophageal cancer: staging system and guidelines for staging and treatment. J Thorac Dis. 2014;(Suppl. 3):S289–97.
6. Gallamini A, Zwarthoed C, Borra A. Positron emission tomography (PET) in oncology. Cancers (Basel). 2014;6(4):1821–89.
7. Flamen P, Lerut A, Van Cutsem E, De Wever W, Peeters M, Stroobants S, et al. Utility of positron emission tomography for the staging of patients with potentially operable esophageal carcinoma. J Clin Oncol. 2000;18(18):3202–10.
8. Kitagawa Y, Ishihara R, Ishikawa H, et al. Esophageal cancer practice guidelines 2022 edited by the Japan esophageal society: part 1. Esophagus. 2023;18:1–30.
9. Rice TW, Patil DT, Blackstone EH. 8th edition AJCC/UICC staging of cancers of the esophagus and esophagogastric junction: application to clinical practice. Ann Cardiothorac Surg. 2017;6(2):119–30.
10. Thakkar S, Kaul V. Endoscopic ultrasound staging of esophageal cancer. Gastroenterol Hepatol (N Y). 2020;16(1):14–20.
11. Pfau PR, Perlman SB, Stanko P, et al. The role and clinical value of EUS in a multimodality esophageal carcinoma staging program with CT and positron emission tomography. Gastrointest Endosc. 2007;65:377–84.
12. Barber TW, Duong CP, Leong T, Bressel M, Drummond EG, Hicks RJ. 18F-FDG PET/CT has a high impact on patient management and provides powerful prognostic stratification in the primary staging of esophageal cancer: a prospective study with mature survival data. J Nucl Med. 2012;53(6):864–71.
13. Munden RF, Macapinlac HA, Erasmus JJ. Esophageal cancer: the role of integrated CT-PET in initial staging and response assessment after preoperative therapy. J Thorac Imaging. 2006;21:137–45.

14. Pennathur A, Gibson MK, Jobe BA, et al. Oesophageal carcinoma. Lancet. 2013;381:400–12.
15. Boellaard R, Delgado-Bolton R, Oyen WJ, Giammarile F, Tatsch K, Eschner W, et al. European Association of Nuclear Medicine (EANM). FDG PET/CT: EANM procedure guidelines for tumour imaging: version 2.0. Eur J Nucl Med Mol Imaging. 2015;42(2):328–54.
16. Kratochwil C, Flechsig P, Lindner T, Abderrahim L, Altmann A, Mier W, Adeberg S, Rathke H, Röhrich M, Winter H, Plinkert PK, Marme F, Lang M, Kauczor HU, Jäger D, Debus J, Haberkorn U, Giesel FL. $^{68}$Ga-FAPI PET/CT: tracer uptake in 28 different kinds of cancer. J Nucl Med. 2019;60(6):801–5.
17. Matthews R, Choi M. Clinical utility of positron emission tomography magnetic resonance imaging (PET-MRI) in gastrointestinal cancers. Diagnostics (Basel). 2016;6(3):35.
18. Lee G, Hoseok I, Kim SJ, Jeong YJ, Kim IJ, Pak K, Park DY, Kim GH. Clinical implication of PET/MR imaging in preoperative esophageal cancer staging: comparison with PET/CT, endoscopic ultrasonography, and CT. J Nucl Med. 2014;55(8):1242–7.
19. Buck A, Prade VM, Thomas KT. Metabolic tumor constitution is superior to tumor regression grading for evaluating response to neoadjuvant therapy of esophageal adenocarcinoma patients. J Pathol. 2022;256:202–13.
20. Tustumi F, Albenda DG, Sallum RAA, Nahas SC, Ribeiro Junior U, Buchpiguel C, et al. 18F-FDG-PET/CT-measured parameters as potential predictors of residual disease after neoadjuvant chemoradiotherapy in patients with esophageal carcinoma. Radiol Brasil. 2022;55:286–92.
21. Marr L, Haller B, Pyka T, Peeken JC, Jesinghaus M, Scheidhauer K, et al. Predictive value of clinical and 18F-FDG-PET/CT derived imaging parameters in patients undergoing neoadjuvant chemoradiation for esophageal squamous cell carcinoma. Sci Rep. 2022;12(1):7148.
22. Makino T, Yamasaki M, Tanaka K, Masuike Y, Tatsumi M, Motoori M, et al. Metabolic tumor volume change predicts long-term survival and histological response to preoperative chemotherapy in locally advanced esophageal cancer. Ann Surg. 2019;270(6):1090–5. https://doi.org/10.1097/SLA.0000000000002808.
23. Hofheinz F, Li Y, Steffen IG, Lin Q, Lili C, Hua W, van den Hoff J, Zschaeck S. Confirmation of the prognostic value of pretherapeutic tumor SUR and MTV in patients with esophageal squamous cell carcinoma. Eur J Nucl Med Mol Imaging. 2019;46(7):1485–94.
24. Soydal C, Yüksel C, Küçük NÖ, Okten I, Ozkan E, Doğanay Erdoğan BE. Prognostic value of metabolic tumor volume measured by 18F-FDG PET/CT in esophageal cancer patients. Mol Imaging Radionucl Ther. 2014;23(1):12–5.
25. van Vliet EP, Eijkemans MJ, Poley JW, et al. Staging of esophageal carcinoma in a low-volume EUS center compared with reported results from high-volume centers. Gastrointest Endosc. 2006;63:938–47.
26. Sakellis CG, Jacene HA, Van den Abbeele AD. Diagnostic applications of nuclear medicine: esophageal cancers. In: Volterrani D, Erba PA, Strauss HW, Mariani G, Larson SM, editors. Nuclear oncology. Springer; 2022. p. 811–26.
27. Salavati A, Basu S, Heidari P, et al. Impact of fluorodeoxyglucose PET on the management of esophageal cancer. Nucl Med Commun. 2009;30:95–116.
28. Dehdashti F, Siegel BA. Neoplasms of the esophagus and stomach. Semin Nucl Med. 2004;34:198–208.
29. Kayani B, Zacharakis E, Ahmed K, Hanna GB. Lymph node metastases and prognosis in oesophageal carcinoma—a systematic review. Eur J Surg Oncol (EJSO). 2011;37(9):747–53.
30. van Westreenen HL, Westerterp M, Bossuyt PM, et al. Systematic review of the staging performance of $^{18}$F-fluorodeoxyglucose positron emission tomography in esophageal cancer. J Clin Oncol. 2004;22:3805–12.
31. Lerut T, Flamen P, Ectors N, et al. Histopathologic validation of lymph node staging with FDG-PET scan in cancer of the esophagus and gastroesophageal junction: a prospective study based on primary surgery with extensive lymphadenectomy. Ann Surg. 2000;232:743–52.
32. Njeh CF. Tumor delineation: the weakest link in the search for accuracy in radiotherapy. J Med Phys. 2008;33:136–40.

33. Mamede M, El Fakhri G, Abreu-e-Lima P, et al. Pre-operative estimation of esophageal tumor metabolic length in FDG-PET images with surgical pathology confirmation. Ann Nucl Med. 2007;21:553–62.
34. Muijs CT, Beukema JC, Pruim J, et al. A systematic review on the role of FDG-PET/ CT in tumour delineation and radiotherapy planning in patients with esophageal cancer. Radiother Oncol. 2010;97:165–71.
35. Sharma P, Jain S, Karunanithi S, et al. Diagnostic accuracy of $^{18}$F-FDG PET/CT for detection of suspected recurrence in patients with oesophageal carcinoma. Eur J Nucl Med Mol Imaging. 2014;41:1084–92.
36. Kato H, Miyazaki T, Nakajima M, et al. Value of positron emission tomography in the diagnosis of recurrent oesophageal carcinoma. Br J Surg. 2004;91:1004–9.
37. Blom RL, Schreurs WM, Belgers HJ, et al. The value of post-neoadjuvant therapy PET-CT in the detection of interval metastases in esophageal carcinoma. Eur J Surg Oncol. 2011;37:774–8.
38. Duong CP, Hicks RJ, Weih L, Drummond E, Leong T, Michael M, Thomas RJ. FDG-PET status following chemoradiotherapy provides high management impact and powerful prognostic stratification in oesophageal cancer. Eur J Nucl Med Mol Imaging. 2006;33(7):770–8.
39. Eisenhauer EA, Therasse P, Bogaerts J, et al. New response evaluation criteria in solid tumours: revised RECIST guideline (version 1.1). Eur J Cancer. 2009;45:228–47.
40. Westerterp M, van Westreenen HL, Reitsma JB, et al. Esophageal cancer: CT, endoscopic US, and FDG PET for assessment of response to neoadjuvant therapy—systematic review. Radiology. 2005;236:841–51.
41. van Rossum PSN, Goense L, Meziani J, Reitsma JB, Siersema PD, Vleggaar FP, van Vulpen M, Meijer GJ, Ruurda JP, van Hillegersberg R. Endoscopic biopsy and EUS for the detection of pathologic complete response after neoadjuvant chemoradiotherapy in esophageal cancer: a systematic review and meta-analysis. Gastrointest Endosc. 2016;83(5):866–79.
42. Vanderhoek M, Perlman SB, Jeraj R. Impact of the definition of peak standardized uptake value on quantification of treatment response. J Nucl Med. 2012;53(1):4–11.
43. Lu HH, Chiu NC, Tsai MH. Prognostic significance of pretreatment staging with 18F-FDG PET in esophageal cancer: a nationwide population-based study. Clin Nucl Med. 2021;46(8):647–53.
44. Lee H, Lee KS, Min YW, Kim HK, Zo JI, Shim YM, Choi JY. Prognostic significance of FDG PET/CT in esophageal squamous cell carcinoma in the era of the 8th AJCC/UICC staging system. Front Oncol. 2022;12:861–7.
45. Shapiro J, van Lanschot JJ, Hulshof MC, et al. Neoadjuvant chemoradiotherapy plus surgery versus surgery alone for oesophageal or junctional cancer (CROSS): long-term results of a randomised controlled trial. Lancet Oncol. 2015;16:1090–8.
46. Gabrielson S, Sanchez-Crespo A, Klevebro F, et al. 18F FDG-PET/CT evaluation of histological response after neoadjuvant treatment in patients with cancer of the esophagus or gastroesophageal junction. Acta Radiol. 2019;60(5):578–85.
47. Hatt M, Krizsan AK, Rahmim A, Bradshaw TJ, Costa PF, Forgacs A, Seifert R, Zwanenburg A, El Naqa I, Kinahan PE, Tixier F, Jha AK, Visvikis D. Joint EANM/SNMMI guideline on radiomics in nuclear medicine: Jointly supported by the EANM Physics Committee and the SNMMI Physics, Instrumentation and Data Sciences Council. Eur J Nucl Med Mol Imaging. 2023;50(2):352–75.
48. van Rossum PSN, Xu C, Fried DV, Goense L, Court LE, Lin SH. The emerging field of radiomics in esophageal cancer: current evidence and future potential. Transl Cancer Res. 2016;5(4):410–23.
49. Hatt M, Tixier F, Le Rest CC, et al. Robustness of intratumour $^{18}$F-FDG PET uptake heterogeneity quantification for therapy response prediction in oesophageal carcinoma. Eur J Nucl Med Mol Imaging. 2013;40:1662–71.

# Anesthesia Management in Esophageal Cancer Surgery

# 13

F. Ferda Kartufan, Erkan Bayram, and Muslum Cicek

In the twentieth century, thoracic surgery was frequently needed for infectious diseases such as lung abscess, empyema, and bronchiectasis. Fortunately, the use of antibiotics for treatment of those illnesses today has reduced the need for surgical treatment. Nowadays, pulmonary, esophageal, and mediastinal cancers are the foremost indications for thoracic surgery procedures [1].

Esophageal cancer (EC) surgery is a thoracic surgery procedure that demands particular assessment and management. With certain distinctions, the anesthetic approach for esophageal surgery corresponds to the management of anesthesia for thoracic surgery. Anesthesia for esophageal surgery necessitates an extensive knowledge of the physiology of the esophagus and the surgical techniques [2]. The anesthetic management of patients going through esophageal surgery can be challenging due to the possibility of either intraoperative or postoperative complications. To assure optimal patient outcomes, anesthesia for esophageal surgery must be carefully planned and administered. With proper care and attention to every detail, esophageal surgery anesthesia can be administered safely and effectively.

In this section, we are going to explore the anesthetic strategy for patients undergoing scheduled EC surgery, including preoperative patient evaluation, perioperative preparation, perioperative anesthesia management, and postoperative pain management.

F. F. Kartufan (✉)
Anesthesiology and Reanimation Department, İzmir Economics University, Medical Point Hospital, İzmir, Turkey
e-mail: ferda.kartufan@ieu.edu.tr

E. Bayram · M. Cicek
Anesthesiology and Reanimation Department, Istinye University Medical Faculty, Medical Park Gaziosmanpasa Hospital, Istanbul, Turkey
e-mail: fatma.kartufan@isu.edu.tr; erkan.bayram@isu.edu.tr; muslum.cicek@isu.edu.tr


O. Engin (ed.), *Risk Factors and Therapy of Esophagus Cancer*,
https://doi.org/10.1007/978-3-031-47024-0_13

## 13.1 Preoperative Evaluation

EC patients should undergo routine but also detailed evaluations and preparations prior to surgery. Despite the consensus that esophagectomy is a high-risk surgical procedure [3], the American Society of Anesthesiologists (ASA) risk factors should be determined for each patient, regardless of the surgical technique.

The most important objective of the preoperative evaluation is to identify potential anesthesia complications brought on by preexisting medical conditions and to enhance the outcome. Evaluation of the patient's cardiac risk is essential for ensuring patient safety. Malignant patients may manifest with anemia and weight loss. EC patients typically have a smoking and alcohol consumption history. These patients need to be evaluated for chronic obstructive pulmonary disease, coronary artery disease, and hepatic dysfunction [4]. In addition, preoperative evaluation is beneficial for ensuring that high-risk patients are stable during the perioperative period. Preparation for potential complications and organizing the necessary monitorizations or resources are essential. The postoperative recovery of patients is aided by the incorporation of preoperative evaluation into the planning of postoperative pain management and the postoperative transfer area.

Here are a few essential components of the preoperative evaluation for EC surgery patients:

### 13.1.1 Medical History

The anesthesiologist should acquire a comprehensive medical history, including any prior surgical procedures, allergies, chronic medical conditions, and medications. An esophageal surgery patient's history of gastroesophageal reflux disease, Barrett's esophagus, achalasia, obesity, obstructive sleep apnea, or pulmonary disease may be especially relevant to anesthetic management [5].

Tobacco and alcohol consumption are significant risk factors for EC. Patients undergoing thoracic surgery who quit smoking more than 4 weeks before surgery have a decreased risk of pulmonary complications [6]. If a person quits smoking for more than 12 h, carboxyhemoglobin levels decline [7]. The anesthesiologist should also consider chemotherapeutic agents for pulmonary toxicity (bleomycin, mitomycin), cardiac toxicity (doxorubicin), and renal toxicity (cisplatin) [8].

### 13.1.2 Physical Examination

The anesthesiologist should perform a comprehensive physical examination, as recommended by the ASA for preoperative evaluation, focusing on the patient's airway, cardiopulmonary function, and fluid status. Any anatomical abnormalities or symptoms of pulmonary congestion may contribute to the selection of an anesthetic technique or fluid management. Patients tend to be malnourished (protein-calorie malnutrition) before and for several months after esophagectomy. Fortunately, over the past decade, regular examinations of patients with Barrett's esophagus has led to the early diagnosis of some esophageal cancers, so these patients are usually scheduled for surgery with a healthy nutritional status. Some patients presenting for esophagectomy may have undergone chemotherapy and/or radiation therapy, which can result in pancytopenia, dehydration, and pulmonary injury [9].

Age is also a factor in EC diagnosis and treatment. EC incidence increases with age. Although last reports showed controversy, it's known that cases are diagnosed in patients older than 50, who are more likely to experience complications from surgery, such as pneumonia, heart attack, or stroke and may require a prolonged period of recovery. Moreover, elderly patients may be more likely to have comorbidities such as chronic obstructive pulmonary disease (COPD), heart disease, or diabetes, which can affect their treatment options and outcomes [10, 11]. Before performing surgery, it is recommended that older patients undergo an in-depth cardiac evaluation, which may include a transthoracic echocardiogram to detect pulmonary hypertension. To optimize the patient's overall health and well-being, it is the responsibility of healthcare providers to evaluate and manage these conditions with great care [11].

### 13.1.3 Laboratory Testing

Depending on the patient's medical history and the planned surgical procedure, laboratory tests may be required. Examination of the patient's baseline blood counts, electrolyte levels, renal and liver functions, coagulation status, as well as metabolic abnormalities (hyponatremia, hyperkalemia), including respiratory or metabolic acid–base disorders can be detected. Additionally, the anesthesiologist may need to identify the patient's blood type and verify that the required blood products are readily accessible for transfusion [6].

### 13.1.4 Imaging Studies

Imaging analyses such as chest X-rays or computed tomography scans are frequently performed to evaluate the extent of the esophageal disease. Involved potential issues, such as mass effects (Obstructive pneumonia, lung abscess, superior vena cava syndrome, tracheobronchial distortion, Pancoast syndrome, recurrent laryngeal nerve or phrenic nerve paralysis, chest wall or mediastinal extension), metastases (mediastinal invasion or lymph nodes), could be detected [6, 12]. Performing these tests could assist the surgical team in deciding the type of surgery and the anesthesiologist to estimate intubation difficulties [13].

### 13.1.5 Consultations

The anesthesiologist may consult with other members of the medical team, such as the gastroenterologist, cardiologist, and pulmonologist, regarding the patient [14]. Several types of surgery can be performed to treat EC. The specific type of surgery suggested for EC patient will depend on a variety of factors, including the size and location of the tumor, the stage of the cancer, the patient's overall health, and the surgeon's field of proficiency [15]. Therefore, it is essential to discuss the surgical plan and any potential obstacles or complications with the surgeon. It should also be remembered that, particularly in high-risk patients, surgical procedures may alter immediately before or even during surgery; thus, the anesthesiologist should not only have information about the surgery but also knowledge and experience with other surgical approaches.

Here are some additional factors that may be taken into account during the preoperative evaluation of these patients:

#### 13.1.5.1 Lung Function Assessment

EC patients planned for surgery may need pulmonary function testing to evaluate their baseline respiratory function and predict their postoperative lung function. These evaluations assess the cardio–respiratory relationship between respiratory mechanics, gas exchange, and lung parenchymal function.

Forced expiratory volume in 1 second (FEV1), forced vital capacity (FVC), maximal voluntary ventilation (MVV), and residual volume/total lung capacity (RV/TLC) are the mostly detected respiratory mechanics tests. Arterial blood gas parameters are mainly used to assess the parenchymal function of the lungs. Cut-off thresholds of partial arterial oxygen pressure ($PaO_2$) below 60 mmHg-hypoxemia or partial arterial carbon dioxide pressure ($PaCO_2$) above 45 mmHg-hypercapnia were taken into account [16].

The measurement of the lung's $CO_2$ diffusion capacity (DLCO) is one of the most essential gas exchange parameters. DLCO is correlated with the lung's functional surface area in terms of lung capacity. Consequently, patients with a postoperative DLCO rate of <40% have a greater incidence of respiratory and cardiac complications. In addition, the National Emphysema Treatment Trial reported that a preoperative FEV1 or DLCO of <20% was an indicator of unacceptable mortality rates in surgery sequence [17].

Ventilation–perfusion scintigraphy is useful for estimating postoperative pulmonary function in pneumonectomy patients. Therefore, this test is advised particularly for patients with FEV1 and/or DLCO values below 80% [18].

The cardiopulmonary exercise test is the "gold standard" procedure for evaluating the VO2max and determining cardiopulmonary function. Consumption of maximal oxygen (VO2max) that is <15 mL/kg/min before surgery may indicate higher risks of postoperative morbidity and mortality. The traditional "climbing stairs" evaluation is one of the greatest indicators of cardiopulmonary interaction for patients whose mobility is not restricted for other reasons. The patient's VO2max is >20 mL/kg/min if he/she ascends "five flights of stairs" at his/her own tempo and without pausing. A patient who is unable to climb "two flights of stairs" without respite, assuming 20 steps on each floor and 6 inches in height for each step, is considered to be at an exceedingly high risk for perioperative and postoperative complications. The "six-minute walking test" (6-MWT) is a VO2max correlation test as well. Less than 15 mL/kg/min of VO2max is associated with walking <610 m at

6-MWT. A decrease in $SpO_2$ of >4% during an exercise sequence, equivalent to two or three flights of stairs, is indicative of high morbidity and mortality in patients [18–20].

In addition, preoperative evaluation and management COPD is important to reduce the risk of complications and optimize outcomes. The severity of COPD is assessed based on the FEV1% of predicted values. The American Thoracic Society categorizes of COPD stage II and III potentialize respiratory complications during and after surgery and risk of postoperative respiratory failure [21].

With the combined evaluation of these methodologies, it is possible to accurately predict the patient's respiratory function prior to thoracotomy. Similarly, based on the estimated levels of these tests after surgery, the extubation and weaning processes of postoperative thoracotomy patients can be determined.

#### 13.1.5.2 Cardiovascular Assessment

EC surgery is associated with hemodynamic alterations and cardiovascular threats; therefore, patients with a history of cardiac ischemia or arrhythmias may be at increased risk for cardiac complications during surgery. Evaluating cardiac function prior to surgery may necessitate additional cardiac evaluation and management prior to and after the procedure, such as electrocardiography, cardiac imaging, echocardiography, or stress testing, as well as consultation with a cardiologist [22, 23].

According to studies, patients undergoing esophagectomy may experience right ventricular dysfunction, which can result in complications such as pulmonary hypertension, right heart failure, and increased mortality. The risk of right ventricular dysfunction is increased in patients with cardiovascular disease or those who have received neoadjuvant therapy (chemotherapy or radiation therapy) before surgery [24].

### 13.1.6 Final Preoperative Evaluation

The EC surgery patients should undergo a final preoperative anesthetic evaluation, prior to the operating theatre admission. At this time, two other specific aspects of anesthesia must be evaluated one of which is the likelihood of challenging lung isolation [25, 26], and the other one is the potential risk of desaturation during one-lung ventilation (OLV) [27, 28].

#### 13.1.6.1 Premedication

The standard procedure is to provide a short-acting benzodiazepine intravenously for mild sedation just before the administration of invasive monitoring lines and catheters. Preoperative administration of H2-receptor blockers, proton pump inhibitors, or metoclopramide can also be considered to avoid common pulmonary complications in the postoperative period. In addition, oral hygiene should also be questioned and ensured before surgery to prevent the patient from developing pulmonary or cardiac infections [29, 30]. An antisialagogue (such as atropine or glycopyrrolate) is traditionally used for the patients with copious secretions [31].

Therefore, administering an antisialagogue just before performing fiberoptic bronchoscopy to place a doublelumen endobronchial tube (DLT) or bronchial blocker (BB) for one-lung ventilation is also advisable. Before the thoracic procedures, it is recommended to administer short-term intravenous antimicrobial prophylaxis, such as a cephalosporin. However for esophageal surgeries, cefepime utilization is also recommended especially for preventing the patient from an anaerobic burden due to perforation [32]. At the initial preoperative evaluation, patients who have penicillin or cephalosporin allergies should be taken into account.

The anesthesiologist should create a "consolidated anesthetic plan," which may require specialized monitoring, additional treatments, and fluid therapies during general anesthesia management, in conjunction with thoracic epidural catheterization for postoperative pain management. The postoperative period, especially for those who have had thoracic surgery, can be characterized by severe pain and nausea. A discussion of pain management techniques with the patient, such as thoracic epidural analgesia (TEA), patient-controlled analgesia, or non-opioid agents, must be a part of the preoperative examination [33].

#### 13.1.6.2 Postoperative Analgesia Planning

During the initial preoperative evaluation, a plan for postoperative analgesia should be planned and discussed with the patient. When it comes to managing pain, there are several methods that are more effective than relying solely on parenteral (intramuscular or intravenous) opioids on demand. These involve combining narcotic-based analgesia with paravertebral blocks, neuraxial blockade, and anti-inflammatory medications. However, in high-risk patients, epidural approaches may minimize post-thoracotomy respiratory problems [34]. The patient should be informed of the advantages and disadvantages of each kind of post-thoracotomy analgesia during the initial preoperative evaluation. It is crucial to identify any potential contraindications to a certain type of analgesia, such as coagulation issues, infections, or neurological conditions. The proper timing of anticoagulant administration and neuraxial catheter insertion must be coordinated if the patient is receiving prophylactic anticoagulants, as if it has been agreed upon to use epidural analgesia. According to American Society of Regional Anesthesia recommendations, prophylactic heparin administration should occur 2–4 h before or 1 h after catheter insertion. Recommendations and warnings for low-molecular-weight heparin (LMWH) are as follows: (1) a minimum of 12 h must pass after taking low-dose LMWH and (2) 24 h must pass after taking higher dose LMWH before catheterization. In addition, LMWH should not be administered until at least 4 h after removal of the epidural catheter [6, 35].

## 13.2 Considering the Procedures

Although multidisciplinary treatments for EC have made encouraging progress in improving patients' survival, surgery is still an irreplaceable intervention. Different surgical approaches, such as the Sweet esophagectomy, the Ivor Lewis esophagectomy, the McKeown esophagectomy, and the transhiatal esophagectomy, have been applied clinically based on specific locations in the esophagus [36]. However, transthoracic approaches and minimally invasive surgery (laparoscopic/thoracoscopic, or robotic esophagectomy) are the most commonly performed techniques of surgical treatments for EC [37].

### 13.2.1 Transthoracic Approach

The transthoracic esophagectomy technique often consists of two phases. A supine laparotomy and the construction of a neoesophageal tube utilizing the stomach reflect the initial stage of the procedure. The second stage involves an esophagus repair through the thoracic route and a right-sided thoracotomy in the left lateral decubitus position (LDP) [38].

An invasive arterial line and a central venous pressure (CVP) catheter implementation are necessary in these patients' anesthetic monitoring and management in order to compensate for the considerable fluid shifts in value, and monitoring beat-by-beat blood pressure is crucial. Esophageal manipulation during thoracotomy may impair venous return, which may result in hypotensive episodes. There is no difficulty in gaining access to the right internal jugular vein, but CVP implementation from the left side is not appropriate because surgical esophageal anastomosis is nearly always performed from the left side of the patient's neck. To provide postoperative analgesia, a thoracic epidural catheter implantation is frequently done. It is recommended to use hydrophilic opioids (such as hydromorphone) in conjunction with epidural anesthesia for pain management due to the number of dermatomes that need to be closed for both incisions. Gastric reflux affects the majority of esophageal cancer patients; as a result, a decent plan for protecting the airway from aspiration is essential [39].

A left-sided DLT or a right-sided BB is administered during the induction of anesthesia for the second stage (right thoracotomy) to induce lung collapse. Since esophagectomy requires longer OLV management than other procedures, it triggers a significant inflammatory response. According to Michelet and colleagues' research, the use of protective ventilatory techniques during OLV lessens the proinflammatory systemic response [39].

### 13.2.2 Minimal Invasive Technique

Minimally invasive esophagectomy (MIE) employs laparoscopic, thoracoscopic, and robotic surgical techniques. These techniques are preferred over traditional open surgery procedures because patients will be able to experience less pain, have shorter hospital stays, and recover more quickly. In addition, their outcomes will be comparable to or superior to those of open surgery. Due to the intragastric pressure generated by carbon dioxide insufflation, distention of the peritoneum during a laparoscopic procedure may result in hemodynamic changes. In these instances, it is essential to modify ventilatory parameters to achieve an optimal $PaCO_2$ level [40]. The thoracoscopic approach requires a left-sided DLT or BB. To achieve OLV during robotic surgery, a lung isolation device is required. The benefits include a shorter hospital stay, less discomfort, and less blood loss. Nevertheless, this procedure requires more time for the surgery [41].

Every patient undergoing an esophagectomy must have a nasogastric tube, which must be properly secured at the end of the procedure. After esophageal surgery, intrathoracic anastomotic leakage is a feared major complication with a high mortality rate of 4%–71% [42, 43].

## 13.3 Intraoperative Monitoring

The majority of these surgeries involve positioning the patient (usually in the left LDP), and stabilizing the patient until the end of the surgery, for 2–6 h [44]. Considering the position of the patient, it is generally accepted to initially place monitoring tools just before the induction of anesthesia with mild sedation or just after the induction of anesthesia while the patient is still in the supine position [45]. The recommendations for intraoperative monitoring involve the standard ASA monitoring protocols (pulse oximetry, noninvasive blood pressure monitoring, and 12-lead electrocardiography), including the monitoring of urine output via bladder catheterization and those mentioned below according to the patient's surgical procedure and condition.

### 13.3.1 Oxygenation

In the majority of thoracotomy patients, direct measurement of arterial $PaO_2$ periodically remains necessary despite the availability of pulse oximetry ($SpO_2$). Although patients potentially displaying $SpO_2$ levels of 99–100% may tend to desaturate during OLV even in the supine position [46]. Demonstrating a $PaO_2 >$ 400 mmHg, or an appropriate $PaO_2/FiO_2$ ratio during total-lung ventilation while administering a $FiO_2$ of 1.0, usually means there is no risk of experiencing desaturation during OLV. Conversely, patients with a $PaO_2$ of 200 mmHg are at risk for desaturation during OLV [47]. Two different studies showed that the left LDP is more beneficial to the $PaO_2$ level even in COPD patients than the supine position [46].

### 13.3.2 Capnometry

The end-tidal $CO_2$ ($ETCO_2$) is a comparatively less dependable marker of the partial pressure of arterial carbon dioxide ($PaCO_2$) in the situation of OLV. Additionally, the gradient between $PaCO_2$ and $ETCO_2$ tends to increase during OLV [48].

The ETCO$_2$ measurement is indicative of both lung perfusion and cardiac output (CO); therefore, relative changes of ETCO$_2$ may differ at OLV during different positions according to perfusion of each lung [49].

A patient who may ultimately desaturate during OLV may show early warning signs, including severe (>5 mmHg) or prolonged declines in PETCO$_2$, which can signify an imbalance in perfusion between ventilated (dependent) and nonventilated (nondependent) lungs [50]. However, permissive hypercapnia is advised for improved PaO$_2$ and O$_2$ carrying capacity, as well as enhanced pulmonary mechanics during OLV, suggesting that it may help to manage oxygenation during OLV [50].

### 13.3.3 Cerebral Oximetry

Cerebral oximetry (SctO$_2$) has been reported as an intraoperative monitoring technique that can be used especially for elderly patients that are in a frail state, who can experience a higher probability of a decrease in SctO$_2$ while undergoing OLV. This occurrence is linked to reductions in SpO$_2$ and cognitive dysfunction after the surgery [51].

### 13.3.4 Continuous Spirometry Monitoring

The monitorization enhances the ventilation strategies success during OLV according to the continuous monitoring of inspiratory and expiratory volumes, pressures, and flow interactions, allowing for the prediction of lung function.

The continuous monitoring of tidal volumes during inspiration and expiration can provide prompt detection of unintentional positional changes in a DLT, which may result in loss of lung isolation. A sudden decrease in expired volume may be taken as a warning sign of such changes [52].

The flow-volume loop can exhibit the emergence of auto-positive end-expiratory pressure (auto-PEEP), which is associated with the establishment of a persistent end-expiratory flow during OLV [53].

### 13.3.5 Temperature

The maintenance of body temperature may become challenging during thoracic surgery due to the potential for heat loss from the exposed hemithorax. Most effective strategies for preventing unintended intraoperative hypothermia include elevating the ambient room temperature, utilizing fluid warmers, and implementing lower and/or upper body forced-air patient warmers.

Hypothermia inhibits the majority of physiological processes in the human body. There is a lack of evidence as to whether this also covers hypoxic pulmonary vasoconstriction (HPV), but a study in animals has shown that HPV is attenuated by hypothermia and enhanced by hyperthermia [54].

### 13.3.6 Fiberoptic Bronchoscopy

Fiberoptic bronchoscopy is a procedure that involves the use of a flexible fiber optic that assures visual examination of the lungs and the positioning of DLTs and BBs that are used for "Lung Isolation." Malpositioning of DLTs and BBs can result in desaturation during OLV, some of those cannot be detected by auscultation or other conventional techniques for verifying placement [55]. The appropriate placement of DLTs or blockers necessitates the use of fiberoptic bronchoscopic guidance and subsequent reconfirmation after the patient has been positioned for surgery. This is because a considerable proportion of these tubes/blockers have been observed to migrate during patient repositioning [56].

### 13.3.7 Hemodynamic Monitoring

Surgical compression of the heart or major vessels during intrathoracic operations has the potential to cause transient, severe hypotension. Therefore, it is important to monitor systemic blood pressure invasively beat-by-beat during the thoracic surgery. The implementation of the arterial catheter in a radial artery can be done to either arm for this purpose. In addition, this line can be used for periodical arterial blood gas evaluation during OLV [39].

The right internal jugular vein is the preferred site for central venous pressure (CVP) measurement unless contraindicated. While there are limitations to measuring CVP in certain conditions and positions, these do not diminish its value as a postoperative monitoring tool, particularly in situations where fluid management is crucial [57]. In certain scenarios, such as surgically caused hypotension, a CVP catheter may be regarded as necessary for the purpose of vascular access or for administering vasopressor/inotrope infusions.

### 13.3.8 Transesophageal Echocardiography

Transesophageal echocardiography (TEE) enables the anesthesiologist to observe an uninterrupted, live display of myocardial performance, and cardiac preload. During controlled ventilation for nonthoracic surgery, the application of positive end-expiratory pressure (PEEP) up to 15 $cmH_2O$ resulted in the development of a right-to-left intracardiac shunt in 9% of the patients. Intraoperative TEE may be indicated in thoracic surgery for various reasons such as hemodynamic instability, pericardial effusions, cardiac involvement by tumor, air emboli, pulmonary thromboendarterectomy, thoracic trauma, lung transplantation, and pleuropulmonary disease. However, the probability of experiencing adverse effects is relatively minimal, unless there is an underlying esophageal ailment or trauma. Therefore, prior to conducting TEE for EC patients, the anesthesiologist must assess whether the advantages of the procedure surpass the potential hazards [58].

## 13.4 Anesthetic Management

The administration of general anesthesia and management of the airway in esophageal surgery necessitate consideration from multiple perspectives, including the patient's cardiopulmonary, hemodynamic, and nutritional status. The mediastinal mass effect, tobacco and alcohol use, and the physical condition of the patient with predisposing conditions like gastroesophageal acid reflux, hiatal hernia, and achalasia may all have an impact on the induction and maintenance of anesthesia during surgery. These factors may increase the risks of possible aspiration and hypoxemia [44].

Prior to induction, it is essential for the anesthesiologist to have knowledge of the anatomical location of the mediastinal mass and to take the necessary precautions. It is crucial to evaluate the mediastinal masses [59] and the dilated esophagus [60] before induction. The trachea is prone to posterior compression due to the absence of cartilaginous support, which can lead to obstruction [61].

The utilization of "rapid sequence induction and intubation" has been commonly recommended for patients who have an increased likelihood of experiencing regurgitation and aspiration. The majority of medical professionals prefer intravenous induction agents, including propofol, thiopental, etomidate, or ketamine, in combination with a quickly acting neuromuscular blocking agent, such as rocuronium. The smooth induction of anesthesia and rapidly performing laryngoscopy and tracheal intubation without any intervening positive pressure ventilation and immediate tracheal intubation while applying cricoid pressure (also known as the Sellick maneuver) are mostly advised [62]. It is not relevant whether the compression is adequate to completely obstruct the lumen or safe. Reducing the duration between the onset of unconsciousness, muscle relaxation, and tracheal intubation can potentially mitigate the risk of passive reflux of gastric contents and subsequent aspiration. This can be achieved through the use of a lubricated cuffed tube and positioning the patient in a head-up or reverse Trendelenburg [63]. If the patient is difficult to intubate according to preoperative evaluation, it is beneficial to make a plan thoroughly and carefully before performing intubation, especially for those patients who are at a heightened risk of aspiration.

It is important to consider potential etiologic and predisposing factors, such as tobacco usage and concomitant factors, when managing patients with EC. Particularly if OLV is required, especially in patients with COPD [62]. To help reduce bronchial irritability, it is recommended to choose anesthetic agents capable of decreasing it. The importance of the issue becomes more vital while implementing a DLT or BB, which could also trigger bronchospasm. Therefore, the anesthetic management of patients undergoing EC surgery and requiring OLV ought to be like the management of patients with asthma. The principles in the present situation are the avoidance of airway manipulation in a lightly anesthetized patient, the use of drugs that do not trigger the release of histamine, and the administration of anesthetic agents that maintain bronchodilator properties or those that reduce bronchospasm. The anesthetics that are recommended for this purpose include propofol, ketamine, and volatile agents, particularly sevoflurane [64].

The maintenance of anesthesia involves the selection of anesthetic agents, which can be achieved through various methods. Researchers recently preferred total intravenous anesthesia during management, which was associated with better postoperative survival rates compared with volatile anesthesia [65]. Chow et al. [66] have reported that both remifentanil infusion and thoracic epidural anesthesia are viable options for providing analgesia during OLV.

If the surgical procedure requires OLV, it is important to take into account HPV which will be explained widely in "Ventilation" section of this chapter. Certain volatile anesthetics have been observed to exhibit a reduction in the presence of HPV. Halothane exhibits the highest potency, followed by enflurane and isoflurane. The amount of 1 minimum alveolar concentration (MAC) isoflurane required to inhibit HPV is generally too minimal to be detected in most clinical studies [67]. In contrast, the utilization of inhalation anesthesia has been shown to maintain intraoperative cardiac function and mitigate postoperative pulmonary complications among individuals undergoing surgery with one-lung ventilation. However, it is not recommended to utilize nitrous oxide/oxygen ($N_2O/O_2$) combinations, as they have been associated with a rise in the incidence of post-thoracotomy radiographic atelectasis (51%) in the ventilated-dependent lung, as compared to the use of air/oxygen mixtures (24%). The administration of nitrous oxide has been found to cause an increase in pulmonary artery pressures among patients who suffer from pulmonary hypertension, blebs, or bullae. Furthermore, apart from the aforementioned volatile agents, it has been observed that N2O also has an inhibitory effect on HPV [68].

## 13.5 Positioning

During a thoracoscopic esophagectomy or a MIE, the patient may be positioned either supine or left lateral decubitus. The majority of surgeons are still performing the thoracic phase in the left LDP [69]. During OLV, additional factors determine the redistribution of blood circulation between the dependent and nondependent lungs. Patient position is an essential factor from a clinical perspective. Gravity tends to enhance the proportion of blood flow (approximately 10%) to the dependent lung when OLV is performed in the LDP. When OLV is required, the most reliable position is the left LDP [67].

The implications of patient positioning for the anesthesiologist are specific. Firstly, monitors will be installed, then anesthesia will be induced while the patient is in supine position, and afterwards he/she will be positioned for the surgery. When changing positions, the anesthesiologist should be in command of the surgical team and be responsible for the head, neck, and airway. After induction and intubation, it is helpful to perform a "head-to-toe" examination of the patient to check for oxygenation, ventilation, hemodynamics, lines, monitors, and any nerve damage. Afterwards, repositioning requires another round of this survey [70]. Therefore, all lines and monitors should be secured, and their functionality reevaluated after positioning.

Repositioning a DLT or BB is almost impossible without causing some movement. Frequently, the margin of error in positioning endobronchial tubes or blockers is so small that even minor alterations can have significant clinical consequences. Therefore, the position of the endobronchial tube/blocker and the adequacy of ventilation must be evaluated again using auscultation and fiberoptic bronchoscopy [71].

### 13.5.1 Ventilation/Perfusion Mismatch in the Lateral Decubitus Position

Ventilation/perfusion matching is maintained during spontaneous ventilation when a supine patient encounters the LDP. Due to gravitational influences on the distribution of blood flow in the pulmonary circulation, the dependent lung (lower lung) obtains greater perfusion than the independent lung (upper lung). The dependent lung also receives more ventilation because the contraction of the dependent hemidiaphragm is more efficient than that of the nondependent [upper] hemidiaphragm; thus, the dependent lung is located on a more favorable portion of the compliance curve. However, the upper (nondependent) lung has better compliance following general anesthetic induction. This is due to the decline in the FRC. The upper nondependent lung is ventilated more than the lower dependent lung, meanwhile the dependent lung continues to have greater perfusion. This ventilation/perfusion mismatching worsens and predisposes the patient to hypoxemia after opening the nondependent side of the thorax for the surgery. This will enhance the difference in compliance between the two sides because the nondependent lung is now less restricted in movement [72].

## 13.6 Ventilation

### 13.6.1 Lung Isolation

Lung isolation techniques are mainly used to facilitate OLV in patients undergoing cardiac, thoracic, mediastinal, vascular, esophageal, or orthopedic chest cavity procedures. Lung isolation and OLV are crucial for thoracoscopic esophageal surgery and are generally accepted as "the gold standard" for transthoracic esophageal procedures. Three different methods, including BB, single-lumen endotracheal tubes (SLT), and DLT, can be used to isolate the lung. DLT and BB are applied frequently, and of those, left-sided DLT is the most commonly used one for transthoracic esophagectomy. Bronchial blockers can be administered via an endotracheal tube or a modified SLT, such as the Univent tube (LMA North America, San Diego, California) [39].

#### 13.6.1.1 Double-Lumen Endotracheal Tubes

The development of the Carlens DLT for lung surgery in 1950 was an evolution for thoracic anesthesia because it allowed anesthesiologists to obtain reliable lung isolation by only performing laryngoscopy and auscultation in the vast majority of patients. Since then, improvements have been made, including radiographic markers and endobronchial cuffs with enhanced visibility (bright blue, low volume, low pressure). Selecting the size of the DLT, implementing the tube properly, and managing its position and depth require technical knowledge and experience.

Here are some useful hints for DLT administration:

(a) Size of the DLT: [39].
   - The bronchial tip of a left-sided DLT should be 1–2 mm smaller than the diameter of the patient's left bronchus.
   - Chest radiographs and computed tomography scans are not only valuable for determining the correct DLT size, but they are also useful for assessing abnormal tracheobronchial anatomy.
   - A simplified method has been found for determining the size of DLT based on gender and height*:

     *For female patients shorter than 160 cm and taller than 160 cm, 35 Fr and 37 Fr, respectively, can be administered.

     *For male patients shorter than 170 cm and taller than 170 cm, 37 Fr and 41 Fr, respectively, can be administered.

(b) Implementation and positioning of the DLT:
   - Implementation: Using direct laryngoscopy, the DLT is rotated 90° counterclockwise (for a left-sided DLT implantation) after the endobronchial cuff has passed beyond the vocal cords.
   - Positioning the tube**:

     **The tube can be inserted until resistance is felt (the average depth of insertion is about 29 cm at the teeth level) [72].

     **The depth can be predicted according to the formula based on the patient's height: [73]

     (12 + [patient height/10]) cm at the teeth level. However, patient height is not a reliable predictor for patients shorter than 155 cm [74].

(c) After the DLT has passed the vocal cords, the head of the endobronchial lumen can also be guided into the correct bronchus using direct vision with a flexible fiberoptic bronchoscope. Boucek and colleagues [75] used laryngoscopy or fiberoptic bronchoscope for DLT implementation and revealed that both techniques resulted in the successful placement of the left mainstem bronchus in all patients, but the fiberoptic bronchoscopy guidance technique required more time (181 vs. 88 s).

Our experiences have taught us that auscultation alone is insufficient to confirm DLT placement. Auscultation and fiberoptic bronchoscopy must be performed whenever a DLT is inserted or relocated.

#### 13.6.1.2 Bronchial Blockers

Another method for lung isolation is occlusion of the main bronchus, which allows lung to collapse from downstream of the occlusion. The use of endobronchial blockers is well described for thoracic procedures, including esophageal surgery, and is preferred by certain researchers due to the perceived reduction in aspiration risk with the use of the SLT and rapid sequence induction, as well as the practicality of managing difficult airways, and similar lung collapse scores with the DLT [76]. When necessary, BBs can be used selectively to induce lobar collapse. Patients who have undergone oral or neck surgery and are diagnosed with a difficult airway and require lung isolation for intrathoracic surgery may benefit from a BB rather than a DLT [77].

### 13.6.2 Ventilation Strategies During One-Lung Ventilation

#### 13.6.2.1 Tidal Volume

The optimal combination of tidal volume, respiratory rate, I:E ratio, and pressure or volume control ventilation for each individual patient during OLV influences the distribution of pulmonary blood flow between the lungs. Hypoxemia, still an intraoperative problem during OLV, has become infrequent due to better lung isolation methods, ventilation techniques, and the use of anesthetic agents with less detrimental effects on HPV [67]. Attention has currently shifted toward the prevention of acute lung injury (VENT). Although ALI seems to occur merely (with an incidence of 2.8% in all lung resections), different studies indicate that the incidence of ALI after esophagectomy is between 4.6% and 9.7%. In addition, the research showed that the lung lobes on the operation side are more likely to be affected by ALI than the nonoperative side [78]. When it occurs, ALI is associated with a 40% risk of mortality. Therefore, it seems that "protective lung ventilation strategy" is the key to protect the patient from complications, especially from ALI.

**Protective Lung Ventilation Strategy**

- use of lower tidal volumes (6–8 mL/kg—ideal body weight),
- the routine use of PEEP (5–10 $cmH_2O$),
- lower $FiO_2$ (0.5–0.8),
- lower ventilatory pressures,
- (plateau pressure < 25 $cmH_2O$; peak airway pressure < 35 $cmH_2O$)
- choose pressure-controlled ventilation for mechanical ventilation mode,
- allow permissive hypercapnia [72].

Although using lower tidal volumes may result in lung atelectasis and hypoxemia, frequent recruitment maneuvers and the application of external PEEP can prevent patients from those problems (except patients who have COPD). Historically, in all surgical procedures, volume-controlled mode was used for ventilation. Therefore, the tidal volume was ought to be under control so that peak airway pressures do not exceed 35 $cmH_2O$. The recent availability of anesthesia ventilators with pressure control modes has enabled the usage and application of "lung protective ventilation" during thoracic surgery. Even though pressure control ventilation prevents thorax from abrupt increases of peak airway pressures during surgical manipulations, the administered tidal volume by the ventilator must be closely monitored due to the rapid changes in lung compliance [79].

#### PEEP and Auto-PEEP

Intraoperative factors such as LDP, paralysis, and opening the nondependent thorax result in a decreased FRC due to the weight of the mediastinum compressing the dependent lung. The combination of hyperinflation and positive end-expiratory pressure, known as auto-PEEP, is commonly observed in COPD patients and complicates the measurement of FRC during OLV [80]. During OLV, occurrence of 4–6 $cmH_2O$ auto-PEEP is enough to reduce the dependent lung's FRC. The application of external PEEP during OLV will improve a patient's gas exchange, but the management of OLV with PEEP in the presence of auto-PEEP will cause complications. Present intensive care ventilators can measure auto-PEEP, whereas ventilators in the operation theatre typically struggle to detect and measure auto-PEEP. However, in the operating room, the most common method for detecting auto-PEEP is actually simple: total end-expiratory pressure is the sum of the auto-PEEP and the extrinsically applied PEEP in the mechanically ventilated patients [81].

### 13.6.3 Hypoxic Pulmonary Vasoconstriction

Hypoxic pulmonary vasoconstriction (HPV) is a physiological response to reduced levels of oxygen in the alveoli of the lungs, in which the pulmonary blood vessels contract. This constriction of intrapulmonary arteries redirects blood to oxygenated pulmonary areas to optimize ventilation/perfusion ratio and systemic oxygen delivery. Therefore, the HPV response is distinct from the systemic response to hypoxia, while the renal, mesenteric, and cerebral arteries dilate to increase tissue oxygen delivery. The time-related exposure of HPV to reduced alveolar oxygen levels is biphasic. The rapid-onset phase begins immediately and reaches to a plateau within 15 min. The second phase begins after 40 min and comes to a stable phase after 2 h [82].

Within OLV, HPV primarily decreases blood circulation of the nonventilated lung, which will facilitate the thoracic surgery. On the other hand, various factors may affect HPV while managing general anesthesia during one-lung ventilation (OLV) and require evaluation. These factors include cardiac output (CO), mixed venous oxygen, medications for comorbidities or administered by the anesthesiologist, duration of hypoxia, $PaCO_2$ levels, body temperature, and iron status [83].

In clinical practice, if the ventilated lung does not develop atelectasis and CO is maintained, the $PaO_2$ will typically reach its lowest level 20–30 minutes after the initiation of OLV and then increase progressively over the following 1–2 h. Notably, it has also been demonstrated that once the second phase of HPV has begun, its offset will be delayed, causing elevated pulmonary vascular resistance, for approximately 2 h [84]. Therefore, anesthesiologists must understand the circumstances and medications that can impact HPV during OLV.

Acid–base status is crucial during OLV because the vessels in the lungs contract and dilate in response to acidosis and alkalosis, respectively. It is unknown whether acidosis enhances HPV, but alkalosis during OLV should be avoided. Considering vasodilation in the nondependent lung attenuates HPV, and supposing the dependent lung has already mostly vasodilated, there can be an indirect relocation of blood flow to the nondependent lung, which can cause complications during surgery [85].

HPV decreases when the CO increases. The effect of the increase in CO is a rise in pulmonary arterial pressure and mixed venous oxygen saturation, causing a decrease in HPV. Similarly, a decrease in CO and a passive decrease in pulmonary arterial pressure will typically increase the efficiency of HPV. However, if CO is decreased during OLV, the concurrent decrease in the oxygen content of the mixed venous blood will result in a net decrease in $PaO_2$ [86].

Temperature is another factor that should be assessed. There is only one animal study that has shown that hypothermia suppresses HPV and hyperthermia amplifies it [87].

The patient's previous iron status influences the HPV response. This was elegantly demonstrated in humans by observing the effect of intravenous iron and the iron chelator desferrioxamine on HPV. Iron attenuates HPV and significantly reduces the enhanced response typically observed following prolonged hypoxic exposure [67].

Essentially, any vasodilator can be used to suppress HPV. All modern volatile anesthetic agents reduce HPV in a dose-dependent way. Halothane has been extensively researched and is a potent HPV inhibitor. Isoflurane is a less potent inhibitor than halothane. A clinical trial showed that changing the anesthetic management from 1 MAC isoflurane to intravenous anesthesia resulted in a nonsignificant increase in $PaO_2$ (from 232 to 234 mmHg) and a decrease in shunt (from 38% to 36%). It seems that there appears to be no difference in HPV inhibition between the modern volatile anesthetics' isoflurane, sevoflurane, and desflurane at equivalent MAC levels. Unlike other current volatile anesthetics, nitrous oxide appears to have vasoconstrictive effects on the pulmonary vasculature. Nitrous oxide may inhibit HPV, according to animal studies, but this has not been observed in humans [88].

The most prevalent intravenous anesthetics do not inhibit HPV. Although propofol induces some systemic vasodilation, it has no inhibitory effect on HPV [89].

There is some evidence that neuraxial blockade with local anesthetics, particularly thoracic epidural analgesia, can inhibit HPV and impair oxygenation during OLV. However, there is no evidence that HPV is subject to neurogenic control at the central level. Rare reports of a decrease in $PaO_2$ associated with epidural analgesia during OLV are more likely attributable to a decrease in CO and a decrease in mixed venous oxygen saturation as a result of vasodilation with epidural neuraxial blockade than an effect on HPV [82].

As a result, it is crucial to maintain stabilized anesthesia administration with adequate CO during OLV. Additionally, the anesthesiologist should be aware of the medications that can inhibit or enhance the HPV response. Acetazolamide, inhaled nitric oxide, steroids, phosphodiesterase inhibitors, prostacyclin, calcium antagonists, angiotensin-converting enzyme inhibitors, and endothelin antagonists are some of the medications that attenuate the HPV response [67]. Inhaled Beta2-agonists, phenylephrine, norepinephrine*, and almitrine**, are examples of pharmaceuticals that enhance the HPV response [90].

* Norepinephrine used in patients with severe ALI showed a reverse effect. There was no improvement in oxygenation in those who received norepinephrine, which the authors attributed to the possibility of nonspecific diffuse vasoconstriction by norepinephrine. In contrast, a study utilizing the pure alpha-1 agonist phenylephrine showed that half of the patients experienced improved oxygenation [91].

** Studies on animals indicate that modest concentrations of almitrine enhance HPV. It is known to improve $PaO_2$ during OLV when used systemically. However, it is not used clinically due to the challenges of the correct dose selection. At high dosages, almitrine also contracts the vessels of the normoxic lung, which causes worse outcomes during OLV [92]. On the other hand, Almitrine's chronic usage has been linked to peripheral neuropathy, which is why it has been withdrawn from the market in many countries [93].

ALI should also be taken into account while understanding the HPV response, while ALI is a merely seen but a mortal situation after eosaphagectomy. The right-to-left shunt is the primary physiological barrier to oxygenation in ALI. The shunt fraction increases when diltiazem or intravenous nitrates are used to inhibit HPV, whereas it decreases when almitrine is used to enhance HPV. Unfortunately, numerous animal studies have shown that endotoxemia, which is frequently present in ALI, can inhibit HPV [85].

### 13.6.4 Hypoxemia Treatment During One-Lung Ventilation

In the first 10 min of OLV, the majority of patients experience a rapid desaturation, which typically achieves its lowest level within the 20–30 min after the beginning of OLV, as stated previously.

The following are the suggested treatments for desaturation during OLV:

- 1.0 supplied $FiO_2$: Increasing the $FiO_2$ level to 1.0 (be cautious with bleomycin that can cause pulmonary oxygen toxicity).
- Use fiberoptic bronchoscopy to confirm the location of the DBT and to ensure the dependent lung is not obstructed.
- Be sure that the patient's hemodynamic functions are optimal and stabilized. If not, investigate the surgical site (compression of the inferior vena cava decreases arterial blood pressure and CO). If needed, reduce volatile anesthetics to below 1 MAC and then administer inotropes or vasopressors.
- It is also possible to apply recruitment to the dependent lung, but if the patient is receiving vasodilator therapy, it must be discontinued prior to recruitment to the dependent lung.

- Administer a PEEP of 5 $cmH_2O$ to the dependent lung (do not administer PEEP to patients with emphysema or COPD, as this will increase their end-expiratory lung capacity; these patients have higher levels of auto-PEEP).
- Apply CPAP 1–2 $cmH_2O$ to the nondependent lung (perform a recruitment technique on this lung prior to CPAP). Administering CPAP to the nondependent lung interrupts the surgical procedure. In contrast, the use of PEEP does not necessitate pausing the operation or reinflating the nonventilated lung.

Only for severe or unexpected desaturation, give attempt to resume bilateral lung ventilation, it will be necessary to interrupt the procedure. After achieving an acceptable level of oxygenation, the cause of the desaturation can be quickly determined [94].

## 13.7 Fluid Management

One of the most controversial topics that comes up with EC operations is fluid management. These concerns include deciding on fluid therapy and how much fluid the patient should consume.

Targeted fluid therapy is the key factor. Numerous indicators, including base deficit, serum lactate, and mixed venous $O_2$ saturation, can be used to direct fluid treatment. The goal of ideal fluid management is to avoid "overload" fluid administration while optimizing oxygen and CO [95]. The results imply that fluid restriction without impairing the CO may also improve surgical outcomes and reduce the incidence of complications after esophagectomy. However, the adverse effects of a severe fluid restriction include hypotension, prerenal failure, and the requirement for inotrope support. Because anastomotic ischemia is a substantial cause of postoperative mortality, there has been concern over the use of vasopressors during esophagectomy. Although norepinephrine has been linked to severe graft hypoperfusion when administered to treat hypotension caused by bleeding in a pig model [96], a small human study demonstrated that the reduction in anastomotic blood flow caused by thoracic epidural bupivacaine may be reversed by administering epinephrine [97]. Similarly, another study determined that phenylephrine infusion may reverse the epidural bolus-induced reduction in blood flow at the anastomotic end of the newly constructed gastric tube [98]. Vasoactive drugs may, therefore, be utilized to counteract hypotension brought on by general or neuraxial anesthesia without endangering the surgical anastomosis [97].

Fluid restriction protects the patient against respiratory problems by providing early extubation following esophagectomy not only as a sole factor but also as a component of a standardized multimodal regimen, with concordance to thoracic epidural analgesia. The "zero balance" fluid management is also advised for esophagectomy because it is known to be a high-risk procedure. To achieve "zero balance," it is recommended to infuse balanced fluid solutions with 1–3 mL/kg/h. dosage until the procedure ends [99]. An increasing amount of research indicates that fluid restriction or multimodal perioperative care regimen may enhance surgical outcomes following gastrointestinal surgery, particularly anastomotic integrity [100].

On the other hand, excessive fluid administration, after following surgery, may have a negative impact on the esophagogastric anastomosis and the pulmonary system. Excessive intravenous fluid administration might progress shunting, which can result in pneumonic edema of the dependent lung, especially after a prolonged surgical procedure. Cardiopulmonary complications and mortality have been linked to a higher perioperative fluid balance [101].

Emerging clinical data suggests that, in addition to the potential importance of the quantity and time of fluid administration, the choice of fluid type also affects the clinical results. Similar to what was said earlier, the majority of studies demonstrated negative outcomes as a result of excessive perioperative fluid administration in patients undergoing EC surgery, supporting the idea of crystalloid overload rather than fluid overload [101].

Dessel et al. [102] studied restrictive and liberal perioperative fluid administration regimes during esophagectomy and correlated the outcomes. Postoperative pulmonary complications were 10 times higher in patients who received fluid overload. Additionally, this research also revealed that the patients perioperatively managed with a restrictive fluid regime who needed to receive a vasopressor agent developed approximately three times higher postoperative complications than the other patients who did not need to receive a vasopressor agent but were managed with a restrictive fluid regime. Another study conducted in 2020 showed nearly the same outcomes regarding perioperative fluid management during MIE with postoperative complications. Patients with a significantly higher fluid balance had a higher incidence of complications than those with a lower fluid balance (46% vs. 18%) [103]. Additionally, higher mortality rates linked to postoperative fluid imbalances above 1900 milliliters might mean that right heart failure is brought on by fluid excess or that renal dysfunction is also linked to problems from esophageal surgery [101].

There is still a lack of evidence about "how to" manage fluid administration during EC surgeries. According to enhanced recovery after surgery-based protocols and recent guidelines for esophagectomy, "restrictive management" is advocated; however, goal-directed treatment may be useful [104].

Our final decision about fluid treatment is that the fluid management during EC surgery should be based on the requirements and medical background of each patient in a restrictive manner. Comorbidities, the surgical approach, and fluid losses during the procedure should all be considered.

## 13.8 Blood and Blood Product Transfusions

Numerous studies have shown a correlation between postoperative complications and mortality after higher risk surgeries and perioperative transfusions of blood products, notably red blood cells (RBC). Therefore, only patients with adequate organ perfusion outcomes, such as blood lactate levels, urine output, and $ScVO_2$, as well as an optimized hemodynamic condition without heart disease, are advised to receive RBCs when hemoglobin (Hb) levels are <7 g/dL. On the other hand, a higher Hb threshold value (8–9 g/dL) should be maintained if there is evidence of poor organ perfusion or a history of cardiovascular disease. Rarely do patients with Hb levels above 10 g/dL need RBC therapy [105].

## 13.9 Postoperative Pain Management

The surgical approach to the esophagus frequently leads the postoperative pain management. Most esophageal endoscopic surgical procedures result in mild to moderate postoperative discomfort, which does not necessitate an intense analgesic strategy. Similarly, laparoscopic surgery often does not result in a high postoperative analgesic demand. However, one of the most painful surgical incisions is the thoracotomy incision, which is used in the majority of transthoracic esophageal procedures [62]. Therefore, intensive anesthetic methods for managing postoperative pain are crucial for enhancing the results of transthoracic esophageal surgeries. Inadequate pain control will primarily cause hypertension and bleeding, and afterwards, due to the inability to cough and clear secretions, airway closure, atelectasis, shunting, and hypoxemia can occur, in these high-risk patients.

The anesthesiologists should develop a detailed pain management strategy. With parenteral opioids alone, it is challenging to achieve a balance between comfort and adequate respiratory function in patients with limited lung function. The incorporation of the additional analgesic administrations that will be described later might lessen the requirement for intravenous opioids, which is definitely beneficial for patients who have undergone thoracotomies [106]. The best way for utilizing parenteral opioids, when used solely, is through a patient-controlled analgesia device.

Thoracic epidural analgesia (TEA), which is superior to parenteral opioid pain therapy in terms of providing analgesia after esophagectomy, is considered by many surgeons and anesthesiologists as "the gold standard" for postoperative pain management following thoracotomy for the last decades [34].

Numerous studies have shown that TEA has perioperative and postoperative adventitious outcomes, such as enabling patients to mobilize more quickly, collaborate easily with respiratory physiotherapists, and achieve satisfactory postoperative lung functions more quickly. The associated sympathetic block has been shown to increase blood flow to the bowel, prevent reductions in gastric conduit perfusion, and improve gastrointestinal mobility [107]. TEA can additionally lower the risk of anastomotic leak after emergency laparotomies, esophageal surgery, and other gastrointestinal procedures.

Intercostal nerve catheters have been compared to TEA with varying degrees of success, and paravertebral blocking has been demonstrated as an alternative promising analgesia treatment [108]. For the management of post-thoracotomy pain, a number of non-neuraxial treatments have been investigated; the most promising of these is the "multimodal anesthesia" approaches, using intrathecal diamorphine, local anesthetic infusion catheters into the paravertebral space and rectus sheaths, and intravenous opioids postoperatively. However, those effects are not proven to alter TEA [109]. Intercostal or paravertebral nerve blocks with long-acting local anesthetics may provide early extubation in the absence of an epidural catheter, but

their duration of action is short, necessitating the use of alternate pain relief techniques. The intercostal nerves can also be frozen intraoperatively by using a cryoanalgesia probe to generate long-lasting anesthesia.
Different types of perioperative pain management (such as continuous infusion of short-acting analgesics, intercostal nerve blocks, paravertebral or transverse abdominis plane blockade, patient-controlled analgesia, continuous wound catheter infusion of local anesthetic) and the multimodal approaches have been encouraged and performed as alternative modalities to TEA, due to the incidence of failed or contraindicated epidurals. However, most centers prefer TEA usage as a part of multimodal analgesic approach to lower the risk of adverse effects or complications, according to its potential of improving outcomes by achieving early extubation, rapid patient mobilization, and quick recovery following esophagectomy [110].

## 13.10 Extubation

Surgeons, anesthesiologists, and intensive care unit (ICU) specialists had previously advised "prophylactic mechanical ventilation" after surgery until it was safe for the patient to undergo extubation. To prevent aspiration, secure the airway, and permit adequate pain management, prolonged mechanical ventilation was administered. This approach was definitely contributed to weakened pulmonary mechanics, pulmonary morbidity, and acute respiratory distress syndrome (ARDS) as a result of fluid shifts caused by substantial perioperative inflammation with lung edema, obstruction of the airway, and aspiration pneumonia [111].
Nowadays, efforts to reduce complications currently focus on anesthesia protocols that enable extubation of EC surgery patients in the operating room. Improvements in surgical technique, surgical time, reduced blood loss, and pain management with TEA have further undermined the "prophylactic mechanical ventilation" procedure. A history of smoking, COPD, difficult airway, hypercarbia, excessive hemorrhage, prolonged operative time, hypothermia, hemodynamic instability, and acidosis are defined as relative contraindications of extubation. If two or more of these parameters are present at the end of the EC surgery, it is appropriate to delay extubation. Multiple studies have shown that extubation in the operating room is feasible, safe, and associated with decreased morbidity. It is safe to transfer the patient to the surgery unit after recovering in the ICU for at least 12–24 h [112].

## 13.11 Perioperative Complications

### 13.11.1 Lateral Decubitus Position-Related Complications

It is crucial to understand why the LDP causes a particular combination of nerve and vascular damage during the operation. It is the anesthesiologist's primary duty to protect the patient from those kinds of nerve damage. The brachial plexus is the site of a sizeable proportion of the LDP's contribution to the incidence of nerve damage sustained during surgery. It is recommended that the patient be positioned with supportive padding below the dependent thorax so that the weight of the upper body is not placed on the brachial plexus of the arm that is dependent while the axilla is free. The arms should not be flexed anteriorly more than 90°, abducted more than 90°, or stretched posteriorly beyond the neutral position. To avoid traction injuries of the suprascapular nerve, the shoulder (circumduction) across the thorax should not be flexed anteriorly or the neck laterally to the opposing site [113].

The dependent leg should be gently bent, and padding should be placed underneath the knee, in order to protect the peroneal nerve. Another padding should be placed between the legs and the other leg should be stretched in a neutral posture. It is essential to check for signs of vascular compression in the limb that is reliant. Strapping that is overly tight at the hip level has the potential to put pressure on the sciatic nerve of the nondependent leg. Additional regions that are particularly susceptible to neurovascular injury in the LDP include the dependent ear pinna and eye [39].

### 13.11.2 Intraoperative Blood Loss

Esophagectomy procedures performed in the thoracic and transhiatal (blunt) positions warrant special care. These operations frequently result in a substantial amount of lost blood. It is recommended to monitor both the arterial pressure and the central venous pressure, with available large-bore intravenous catheter lines, fluid warmers, and body warmers. Patients suspected of continued bleeding need to be monitored closely; urine output and chest aspiration or drainage and arterial blood gas measurements including hemoglobin concentration should be checked intermittently. Nowadays, the intraoperative excessive blood loss has been reduced to approximately <300 mL per-operation according to the procedures such as MIE and video-assisted thoracoscopic surgery (VATS). However, additional attention should be given, especially while performing abdominal laparotomy, thoracic duct resection, and division of the azygos arch. These are the procedures that are strongly associated with high volumes of blood loss during VATS [114].

### 13.11.3 Hypotension

Inadequate intraoperative plasma volume expansion, bleeding, cardiac dysrhythmias (most often atrial tachyarrhythmias), pneumothorax, and sympathectomy as a result of the use of TEA are some of the causes of this complication. The epidural-associated sympathectomy is the most prevalent cause, and it may be treated in the same way that was described earlier. As a result of hypotension, the decrease of the blood flow to the esophagogastric anastomosis can cause respiratory symptoms and shock findings in the early postoperative phase. Multimodal anesthetic management that involves restrictive fluid intake, early extubation, thoracic epidural analgesia, and administering infusions of vasopressors and inotropes to stabilize blood pressure if needed will improve the outcomes [115].

### 13.11.4 Cardiovascular Complications

A significant proportion of morbidity and mortality following esophagectomy can be attributed to cardiovascular issues, particularly arrhythmias; specifically atrial dysrhythmias such as atrial fibrillation, atrial flutter, and paroxysmal supraventricular tachycardia. Risk factors for the development of atrial dysrhythmias after esophagectomy include older age, perioperative theophylline use, a low diffusion capacity, COPD, and male sex. Furthermore, a history of cardiac disease (such as peripheral vascular disease), mediastinal tumor or pulmonary resection, esophagectomy, and intraoperative blood transfusion could also increase the risk. Patients who are at a greater risk of developing atrial tachyarrhythmias after esophagectomy may benefit from calcium channel blockers or beta blockers as a preventative measure. However, it is essential to remember that beta blockers have the potential to cause adverse effects [116].

### 13.11.5 Pulmonary Complications

It is common for patients to experience respiratory complications following thoracic surgery and esophagectomy. Variables that increased the risk are a low body mass index, a history of smoking, the experience of the surgeon, the duration of the operation and OLV, anastomotic leakage, and cardiorespiratory instability. Age, the proximal location of the esophageal tumor, and the length of surgery have all been shown to predict pulmonary complications following esophagectomy. In addition, FEV1 has been shown to predict pulmonary complications in COPD patients [62].

Insufficient reversal of neuromuscular blockade may be to blame for the weakness that leads to respiratory insufficiency, which occurs most frequently in individuals with decreased respiratory function history. These individuals tend to retain carbon dioxide, which may lead to hypercapnia and stupor. Inadequately treated pain is a consequence of upper airway obstruction. In the majority of cases, the remarkable improvement in respiratory function follows by the effective treatment of incisional pain [117].

In addition, bronchospasm, aspiration pneumonitis, pulmonary edema, pneumothorax, ALI, ARDS, bronchopleural fistula, atelectasis, and pulmonary embolism may contribute to hypoventilation. Any one of these conditions alone, or a combination of them, may cause respiratory failure. If this occurs, the patient may require specialized treatment, such as continued or reinstitution of mechanical ventilation. In a large cohort of esophagectomy patients, the incidence of ARDS and ALI was 23.8% and 14.5%, respectively. These are two of the most serious pulmonary complications associated with esophagectomy. In a particular research, ARDS was associated with a 50% mortality rate [118].

### 13.11.6 Acute Renal Failure

Postoperative acute renal failure occurrence is 2.4% in patients after esophageal surgery. Age, gender(male), increased BMI, dyslipidemia, high preoperative serum creatinine level, duration of surgery, smoking history, hypertension, and the usage of angiotensin II receptor antagonists were defined as independent risk factors for postoperative acute renal failure. The administration of hydroxyethyl starch is another predictor of renal failure following esophagectomy [119]. Open thoracotomies may also be associated with a greater risk of renal failure than minimally invasive procedures.

### 13.11.7 Consequences of Esophagectomy

Esophageal anastomotic leakage is one of the potential adverse effects of an esophagectomy. The mortality rates associated with intrathoracic leakage ranged from 3.3% to 71% [120]. Even though it is still considered a surgical complication, intraoperative and postoperative care may reduce its incidence. Through their effects on oxygen delivery and blood flow, fluid state, hemodynamics, and oxygenation can affect anastomotic integrity. Esophageal anastomotic leakage was associated with preoperative comorbidities such as diabetes, pulmonary disease, and cardiovascular disease, and postoperative comorbidities such as gastric distension, prolonged ventilatory support, and hypoxia [121].

In summary, the success of esophagectomy procedures greatly depends on the expertise of the surgical team and the resources available at the center where the surgery is performed. Patients undergoing this surgery are at high risk of complications, and proper preoperative and intraoperative care is crucial for achieving the best possible outcomes. Therefore, patients must be referred to high-volume centers with experienced teams and well-established protocols for managing the perioperative period. With meticulous attention to detail in all aspects of care, including lung protective ventilation, fluid management, pain control, and nutritional support, patients can have the best chance for a successful recovery.

## References


1. Chen-Yoshikawa TF, Fukui T, Nakamura S, et al. Current trends in thoracic surgery. Nagoya J Med Sci. 2020;82(2):161–74.
2. Atkins BZ, Shah AS, Hutcheson KA, et al. Reducing hospital morbidity and mortality following esophagectomy. Ann Thorac Surg. 2004;78(4):1170–6.
3. Swisher SG, Deford L, Merriman KW, et al. Effect of operative volume on morbidity, mortality, and hospital use after esophagectomy for cancer. J Thorac Cardiovasc Surg. 2000;119(6):1126–32.
4. Hawkins NM, Petrie MC, Jhund PS, Chalmers GW, Dunn FG, McMurray JJ. Heart failure and chronic obstructive pulmonary disease: diagnostic pitfalls and epidemiology. Eur J Heart Fail. 2009;11(2):130–9.
5. Hadi YB, Khan AA, Naqvi SFZ, Kupec JT. Independent association of obstructive sleep apnea with Barrett's esophagus. J Gastroenterol Hepatol. 2020;35(3):408–11.
6. Committee on Standards and Practice Parameters; Apfelbaum JL, Connis RT, Nickinovich DG; American Society of Anesthesiologists Task Force on Preanesthesia Evaluation; Pasternak LR, Arens JF, Caplan RA, Connis RT, Fleisher LA, Flowerdew R, Gold BS,

Mayhew JF, Nickinovich DG, Rice LJ, Roizen MF, Twersky RS. Practice advisory for preanesthesia evaluation: an updated report by the American Society of Anesthesiologists Task Force on Preanesthesia Evaluation. Anesthesiology. 2012;116(3):522–38. https://doi.org/10.1007/10.1097/ALN.0b013e31823c1067.
7. Boehm RE, Arbo BD, Leal D, et al. Smoking fewer than 20 cigarettes per day and remaining abstinent for more than 12 hours reduces carboxyhemoglobin levels in packed red blood cells for transfusion. PLoS One. 2018;13(9):e0204102.
8. Cohen NH, Eriksson LI, Fleisher LA, Leslie K, Wiener-Kronish JP. Millers anesthesia. In: Miller RD, editor. Preoperative evaluation; 2020. p. 1085–115.
9. Dionigi G, Rovera F, Boni L, et al. Cancer of the esophagus: the value of preoperative patient assessment. Expert Rev Anticancer Ther. 2006;6(4):581–93.
10. Clermont M, Falk GW. Clinical guidelines update on the diagnosis and management of Barrett's esophagus. Dig Dis Sci. 2018;63(8):2122–8.
11. Strauss A, Min EJ, Long Q, Gabriel P, Yang YX, Falk GW. Is the age of diagnosis of esophageal adenocarcinoma getting younger? Analysis at a tertiary care center. Dis Esophagus. 2020;33(9):doz112.
12. Whyte RI. Preoperative preparation of patients for thoracic surgery. Thorac Surg Clin. 2005;15(2):xi. https://doi.org/10.1016/j.thorsurg.2005.03.008.
13. Congedo E, Aceto P, Petrucci R, Mascia A, Gualtieri E, De Cosmo G. Preoperative anesthetic evaluation and preparation in patients requiring esophageal surgery for cancer. Rays. 2005;30(4):341–5.
14. Stephens MR, Lewis WG, Brewster AE, et al. Multidisciplinary team management is associated with improved outcomes after surgery for esophageal cancer. Dis Esophagus. 2006;19(3):164–71.
15. Takahashi C, Shridhar R, Huston J, Meredith K. Esophagectomy from then to now. J Gastrointest Oncol. 2018;9(5):903–9.
16. Shebl E, Mirabile VS, Sankari A, et al. Respiratory failure. [Updated 2023 Feb 15]. In: StatPearls. Treasure Island (FL): StatPearls Publishing; 2023. Available from: https://www.ncbi.nlm.nih.gov/books/NBK526127/.
17. Weinmann GG, Chiang YP, Sheingold S. The National Emphysema Treatment Trial (NETT): a study in agency collaboration. Proc Am Thorac Soc. 2008;5(4):381–4.
18. Criner GJ, Sternberg AL. National Emphysema Treatment Trial: the major outcomes of lung volume reduction surgery in severe emphysema. Proc Am Thorac Soc. 2008;5(4):393–405.
19. Weisman IM. Cardiopulmonary exercise testing in the preoperative assessment for lung resection surgery. Semin Thorac Cardiovasc Surg. 2001;13(2):116–25.
20. Banki F. Pulmonary assessment for general thoracic surgery. Surg Clin North Am. 2010;90(5):969–84.
21. Carter R, Holiday DB, Stocks J, Grothues C, Tiep B. Predicting oxygen uptake for men and women with moderate to severe chronic obstructive pulmonary disease. Arch Phys Med Rehabil. 2003;84(8):1158–64.
22. Winkler C, Funk M, Schindler DM, Hemsey JZ, Lampert R, Drew BJ. Arrhythmias in patients with acute coronary syndrome in the first 24 hours of hospitalization. Heart Lung. 2013;42(6):422–7.
23. Creswell LL. The problem of atrial arrhythmias after noncardiac thoracic surgery. J Thorac Cardiovasc Surg. 2004;127(3):629–30.
24. Pedoto A, Amar D. Perioperative arrhythmias and acute right heart failure in noncardiac thoracic surgery. Curr Anesthesiol Rep. 2014;4(2):142–9.
25. Campos JH. Lung isolation techniques for patients with difficult airway. Curr Opin Anaesthesiol. 2010;23(1):12–7.
26. Collins SR, Titus BJ, Campos JH, Blank RS. Lung isolation in the patient with a difficult airway. Anesth Analg. 2018;126(6):1968–78.
27. Karzai W, Schwarzkopf K. Hypoxemia during one-lung ventilation: prediction, prevention, and treatment. Anesthesiology. 2009;110(6):1402–11.

28. Ng A, Swanevelder J. Hypoxaemia during one-lung anaesthesia. Contin Educ Anaesth Criti Care Pain. 2010;10(4):117–22.
29. Gothard JW. Anesthetic considerations for patients with anterior mediastinal masses. Anesthesiol Clin. 2008;26(2):305–vi.
30. Güldner A, Pelosi P, de Abreu MG. Nonventilatory strategies to prevent postoperative pulmonary complications. Curr Opin Anaesthesiol. 2013;26(2):141–51.
31. Grønnebech H, Johansson G, Smedebøl M, Valentin N. Glycopyrrolate vs. atropine during anaesthesia for laryngoscopy and bronchoscopy. Acta Anaesthesiol Scand. 1993;37(5):454–7.
32. Chang SH, Krupnick AS. Perioperative antibiotics in thoracic surgery. Thorac Surg Clin. 2012;22(1):35–vi.
33. American Society of Anesthesiologists Task Force on Acute Pain Management. Practice guidelines for acute pain management in the perioperative setting: an updated report by the American Society of Anesthesiologists Task Force on Acute Pain Management. Anesthesiology. 2012;116(2):248–73.
34. Ng A, Swanevelder J. Pain relief after thoracotomy: is epidural analgesia the optimal technique? Br J Anaesth. 2007;98(2):159–62.
35. Horlocker TT, Vandermeuelen E, Kopp SL, Gogarten W, Leffert LR, Benzon HT. Regional anesthesia in the patient receiving antithrombotic or thrombolytic therapy: American Society of Regional Anesthesia and Pain Medicine Evidence-Based Guidelines (Fourth Edition) [published correction appears in Reg Anesth Pain Med. 2018 Jul;43(5):566. Vandermeuelen, Erik [corrected to Vandermeulen, Erik]]. Reg Anesth Pain Med. 2018;43(3):263–309.
36. Feng Y, Wu N, Yan S, Wang X, Yang Y. Comparison of Ivor Lewis esophagectomy and Sweet esophagectomy for the treatment of middle-lower esophageal squamous cell carcinoma. J Thorac Dis. 2019;11(8):3584–92.
37. Smithers BM, Gotley DC, Martin I, Thomas JM. Comparison of the outcomes between open and minimally invasive esophagectomy. Ann Surg. 2007;245(2):232–40.
38. Biere SS, Maas KW, Bonavina L, et al. Traditional invasive vs. minimally invasive esophagectomy: a multi-center, randomized trial (TIME-trial). BMC Surg. 2011;11:2.
39. Miller RD, Eriksson LI, Fleisher LA, et al. Miller's anesthesia, 2-volume set. In: Anesthesia for thoracic surgery, vol. 2; 2014. p. 1954–5.
40. Chen H, Liu Y, Peng H, Wang R, Wang K, Li D. Robot-assisted minimally invasive esophagectomy versus video-assisted minimally invasive esophagectomy: a systematic review and meta-analysis. Transl Cancer Res. 2021;10(11):4601–16.
41. Hosoda K, Niihara M, Harada H, Yamashita K, Hiki N. Robot-assisted minimally invasive esophagectomy for esophageal cancer: Meticulous surgery minimizing postoperative complications. Ann Gastroenterol Surg. 2020;4(6):608–17.
42. Kassis ES, Kosinski AS, Ross P Jr, Koppes KE, Donahue JM, Daniel VC. Predictors of anastomotic leak after esophagectomy: an analysis of the society of thoracic surgeons general thoracic database. Ann Thorac Surg. 2013;96(6):1919–26.
43. Schuchert MJ, Abbas G, Nason KS, et al. Impact of anastomotic leak on outcomes after transhiatal esophagectomy. Surgery. 2010;148(4):831–40.
44. Carney A, Dickinson M. Anesthesia for esophagectomy. Anesthesiol Clin. 2015;33(1):143–63.
45. Muñoz de Cabo C, Hermoso Alarza F, Cossio Rodriguez AM, Martín Delgado MC. Perioperative management in thoracic surgery. Manejo perioperatorio en cirugía torácica. Med Intensiva (Engl Ed). 2020;44(3):185–91.
46. Watanabe S, Noguchi E, Yamada S, Hamada N, Kano T. Sequential changes of arterial oxygen tension in the supine position during one-lung ventilation. Anesth Analg. 2000;90(1):28–34.
47. Guenoun T, Journois D, Silleran-Chassany J, et al. Prediction of arterial oxygen tension during one-lung ventilation: analysis of preoperative and intraoperative variables. J Cardiothorac Vasc Anesth. 2002;16(2):199–203.
48. Cox P, Tobias JD. Noninvasive monitoring of PaCO(2) during one-lung ventilation and minimal access surgery in adults: end-tidal versus transcutaneous techniques. J Minim Access Surg. 2007;3(1):8–13.

49. Fujii S, Kikura M, Takada T, Katoh S, Aoyama N, Sato S. A noninvasive partial carbon dioxide rebreathing technique for measurement of pulmonary capillary blood flow is also a useful oxygenation monitor during one-lung ventilation. J Clin Anesth. 2004;16(5):347–52.
50. Lee JH, Kim Y, Mun J, Lee J, Ko S. Effects of hypercarbia on arterial oxygenation during one-lung ventilation: prospective randomized crossover study. Korean J Anesthesiol. 2020;73(6):534–41.
51. Tang L, Kazan R, Taddei R, Zaouter C, Cyr S, Hemmerling TM. Reduced cerebral oxygen saturation during thoracic surgery predicts early postoperative cognitive dysfunction. Br J Anaesth. 2012;108(4):623–9.
52. Bardoczky GI, Levarlet M, Engelman E, deFrancquen P. Continuous spirometry for detection of double-lumen endobronchial tube displacement. Br J Anaesth. 1993;70(5):499–502.
53. Spaeth J, Ott M, Karzai W, et al. Double-lumen tubes and auto-PEEP during one-lung ventilation. Br J Anaesth. 2016;116(1):122–30.
54. Benumof JL, Wahrenbrock EA. Dependency of hypoxic pulmonary vasoconstriction on temperature. J Appl Physiol Respir Environ Exerc Physiol. 1977;42(1):56–8.
55. Klein U, Karzai W, Bloos F, et al. Role of fiberoptic bronchoscopy in conjunction with the use of double-lumen tubes for thoracic anesthesia: a prospective study. Anesthesiology. 1998;88(2):346–50.
56. de Bellis M, Accardo R, Di Maio M, et al. Is flexible bronchoscopy necessary to confirm the position of double-lumen tubes before thoracic surgery? [published correction appears in Eur J Cardiothorac Surg. 2012;41(6):1411. Lamanna, Carmine [corrected to La Manna, Carmine]]. Eur J Cardiothorac Surg. 2011;40(4):912–6.
57. Song IK, Ro S, Lee JH, et al. Reference levels for central venous pressure and pulmonary artery occlusion pressure monitoring in the lateral position. J Cardiothorac Vasc Anesth. 2017;31(3):939–43.
58. Zambouri A. Preoperative evaluation and preparation for anesthesia and surgery. Hippokratia. 2007;11(1):13–21.
59. Tan JC, Lin PS, He LX, Lin Y, Yao YT. Evidence in Cardiovascular Anesthesia(EICA) Group. Anesthetic management of patients undergoing mediastinal mass operation. Front Surg. 2022;9:1033349.
60. Parker JD. Acute airway obstruction from megaoesophagus secondary to achalasia evaluated with flexible bronchoscope. Case Rep Anesthesiol. 2021;2021:8815376.
61. Shen T, Bao X, Alfille PH. Perioperative complications in adults with a posterior mediastinal mass: a retrospective observational cohort study. Can J Anaesth. 2016;63(4):454–60.
62. Slinger P, editor. Principles and practice of anesthesia for thoracic surgery. Springer; 2019. https://doi.org/10.1007/978-3-030-00859-8.
63. Zdravkovic M, Berger-Estilita J, Sorbello M, Hagberg CA. An international survey about rapid sequence intubation of 10,003 anaesthetists and 16 airway experts. Anaesthesia. 2020;75(3):313–22.
64. Bayable SD, Melesse DY, Lema GF, Ahmed SA. Perioperative management of patients with asthma during elective surgery: a systematic review. Ann Med Surg (Lond). 2021;70:102874.
65. Jun IJ, Jo JY, Kim JI, et al. Impact of anesthetic agents on overall and recurrence-free survival in patients undergoing esophageal cancer surgery: a retrospective observational study. Sci Rep. 2017;7(1):14020.
66. Chow MY, Goh MH, Boey SK, Thirugnanam A, Ip-Yam PC. The effects of remifentanil and thoracic epidural on oxygenation and pulmonary shunt fraction during one-lung ventilation. J Cardiothorac Vasc Anesth. 2003;17(1):69–72.
67. Lumb AB, Slinger P. Hypoxic pulmonary vasoconstriction: physiology and anesthetic implications. Anesthesiology. 2015;122(4):932–46.
68. Ismail-Zade IA, Vuylsteke A, Ghosh S, Latimer RD. Inhaled nitric oxide and one-lung ventilation in the lateral decubitus position. J Cardiothorac Vasc Anesth. 1997;11(7):926–7.
69. Sohda M, Kuwano H, Saeki H, et al. Nationwide survey of neuroendocrine carcinoma of the esophagus: a multicenter study conducted among institutions accredited by the Japan Esophageal Society. J Gastroenterol. 2021;56(4):350–9.

70. Cassorla L. Miller's anesthesia. In: Patient Positioning, and associated risks, vol. 41. Elsevier Churchill Livingstone; 2020. p. 1240–65.
71. Zhang X, Wang DX, Wei JQ, Liu H, Hu SP. Recent advances in double-lumen tube malposition in thoracic surgery: a bibliometric analysis and narrative literature review. Front Med (Lausanne). 2022;9:1071254.
72. Butterworth. Morgan and Mikhail's clinical anesthesiology. In: Anesthesia for thoracic surgery. 5th ed. McGraw Hill Medical; 2022. p. 545–73.
73. Bahk JH, Oh YS. Prediction of double-lumen tracheal tube depth. J Cardiothorac Vasc Anesth. 1999;13(3):370–1.
74. Yasumoto M, Higa K, Nitahara K, Shono S, Hamada T. Optimal depth of insertion of left-sided double-lumen endobronchial tubes cannot be predicted from body height in below average-sized adult patients. Eur J Anaesthesiol. 2006;23(1):42–4.
75. Boucek CD, Landreneau R, Freeman JA, Strollo D, Bircher NG. A comparison of techniques for placement of double-lumen endobronchial tubes. J Clin Anesth. 1998;10(7):557–60.
76. Angie Ho CY, Chen CY, Yang MW, Liu HP. Use of the Arndt wire-guided endobronchial blocker via nasal for one-lung ventilation in patient with anticipated restricted mouth opening for esophagectomy. Eur J Cardiothorac Surg. 2005;28(1):174–5.
77. Vanner R. Arndt endobronchial blocker during oesophagectomy. Anaesthesia. 2005;60(3):295–6.
78. Jin Z, Chun Suen K, Ma D. Perioperative "remote" acute lung injury: recent update. J Biomed Res. 2017;31(3):197–212.
79. Tuğrul M, Camci E, Karadeniz H, Sentürk M, Pembeci K, Akpir K. Comparison of volume controlled with pressure controlled ventilation during one-lung anaesthesia. Br J Anaesth. 1997;79(3):306–10.
80. Ranieri VM, Giuliani R, Cinnella G, et al. Physiologic effects of positive end-expiratory pressure in patients with chronic obstructive pulmonary disease during acute ventilatory failure and controlled mechanical ventilation. Am Rev Respir Dis. 1993;147(1):5–13.
81. Lapinsky SE. Auto-PEEP encyclopedia of trauma care; 2015. p. 182–5.
82. Nagendran J, Stewart K, Hoskinson M, Archer SL. An anesthesiologist's guide to hypoxic pulmonary vasoconstriction: implications for managing single-lung anesthesia and atelectasis. Curr Opin Anaesthesiol. 2006;19(1):34–43.
83. Dunham-Snary KJ, Wu D, Sykes EA, et al. Hypoxic pulmonary vasoconstriction: from molecular mechanisms to medicine. Chest. 2017;151(1):181–92.
84. Talbot NP, Balanos GM, Dorrington KL, Robbins PA. Two temporal components within the human pulmonary vascular response to approximately 2 h of isocapnic hypoxia. J Appl Physiol (1985). 2005;98(3):1125–39.
85. Sylvester JT, Shimoda LA, Aaronson PI, Ward JP. Hypoxic pulmonary vasoconstriction [published correction appears in Physiol Rev. 2014 Jul;94(3):989]. Physiol Rev. 2012;92(1):367–520.
86. Marongiu I, Spinelli E, Mauri T. Cardio-respiratory physiology during one lung ventilation: complex interactions in need of advanced monitoring. Ann Transl Med. 2020;8(8):524.
87. Schwarzkopf K, Schreiber T, Gaser E, et al. The effects of xenon or nitrous oxide supplementation on systemic oxygenation and pulmonary perfusion during one-lung ventilation in pigs. Anesth Analg. 2005;100(2):335–9.
88. Van Keer L, Van Aken H, Vandermeersch E, Vermaut G, Lerut T. Propofol does not inhibit hypoxic pulmonary vasoconstriction in humans. J Clin Anesth. 1989;1(4):284–8.
89. Ozcan PE, Sentürk M, Sungur Ulke Z, et al. Effects of thoracic epidural anaesthesia on pulmonary venous admixture and oxygenation during one-lung ventilation. Acta Anaesthesiol Scand. 2007;51(8):1117–22.
90. Doering EB, Hanson CW 3rd, Reily DJ, Marshall C, Marshall BE. Improvement in oxygenation by phenylephrine and nitric oxide in patients with adult respiratory distress syndrome. Anesthesiology. 1997;87(1):18–25.
91. Dalibon N, Moutafis M, Liu N, Law-Koune JD, Monsel S, Fischler M. Treatment of hypoxemia during one-lung ventilation using intravenous almitrine. Anesth Analg. 2004;98(3):590–4.

92. Gherardi R, Louarn F, Benvenuti C, et al. Peripheral neuropathy in patients treated with almitrine dimesylate. Lancet. 1985;1(8440):1247–50.
93. Miller RD, Eriksson LI, Fleisher LA, Wiener-Kronish JP, Cohen NH, Young WL. Miller's anesthesia. In: Miller, editor. Anesthesia for thoracic surgery, vol. 2; 2014. p. 1942–2004.
94. Ashes C, Slinger P. Volume management and resuscitation in thoracic surgery. Curr Anesthesiol Rep. 2014;4:386–96.
95. Theodorou D, Drimousis PG, Larentzakis A, Papalois A, Toutouzas KG, Katsaragakis S. The effects of vasopressors on perfusion of gastric graft after esophagectomy. An experimental study. J Gastrointest Surg. 2008;12(9):1497–501.
96. Al-Rawi OY, Pennefather SH, Page RD, Dave I, Russell GN. The effect of thoracic epidural bupivacaine and an intravenous adrenaline infusion on gastric tube blood flow during esophagectomy. Anesth Analg. 2008;106(3):884–7.
97. Pathak D, Pennefather SH, Russell GN, et al. Phenylephrine infusion improves blood flow to the stomach during oesophagectomy in the presence of a thoracic epidural analgesia. Eur J Cardiothorac Surg. 2013;44(1):130–3.
98. Perez Nieto OR, Wong A, Lopez Fermin J, et al. Aiming for zero fluid accumulation: First, do no harm. Anaesthesiol Intensive Ther. 2021;53(2):162–78.
99. Lobo DN, Bostock KA, Neal KR, Perkins AC, Rowlands BJ, Allison SP. Effect of salt and water balance on recovery of gastrointestinal function after elective colonic resection: a randomised controlled trial. Lancet. 2002;359(9320):1812–8.
100. Wei S, Tian J, Song X, Chen Y. Association of perioperative fluid balance and adverse surgical outcomes in esophageal cancer and esophagogastric junction cancer. Ann Thorac Surg. 2008;86(1):266–72.
101. Hikasa Y, Suzuki S, Mihara Y, et al. Intraoperative fluid therapy and postoperative complications during minimally invasive esophagectomy for esophageal cancer: a single-center retrospective study. J Anesth. 2020;34(3):404–12.
102. Van Dessel E, Moons J, Nafteux P, et al. Perioperative fluid management in esophagectomy for cancer and its relation to postoperative respiratory complications. Dis Esophagus. 2021;34(7):doaa111.
103. Buise MP. Proper volume management during anesthesia for esophageal resection. J Thorac Dis. 2019;11(Suppl. 5):S702–6.
104. Kaufmann KB, Baar W, Glatz T, et al. Epidural analgesia and avoidance of blood transfusion are associated with reduced mortality in patients with postoperative pulmonary complications following thoracotomic esophagectomy: a retrospective cohort study of 335 patients. BMC Anesthesiol. 2019;19(1):162.
105. Behera BK, Puri GD, Ghai B. Patient-controlled epidural analgesia with fentanyl and bupivacaine provides better analgesia than intravenous morphine patient-controlled analgesia for early thoracotomy pain. J Postgrad Med. 2008;54(2):86–90.
106. Zoumprouli A, Chatzimichali A, Papadimitriou S, Papaioannou A, Xynos E, Askitopoulou H. Gastrointestinal motility following thoracic surgery: the effect of thoracic epidural analgesia. A randomised controlled trial. BMC Anesthesiol. 2017;17(1):139.
107. Casati A, Alessandrini P, Nuzzi M, et al. A prospective, randomized, blinded comparison between continuous thoracic paravertebral and epidural infusion of 0.2% ropivacaine after lung resection surgery. Eur J Anaesthesiol. 2006;23(12):999–1004.
108. Donohoe CL, Phillips AW, Flynn E, et al. Multimodal analgesia using intrathecal diamorphine, and paravertebral and rectus sheath catheters are as effective as thoracic epidural for analgesia post-open two-phase esophagectomy within an enhanced recovery program. Dis Esophagus. 2018;31(6) https://doi.org/10.1093/dote/doy006.
109. Li Y, Dong H, Tan S, Qian Y, Jin W. Effects of thoracic epidural anesthesia/analgesia on the stress response, pain relief, hospital stay, and treatment costs of patients with esophageal carcinoma undergoing thoracic surgery: a single-center, randomized controlled trial. Medicine (Baltimore). 2019;98(7):e14362.
110. Nishino I. Centronuclear myopathy. Ryoikibetsu Shokogun Shirizu. 2001;(35):414–7.

111. Rocker M, Havard TJ, Wagle A. Early extubation after two-stage oesophagectomy. Br J Anaesth. 2003;91(5):760.
112. Urabe M, Ohkura Y, Haruta S, Ueno M, Udagawa H. Factors affecting blood loss during thoracoscopic esophagectomy for esophageal carcinoma. J Chest Surg. 2021;54(6):466–72.
113. Basta M, Sanganeria T, Varacallo M. Anatomy, shoulder and upper limb, suprascapular nerve. [updated 2022 Oct 3]. In: StatPearls. Treasure Island (FL): StatPearls Publishing; 2023.
114. Hölscher AH, Fetzner UK, Bludau M, Leers J. Komplikationen und Komplikationsmanagement in der Ösophaguschirurgie [complications and management of complications in oesophageal surgery]. Zentralbl Chir. 2011;136(3):213–23.
115. Sedrakyan A, Treasure T, Browne J, Krumholz H, Sharpin C, van der Meulen J. Pharmacologic prophylaxis for postoperative atrial tachyarrhythmia in general thoracic surgery: evidence from randomized clinical trials. J Thorac Cardiovasc Surg. 2005;129(5):997–1005.
116. Law S, Wong KH, Kwok KF, Chu KM, Wong J. Predictive factors for postoperative pulmonary complications and mortality after esophagectomy for cancer. Ann Surg. 2004;240(5):791–800.
117. Tandon S, Batchelor A, Bullock R, et al. Peri-operative risk factors for acute lung injury after elective oesophagectomy. Br J Anaesth. 2001;86(5):633–8.
118. Jo JY, Kim WJ, Choi DK, Kim HR, Lee EH, Choi IC. Effect of restrictive fluid therapy with hydroxyethyl starch during esophagectomy on postoperative outcomes: a retrospective cohort study. BMC Surg. 2019;19(1):15.
119. Martin LW, Swisher SG, Hofstetter W, et al. Intrathoracic leaks following esophagectomy are no longer associated with increased mortality. Ann Surg. 2005;242(3):392–402.
120. Isomoto H, Yamaguchi N, Minami H, Nakao K. Management of complications associated with endoscopic submucosal dissection/endoscopic mucosal resection for esophageal cancer. Dig Endosc. 2013;25(Suppl. 1):29–38.
121. Townsend AN, Denton A, Gohel N, et al. An association between comorbidities and postsurgical complications in adults who underwent esophagectomy. Cureus. 2023;15(3):e36395.

# Postoperative Critical Care for Esophageal Surgery

# 14

Erkan Bayram, Sukru Ciftci, and Muslum Cicek

## 14.1 Introduction

Esophageal cancer is the eighth most common cancer and the sixth leading cause of death from cancer [1]. Despite advances and improvements in patient care and techniques, the incidence of esophageal adenocarcinoma is still high and survival remains poor in Western countries in comparison to other same-stage malignancies. Postoperative management of patients undergoing esophagectomy due to esophageal cancer is crucial in terms of the surgical outcomes and survival [2]. Postoperative critical care for patients undergoing esophageal surgery includes admission to the intensive care unit, extubation, weaning from mechanical ventilation, parenteral, enteral and oral nutrition, fluid management and postoperative respiratory and anastomotic complications including acute lung injury (ALI) and acute respiratory distress syndrome (ARDS) [3]. In this chapter, above-mentioned issues are discussed in light of the current literature.

## 14.2 Esophageal Surgery

Globally, esophageal cancer is the eighth most common cancer and the sixth leading cause of death from cancer [4]. Despite advances and improvements in patient care and techniques, the incidence of esophageal adenocarcinoma is still high, and survival remains poor in Western countries in comparison to other same-stage malignancies [5]. Today, esophagectomies are associated with significant morbidity and mortality of 39% and 11%, respectively [6]. Interval esophagectomy after adjuvant

E. Bayram (✉) · S. Ciftci · M. Cicek
Anesthesiology and Reanimation Department, Istinye University Medical Faculty, Medical Park Gaziosmanpasa Hospital, Istanbul, Turkey
e-mail: erkan.bayram@isu.edu.tr; sukru.ciftci@isu.edu.tr; muslum.cicek@isu.edu.tr



O. Engin (ed.), *Risk Factors and Therapy of Esophagus Cancer*, https://doi.org/10.1007/978-3-031-47024-0_14

chemotherapy remains the gold standard for the treatment of resectable esophageal cancer patients up to stage II [7]. In esophageal surgery, gastrointestinal integrity is achieved by the transposition and anastomosis of a gastric conduit into the posterior mediastinum of the left latero-cervical compartment.

Currently, the main radical surgical methods for esophageal cancer include sweet esophagectomy, Ivor Lewis surgery, and minimally invasive esophagectomy (MIE) [8]. The choice of approach depends on the experience of the surgeon and the anatomy of the patient. MIE has become a widely adopted approach for the treatment of esophageal carcinoma. In comparison with open esophagectomy, MIE reduces duration of hospitalization, blood loss, and complications. Almost all patients can be considered for MIE with reduction in complication rates and rapid recovery. The three commonly used approaches for MIE include McKeown or three-field, Ivor Lewis (IL-MIE), and transhiatal (TH-MIE) [9]. Esophagectomy consists of two phases: abdominal phase and thoracic phase. In conclusion, MIE is a complex technical operation with steep learning curves, but currently is the surgical treatment of choice for esophageal carcinomas.

## 14.3 Postoperative Critical Care for Esophageal Surgery

### 14.3.1 Admission to Intensive Care Unit

Since esophageal cancer surgery is invasive in nature, patients are routinely admitted to the intensive care unit (ICU) for hemodynamic support, respiratory support, and pain management [10]. After the introduction of MIE and enhanced recovery after surgery (ERAS), the value of routine ICU admission has been questioned [11]. Studies have reported that routine ICU admission following esophagectomy varied between hospitals, with no effect on short-term mortality rates [10, 12]. Patients who require invasive mechanical ventilation or continuous infusion of vasoactive medications or for whom anesthesiologist deem ICU care mandatory because of intraoperative course and comorbidities are admitted to the ICU. An anesthesiologist-led multidisciplinary critical care team is mainly responsible for the care of the patients in ICU in cooperation with the surgical team [13]. Therefore, traditional postoperative management after esophagectomy frequently requires ICU admission. Some patients who underwent MIE are ventilated and intubated for up to 2 days. Sedation, which is applied for comfort sometimes, leads to hypotension. With facilities of better pain relief including minimally invasive approaches and thoracic epidurals, immediate extubation has become more common [14]. Avoiding routine ventilation and admission to ICU have significant economic implications.

#### 14.3.1.1 Extubation and ICU

Immediate extubation after esophagectomy has been the norm except for patients who are at low risk, owing to minimally invasive surgery, judicious administration fluids intraoperatively, and new techniques used to relief pain [15]. Elective ventilation can be applied in patients at a high risk, those on pressor support and hypothermic patients. After extubation, ICU should be considered for high-risk patients who require intensive monitoring and support and patients who are at low risk can be managed in another unit [16].

Weaning mechanic ventilation within the first 24 h after esophagectomy and rehabilitation of respiration are needed based on the recommendations of postoperative recovery [17]. In a study by Patti et al., postoperative mechanical ventilation was given for a mean of 49 h [18].

### 14.3.2 Pulmonary Complications

#### 14.3.2.1 Acute Lung Injury

Following esophagectomy, among pulmonary complications acute lung injury (ALI), which is defined as the acute-onset hypoxemia with radiographic pulmonary infiltrates findings without a detectable cause, has been reported [19, 20]. Studies have reported that 25–38% of patients undergoing esophagectomy for esophageal cancer develop ALI [21, 22].

Because ALI following esophagectomy is clinically significant, several studies have investigated its pathophysiology. The release of inflammatory mediators and pulmonary cytokines and ventilator-induced lung injury have been proposed as possible mechanisms [23, 24]. In addition, systematic and pulmonary inflammation has been associated with ALI following esophagectomy [25]. Furthermore, one lung ventilation (OLV) during esophagectomy has been suggested as a significant factor underlying ALI [26]. High airway pressure and large tidal volume during OLV have been correlated with an increase in the risk of developing ALI postoperatively [27]. Using corticosteroids in patients who develop ALI after esophageal surgery requires attention to the development of surgery site complications to determine infections and treat them timely.

#### 14.3.2.2 Acute Respiratory Distress Syndrome

The roles of corticosteroids in acute respiratory distress syndrome (ARDS) have been comprehensively investigated. The useful effects of corticosteroids are in compliance with the hypothesis suggesting that fibroproliferation is an early reaction to pulmonary injury, which is inhibited by early administration of low-dose corticosteroids [28]. Nevertheless, despite these benefits, the suppressant effect of corticosteroids on wound healing and the immune response raises concerns in patients undergoing esophagectomy.

Recent studies have reported that vitamin C was applied to various conditions such as ARDS and septic shock [29, 30]. It has been stated that the combination of vitamin C and corticosteroids has therapeutic effects on postoperative lung function following esophagectomy [31]. However, large-scale prospective studies are needed on this issue. Gas inhalation therapy may exhibit the potential to reduce pulmonary morbidity following esophagectomy. Inhalation of β-agonists treats ARDS effectively through decreasing infiltration of inflammatory cells and cytokine release, increasing alveolar fluid clearance, and improving alveolar capillary barrier function [32].

### 14.3.3 Anastomotic Leak

Regardless of surgical method used, esophageal surgery is associated with high rates of mortality and morbidity. Esophagogastric anastomotic leak is one of the most common complications following esophagectomy [33]. The rates of anastomotic leakage following thoracic and cervical anastomoses have been reported as 6.6–17.2% and 2–15.9% in the literature [34, 35]. Anastomotic leakage following esophagectomy causes prolonged stay in the ICU and hospital, increased postoperative mortality, and reduced quality of life (QoL) [36]. Risk factors for developing anastomotic leakage include cervical localization of the anastomosis, preoperative external beam, technical mistakes, and comorbidities including, diabetes mellitus, obesity, malnutrition, smoking, and use of corticosteroids [37].

Both nonoperative and operative methods have been utilized in order to manage anastomotic leakage after esophageal surgery. Although traditional approach is excision of the conduit and diversion of the patients with delayed reconstruction, today most surgeons prefer to salvage the conduit, if possible. When making decisions for optimal treatment strategy, the surgeon usually assesses the general status of the patient, absence or presence of multi-organ failure, severity of the leakage, and conduit viability.

### 14.3.4 Postoperative Nutrition

Patients who undergo surgery for esophageal cancer have a high risk for developing malnutrition. The disease itself can potentially decrease oral food intake. The risk of malnutrition is also increased due to chemotherapy, the physiological influence of a constructed upper gastrointestinal tract, the extent of the surgery, and inadequate nutrition in the perioperative period. Thus, support for nutrition may be needed over months after esophageal surgery [38].

Enteral feeding has been correlated with a decrease in the duration of hospitalization and rate of complications compared to parenteral feeding [39]. The incidence of significant complications and duration of hospitalization after esophagectomy have been reported to be reduced with the establishment of enteral nutrition in the early postoperative period [40].

Patients are at a high risk of malnutrition following esophageal cancer surgery, particularly those who have undergone neoadjuvant therapy. Establishment of early enteral nutrition is crucial, but the ideal way of food intake is yet to be elucidated. Further studies are needed to evaluate the long-term patient satisfaction related to nutritional outcomes [41].

#### 14.3.4.1 Oral Nutrition

Starting oral feeding in the postoperative early period has been stated to result in positive outcomes in patients undergoing gastrointestinal tract procedures. However, it is correlated with an increase in the risk of aspiration pneumonia and vomiting [42]. Oral nutrition in the existence of significant complications may be impossible and may be associated with high rates of morbidity and mortality. On the other hand, two randomized controlled trials compared late versus early oral nutrition in patients who underwent gastrointestinal procedures and reported reduced hospitalization with no increase in major complications and morbidity in patients who administered early oral feeding.

Randomized controlled studies evaluating early oral feeding following upper gastrointestinal resections have reported no benefit in delaying oral intake beyond 48 h. Early oral feeding has been associated with fewer complications and early discharge, but no data analysis have been conducted for esophageal anastomoses that present unique challenges [43]. The modalities to ascertain anastomotic integrity involve contrast swallow, endoscopy, and computerized tomography (CT) scan with oral contrast agent. There is no adequate evidence to justify the routine use of these modalities before starting oral feeding or the superiority of one of them over others [44]. A recently published study assessing early establishment of oral food intake as liquids on postoperative day 1 and solid foods on postoperative day 2 following esophageal surgery observed no increased postoperative complications, an earlier correction of intestinal functioning, and improved QoL. In the mentioned study, the patients underwent endoscopic assessment on postoperative day 1 to evaluate functioning of the vocal cords before initiating oral nutrition [45]. In patients who have laryngeal nerve palsy, assessment of the swallowing through video endoscopy is recommended before starting oral feeding [46].

### 14.3.5 Early Mobilization

Early mobilization is one of the significant components of all ERAS protocols. Prolonged bed resting causes increased muscle weakness and loss, developed insulin resistance, tissue oxygenation and lung functioning, and an increase in the risk of developing thromboembolic and pulmonary complications [47, 48]. Early mobilization prevents major complications and preserves muscle functions as well as promotes patients to have an active involvement in the recovery from esophageal surgery. However, this is challenging in patients undergoing esophagectomy due to pain-related restrictions and various medical instruments including drains, pumps, and nutritional apparatus.

Timing and pattern of mobilization after esophagectomy are unclear, although in a review of nine non-randomized trials, early mobilization reduced the frequency of venous thromboembolism, accelerating functional recovery after esophageal surgery. In conclusion, postoperative mobilization should be initiated on the day of surgery whenever feasible [11].

### 14.3.6 Fluid Management

#### 14.3.6.1 Liberal Fluid Management

Liberal fluid management involves maintenance and conservation of sufficient tissue and organ perfusion. Loss of fluid is determined by taking into account the influence of starvation, blood loss, and insensible loss that led to edema. Fluids are given based on urinary output, heart rate, systemic blood pressure, and skin temperature but are mostly directed by the supervision and the anesthetist's experience [49].

Conventionally, surgeons have avoided using vasopressors such as vasopressin and nor-epinephrine in the perioperative stage of esophageal surgery due to the subtle gastroesophageal anastomoses. After the resection, the gastric conduit is reconstructed and the arterial delivery is based only on the right gastroepiploic arterial arcade [50]. In cervical anastomoses, the top side of the gastric conduit depends on microcirculation and there is an increased risk of developing ischemia. Studies regarding tissue perfusion have shown a significant reduction in tissue oxygenation and blood flow in the gastric side of the anastomosis. Despite the cause of these major complications is yet to be understood, hypoxia of the gastric tube and impaired microvascular blood flow have been stated as the most crucial factors causing failure of the gastroesophageal junction [51].

#### 14.3.6.2 Restrictive Fluid Management

Pulmonary complications are often seen after esophageal surgery with an incidence up to 60%. Interstitial edema is one of the underlying factors of these pulmonary complications. Restrictive fluid management aims at avoiding interstitial edema via the maintenance of a balance of zero fluid. Sensible loss, starvation, and third spacing are accepted to be less crucial and thus are not corrected with the administration of fluid boluses. Besides respiratory complications, interstitial edema may also result in anastomotic failure and disrupted wound healing. Some anesthetists have considered the term "restrictive" as frightening due to the belief that restrictive fluid management causes microcirculatory disturbance, intravascular hypovolemia, and dehydration. Particularly, the potential for developing acute kidney injury (AKI) and the influence of hypoperfusion on renal perfusion are issues of concern. However, studies promoting restrictive fluid management have demonstrated that most of the fluid regimens used were not restrictive but represented a sufficient substitution of the need for fluids [52]. Restrictive fluid management has become a major component of ERAS protocols in esophageal surgery as well as some types of abdominal surgery. Various authors have reported the useful influences of restrictive fluid management on pulmonary recovery following esophageal surgery [53, 54]. A recent protocol of restrictive fluid management was recommended as part of ERAS guidelines in esophageal surgery due to cancer [11].

**Goal-Directed Therapy**

Goal-directed therapy (GDT) may offer a balanced management of fluids via a care algorithm mainly utilized perioperatively in high-risk or septic shock patients. GDT aims optimization of tissue oxygen delivery and total blood flow through vasoactive medications including inotropes, vasopressors and vasodilators, and supplemental fluids. Today, GDT is utilized in cardiothoracic surgery, general surgery, vascular, and orthopedic surgeries. Shoemaker et al. evaluated GDT in high-risk surgical patients for the first time in 1988 [55]. In the mentioned study, a pulmonary artery catheter was utilized to direct supportive treatment in order to obtain optimal oxygen delivery and cardiac output. Since the application of this catheter was invasive and complex, it has been subsequently replaced by various, less invasive methods such as pulse pressure variation and pulse contour analysis.

### 14.3.7 Nasogastric Tube and Decompression

The decompression of gastric conduit has been thought to be more crucial compared with other abdominal resection operations. Several factors have been implicated, including decreasing the incidence of nausea and or vomiting, reducing the risk of anastomotic complications, reducing respiratory complications, and avoiding conduit distension through the use of nasogastric tubes for postoperative conduit decompression [44]. Nonrandomized studies that compared nasogastric tube decompression with the absence of nasogastric tube and a perioperatively inserted gastrostomy reported an increase in the risk of developing anastomotic or pulmonary complications in patients with nasogastric tubes [43]. On the other hand, two randomized controlled studies compared nasogastric decompression with early removal on postoperative day 2 and the absence of nasogastric tube and reported that the incidence of respiratory complications was higher in the group which had no nasogastric tube decompression [56, 57]. But no significant difference was found between the delayed and early removal of the nasogastric tube. In conclusion, nasogastric tube decompression is recommended at the time of esophagectomy, considering early removal postoperatively if it is clinically appropriate.

### 14.3.8 Early Removal of Tubes and Drains

Insertion of peri-anastomotic drains (thorax or neck) is not routinely recommended because this has not been proven to increase identification of leakage [11]. A chest drain is inserted following esophageal surgery to ensure expansion of the lungs and to detect anastomotic leakage, bleeding, and air. Using a single central chest drain is recommended by the ERAS guidelines [11].

In the immediate postoperative period, a patient who underwent esophagectomy in general has a nasogastric tube, a jejunostomy or nasojejunal tube, an arterial i.v. access, an intravenous catheter, a chest tube, an epidural catheter, and a urinary catheter. These make early mobilization difficult. The nasogastric tube should be withdrawn on postoperative day 2 if the gastric tube is not dilated [56]. Once the diuretic stage is reached or after 48 h the urinary catheter can be removed, but especially in elderly males, removal of the urinary catheter while the epidural catheter is still in its place leads to a 26% probability of replacement [58]. It is important to monitor urinary retention after removal of the catheter. Chest drains are related with immobilization and pain [59]. Although in most centers, chest drains are removed when their output is 100–150 mL/day, there is no data to support this [60]. In clinical practice, the chest drain can be withdrawn after complete lung expansion is confirmed by chest radiogram, which can typically be observed by postoperative day 2 [11].

### 14.3.9 Multidisciplinary Standardized Clinical Pathways

Utilization of multidisciplinary care requires appropriate use of skills, knowledge, and best practices from various professions and disciplines for optimization of care and outcomes of patients who underwent esophagectomy. In the last decades, goal-directed, standardized clinical pathways that function as templates for all medical staff have been developed in order to coordinate interventions from different disciplines. Such pathways have been introduced to clinical practice successfully for patients undergoing esophagectomy with reduced morbidity, duration of hospitalization, and costs [61]. An analysis of nine studies including 1240 patients with 661 undergoing the conventional pathway and 579 a standard pathway following esophageal surgery demonstrated a reduction in pulmonary complications, anastomotic leak, and length of stay in hospital in patients managed by the standardized pathway [61].

## 14.4 Conclusion

Esophagectomy is one of the most demanding procedures in gastrointestinal surgery. Postoperative critical care of patients undergoing esophagectomy due to esophageal cancer is of paramount importance in terms of morbidity and mortality. Postoperative care includes admission to ICU, extubation, weaning from mechanical ventilation, fluid management, and management of postoperative complications. Studies on postoperative care of patients undergoing esophagectomy are limited in the literature. Therefore, there is a need for especially randomized controlled studies on this subject.

## References

1. Liu CQ, Ma YL, Qin Q, et al. Epidemiology of esophageal cancer in 2020 and projections to 2030 and 2040. Thorac Cancer. 2023;14(1):3–11.
2. D'Amico TA. Outcomes after surgery for esophageal cancer. Gastrointest Cancer Res. 2007;1(5):188–96.
3. Kita T, Mammoto T, Kishi Y. Fluid management and postoperative respiratory disturbances in patients with transthoracic esophagectomy for carcinoma. J Clin Anesth. 2002;14(4):252–6.

4. Malhotra GK, Yanala U, Ravipati A, et al. Global trends in esophageal cancer. J Surg Oncol. 2017;115(5):564–79.
5. International Agency for Research on Cancer. GLOBOCAN-2012. Estimated cancer incidence, mortality and prevalence in 2012. http://globocan.iarc.fr/Pages/fact_sheets.population.aspx.
6. Walters DM, McMurry TL, Isbell JM, Stukenborg GJ, Kozower BD. Understanding mortality as a quality indicator after esophagectomy. Ann Thorac Surg. 2014;98:506–12.
7. Kitagawa Y, Uno T, Oyama T, et al. Esophageal cancer practice guidelines 2017 edited by the Japan Esophageal Society: Part 1. Esophagus. 2019;16:1–24.
8. Ding Q, Zhou W, Xue Y, et al. Comparison of postoperative complications between different operation methods for esophageal cancer. Thorac Cancer. 2019;10(8):1669–72.
9. Takahashi C, Shridhar R, Huston J, Meredith K. Esophagectomy from then to now. J Gastrointest Oncol. 2018;9(5):903–9.
10. Wunsch H, Gershengorn HB, Cooke CR, et al. Use of intensive care services for Medicare beneficiaries undergoing major surgical procedures. Anesthesiology. 2016;124(4):899–907.
11. Low DE, Allum W, De Manzoni G, et al. Guidelines for perioperative care in esophagectomy: enhanced recovery after surgery (ERAS®) society recommendations. World J Surg. 2019;43(2):299–33.
12. Gemmill EH, Humes DJ, Catton JA. Systematic review of enhanced recovery after gastro-oesophageal cancer surgery. Ann R Coll Surg Engl. 2015;97(3):173–9.
13. Iscimen R, Brown DR, Cassivi SD, Keegan MT. Intensive care unit utilization and outcome after esophagectomy. J Cardiothorac Vasc Anesth. 2010;24(3):440–6.
14. Robertson SA, Skipworth RJ, Clarke DL, et al. Ventilatory and intensive care requirements following oesophageal resection. Ann R Coll Surg Engl. 2006;88:354–7.
15. Ashok A, Niyogi D, Ranganathan P, et al. The enhanced recovery after surgery (ERAS) protocol to promote recovery following esophageal cancer resection [published correction appears in Surg Today. 2020 Mar 25]. Surg Today. 2020;50(4):323–34.
16. Chandrashekar MV, Irving M, Wayman J, Raimes SA, Linsley A. Immediate extubation and epidural analgesia allow safe management in a high-dependency unit after two-stage oesophagectomy. Results of eight years of experience in a specialized upper gastrointestinal unit in a district general hospital. Br J Anaesth. 2003;90:474–9.
17. Vrba R, Vrána D, Neoral Č, et al. Respiratory complications following mini-invasive laparoscopic and thoracoscopic esophagectomy for esophageal cancer. Experience in 215 patients. Wideochir Inne Tech Maloinwazyjne. 2019;14(1):52–9.
18. Patti MG, Wiener-Kronish JP, Way LW, Pellegrini CA. Impact of transhiatal esophagectomy on cardiac and respiratory function. Am J Surg. 1991;162(6):563–7.
19. Park SY, Lee HS, Jang HJ, et al. Efficacy of intraoperative, single-bolus corticosteroid administration to prevent postoperative acute respiratory failure after oesophageal cancer surgery. Interact Cardiovasc Thorac Surg. 2012;15:639–43.
20. Tandon S, Batchelor A, Bullock R, et al. Peri-operative risk factors for acute lung injury after elective oesophagectomy. Br J Anaesth. 2001;86:633–8.
21. Boshier PR, Marczin N, Hanna GB. Pathophysiology of acute lung injury following esophagectomy. Dis Esophagus. 2015;28:797–804.
22. Howells P, Thickett D, Knox C, et al. The impact of the acute respiratory distress syndrome on outcome after oesophagectomy. Br J Anaesth. 2016;117:375–81.
23. Jordan S, Mitchell JA, Quinlan GJ, et al. The pathogenesis of lung injury following pulmonary resection. Eur Respir J. 2000;15:790–9.
24. Choi H, Cho JH, Kim HK, et al. Prevalence and clinical course of postoperative acute lung injury after esophagectomy for esophageal cancer. J Thorac Dis. 2019;11(1):200–5.
25. Morita M, Yoshida R, Ikeda K, et al. Acute lung injury following an esophagectomy for esophageal cancer, with special reference to the clinical factors and cytokine levels of peripheral blood and pleural drainage fluid. Dis Esophagus. 2008;21:30–6.
26. Baudouin SV. Lung injury after thoracotomy. Br J Anaesth. 2003;91:132–42.

27. Jeon K, Yoon JW, Suh GY, et al. Risk factors for post-pneumonectomy acute lung injury/acute respiratory distress syndrome in primary lung cancer patients. Anaesth Intensive Care. 2009;37:14–9.
28. Meduri GU, Muthiah MP, Carratu P, et al. Nuclear factor-kappaB- and glucocorticoid receptor alpha-mediated mechanisms in the regulation of systemic and pulmonary inflammation during sepsis and acute respiratory distress syndrome. Evidence for inflammation-induced target tissue resistance to glucocorticoids. Neuroimmunomodulation. 2005;12:321–38.
29. Marik PE. Hydrocortisone, ascorbic acid and thiamine (HAT Therapy) for the treatment of sepsis. Focus on ascorbic acid. Nutrients. 2018;10:1762.
30. Marik PE, Long A. ARDS complicating pustular psoriasis: treatment with low-dose corticosteroids, vitamin C and thiamine. BMJ Case Rep. 2018;2018:bcr2017223475.
31. Matsuoka T, Shinozaki H, Ozawa S, Izawa Y, Koyanagi K, Kawarai Lefor A, et al. Administration of corticosteroids, ascorbic acid, and thiamine improves oxygenation after thoracoscopic esophagectomy. Ann Thorac Cardiovasc Surg. 2020;26:133–9.
32. Perkins GD, McAuley DF, Richter A, Thickett DR, Gao F. Bench-to-bedside review: beta2-agonists and the acute respiratory distress syndrome. Crit Care. 2004;8:25–32.
33. Raymond D. Complications of esophagectomy. Surg Clin N Am. 2012;92:1299–313.
34. Brown AM, Pucci MJ, Berger AC, et al. A standardized comparison of peri-operative complications after minimally invasive esophagectomy: Ivor Lewis versus McKeown. Surg Endosc. 2018;32:204–11.
35. Fumagalli U, Baiocchi G, Celotti A, et al. Incidence and treatment of mediastinal leakage after esophagectomy: insights from the multicenter study on mediastinal leaks. World J Gastroenterol. 2019;25:356–66.
36. Kassis ES, Kosinski AS, Ross P, et al. Predictors of anastomotic leak after esophagectomy: an analysis of The Society of Thoracic Surgeons General Thoracic Database. Ann Thorac Surg. 2013;96:1919–26.
37. Van Daele E, Van de Putte D, Ceelen W, et al. Risk factors and consequences of anastomotic leakage after Ivor Lewis oesophagectomy. Interact Cardiovasc Thorac Surg. 2016;22:32–7.
38. Ryan AM, Rowley SP, Healy LA, et al. Post-oesophagectomy early enteral nutrition via a needle catheter jejunostomy: 8-year experience at a specialist unit. Clin Nutr. 2006;25:386–93.
39. Xiao-Bo Y, Qiang L, Xiong Q, et al. Efficacy of early postoperative enteral nutrition in supporting patients after esophagectomy. Minerva Chir. 2014;69:37–46.
40. Fujita T, Daiko H, Nishimura M. Early enteral nutrition reduces the rate of life-threatening complications after thoracic esophagectomy in patients with esophageal cancer. Eur Surg Res. 2012;48:79–84.
41. Steenhagen E. Preoperative nutritional optimization of esophageal cancer patients. J Thorac Dis. 2019;11(Suppl 5):S645–53.
42. Mazaki T, Ebisawa K. Enteral versus parenteral nutrition after gastrointestinal surgery: a systematic review and metaanalysis of randomized controlled trials in the English literature. J Gastrointest Surg. 2008;12:739–55.
43. Lassen K, Kjaeve J, Fetveit T, et al. Allowing normal food at will after major upper gastrointestinal surgery does not increase morbidity: a randomized multicenter trial. Ann Surg. 2008;247(5):721–9.
44. Findlay JM, Gillies RS, Millo J, Sgromo B, Marshall RE, Maynard ND. Enhanced recovery for esophagectomy: a systematic review and evidence-based guidelines. Ann Surg. 2014;259:413–31.
45. Sun HB, Li Y, Liu XB, et al. Early oral feeding following McKeown minimally invasive esophagectomy: an open-label, randomized, controlled noninferiority trial. Ann Surg. 2018;267:435–42.
46. Kato H, Miyazaki T, Sakai M, et al. Videofuoroscopic evaluation in oropharyngeal swallowing after radical esophagectomy with lymphadenectomy for esophageal cancer. Anticancer Res. 2007;27:4249–54.
47. Pashikanti L, Von Ah D. Impact of early mobilization protocol on the medical-surgical inpatient population: an integrated review of literature. Clin Nurse Spec. 2012;26:87–94.

48. Brower RG. Consequences of bed rest. Crit Care Med. 2009;37:422–8.
49. Hulscher JB, Van Sandick JW, De Boer AGEM, et al. Extended transthoracic resection compared with limited transhiatal resection for adenocancinoma of the esophagus. N Engl J Med. 2002;347:1662–9.
50. Al-Ghamdi AA. Intraoperative fluid management: past and future, where is the evidence? Saudi J Anaesth. 2018;12(2):311–7.
51. Theodorou D, Drimousis PG, Larentzakis A, et al. The effect of vasopressors on perfusion of gastric graft after esophagectomy. An experimental study. J Gastrointest Surg. 2008;12:1497–501.
52. Corcoran T, Rhodes JE, Clarke S, et al. Perioperative fluid management strategies in major surgery: a stratified metaanalysis. Anesth Analg. 2012;114:640–51.
53. Casado D, Lopez F, Marti R. Perioperative fluid management and major respiratory complications in patients undergoing esophagectomy. Dis Esophagus. 2010;23:523–8.
54. Wei S, Tian J, Song X, et al. Association of perioperative fluid balance and adverse surgical outcomes in esophageal cancer and esophagogastric junction cancer. Ann Thorac Surg. 2008;86:266–72.
55. Shoemaker WC, Appel PL, Kram HB, et al. Prospective trial of supranormal values of survivors as therapeutic goals in high-risk surgical patients. Chest. 1988;94:1176–86.
56. Mistry RC, Vijayabhaskar R, Karimundackal G, et al. Effect of short-term vs prolonged nasogastric decompression on major postesophagectomy complications: a parallel-group, randomized trial. Arch Surg. 2012;147:747–51.
57. Shackcloth MJ, McCarron E, Kendall J, et al. Randomized clinical trial to determine the effect of nasogastric drainage on tracheal acid aspiration following oesophagectomy. Br J Surg. 2006;93:547–52.
58. Hu Y, Craig SJ, Rowlingson JC, et al. Early removal of urinary catheter after surgery requiring thoracic epidural: a prospective trial. J Cardiothorac Vasc Anesth. 2014;28:1302–6.
59. Refai M, Brunelli A, Salati M, Xiumè F, Pompili C, Sabbatini A. The impact of chest tube removal on pain and pulmonary function after pulmonary resection. Eur J Cardiothorac Surg. 2011;41:820–3.
60. Lagarde SM, Omloo JM, Ubbink DT, Busch OR, Obertop H, Van Lanschot JJ. Predictive factors associated with prolonged chest drain production after esophagectomy. Dis Esophagus. 2007;20:24–8.
61. Schmidt HM, El Lakis MA, Markar SR, et al. Accelerated recovery within standardized recovery pathways after esophagectomy: a prospective cohort study assessing the effects of early discharge on outcomes, readmissions, patient satisfaction, and costs. Ann Thorac Surg. 2016;102:931–9.

# Perioperative Evaluation for the Respiratory System

# 15

Sertac Arslan

## 15.1 General Principles

Advances in surgery and anesthesia have increased the research for operable patients with comorbid diseases. Nowadays, perioperative complications can be seen more frequently and vary due to the fact that more difficult cases are operated.

There are three main purposes in preoperative evaluation: To determine the risk of preoperative complications, to reduce the risk of perioperative complications, and to eliminate the risk factors in the patient at risk of complications in the postoperative period. For this purpose, a correct preoperative evaluation will ensure that the patient is operated with the least risk. An overprotective approach may cause the patient not to have the operation that should be absolutely necessary or cause delays in the operation. For this reason, accurate and complete preoperative evaluation are of great importance for both the patient and the surgeon.

Postoperative pulmonary complications increase mortality and morbidity, prolong hospital stay, increase the need for intensive care, and consequently increase health expenditure [1–3].

The most important postoperative pulmonary complications are

1. Atelectasis
2. Infection
3. Respiratory failure and prolonged mechanical ventilation
4. Exacerbation of underlying lung disease/Bronchospasm [4–6]

The risk of postoperative pulmonary complications varies according to cardiothoracic surgery and non-thoracic surgery approaches. It has been reported that the

S. Arslan (✉)
Department of Pulmonary Medicine, Acibadem Atasehir Hospital, Istanbul, Turkey


O. Engin (ed.), *Risk Factors and Therapy of Esophagus Cancer*,
https://doi.org/10.1007/978-3-031-47024-0_15

risk of postoperative pulmonary complications in non-thoracic surgery is 2–29%, and the risk of complications in cardiothoracic surgery is 8–39% [7].

### 15.1.1 Atelectasis

It is the most common postoperative pulmonary complication. Although the incidence varies, there are reported rates of 6–75%. Possible causes of atelectasis such as: Decreased ventilation depth during and after general anesthesia, shallow breathing due to insufficient pain control, increased secretion and inability to be excreted, decreased flexibility, and expansion ability of the thoracic wall and lungs. Most patients who are operated under general anesthesia develop atelectasis that is not clinically significant [5]. Severe atelectasis is a facilitating cause for pneumonia. Prevention of atelectasis is important because the development of pneumonia will increase mortality rates. It has been found that 20–25% of the basal regions undergo atelectasis after major surgical interventions [4]. The surgical intervention performed, the risk factors are related to the patient, and the variety of anesthesia applications cause changes in the rates and areas of atelectasis.

### 15.1.2 Infection

Among the postoperative pulmonary complications, pneumonia is an important cause of morbidity and mortality. The incidence of postoperative pneumonia is reported to be around 67% [8]. Changes in diagnosis rates may be due to changes in criteria for diagnosing pneumonia.

In the postoperative period, the suppression of the cough reflex and the inability to cough due to pain cause the secretions to accumulate in the lungs. At the same time, in the postoperative period, a suitable environment develops for the causative pathogens to reach the lungs and initiate the infection due to the increased risk of aspiration [5].

### 15.1.3 Respiratory Failure and Prolonged Mechanical Ventilation

Mild hypoxemia may be encountered in healthy adults in the postoperative period. Superficial breathing, atelectasis, and impaired ventilation/perfusion ratio due to anesthesia may deepen hypoxemia. The presence of an underlying lung disease may lead to further deepening of hypoxemia and prolongation of mechanical ventilation in the postoperative period. Surgical intervention and anesthesia technique as well as patient-specific parameters contribute to the development of respiratory failure. Underlying causes of respiratory failure may include pulmonary embolism and aspiration of gastric contents. Intraoperative and postoperative immobilization and presence of underlying malignancy increase the risk of pulmonary embolism [8].

### 15.1.4 Exacerbation of Underlying Lung Disease

The presence of chronic obstructive pulmonary disease (COPD) increases the risk of respiratory complications 2.7–4.7 times [6]. The presence of bronchospasm before the operation and further deterioration of impaired mucociliary clearance with the operation increase the frequency of COPD exacerbations in the postoperative period. Patients with COPD are more sensitive to the respiratory depressant effects of anesthetic substances, and the risk of developing hypercapnia and hypoxemia is high due to these substances [4].

In asthmatic patients, disease control before the operation is important. The risk of postoperative pulmonary complications in patients with controlled asthma is equal to that of healthy adults. In cases with symptoms, the risk of bronchospasm in the perioperative period was found to be 2% [4].

## 15.2 Risk Factors for Postoperative Pulmonary Complications (POPCs)

### 15.2.1 Patient-Related Risk Factors

#### 15.2.1.1 Age

Postoperative pulmonary complication rates were found to be higher in cases aged 65 and over. In a prospective cohort study, multiple regression analyzes showed three independent factors related to POPCs. These are age >65 and smoking are two of them [9]. In ten separate studies, age was found to be the second most common risk factor (Odds ratio was 2.09 for 60–69 years and 3.04 for 70–79 years of age) [10].

#### 15.2.1.2 Chronic Obstructive Pulmonary Disease (COPD)

In the presence of COPD, POPC rates increase approximately twofold [11, 12]. Lawrence et al. investigated pulmonary complications in patients who underwent elective abdominal surgery, found that POPC increased six times if there was a decrease in breath sounds, prolonged expiration, ral, rhonchi, and wheezing [13]. In addition, Fuster et al., investigated the prognostic value of COPD in patients undergoing coronary artery bypass surgery and evaluated the presence of COPD as a poor prognostic factor. According to this study, FEV1 below 60% should be considered as the primary prognostic factor [14].

According to another opinion, although COPD is a serious risk factor for POPC, there is no pulmonary function parameter that would constitute an absolute contraindication for surgery.

For example, in 15 surgical interventions performed on 12 patients with a FEV1 value below 1 L, no death was observed, whereas POPC was detected in only three cases [15]. Complications related to the type and duration of surgery (higher in patients who underwent coronary bypass and major abdominal surgery) were found in 31 (29%) of 107 surgical interventions performed in 89 patients with severe

COPD (FEV1 < 50%). While five out of ten patients who underwent coronary bypass died, only 1 death was observed in 97 noncoronary surgeries [16]. As can be seen from this study, POPC rates in non-coronary surgeries in patients with COPD are within acceptable limits, even in advanced stages. Nevertheless, the benefit of surgery in these cases should be well evaluated.

#### 15.2.1.3 Asthma

The presence of asthma has always worried surgeons in terms of POPC. In a retrospective analysis by Warner et al., none of 706 patients with asthma died, while 1.7% developed bronchospasm, 0.1% respiratory failure, and 0.3% laryngospasm. Complication rates were found more frequently in elderly patients and those with uncontrolled asthma [17]. While asthma is not a problem in elective surgeries, life-threatening bronchospasm may develop in emergency interventions if the disease is not under control [18].

In patients with bronchial hyperreactivity, bronchospasm may develop after tracheal intubation. Such cases will benefit from administration of short-acting bronchodilators and systemic corticosteroids for 5 days preoperatively [7].

#### 15.2.1.4 Smoking

Even if there is no accompanying chronic lung disease, smoking is an important risk factor for pulmonary complications. The risk of complications was found to be 1.4–4.3 times higher in smokers [19, 20]. Smoking cessation before surgery is a rule that must be followed, but there is no consensus on when to quit. It is generally recommended to quit 8 weeks beforehand. The 8-week period is a logical approach, as it will take weeks/months for improvement in ciliary function, macrophage activity, and small airway function and reduction in mucus secretion. Among 200 patients who underwent elective coronary artery bypass surgery, pulmonary complication rates were four times higher in patients who smoked in the last 2 months compared to those who quit smoking 2 months or before (57.1% vs. 14.5%, respectively). Complication rates in those who quit smoking 6 months ago were similar to those who never smoked (11.9% vs. 11.1%) [21].

#### 15.2.1.5 Health Status

American Society of Anesthesiologists (ASA) classification is generally used to evaluate general health status. There is a good correlation between the ASA classification and POPC, and it is one of the most important indicators of pulmonary risk. While the odds ratio was 7.1 in patients with ASA Class II and above, it was found as 3.34 in ASA Class I patients [10]. In a study investigating POPCs seen after thoracic and major abdominal surgeries in patients with and without COPD, ASA classification by logistic regression analysis and, to a lesser extent, age were found to be independent predictive factors ($p$ = 0.0003 and 0.08, respectively) [12]. In this study, 4 (15%) of 27 patients in ASA Class II, 16 (28%) of 57 patients in Class III, and 27 (59%) of 46 patients in Class IV. Serious POPC or cardiac complications were detected [12]. In addition to the ASA classification, the cardio-pulmonary risk index (CPRI) obtained with the Goldman Cardiac Risk Index and Pulmonary Risk Index is often sufficient in assessing pulmonary risk [22].

Complications were found 17 times more in patients with a CPRI score of more than 4 compared to those with a CPRI score of less than 4. However, no complications were found in scores of 2 and below [7]. In a later study, pulmonary complications were found in all eight patients with CPRI >3 out of 43 patients who underwent thoracic and upper abdominal surgeries [23]. On the other hand, in a review of 180 cases who underwent thoracic surgery, it was found that CPRI scoring was not sufficient to predict complications, and it was necessary to add pulmonary function test (PFT) and blood gases to these indices [7, 24].

#### 15.2.1.6 Sleep Apnea

The importance of obstructive sleep apnea (OSA) has been better understood by studies conducted in recent years. It has also been shown to be a serious risk factor for postoperative pulmonary complications [25]. A patient with OSA should be followed carefully preoperatively, intraoperatively, and postoperatively. Continuous positive airway pressure (CPAP) should be applied preoperatively, especially if OSA is severe [25]. Intraoperatively, sedatives, opioids, and inhaled anesthetics should be used with extreme caution, due to the tendency of the airways to collapse and sleep disturbance. For minor interventions, local anesthesia with or without moderate sedation or peripheral nerve blockade will be appropriate. CPAP or an oral device should be used during sedation. Postoperatively, regional analgesia techniques should be considered to reduce the need for systemic opioids. Nonsteroidal anti-inflammatory drugs can also be tried to reduce the need for opioids. It should be taken into account that sedatives might cause respiratory depression. These patients might need continuous oxygen support; however, oxygen can prolong apnea periods and mask atelectasis, transient apnea, and hypoventilation. Therefore, CPAP or NIPPV with oxygen should be applied if needed. If possible, these patients should be placed in non-supine position [25].

#### 15.2.1.7 Pulmonary Hypertension

In patients with pulmonary hypertension (PH) (right ventricular systolic pressure > 35 mmHg) who underwent noncardiac surgery, New York Heart Association (NYHA) functional class >2, OSA or a history of pulmonary embolism, risks such as postoperative congestive heart failure, cardiac ischemic events, arrhythmias, stroke, respiratory failure (the most common cause of morbidity), hepatic dysfunction, renal dysfunction, or postoperative positive inotropic or vasopressor requirement found increased [7].

In a series of 145 patients with a mean right ventricular systolic pressure of 68 ± 21 mmHg on echocardiography, one or more morbidities were found in 60 patients (42%) [26]. History of pulmonary embolism ($p = 0.01$), NYHA class ≥II ($p = 0.02$), moderate-high-risk surgery ($p = 0.04$), and anesthesia duration >3 h ($p = 0.04$) were found to be independent predictors of morbidity in the early stage. Early death occurred in ten cases (7%) in the study. Factors associated with postoperative mortality are pulmonary embolism ($p = 0.04$), right axis deviation ($p = 0.02$), right ventricular hypertrophy ($p = 0.04$), right ventricular systolic pressure (RVSP)/systolic blood pressure ≥0.66 ($p = 0.01$), intraoperative vasopressor use ($p < 0.01$), and anesthesia ($p < 0.01$) when nitrous oxide was not used [26]. As a result, in patients with PH who underwent non-cardiac surgery under general anesthesia, specific clinical, diagnostic, and intraoperative factors may predict poor outcomes.

#### 15.2.1.8 Heart Failure

The risk of POPC in patients with congestive heart failure is higher than in normal population. The odds ratio for POPC was 2.93 (95% CI 1.02–8.43) in patients with heart failure [27].

#### 15.2.1.9 Metabolic Status

Serum albumin and blood urea nitrogen (BUN) levels can be used to evaluate the risk of POPC [28]. Both low albumin value (<3 g/dL) (odds ratio = 2.53) and high BUN (>30 mg/dL) (odds ratio = 2.29) were found to be important markers for pulmonary complications [28].

### 15.2.2 Procedure Related Risk Factors: Respiratory Physiology Perspective

Depending on the situation, changes in respiratory functions may occur:

1. According to anesthesia
2. According to the type of surgery [29]

#### 15.2.2.1 Anesthesia-Induced Changes in Pulmonary Function

Anesthetic agents cause a decrease in respiratory muscle tone. This reduction causes up to 20% reduction in functional residual capacity (FRC). This decrease in the early postoperative period is mostly correlated with the decrease in $PaO_2$. The reasons for the decrease in FRC include pain, abdominal distension, pulmonary venous congestion, and posture [30]. Abdominal incision pain causes reflex movement in muscle tone. Because of this pain, the patient reduces the postoperative respiratory depth. At the same time, loss of tone and motility, especially after abdominal surgery, causes an increase in intra-abdominal pressure and elevation in the diaphragm. All these factors might cause a decrease in FRC [30].

Anesthetic agents may cause POPC development by reducing respiratory muscle tone or creating atelectasis due to the closure of the airways [31]. The developing atelectasis causes the ventilation/perfusion balance to deteriorate. The shunt fraction and alveolar–arterial gradient increase. Inhalation anesthetics also desensitize the response to hypoxia and hypercarbia. With general anesthesia, the number and functions of alveolar macrophages decrease, mucociliary clearance decreases, alveolocapillary permeability increases, surfactant secretion decreases, and the response of pulmonary vessels to neurohumoral mediators decreases. Anesthetic administration causes decreased tone in the diaphragm and intercostal muscles, resulting in a reduction in the transverse diameter of the thorax. Ventilation/perfusion balance changes due to decreased functional residual capacity, upward displacement of the diaphragm, and inhibition of hypoxic pulmonary vasoconstriction response. The upward displacement of the diaphragm facilitates the development of atelectasis in adjacent lung regions. In addition, inadequate secretion clearance, replacement of nitrogen by inhalation anesthetics, and high oxygen concentration during general anesthesia lead to the development of resorption atelectasis after general anesthesia. With the application of anesthesia, the shape and type of chest wall movements may change, which may cause changes in the elastic properties of the lung and the distribution of inspired gas [32].

Supine position causes a decrease in all lung volumes due to the loss of gravity. The decrease in respiratory muscle tone due to anesthetic agents worsens the decrease in FRC. Dysfunction of the diaphragm and basal atelectasis persist for some time after the surgical procedure. Diaphragmatic dysfunction occurs more commonly after abdominal and thoracic surgery [33].

The depth of anesthesia affects the breathing pattern. Tidal volume is higher in superficial anesthesia. Respiration is faster in moderate anesthesia. In deep anesthesia, respiratory depression is very pronounced, and the activity of the intercostal muscles disappears [34].

Hypoxia may develop due to various reasons during anesthesia. Mechanical reasons such as insufficient oxygen delivery of the anesthesia device or kinking of the endotracheal tube are the first areas to be checked. Decrease in tidal volume and FRC, which become more evident with an increase in the depth of anesthesia, and an increase in the tendency to atelectasis cause hypoventilation, which in turn causes hypoxia [34].

The reduction in all components of lung volume during anesthesia results in a reduction in airway diameter. The tendency to collapse increases due to increased airway resistance. The presence of an endotracheal tube also contributes to an increase in airway resistance. Mucociliary clearance decreases with low inspired air temperature, inflated endotracheal tube cuff, and use of anesthetic agents such as halothane. All these changes contribute to the formation of hypoxia [35].

Supine position and prolonged immobilization during the operation cause dependent changes in the lung. This contributes to the reduction in FRC. During general anesthesia, high-concentration oxygen inhalation is generally used. As a result of low-ventilated areas, encountering high concentrations of oxygen, atelectatic lung areas due to adsorption occurs. These areas cause a decrease in FRC [36].

Oxygen inhalation should be used with caution during anesthesia. Hyperoxia may cause pulmonary damage. It might vary from tracheobronchitis to pulmonary fibrosis. High oxygen administration may also cause respiratory depression by inhibiting the respiratory center's response to hypoxia [37].

The increase in dead space ventilation because of the anesthesia may cause hypercarbia. Due to the release of catecholamines in superficial anesthesia, oxygen consumption increases and might increase the formation of carbon dioxide [38, 39].

Hypercarbia causes an increase in catecholamine release. This causes a rise in blood pressure. Pulmonary arterial pressure rises and pulmonary vascular resistance increases. An increase in the partial pressure of arterial carbon dioxide ($PaCO_2$) depresses respiration. It increases intracranial pressure by causing cerebral vasodilation. Hypercarbia that develops during general anesthesia, especially during the use of halothane, causes serious arrhythmias [39].

General anesthesia with tracheal intubation may trigger life-threatening bronchospasm in patients with bronchial hyperreactivity; therefore, epidural anesthesia is often preferred in this group of patients. However, segmental high thoracic epidural anesthesia is thought to cause pulmonary sympathetic and respiratory motor blockade. In a study investigating the feasibility of the technique, it was reported that despite sympathetic blockade, high thoracic epidural anesthesia did not increase airway obstruction and caused a slight decrease in FEV1 level; therefore, it could be used as an alternative to general anesthesia in patients with severe COPD [40]. No change was detected in peripheral airway resistance in dogs who underwent thoracic epidural anesthesia, but it has been reported that airway reactivity that occurs with acetylcholine or histamine administration is prolonged, which is due to a decrease in cardiac output [41].

In a meta-analysis evaluating patients who underwent surgery for hip fracture, the effects of general anesthesia and regional anesthesia were compared. As a result of the study, it was determined that there was a decrease in 1-month mortality and the incidence of deep vein thrombosis in patients who underwent regional anesthesia [42]. In a study, patients with severe COPD (FEV1 ≤50%) who were operated for an infrarenal aortic aneurysm were divided into two groups as those who underwent epidural anesthesia and those who received general anesthesia; mortality found higher in general anesthesia group [43]. It has been stated that when epidural and spinal anesthesia are applied together, it is an anesthesia option that can be recommended in the conventional abdominal aortic aneurysm operation because of the preservation of spontaneous breathing in patients with severe COPD [44]. In a study evaluating 7306 patients who underwent gastrointestinal, urological, gynecological, and orthopedic surgery, it was reported that the frequency of pulmonary complications were associated with major surgery and general anesthesia with muscle relaxants [45].

In a study conducted with patients with COPD, mortality was found to be 8% in 464 patients who were administered general anesthesia, while death did not occur in any of 121 patients who underwent spinal and epidural anesthesia [46]. It has been reported that epidural analgesia application in the perioperative period reduces both the need for postoperative mechanical ventilator and the length of stay in the intensive care unit in patients with COPD who underwent elective surgery for abdominal aortic aneurysm [47].

It has been reported that epidural analgesia accelerates postoperative recovery by providing adequate pain control in patients undergoing thoracotomy [48]. In a study comparing the effectiveness of ropivacaine and levobupivacaine for epidural analgesia to be applied during thoracotomy, it was found that both agents produced similar sensory block, morphine consumption was at the same rate, and the incidence of minor side effects was similar [49].

#### 15.2.2.2 Surgery-Related Changes in Pulmonary Function

The location, duration, and technique of the surgical intervention have different effects on respiratory functions. While lower abdomen interventions cause a decrease of up to 25% in vital capacity, upper abdomen interventions cause a 50% decrease, sometimes lasting up to 1 week [50].

The POPC rate is inversely proportional to the distance from the incision to the diaphragm. The incidence of POPC is 10–40% in thoracic surgery, 13–33% in upper abdominal surgery, and 0.16% in lower abdominal surgery [51].

Postoperative pain and dissection of the muscles have a role in the basis of the restrictive type of functional disorder that occurs following the operation and the decrease in lung volumes [52]. Vital capacity (VC) is the lung capacity most affected by surgery, and the decrease in VC varies according to the location of the surgery. The greatest reduction in VC occurs in upper abdominal surgery (down to 37–53% of preoperative values), followed by lower abdominal surgery and non-resectional thoracotomy [52].

In upper abdominal and thoracic surgeries, lung volumes decrease, causing atelectasis and hypoxia. Transdiaphragmatic pressures decrease due to several reasons such as inflammation, surgical trauma, pain, and phrenic nerve inhibition [50, 53].

In a meta-analysis evaluating 43 studies, the rate of POPC was 19.7% for upper abdominal surgery, 7.7% for lower abdominal surgery, 14.2% for any abdominal surgery, 10.3% for head and neck surgery, 5.1% for hip surgery, 5.1% for gynecologic surgery and 1.8% for urological surgery [27]. The incidence of pulmonary complications is highest in patients undergoing major abdominal surgery [54]. In another study, it was reported that the most common postoperative pulmonary complications were seen in coronary artery bypass surgery (60%) and major abdominal surgery (56%) [16].

The rate of POPC in esophageal surgery is very high. In a multicenter study including 1777 patients who underwent esophageal resection, the incidence of pneumonia was found to be 21%, and the incidence of respiratory failure was found to be 16% [55]. Patients with mid-distal esophageal adenocarcinoma or gastric cardia adenocarcinoma invading the distal esophagus were randomized to undergo esophagectomy with the transhiatal or transthoracic approach, and it was reported that the rate of postoperative pulmonary complications was lower with the transhiatal approach (57% vs. 27%) [55].

The deterioration in respiratory functions is more pronounced in cardiac surgery. A 30% decrease in lung volumes is detected. Opening the sternum, trauma to the costal joints, and retraction of the lung during the operation cause decreased chest wall compliance and development of atelectasis, resulting in hypoxia and an increase in the alveolar–arterial gradient [50].

For example, in surgical applications other than thorax and abdomen, significant changes in FRC do not occur. After upper abdomen surgery, there is a decrease in the stimulation of the phrenic nerve by the central nervous system as a result of inhibitory reflexes originating from sympathetic, vagal, and splanchnic receptors. In patients who underwent cholecystectomy, the contribution of the diaphragm to tidal breathing decreases after surgery [29].

The rate of development of pulmonary complications was found to be 3.24 times higher in patients who underwent surgery due to malignant tumor [56].

After lung surgery, atelectasis and oxygenation disorders are common. It is possible to predict the lung volumes that will remain in the postoperative period after resection surgery. After lung resection, a 30% loss in the forced expiratory volume (FEV1) and forced vital capacity (FVC) values in the first second can be observed in the early postoperative period [4].

The type of incision is as important as the type of surgery in predicting the development of POPC. In a study that included patients with COPD and normal lung functions who underwent aorto-iliac surgery, it was stated that the incision type affected the development of postoperative complications. In this study, it was found that increased bronchopneumonia rates in patients who had a midline incision and the FEV1 values of patients with COPD were more impaired with the midline incision, but the incision type did not make any difference in the group with normal lung functions. It was found that the vital capacity decreased similarly in both incisions on the second postoperative day, but the recovery was less in those who underwent a midline incision on the fifth day, and the authors emphasized that laparotomy performed with a transverse incision in patients with COPD caused less pulmonary complications and had better postoperative lung functions [57]. In another study that included patients who underwent abdominal aortic surgery, it was stated that although the rate of pulmonary complications was low in the group that underwent transverse incision, there was no difference in morbidity and analgesia need in general with those who underwent midline incision [58]. It has been reported that vertical incisions have a higher incidence of atelectasis and hypoxemia than horizontal incisions [59].

In a study of 7306 cases [60], it has been reported that emergency surgery is an important risk factor in the development of POPC in elderly patients [61]. In a meta-analysis evaluating six studies, the odds ratio (OR) for emergency surgery was reported as 2.21, and it was stated that patients who underwent emergency surgery were at moderate risk for the development of POPC [27].

In a study, it was reported that the presence of atelectasis detected by the radiologist was less in patients who underwent laparoscopic cholecystectomy compared to those who underwent open surgery (29% vs. 63%) [62].

In a meta-analysis evaluating patients who underwent laparoscopic/open surgery for colorectal cancer, overall mortality was not different between the groups, some complications were less in those who underwent laparoscopic surgery, the laparoscopic method was more reliable in terms of pulmonary complications, although it was not statistically significant, respiratory function parameters defined by spirometry improved faster in patients who underwent laparoscopic surgery. It has been reported that the duration of stay is shorter [63]. In another study conducted in patients who underwent colorectal resection, the rate of pneumonia was found to be less (1.8% vs. 3.5%) in the laparoscopic group, although it did not reach statistical significance [64]. In retrospective cohort studies in which a large number of patients were included, the rate of atelectasis was reported as 2% in those who underwent laparoscopic cholecystectomy, 4% in those who underwent open surgery (36%), and as 2.5% in those who underwent laparoscopic sigmoid resection, and 6% in those who underwent open surgery [46].

In operations lasting longer than 3–4 h, the risk of postoperative complications increases 1.6–5.2 times [65]. Surgery time longer than 210 min is an important indicator for the development of POPC [66]. In a study [67], it was reported that reducing the operation time from 303 ± 72 min to 202 ± 53 min in patients with stage 1 lung cancer who underwent lobectomy decreased the complication rate. In another study that included 1082 patients, one of the most important factors in the development of POPC was defined as an operation time longer than 2 h [68]. In another study evaluating patients who underwent elective abdominal aortic surgery, it was reported that an operation time longer than 5 h caused major pulmonary complications [69].

The duration of surgery and complication development rates were classified in 89 patients with severe COPD. The complication rate was reported to be 4% in patients with a surgical duration of <1 h, 23% in patients with 1–2 h, 38% in patients with 2–4 h, and 73% in patients with >4 h [54].

## 15.3 Evaluation of the Patient

The physical examination should focus on the information obtained during the anamnesis. Cardiovascular and respiratory system examination should be performed in all patients, and if there is excessive secretion, obstruction, emphysema, respiratory failure findings, hypertension, rhythm disturbance, and tachycardia, the underlying disease should be investigated. Obtained abnormal findings should be fully evaluated and examined in detail before elective surgery [13, 70].

In a study evaluating 82 cases with postoperative pulmonary complications, it was found that preoperative respiratory system abnormalities increased the risk of postoperative pulmonary complications 5.8 times after elective abdominal surgery [71].

### 15.3.1 Radiology and Laboratory

In patients without risk factors, the contribution of chest X-ray in preventing the decision to operate is minimal, but it is recommended to be taken because it allows the determination of an underlying silent disease state and a comparative evaluation in the postoperative period [72].

Chest radiography is definitely recommended in the preoperative period for those over 60 years of age, with cardiac or pulmonary problems, and for those in the high-risk group for postoperative pulmonary complications [72]. Chest X-ray is useful in the preoperative period, especially in the presence of new or unexplained symptoms and signs, when a sudden worsening of the symptoms and signs of the underlying disease is detected or if thoracic surgery is to be performed [73].

In a meta-analysis in which eight studies ($n$ = 14,650) were evaluated, an abnormality was found in the chest X-ray taken routinely in the preoperative period in 23.1% of the cases, and only 3% of them required treatment [74]. In another meta-analysis ($n$ = 14,390), in which 21 studies were evaluated, 10% of the cases were found to be abnormal in chest X-ray and only 0.1% required treatment [73].

The most common abnormal findings in the preoperative chest X-ray are findings related to a chronic process, consisting of 15–65% cardiomegaly and 7–30% findings related to COPD. There are publications stating that the acute form of pulmonary congestion and congestive heart failure is also detected at a rate of 6–25% [75].

In American College of Chest Physicians (ACCP) guidelines, chest X-ray has been recommended for patients with cardiopulmonary disease, over 50 years of age, who will undergo upper abdominal, thoracic, or abdominal aortic aneurysm surgery [27].

In patients undergoing cardiovascular, thoracic, or abdominal surgery, arterial blood gas analysis is recommended in the presence of dyspnea or smoking [15, 76]. Patients with hypercapnia ($PaCO_2$ > 45 mmHg) are considered to be at high pulmonary risk for surgical intervention [72].

Hypercapnia and hypoxemia should be a warning in terms of preoperative support, close monitoring in the perioperative and postoperative period, and intensive care support [77].

The most frequently used parameters for preoperative evaluation in spirometric examination are forced expiratory volume in 1 s (FEV1) and forced vital capacity (FVC). It was found that the detection of FEV1 <70%, FVC <70%, and FEV1/FVC <65% increased the risk of postoperative pulmonary complications [15, 77]. However, according to other opinion, spirometry alone is not an independent risk factor for postoperative pulmonary complications [51].

Cardiopulmonary exercise test gives information about the patients' metabolic, ventilatory, gas exchange, blood pressure and ECG measurements, measuring their capacity to increase oxygen delivery during exercise, and the state of maintaining end-organ perfusion after surgery. In elderly patients with heart or lung disease, this test may be useful in predicting whether the patient will tolerate surgery [78].

Measurement of maximal oxygen consumption ($VO_2$ max) with the exercise test is the most useful test for determining postoperative morbidity and mortality. It has been shown that perioperative mortality and risks do not increase in cases where $VO_2$ max is above 15 mL/kg/min in lung resection surgery. In cases where the $VO_2$ max is below 15 mL/kg/min, the risk of postoperative complications increases significantly, and the patient is considered to be at high risk for the operation [79, 80].

## 15.4 Preoperative and Postoperative Risk-Reducing Strategies

Taking the necessary precautions to make the preoperative patient suitable for anesthesia and taking measures to prevent postoperative pulmonary complications constitute risk reduction strategies.

Risk reduction strategies generally include

1. Smoking cessation
2. COPD/Asthma control
3. Preoperative antibiotics, mucolytics (if needed)
4. Patient education
5. Prophylaxis against thrombosis
6. Pulmonary rehabilitation and respiratory exercises

### 15.4.1 Smoking Cessation

Smoking increases the risk of pulmonary complications after surgery. Smoking causes mucus hypersecretion, decrease in ciliary activity, and deterioration in mucociliary clearance. In the postoperative period, increased secretions, pulmonary ventilation disorders, atelectasis, hypoxemia, and lung infections are the main complications that may develop due to smoking. On the other hand, physiological changes such as blood pressure, heart rate, and increased oxygen demand, which are caused by the pharmacological effects of tobacco products such as carbon monoxide (CO) and nicotine, contribute to complications [81]. It has been shown that the duration of mechanical ventilator requirement is prolonged after the operation in patients who continue to smoke before the surgical operation. For this reason, in order to prevent the complications that may occur due to smoking, it is recommended that the patient who has decided to have an operation stop smoking must be abandoned. If necessary, the patient should be given medical support to quit smoking [81].

The idea of quitting smoking at least 8 weeks before the operation in order to reduce the complication rate of the patient who is planned for elective surgery has been supported by many studies [82, 83].

### 15.4.2 COPD/Asthma Control

Appropriate bronchodilators and inhaled corticosteroid treatments should be administered to COPD cases as recommended by the GOLD guideline [84]. Breathing exercises and respiratory physiotherapy should be applied to the appropriate patient. It may be appropriate for patients with moderate or severe respiratory function test disorder to switch to the nebulizer form before the operation and receive their treatment. If there is an acute exacerbation of COPD or a lung infection, the operation is postponed. For respiratory tract infection, treatment with antibiotics in the appropriate spectrum should be given in an appropriate time. If the patient has hypoxemia, oxygen should be given, and if the $PaCO_2$ is high, especially in the patient with type 2 respiratory failure, noninvasive mechanical ventilation should be applied if necessary [11].

In cases with high risk of atelectasis and infection in the postoperative period, regular administration of *N*-acetyl cysteine and effective physiotherapy is important for easier removal of secretions [11]. In the postoperative period, pain relief, early extubation, early mobilization, bronchodilator, and oxygen therapy should be continued in order to use the diaphragm comfortably [11].

In studies conducted with asthmatic patients who underwent surgery, bronchospasm was found in 1.7%, respiratory failure in 0.1%, and laryngospasm in 0.3% [11, 17]. Optimal treatment should be arranged to keep the FEV1 or peak flow rate (PEF) value above 80% in asthmatic patients undergoing elective surgery. In asthmatic patients, the use of inhaler bronchodilators should continue until just before the operation. In patients with asthma who have not been fully controlled, it may be considered that the drugs they use in inhaler form should be switched to nebule form 1–2 days before the operation and receive their treatment. Provided that it is evaluated on a case-by-case basis, intravenous steroids may be helpful in reducing perioperative bronchospasm [84]. Treatment with drugs in the form of nebules can be continued after the operation [84, 85].

### 15.4.3 Preoperative Antibiotics/Mucolytics

Pneumonia is common after long-term endotracheal intubation, thorax, and upper abdomen surgical operations. For this purpose, treatment is planned against agents with the highest potential for infection [86]. Indiscriminate use of prophylactic antibiotics should be avoided as it does not reduce pulmonary complications. Preoperative routine antibiotic use is not recommended for the prevention of pneumonia in patients with stable COPD or controlled asthma, unless other disorders such as acute bronchitis, bronchiectasis, or immunodeficiency are present [84]. Postponement of elective surgery should be considered in patients with purulent sputum or changes in sputum character and those with underlying disease such as COPD [84].

### 15.4.4 Patient Education

The main purpose of patient education is to prevent complications that may occur in cooperation with the patient before and after the operation and to inform the patient about these complications. Patient education should be given 2–3 days before surgery if possible. The risk profile of the patient should be prepared and the patient should be told about the condition and the risks that may develop after the operation, the effect of the planned operation on the respiratory system, the procedures to be performed, and the operation process. The importance of coughing, respiratory physiotherapy, and patient compliance during the period of weaning from the ventilator should be explained to the patient. Postural drainage, vibration, percussion, coughing, mucus clearence and lung expansion device use, huffing, and humidification techniques should be taught in patients with high secretion before surgery, and secretion drainage should be provided with these techniques. Postoperative rapid mobilization should be provided [87].

### 15.4.5 Prophylaxis Against Thrombosis

Pulmonary thromboembolism (PTE) secondary to deep venous thrombosis (DVT) is defined as one of the most serious pulmonary problems that can develop after the operation [88]. Underlying malignancies, advanced age, and prolonged immobilization increase the risk of PTE [89]. Prophylactic interventions to prevent the development of DVT after surgery, leg elevation, elastic bandage, compression stockings, use of pressurized compressor devices, lower extremity exercises, and early mobilization. In addition, attention should be paid to linen-clothing folds, cross-positioning of the legs, catheter contacts and pressures that impair blood circulation. Lower extremity exercises and early mobilization are contraindicated in patients with DVT [90].

### 15.4.6 Pulmonary Rehabilitation and Respiratory Exercises

The active return of the patient to his/her functional life after the surgical operation and the absence of additional surgical problems depend on well-planned pulmonary rehabilitation programs to be applied in the preoperative and postoperative periods, as well as a good surgical intervention. Pulmonary rehabilitation is created individually depending on the risk profile of the patient and the operation [81, 85].

Analysis of the patient's risk profile, evaluation of respiratory system symptoms such as shortness of breath, cough, sputum, chest pain, arterial blood gas analysis, chest X-ray, pain evaluation, functional capacity and quality of life evaluation, and posture analysis of the patient to establish the right exercise program, measurement of joint range of motion, peripheral and respiratory muscle strength are included in the scope of pulmonary rehabilitation [91].

#### 15.4.6.1 Preoperative Pulmonary Rehabilitation

Appropriate chest physiotherapy, aerobic exercise program, and smoking cessation should be included in the preoperative pulmonary rehabilitation program in order to reduce postoperative pulmonary complications and thus morbidity and mortality rates, to minimize possible risks, and to shorten the healing process [91].

In order to use applications to improve respiratory capacity in the preoperative period in patients with respiratory tract infection, bronchiectasis, and COPD, information and training should be provided about pursed-lip breathing, diaphragmatic breathing, deep breathing exercises, and the use of incentive spirometry [91]. In studies, it was found that inspiratory muscle strength and respiratory functions of the patients improved with preoperative incentive spirometry and inspiratory muscle training, and inspiratory muscle strength training applied in the preoperative period reduced postoperative complications and hospital stay of the patients [91].

#### 15.4.6.2 Postoperative Pulmonary Rehabilitation

The first aim after extubation is to increase optimal alveolar ventilation, increase lung volume and capacity (especially FRC), improve effective coughing, and provide ventilation of suspected atelectatic areas that receive mechanical compression during surgery [92]. If there is no contraindication, early mobilization with respiratory control should be performed to ensure normal FRC and alveolar ventilation from the earliest period. Also coughing and deep breathing exercises should be performed hourly to increase alveolar volume and to regulate ventilation distribution [92, 93].

One of the methods frequently used in the pulmonary rehabilitation program is early mobilization and general body exercises. The patient should be mobilized with increasing intensity in accordance with his/her condition. In patients undergoing abdominal surgery, it is recommended to mobilize themselves in the bed as soon as possible with a rope tied to the end of the bed, to sit on the edge of the bed with their feet hanging off the bed, and to increase the walking distance according to the patient's clinic. Patients undergoing thoracic surgery should perform postural correction and upper extremity exercises to increase thoracic mobility [93, 94]. Especially in patients with thoracotomy, from the first postoperative day, exercises that increase shoulder, head–neck, rib cage mobility and provide postural smoothness can prevent the operated side shoulder depression and trunk lateral flexion tendency [95, 96]. Since pain, cardiopulmonary limitations, peripheral muscle weakness, and fatigue reduce the exercise capacity of patients in the postoperative period, exercise bands and exercises that improve muscle strength, endurance, and aerobic capacity should be included in the exercise program, as well as early mobilization. It is important to gradually increase the intensity of the exercise program and to perform all exercises with respiratory control [95].

In cases where mobilization of the patient cannot be performed or delayed due to the type of surgery, clinical condition of the patient or pain, it is important to position the patient correctly in the earliest period. The high-head lying position given to the patients prevents the formation of micro atelectasis by reducing the risk of aspiration of stomach contents, ensures that the diaphragm functions more effectively due to the loose abdominal muscles and increases FRC [95].

In cases that mobilization is delayed and positioning cannot be performed exactly, respiratory exercise techniques that increase ventilation and provide bronchial hygiene should be performed in order to prevent the development of pulmonary complications. Thoracic expansion exercises are techniques that can also be used with devices that stimulate coughing by providing secretion drainage. In appropriate cases, aspiration should also be used [96]. It is recommended that applications aimed at providing bronchial hygiene should be repeated after the operation, frequently with 15–30 min intervals, as soon as the patient wakes up [96].

Pursed-lip breathing to increase ventilation prevents airway collapse. By holding the breath for a few seconds at the end of the inspiration, thoracic expansion breathing exercises performed with at least five repetitions three times a day, and diaphragmatic breathing exercises increase regional ventilation, provide ventilation of collapsed alveoli, and facilitate coughing by increasing inspiratory capacity [92, 97].

The development of postoperative hypoxemia and atelectasis can be prevented with the incentive spirometer device, which improves the inspiratory capacity and enables effective coughing. Incentive spirometry is recommended to be used especially in patients who cannot perform respiratory exercises and who are at risk of atelectasis. In addition, the fact that the incentive spirometer can be used independently by the patient is an important advantage in terms of ensuring the active participation of the patient in the treatment [98]. In general, the patient is asked to work with an incentive spirometer in the form of ten repetitions with an interval of 1–2 h at the earliest postoperative period [98]. It consists of holding the breath for 3–5 s after a slow, long, and deep inspiration, starting from the functional residual capacity until the total lung capacity is reached. Thus, it provides collateral ventilation in the alveoli and strengthens the inspiratory muscles. The use of percussion providing secretion excretion and chest wall vibration in cases where coughing and breathing exercises are ineffective in secretion excretion will contribute to bronchial hygiene [98].

The use of percussion providing secretion excretion and chest wall vibration in cases where coughing and breathing exercises are ineffective in secretion excretion will contribute to bronchial hygiene [98].

According to the patient's clinic, the use of postoperative positive airway therapy (PAP) increases vital capacity, decreases respiratory frequency and minute ventilation, increases FRC, decreases respiratory workload by improving lung compliance and collateral ventilation [99]. PAP is important in terms of preventing complications, especially in the first 4 h postoperatively [98]. It has been proven that the use of PAP prevents the development of atelectasis and pneumonia more than deep breathing exercises, incentive spirometry, and coughing techniques. In the study performed, the rate of atelectasis development on the third postoperative day was found to be 23% in the PAP group, whereas 42% in the group given deep breathing exercises and coughing training, and 41% in the group working with incentive spirometry [99].

## References


1. Brooks-Brunn JA. Predictors of postoperative pulmonary complications following abdominal surgery. Chest. 1997;111:564–71.
2. Ferguson MK. Preoperative assessment of pulmonary risk. Chest. 1999;115:58–63.
3. Mitchell CK, Smoger SH, Pfeifer MP, et al. Multivariate analysis of factors associated with postoperative pulmonary complications following general elective surgery. Arch Surg. 1998;133:194–8.

4. O'Donohue WJ Jr. Postoperative pulmonary complications. When are preventive and therapeutic measures necessary? Postgrad Med. 1992;91:167–75.
5. Hall JC, Tarala RA, Hall JL, Mander J. A multivariate analysis of the risk of pulmonary complications after laparotomy. Chest. 1991;99:923–7.
6. Gracey DR, Divertie MB, Didier EP. Preoperative pulmonary preparation of patients with chronic obstructive pulmonary disease: a prospective study. Chest. 1979;76:123–9.
7. Bapoje S, Whitaker J, Schulz T, et al. Preoperative evaluation of the patient with pulmonary disease. Chest. 2007;132:1637–45.
8. Stéphan F, Boucheseiche S, Hollande J, et al. Pulmonary complications following lung resection: a comprehensive analysis of incidence and possible risk factors. Chest. 2000;118:1263–70.
9. McAlister FA, Khan NA, Straus SE, et al. Accuracy of the pre-operative assessment in predicting pulmonary risk after nonthoracic surgery. Am J Respir Crit Care Med. 2003;167:741–4.
10. Qaseem A, Snow V, Fitterman N, et al. Risk assessment for and strategies to reduce perioperative pulmonary complications for patients undergoing noncardiothoracic surgery: a guideline from the American College of Physicians. Ann Intern Med. 2006;144:575–80.
11. Smentana GW. Preoperative pulmonary evaluation: identifying and reducing risks for pulmonary complications. Cleve Clin J Med. 2006;73:36–41.
12. Kroenke K, Lawrence VA, Theroux JF, et al. Postoperative complications after thoracic and major abdominal surgery in patients with and without obstructive lung disease. Chest. 1993;104:1445–51.
13. Lawrence VA, Dhanda R, Hilsenbeck SG, Page CP. Risk of pulmonary complications after elective abdominal surgery. Chest. 1996;110:744–50.
14. Fuster RG, Argudo JAM, Albarova OG, et al. Prognostic value of chronic obstructive pulmonary disease in coronary artery bypass grafting. Eur J Cardiothorac Surg. 2006;29:202–9.
15. Milledge JS, Nunn JF. Criteria of fitness for anesthesia in patients with chronic obstructive lung disease. BMJ. 1975;3:670–3.
16. Kroenke K, Lawrence VA, Theroux JF, Tuley MR. Operative risk in patients with severe obstructive pulmonary disease. Arch Intern Med. 1992;152:967–71.
17. Warner DO, Warner MA, Barnes RD, et al. Perioperative respiratory complications in patients with asthma. Anesthesiology. 1996;85:460–7.
18. Woods BD, Sladen RN. Perioperative considerations for the patient with asthma and bronchospasm. Br J Anaesth. 2009;103(Suppl 1):57–65.
19. Barrera R, Shi W, Amar D, et al. Smoking and timing of cessation. Impact on pulmonary complications after thoracotomy. Chest. 2005;127:1977–83.
20. Wetterslev J, Hansen EG, Kamp-Jensen M, et al. $PaO_2$ during anaesthesia and years of smoking predict late postoperative hypoxaemia and complications after upper abdominal surgery in patients without preoperative cardiopulmonary dysfunction. Acta Anaesthesiol Scand. 2000;44:9–16.
21. Warner MA, Offort KP, Wamer ME, et al. Role of preoperative cessation of smoking and other factors in postoperative pulmonary complications: a blinded prospective study of coronary artery bypass patients. Mayo Clin Proc. 1989;64:609–16.
22. Pasulka PS, Bistrian BR, Benotti PN, Blackburn GL. The risk of surgery in obese patients. Ann Intern Med. 1986;104:540–6.
23. Trayner EM, Girish M, Gottleib S, et al. Symptom limited stair climbing and the cardiopulmonary risk index as predictors of post operative pulmonary complications after high risk surgery—a multicenter trial. Am J Respir Crit Care Med. 1995;151:292.
24. Arslan V, Barrera R, Ginsberg R, et al. Cardiopulmonary risk index (CPRI) does not predict complications after thoracic surgery. Am J Respir Crit Care Med. 1996;153:676.
25. Gross JB, Bachenberg KL, Benumof JL, et al. Practice guidelines for the perioperative management of patients with obstructive sleep apnea: a report by the American Society of Anesthesiologists Task Force on Perioperative Management of patients with obstructive sleep apnea. Anesthesiology. 2006;104:1081–93.

26. Ramakrishna G, Sprung J, Ravi BS, et al. Impact of pulmonary hypertension on the outcomes of noncardiac surgery: predictors of perioperative morbidity and mortality. J Am Coll Cardiol. 2005;45:1691–9.
27. Smentana GW, Lawrence VA, Cornell JE, American College of Physicians. Preoperative pulmonary risk stratification for non-cardiothoracic surgery: systematic review for the American College of Physicians. Ann Intern Med. 2006;144:581–95.
28. Arozullah AM, Daley J, Henderson WG, Khuri SF. Multifactorial risk index for predicting postoperative respiratory failure in men after major noncardiac surgery. The National Veterans Administration Surgical Quality Improvement Program. Ann Surg. 2000;232:242–53.
29. DeLisser HM, Grippi MA. Perioperative respiratory considerations in the surgical patient. In: Fishman AP, editor. Fishman's pulmonary diseases and disorders. 3rd ed. New York: McGraw-Hill; 1998. p. 619–29.
30. Spence AA. Postoperative complications. In: Nunn JF, Utting JE, Brown Jr BR, editors. General anaesthesia. 5th ed. London: Butterworths; 1989. p. 1149–60.
31. Hedenstierna G, Edmark L. The effects of anesthesia and muscle paralysis on the respiratory system. Intensive Care Med. 2005;31:1327–35.
32. Warner DO, Rehder K. Infuence of anesthesia on the thorax. In: Roussos C, editor. The thorax. 2nd ed. New York: Marcel Dekker; 1995. p. 1585–98.
33. Simonneau G, Vivien A, Sartene R, et al. Diaphragm dysfunction induced by upper abdominal surgery. Role of postoperative pain. Am Rev Respir Dis. 1983;128:899–903.
34. Wiener-Kronish JP, Albert RK. Preoperative evaluation. In: Murray JF, Nadel JA, editors. Textbook of respiratory medicine, vol. 1. W.B. Saunders Company; 2000. p. 883–94.
35. Wynne R, Botti M. Postoperative pulmonary dysfunction in adults after cardiac surgery with cardiopulmonary by-pass: clinical significance and implications for practice. Am J Crit Care. 2004;13:384–93.
36. Owens MW, Milligan SA, Eggerstedt JM. Thoracic trauma, surgery, and perioperative management. In: George RB, Light RW, Matthay MA, Matthay RA, editors. Chest medicine. Essential of pulmonary and critical care medicine. 5th ed. Lippincott Williams & Wilkins; 2005. p. 564–88.
37. Allardet-Servent J, Sicard G, Metz V, Chiche L. Benefits and risks of oxygen therapy during acute medical illness: just a matter of dose! Rev Med Interne. 2019;40(10):670–6.
38. Bigatello L, Pesenti A. Respiratory physiology for the anesthesiologist. Anesthesiology. 2019;130(6):1064–77.
39. Davenport HT, Auld PA, Sekelj P, Jegıer W, Mcgregor M. Hypercarbia during light halothane anesthesia with neuromuscular block. Anesthesiology. 1964;25:307–11.
40. Groeben H, Schäfer B, Pavlakovic G, et al. Lung function under high thoracic segmental epidural anesthesia with ropivacaine or bupivacaine in patients with severe obstructive pulmonary disease undergoing breast surgery. Anesthesiology. 2002;96:536–41.
41. Yuan HB, Tang GJ, Kou YR, Lee TY. Effects of high thoracic epidural anaesthesia on the peripheral airway reactivity in dogs. Acta Anaesthesiol Scand. 1998;42:85–90.
42. Urwin SC, Parker MJ, Griffiths R. General versus regional anaesthesia for hip fracture surgery: a meta-analysis of randomized trials. Br J Anaesth. 2000;84:450–5.
43. Kalko Y, Ugurlucan M, Basaran M, et al. Epidural anaesthesia and minilaparotomy for the treatment of abdominal aortic aneurysms in patients with severe chronic obstructive pulmonary disease. Acta Chir Belg. 2007;107:307–12.
44. Flores JA, Nishibe T, Koyama M, et al. Combined spinal and epidural anesthesia for abdominal aortic aneurysm surgery in patients with severe chronic pulmonary obstructive disease. Int Angiol. 2002;21:218–21.
45. Pedersen T, Eliasen K, Henriksen E. A prospective study of risk factors and cardiopulmonary complications associated with anaesthesia and surgery: risk indicators of cardiopulmonary morbidity. Acta Anaesthesiol Scand. 1990;34:144–55.
46. Guller U, Jain N, Hervey S, et al. Laparoscopic vs open colectomy: outcomes comparison based on large nationwide databases. Arch Surg. 2003;138:1179–86.

47. Bush RL, Lin PH, Reddy PP, et al. Epidural analgesia in patients with chronic obstructive pulmonary disease undergoing transperitoneal abdominal aortic aneurysm—a multiinstitutional analysis. Cardiovasc Surg. 2003;11:179–84.
48. Dango S, Offner K, Kirschbaum A, et al. Epidural analgesia in thoracic surgery optimising postoperative rehabilitation. Zentralbl Chir. 2008;133:491–7.
49. De Cosmo G, Congedo E, Lai C, et al. Ropivacaine vs. levobupivacaine combined with sufentanil for epidural analgesia after lung surgery. Eur J Anaesthesiol. 2008;25:1020–5.
50. Dureuil B, Cantineau JP, Desmonts JM. Effects of upper or lower abdominal surgery on diafragmatic functions. Br J Anaesth. 1987;59:1230–5.
51. Smentana GW. Preoperative pulmonary evaluation. N Engl J Med. 1999;340:937–44.
52. Ali J, Weisel RD, Layug AB, et al. Consequences of postoperative alterations in respiratory mechanism. Am J Surg. 1974;128:376–82.
53. Hall JC, Tarala RA, Tappert J, Hall JL. Prevention of respiratory complications after abdominal surgery: a randomised clinical trial. BMJ. 1996;312:148–52.
54. Pedersen T. Complications and death following anesthesia. A prospective study with special reference to the influence of patient, anesthesia, and surgery related risk factors. Dan Med Bull. 1994;41:319–31.
55. Bailey SH, Bull DA, Harpole DH, et al. Outcomes after esophagectomy: a ten year prospective cohort. Ann Thorac Surg. 2003;75:217–22.
56. Fuso L, Cisternino L, Di Napoli A, et al. Role of spirometric and arterial gas data in predicting pulmonary complications after abdominal surgery. Respir Med. 2000;94:1171–6.
57. Becquemin JP, Piquet J, Becquemin MH, et al. Pulmonary function after transverse or midline incision in patients with obstructive pulmonary disease. Intensive Care Med. 1985;11:247–51.
58. Lacy PD, Burke PE, O'Regan M, et al. The comparison of type of incision for transperitoneal abdominal aortic surgery based on postoperative respiratory complications and morbidity. Eur J Vasc Surg. 1994;8:52–5.
59. Halasz NA. Vertical vs. horizontal laparotomies—early postoperative comparisons. Arch Surg. 1964;88:911–4.
60. Pedersen T, Eliasen K, Henriksen E. A prospective study of mortality associated with anaesthesia and surgery: risk indicators of mortality in hospital. Acta Anaesthesiol Scand. 1990;34:176–82.
61. Smentana GW. Preoperative pulmonary assessment of the older adult. Clin Geriatr Med. 2003;19:35–55.
62. Karayiannakis AJ, Makri GG, Mantzioka A, et al. Postoperative pulmonary function after laparoscopic and open cholecystectomy. Br J Anaesth. 1996;77:448–52.
63. Abraham NS, Young JM, Solomon MJ. Meta-analysis of short term outcomes after laparoscopic resection for colorectal cancer. Br J Surg. 2004;91:1111–24.
64. Vignali A, Braga M, Zuliani W, et al. Laparoscopic colorectal surgery modifies risk factors for postoperative morbidity. Dis Colon Rectum. 2004;47:1686–93.
65. Tarhan S, Moffitt EA, Sessler AD, et al. Risk of anesthesia and surgery in patients with chronic bronchitis and chronic obstructive pulmonary disease. Surgery. 1973;74:720–6.
66. Filardo Fde A, Faresin SM, Fernandes AL. Index for a pulmonary postoperative complication after upper abdominal surgery: a validation study. Rev Assoc Med Bras. 2002;48:209–16.
67. Haraguchi S, Koizumi K, Hatori N, et al. Prediction of the postoperative pulmonary function and complication rate in elderly patients. Surg Today. 2001;31:860–5.
68. Iannuzzi C, Terracciano CA, Santangelo E, et al. Multifactorial surgical risk index of the development of respiratory complications. Ann Ital Chir. 1992;63:439–42.
69. Calligaro KD, Azurin DJ, Dougherty MJ, et al. Pulmonary risk factors of elective abdominal aortic surgery. J Vasc Surg. 1993;18:914–20.
70. Pratter MR, Curley FJ, Dubois J. Cause and evaluation of chronic dyspnea in a pulmonary disease clinic. Arch Intern Med. 1989;149:2277–82.
71. Sweitze BJ, Smetana GW. Identification and evaluation of the patient with lung disease. Anesthesiol Clin. 2009;27:673–86.

72. Doyle RL. Assessing and modifying the risk of postoperative pulmonary complications. Chest. 1999;115:77–81.
73. Archer C, Levy AR, McGregor M. Value of routine preoperative chest x-rays: a metaanalysis. Can J Anesth. 1993;40:1022–7.
74. Smentana GW, Macperson DS. The case against routine preoperative laboratory testing. Med Clin North Am. 2003;87:7–40.
75. Joo HS, Wong J, Naik VN, Savoldelli GL. The value of screening preoperative chest x-rays: a systematic review. Can J Anesth. 2005;52:568–74.
76. Powell NB, Riley RW, Guilleminault C, Murcia GN. Obstructive sleep apnea, continuous positive airway pressure, and surgery. Otolaryngol Head Neck Surg. 1988;99:362–9.
77. Gass GD, Olsen GN. Preoperative pulmonary function testing to predict postoperative morbidity and mortality. Chest. 1986;89:127–35.
78. Vintch JRE, Hansen JE. Preoperative evaluation and relation to postoperative complications. In: Crapo JD, Glassroth J, Karlinsky J, King TE, editors. Baum's textbook of pulmonary disease. 7th ed. Lippincot Williams & Wilkins; 2004. p. 113–32.
79. Pate P, Tenholder MF, Griffin JP. Preoperative assesment of high risk patient for lung resection. Ann Thorac Surg. 1996;61:1494–500.
80. Larsen KR, Svedsen UG, Milman N. Exercise testing in the preoperative evaluation of patients with bronchogenic carcinoma. Eur Respir J. 1997;10:1559–65.
81. Moores LK. Smoking and postoperative pulmonary complications. An evidence-based review of the recent literature. Clin Chest Med. 2000;21:139–46.
82. Theodoma A, Cropley M, Prevettoni G, Webb G. The effectiveness of smoking cessations interventions prior to surgery: a systemic review. Nicotine Tob Res. 2008;10:407–12.
83. Zaki A, Abrishami A, Wong J, Chung FF. Interventions in the perioperative clinic for long term smoking cessation: a quantitative systemic review. Can J Anesth. 2008;55:11–21.
84. Stoller JK. Clinical practice. Acute exacerbations of chronic obstructive pulmonary disease. N Engl J Med. 2002;346:988–94.
85. Mercado DL, Petty BG. Perioperative medication management. Med Clin North Am. 2003;87:41–57.
86. Weed HG. Antimicrobial prophylaxis in the surgical patient. Med Clin North Am. 2003;87:59–75.
87. Carrie LES, Simpson PJ, Popat MT. Preoperative preparation. Practical procedures. Update Anesth. 1997;7:2–12.
88. Kaboli P, Henderson MC, White RH. DVT prophylaxis and anticoagulation in the surgical patient. Med Clin North Am. 2003;87:77–110.
89. Chan AT, Atiemo A, Diran LK, et al. Venous thromboembolism occurs frequently in patients undergoing brain tumor surgery despite prophylaxis. J Thromb Thrombolysis. 1999;8:139–42.
90. Cohen AT, Davitson BL, Gallus AS, et al. Efficacy and safety of fondaparinux for the prevention of VTE in older acute medical patients. BMJ. 2006;332:325–9.
91. Hulzebos EHJ, Helders PJM, Favie NJ, et al. Preoperative intensive inspiratory muscle training to prevent postoperative pulmonary complications in high risk patients undergoing CABG surgery: a randomized clinical trial. JAMA. 2006;296:1851–7.
92. Takaoka ST, Weinacker AB. The value of pulmonary rehabilitation. Thorac Surg Clin. 2005;15:203–11.
93. Sekine Y, Chiyo M, Lwata T, et al. Perioperative rehabilitation and physiotherapy for lung cancer patient with chronic obstructive pulmonary disease. Jpn J Thorac Cardiovasc Surg. 2005;53:237–43.
94. Varella G, Ballesteros E, Jimenes MF, et al. Cost effectiveness analysis of prophylactic respiratory physiotherapy in pulmonary lobectomy. Eur J Cardiothorac Surg. 2006;29:216–20.
95. Rochester CL. Pulmonary rehabilitation for patients who undergo lung volume reduction surgery or lung transplantation. Respir Care. 2008;53:1196–202.
96. Reeve J, Denehy L, Stiller K. The physiotherapy management of patients undergoing thoracic surgery: a survey of current practice in Australia and New Zealand. Physiother Res Int. 2007;12:59–71.

97. Ries AL, Bouldoff GS, Carlin BW, et al. Pulmonary rehabilitation: joint ACCP/AACVPR evidence-based clinical practice guidelines. Chest. 2007;13:4–42.
98. Overand TJ, Anderson CM, Lucy SD, et al. The effect of incentive spirometry on postoperative pulmonary complications: a systematic review. Chest. 2001;120:971–8.
99. Denehy L, Berney S. The use of positive pressure devices by physiotherapy. Eur Resp J. 2001;17:821–9.

# Preoperative Cardiovascular Assessment and Perioperative Management of Patients with Esophageal Cancer

16

Bektas Murat, Selda Murat, and Tolga Sinan Guvenc

## Abbreviations

| | |
|---|---|
| 6MWT | 6-min walking test |
| ACS | Acute coronary syndrome |
| AF | Atrial fibrillation |
| AR | Aortic regurgitation |
| AS | Aortic stenosis |
| ASA | Acetylsalicylic acid |
| ASA-PS | American Society of Anesthesiologists Physical Status |
| ATP | Antiplatelet therapy |
| AVR | Aortic valve replacement |
| BB | Beta-blocker |
| BMS | Bare-metal stents |
| BNP | Brain natriuretic peptide |
| CAD | Coronary artery disease |
| CARP | Coronary artery revascularization prophylaxis |
| CCTA | Coronary computed tomography angiography |
| CPET | Cardiopulmonary exercise test |
| CV | Cardiovascular |
| DAPT | Dual antiplatelet therapy |

B. Murat
Cardiology Department, Eskisehir City Hospital, Eskisehir, Turkey

S. Murat
Cardiology Department, Eskisehir Osmangazi University Faculty of Medicine, Eskisehir, Turkey

T. S. Guvenc (✉)
Cardiology Department, Istinye University School of Medicine, Istanbul, Turkey
e-mail: tolgasinan.guvenc@istinye.edu.tr


O. Engin (ed.), *Risk Factors and Therapy of Esophagus Cancer*,
https://doi.org/10.1007/978-3-031-47024-0_16

| | |
|---|---|
| DES | Drug-eluting stents |
| EC | Esophageal cancer |
| ECG | Electrocardiography |
| ESC | European Society of Cardiology |
| ESCC | Esophageal squamous cell cancer |
| HF | Heart failure |
| Hs-cTn T/I | High-sensitivity cardiac troponin |
| HT | Hypertension |
| ICV | Invasive coronary angiography |
| LMWH | Low molecular weight heparin |
| MACE | Major adverse cardiac events |
| MI | Myocardial infarction |
| MINS | Myocardial injury after noncardiac surgery |
| MR | Mitral regurgitation |
| MS | Mitral stenosis |
| NCS | Noncardiac surgery |
| NOAC | Non-vitamin K antagonist oral anticoagulant |
| NSQIP | National Surgical Quality Improvement Program |
| NT-proBNP | N-terminal fragment of the prohormone BNP |
| OAC | Oral anticoagulant |
| PCI | Percutaneous coronary intervention |
| PER | Pre-operative esophagectomy risk |
| RCRI | Revised Cardiac Risk Index |
| TAVI | Transcatheter aortic valve implantation |
| TTE | Transthoracic echocardiography |
| VHD | Valvular heart disease |
| VKA | Vitamin K antagonists |
| VTE | Venous thromboembolism |

## 16.1 Introduction

Esophageal cancer (EC) is the sixth leading cause of cancer death and the eighth most common cancer worldwide [1]. Advances in the management and treatment of EC patients have improved over the years. However, the 5-year survival rate is still around 10%. The 5-year survival rate after esophagectomy varies between 15% and 40% [2]. The current main standard of care for resectable EC is multimodality therapy, combining perioperative chemotherapy or chemoradiotherapy with surgery [3, 4]. This multimodality approach has resulted in a 5-year overall survival rate of 50% [5]. However, esophagectomy remains the most effective treatment modality for EC. Esophagectomy is associated with several serious postoperative cardiac and non-cardiac complications, including pulmonary complications, anastomotic leakage, new-onset atrial fibrillation (AF), venous thromboembolism, and myocardial infarction (MI) [6–9]. While esophageal surgery can be performed using open techniques, minimally invasive, hybrid, or robotic techniques have also been used in recent years. Regardless of the surgical technique, esophagectomy is associated with high morbidity of 17–74% and mortality in up to 3–5% of cases, even when performed in high-volume centers [10, 11].

According to the European Society of Cardiology (ESC) guidelines for non-cardiac surgery (NCS), esophagectomy is considered a high-risk procedure for postoperative cardiovascular (CV) complications, with an expected 1-month CV death or MI risk >5% [12]. In addition to the stage of EC, surgical challenge and perioperative CV complications are important causes of morbidity and mortality associated with EC surgery. For patient safety, CV risk should be assessed before surgery. Perioperative management is another important step to reduce postoperative risk and improve patient survival and care. In this section, preoperative cardiac risk assessment scores, ischemic and non-ischemic cardiac risk assessment, preoperative cardiac testing, and management of postoperative outcomes in EC patients are reviewed in detail [12].

## 16.2 Definitions of Perioperative Cardiac Risk and Urgency

Definitions of surgical risk, timing of surgery, and patient-related factors should be considered in the perioperative evaluation. Surgical risk is determined by the type and duration of surgery and the urgency of the procedure or intervention. In addition, perioperative cardiac risk is variably defined and may include the risk of myocardial ischemia and injury, myocardial infarction (MI), heart failure (HF), arrhythmias, stroke, and death. The definition of perioperative cardiac events often includes MI and cardiac arrest or death as major adverse cardiac events (MACE). Another definition is myocardial injury after noncardiac surgery (MINS). MINS is defined as an elevated troponin during the first 30 days after NCS, presumed to be of ischemic etiology. MINS occurs in 10–20% of patients and is associated with worse outcomes 30 days after surgery [12].

### 16.2.1 Surgical Risk Definition

Surgical risk definitions are based on one-month risk rates of CV death, MI, and stroke that consider only the specific surgical procedure without regard to the patient's comorbidities as follows: high risk >5%, intermediate risk ≥1% to ≤5%, low risk <1% [12].

#### 16.2.1.1 Definitions for Timing of Surgery

According to urgency, the ESC guideline on NCS and the American College of Cardiology/American Heart Association (ACC/AHA) perioperative clinical practice guideline classify procedures into immediate (emergent), urgent, time-sensitive, and elective categories as follows [12, 13]:

1. **Emergent/Immediate**: A procedure should be performed in an emergency to save life or organ function (within 6 h).
2. **Urgent**: A procedure should be performed without unnecessary delay to save life, limb, or organ function (6–24 h).
3. **Time-sensitive**: A procedure should be performed as soon as possible as there is a time-dependent risk of losing limb or organ function or increased risk of complications (1–6 weeks). Cancer surgery is typically time-sensitive.
4. **Elective**: A procedure can be performed electively (not further defined) without significant risk of losing limb, or organ function, or increased risks of complications (for up to 12 months).

## 16.3 Preoperative Cardiac Risk Assessment and Risk Reduction

Risk prediction is fundamental to determine eligibility for EC surgery, promote a care-related quality improvement process, assist patients, guide treatment decisions, and reduce perioperative cardiac risk. Preoperative risk stratification is based on patient-related factors such as age and presence or absence of comorbidities, as well as other factors such as center surgical expertise, timing of surgery, and pathological findings related to EC [12, 13].

While several models are available to predict mortality after esophagectomy, none of these risk prediction models have sufficient accuracy to predict postoperative morbidity and mortality and therefore should not be considered as a stand-alone tool to evaluate a given patient's eligibility for surgery. In addition, most of these tools predict all-cause mortality and are not calibrated to predict cardiac risk after EC surgery. However, as objective measures of postoperative events, these tools can be used in the preoperative evaluation of EC patients (Table 16.1) [12–14].

## 16.4 Cardiac Risk Assessment Scores

All patients scheduled to undergo NCS should have an initial assessment of the risk (in percent) of a perioperative CV cardiac event using validated models that typically incorporate information from the patient's medical history, physical examination, electrocardiography (ECG), and surgical approach and timing [13, 14]. As noted above, patients undergoing esophagectomy are at high risk for postoperative cardiac complications regardless of a given patient's baseline characteristics [12]. The American Society of Anesthesiologists Physical Status (ASA-PS) classification system and clinical risk assessment models such as the Revised Cardiac Risk Index (RCRI) or the National Surgical Quality Improvement Program (NSQIP) are recommended to quantify risk in patients with CV disease [12–14].

**Table 16.1** Available risk assessment tools that can be used to predict postoperative adverse events (including cardiovascular events) following esophagectomy

| Scores | Definitions and variables |
|---|---|
| American Society of Anesthesiologists Physical Status | Class I: A normal healthy patient |
| | Class II: A patient with mild systemic disease |
| | Class III: A patient with severe systemic disease |
| | Class IV: A patient with severe systemic disease that is a constant threat to life |
| | Class V: A moribund patient who is not expected to survive without operation |
| | Class VI: A declared brain-dead patient whose organs are being removed for donation |
| Revised Cardiac Risk Index | Ischemic heart disease |
| | Cerebrovascular disease |
| | History of congestive heart failure |
| | Insulin therapy for diabetes |
| | Chronic renal insufficiency (serum creatinine level ≥2 mg/dL) |
| | High-risk surgical procedures |
| The American College of Surgery National Surgical Quality Improvement Program | Age and sex |
| | Functional status |
| | Emergency case |
| | American Society of Anesthesiologists Physical Status |
| | Current steroid use |
| | Ascites within 30 days |
| | Systemic sepsis within 48 h |
| | Ventilator dependence |
| | Disseminated cancer |
| | Diabetes mellitus |
| | Hypertension on treatment |
| | Congestive heart failure |
| | Dyspnea |
| | Current smoker |
| | History of severe chronic obstructive pulmonary disease |
| | Dialysis |
| | Acute renal failure |
| | Body mass index |
| | Surgery code |

### 16.4.1 American Society of Anesthesiologists Physical Status Classification for Esophagectomy

The ASA PS Classification System is a grading system that has been used for over half a century to assess a patient's preoperative physical status. The original purpose of the system is to assess and communicate a patient's medical comorbidities prior to anesthesia. The classification system alone does not predict perioperative risks; however, when used with other factors (e.g., type of surgery, frailty, degree of deconditioning), it may be helpful in predicting postoperative events. There are insufficient data on the usefulness of using ASA-PS as a risk prediction tool in patients undergoing esophagectomy [15, 16]. Recently, some studies have reported that worse ASA-PS is associated with poor long-term prognosis in patients with EC [17, 18]. A recent study evaluating the effect of ASA-PS on the management of EC indicates that ASA-PS is a highly effective clinical tool for preoperative classification of a patient's status. This study also highlighted that ASA-PS may be a valuable long-term prognostic factor for patients with EC undergoing esophagectomy [16].

### 16.4.2 Revised Cardiac Risk Index for Esophagectomy

The RCRI is a scoring system used to estimate the risk of cardiac arrest, MI, or 30-day mortality. This index includes six variants (i.e., cerebrovascular disease, history of ischemic heart disease, preoperative insulin use, preoperative creatinine >177 mmol/L, high-risk surgery, and congestive HF) that contribute equally to the risk. While the postoperative risk after major noncardiac surgery is 4% in patients with a score of 0, the risk increases up to 15% in patients with a score of ≥3 [19]. In a recent report from the United States, 7.7% of individuals ≥45 years of age who underwent major NCS had an RCRI score ≥3 [20]. Specific data on the utility of RCRI for esophagectomy are insufficient to recommend it as a stand-alone tool for preoperative cardiac evaluation. However, there is evidence that RCRI may be useful in predicting short-term outcomes after esophagectomy when used in combination with other organ-specific risk assessment tools as part of a broader risk score (Preoperative Esophagectomy Risk score) [21]. The RCRI has the advantage of being specific to postoperative cardiovascular events compared to other risk assessment tools that allow prediction of total events.

### 16.4.3 The American College of Surgery National Surgical Quality Improvement Program (ACS NSQIP) for Esophagectomy

ACS-NSQIP is a risk calculator developed by reviewing data from more than four million surgeries in the United States [22, 23]. The risk calculator is a model that includes 20 patient-specific variables, including CV variables such as hypertension (HT), dyspnea, and presence of HF [22, 23]. The ACS-NSQIP has been shown to be an effective tool for improving the quality of surgical care and reducing complications. As with the other risk assessment tools, there is little evidence that ACS-NSQIP is specific to patients undergoing esophagectomy for EC. The ACS-NSQIP Surgical Risk Calculator can be used to preoperatively identify patients at higher risk of conversion to open esophagectomy during minimally invasive esophagectomy [24].

### 16.4.4 Preoperative Assessment of Functional Capacity and Frailty

Assessing functional capacity before surgery is a critical step in ensuring better outcomes [12]. Good physical function is associated with improved quality of life, treatment tolerance, and survival in cancer patients. Functional capacity is typically expressed in metabolic equivalents (METs), and a MET value of less than 4 indicates poor functional capacity [12]. The cardiopulmonary exercise test (CPET) is the gold standard for assessing physical function, although its use is somewhat limited [25–27]. Recent studies have suggested a role for CPET in assessing perioperative risk and improving management, especially for high-risk patients undergoing high-risk surgery [28, 29]. Direct evidence for patients with EC undergoing surgery is somewhat limited, and available evidence from at least one observational study does not suggest a role for CPET [30]. Therefore, surgical decisions should not be based solely on CPET findings, although CPET can be considered as a supportive method for preoperative assessment of a patient's functional status [31].

Functional capacity can be assessed in several ways, including patient self-reported activities of daily living, the 6-min walk test (6MWT), metabolic equivalents, and the Duke Activity Status Index [12, 27]. The 6MWT is a simple method to assess exercise capacity and has been shown to predict postoperative complications in patients undergoing EC surgery when performed preoperatively [32, 33]. In addition, a study investigating the effect of the 6MWT on postoperative survival before EC surgery found that the 6MWT was associated with 5-year survival [34]. These findings highlight the importance of preoperative 6MWT in assessing exercise capacity and predicting long-term outcomes in patients undergoing esophagectomy. Furthermore, they suggest that a preoperative exercise program may improve long-term prognosis [34].

Frailty is a complex and dynamic clinical syndrome that includes impaired physical reserve and function typically associated with aging. Frailty has also been shown to correlate with poor outcomes after surgery [35, 36]. A study examining the impact of frailty on clinical outcomes in patients undergoing esophagectomy found that frailty was associated with worse outcomes after surgery. In addition, the study reported a higher prevalence of HF in frail patients compared to non-frail patients [36]. Given these findings, frailty may serve as a useful tool to improve risk assessment and patient selection for esophagectomy.

The 2022 ESC guidelines on NCS have highlighted the importance of frailty assessment [12]. The guideline recommends frailty screening for elderly patients (≥70 years) scheduled for high-risk non-cardiac surgery (NCS). In addition, for patients being evaluated for high-risk NCS, the guideline suggests that the ability to climb two flights of stairs should be considered when adjusting the risk assessment [12].

## 16.5 Initial Evaluation

### 16.5.1 Past Medical History and Physical Examination

The preoperative evaluation should include a history and physical examination focusing on the presence of prior cardiac disease and/or cardiac procedures, prior cardiac testing (diagnostic tests), risk factors for coronary artery disease (CAD), comorbidities, current symptoms, and medications. Depending on the patient's specific medical history and cardiac examination findings, more detailed testing and medical treatment may be required [12].

## 16.6 Preoperative Testing

### 16.6.1 Electrocardiography

The 12-lead ECG is the most widely used test to assess CV risk in the preoperative period. In patients undergoing major NCS, preoperative ECG can predict perioperative adverse events. The 2022 ESC guidelines for preoperative cardiovascular evaluation of patients undergoing NCS recommend obtaining a preoperative 12-lead ECG in the following situations:

1. Patients with known CV disease history
2. Presence of CV risk factors in a given patient
3. Presence of symptoms or signs suggestive of CV disease in patients undergoing intermediate or high-risk surgery [12]

Given that EC shares many risk factors with CV disease, virtually all patients undergoing esophagectomy would qualify for ECG according to these guidelines. Obtaining a preoperative baseline ECG is also important to evaluate ECG changes in the perioperative and postoperative periods [12].

### 16.6.2 Laboratory Testing

Preoperative laboratory testing should be based on the clinical history and risk factors for CV disease. There are no routine screening blood tests specifically indicated for cardiac risk assessment, but in patients with known risk factors (age > 65 years, BMI > 30, diabetes, HT, hyperlipidemia, CV disease, or smoking) undergoing intermediate- or high-risk NCS, it is recommended to screen for preoperative renal disease by measuring serum creatinine and glomerular filtration rate [12–14].

#### 16.6.2.1 Cardiac Biomarkers

B-type natriuretic peptide (BNP; or brain natriuretic peptide) and the N-terminal prohormone of BNP (NT-proBNP) are released from cardiac myocytes in response to mechanical stress and wall stress. Routine use of BNP or NT-proBNP for preoperative risk stratification is not currently recommended. However, BNP/NT-proBNP is complementary to clinical assessment and ECG in risk stratification in patients whose decision to undergo preoperative cardiac testing is unclear [12, 37–39]. The concentration of these biomarkers may have prognostic value for perioperative cardiac risk stratification, but it should be kept in mind that both BNP and NT-proBNP are elevated in many pathological conditions such as HF, valvular heart disease (VHD), myocarditis, CAD, arrhythmias (especially AF), acute pulmonary embolism, and pulmonary hypertension [12].

The optimal cut-off values for BNP and NT-proBNP for perioperative risk stratification are not clear. A meta-analysis evaluating BNP/NT-proBNP in noncardiac surgery showed that BNP ≥92 ng/L and NT-proBNP ≥300 ng/L were associated with an increased risk of MACE [40]. The 2022 ESC guidelines recommend measurement of BNP or NT-proBNP before intermediate- and high-risk NCS in patients with known CV disease, CV risk factors (including age ≥65 years), or symptoms suggestive of CV disease (class IIa) [12].

Postoperative atrial fibrillation (AF) is associated with increased short- and long-term morbidity and mortality in patients undergoing NCS [12]. Several studies have focused on the predictive value of BNP/NT-proBNP for identifying patients at risk of postoperative AF. Some studies have reported that preoperative high BNP indicates an increased risk of postoperative AF in patients undergoing major thoracic surgery, such as esophageal and pulmonary surgery. Therefore, natriuretic peptides may be useful in selecting candidates for prophylactic antiarrhythmic treatment prior to NCS to reduce the risk of AF [41–44].

Routine preoperative troponin measurement is not recommended. The value of troponin in risk stratification and its significance in asymptomatic patients with high troponin levels is not clear. The 2022 ESC guidelines recommend measuring high-sensitivity cardiac troponin (hs-cTn) in patients with known CV disease, CV risk factors (including age ≥65 years), or symptoms suggestive of CV disease before and at 24 and 48 h after intermediate- and high-risk NCS [12]. This suggestion is based on the presumed usefulness of troponin in predicting major cardiovascular events and mortality in patients undergoing NCS, but it should be emphasized that troponin is a nonspecific marker of myocardial injury that is often misinterpreted as a biomarker of underlying ischemic heart disease. Given that virtually all patients undergoing esophagectomy would qualify for preoperative troponin testing according to these recommendations, "routine" troponin measurement may lead to an increase in unnecessary delays due to further downstream testing for coronary artery disease, with potentially devastating consequences for the patient due to postponement of potentially life-saving surgery. Perhaps because of these concerns, the ACC/AHA guidelines do not include a similar recommendation [13, 14].

### 16.6.3 Transthoracic Echocardiography

Preoperative transthoracic echocardiography (TTE) is useful to evaluate left ventricular dysfunction, cardiomyopathies, and VHDs, which are important in predicting postoperative cardiac outcomes [12, 45]. Routine preoperative TTE before high-risk NCS does not reduce the risk of postoperative MACE or provide more information than clinical risk models. Therefore, routine echocardiography before NCS is not recommended [12]. The indications for TTE are as follows [12–14]:

1. Poor functional capacity
2. High NT-proBNP/BNP
3. Presence of murmurs
4. Suspected new CV disease
5. Abnormal ECG
6. Unexplained signs or symptoms

Although echocardiography has limited utility in predicting overall adverse CV events in patients undergoing NCS, several studies have shown that preoperative TTE may predict the development of postoperative AF, particularly in cases undergoing thoracic surgery (lung or EC surgery). In particular, it has been reported that risk stratification using left atrial diameter, left atrial diastolic volume index, and $E/e'$ parameters may allow the identification of patients at high risk for postoperative AF prior to major thoracic surgery [46–48].

### 16.6.4 Stress Testing for Ischemic Heart Disease

Stress testing is designed to induce ischemia and provide indirect evidence of epicardial CAD. This can be done either with exercise (with or without imaging) or with pharmacological agents in patients scheduled for NCS. Alternatives for imaging include myocardial perfusion imaging with SPECT or stress echocardiography, and both modalities have comparable accuracy for diagnosing angiographically proven epicardial CAD. Routine stress testing is discouraged because revascularization of stable CAD (with the exception of severe CAD with extensive ischemia) does not improve postoperative outcomes but causes unnecessary delays in potentially life-saving surgery. Therefore, preoperative stress imaging should not be performed in the vast majority of patients with EC. In the minority of patients in whom an acute coronary event is suspected at the time of evaluation, or in those with a very high likelihood of severe CAD in whom surgery can be postponed for a short time, preoperative stress testing may be appropriate [12–14].

For patients undergoing high-risk surgery, the 2022 ESC guidelines for preoperative evaluation recommend stress testing in patients with poor functional capacity if the patient has a high likelihood of severe CAD and/or a history of revascularization [12]. Similarly, the ACC/AHA guidelines recommend stress testing only when the patient has poor functional capacity, is at high risk for major adverse cardiac events, and the results of stress testing would change clinical decision making [13, 14].

### 16.6.5 Coronary Angiography

#### 16.6.5.1 Coronary Computed Tomography Angiography

Coronary artery computed tomography has a high negative predictive value for excluding coronary artery disease, but limited specificity for excluding significant CAD. There are insufficient data to recommend the routine use of coronary computed tomography angiography (CCTA) for preoperative evaluation. However, it can be considered a noninvasive alternative to invasive coronary angiography (ICA) for preoperative cardiac risk assessment. Current guidelines recommend CCTA (instead of ischemia testing or invasive angiography) when the clinical likelihood of CAD is low or intermediate and/or noninvasive functional testing could not be performed for any reason [12].

#### 16.6.5.2 Invasive Coronary Angiography

Despite the availability of noninvasive modalities, invasive coronary angiography (ICA) remains the gold standard for the diagnosis of epicardial CAD. Recommendations for preoperative ICA are similar to those for patients with suspected or known CAD and are beyond the scope of this chapter. However, it should be emphasized that there are no data to suggest that revascularization prior to NCS improves postoperative outcomes, and the need for anticoagulation after revascularization (particularly after percutaneous procedures) may cause significant delays in the treatment of EC. Therefore, "frequent" or "routine" use of ICA for preoperative evaluation is discouraged [12–14].

An algorithm for the preoperative evaluation of patients undergoing esophagectomy is given in Fig. 16.1.

## 16.7 Management of Cardiac Disease for Reducing Perioperative Risk

### 16.7.1 Management of Hypertension

The prevalence of arterial HT is common (30–45%) in adults, and only 40% of these patients have well-controlled blood pressure [12, 49, 50]. Hypertension is a determinant of postoperative outcomes after high-risk surgery. Therefore, hypertensive patients scheduled for elective high-risk NCS should be evaluated preoperatively for CV risk factors and end-organ damage [12–14]. The presence of uncontrolled HT before surgery is associated with an increased risk of death after NCS [51]. The general preoperative approach to HT is as follows:

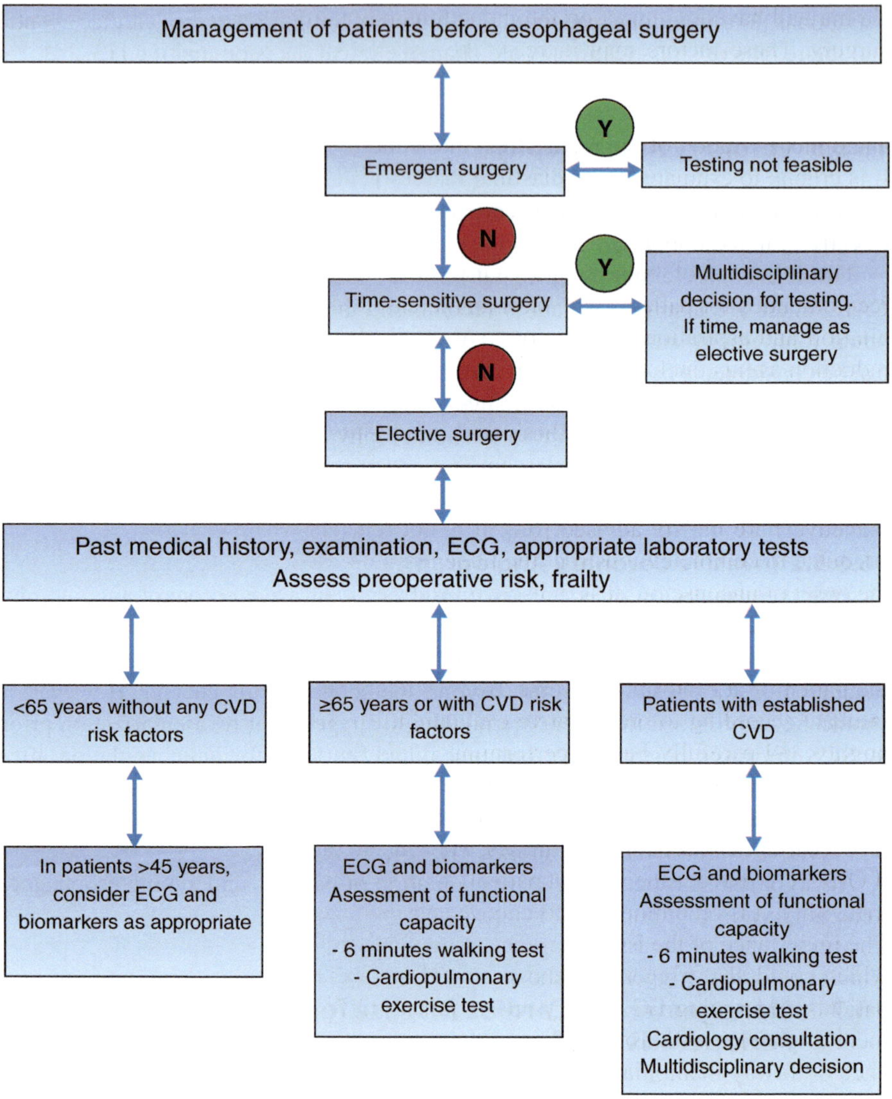


**Fig. 16.1** Recommended algorithm for preoperative cardiac evaluation before esophageal surgery. *NCS* noncardiac surgery, *CV* cardiovascular, *CVD* cardiovascular disease, *ECG* electrocardiography. (Modified from the 2022 European Society of Cardiology Guidelines on non-cardiac surgery [12])

1. In patients with grade 1 or 2 HT; postponing the surgery is generally not recommended [12].
2. In patients with systolic blood pressure (BP) ≥180 mmHg and/or diastolic BP ≥110 mmHg, it is recommended that the intervention should be delayed until BP is under control, except in emergency surgery [12].

3. For patients with chronic HT; it is suggested to avoid fluctuations in BP, especially hypotension [12].

In patients undergoing esophagectomy for EC, the relationship between preoperative HT and prognosis was evaluated, and HT was associated with poor long-term prognosis [52].

HT management prior to elective NCS should be in accordance with guideline recommendations. The 2018 ESC guidelines for HT recommend the use of calcium channel blockers or renin-angiotensin-aldosterone system inhibitors, alone or in combination [53]. While beta-blockers (BBs) are not recommended as first-line agents, third-generation BBs such as carvedilol, nebivolol, and labetalol can be used in patients with HT and an indication for BBs [53]. Beta-blockers have some practical advantages and disadvantages over other classes of antihypertensives in patients undergoing major NCS. Indeed, one-month mortality after NCS is lower in patients with multiple CV risk factors, whereas the risk of death is increased in those undergoing NCS but without CV risk factors [54]. Therefore, when considering an antihypertensive agent, BBs are more appropriate for those with multiple risk factors for CV disease.

### 16.7.2 Management of Coronary Artery Disease

It has been reported that almost half of the cases aged >45 years undergoing NCS have ≥2 CV risk factors and 18% have CAD [12–14]. Therefore, it is important to focus on preoperative CV risk assessment and perioperative CV disease management of CAD patients undergoing NCS [12–14]. Management of concomitant CAD in patients undergoing NCS includes evaluation of the following conditions in patients on antiplatelet therapy and risk assessment [55]:

1. Appropriate time and duration of interruption of antiplatelet preoperatively
2. Dual antiplatelet therapy requirement
3. Resuming antiplatelet after surgery
4. Option to bridge with other antithrombotic drugs
5. Preoperative ICA requirement
6. Preoperative PCI requirement

#### 16.7.2.1 Perioperative Management of Antiplatelet Agents

In the management of patients on antithrombotic therapy undergoing NCS, the dual risk of bleeding and thrombosis should be considered prior to the procedure. Major thoracic surgery, including esophagectomy, is a difficult, complex, and lengthy procedure that carries a high risk of bleeding during or after the procedure. Unfortunately, major thoracic NCS also carries a high risk of postoperative ischemic events, and therefore the risk of bleeding and thrombosis should be assessed individually [12–14, 56]. The risk of coronary stent thrombosis is particularly pronounced in patients with a recent percutaneous intervention. A multidisciplinary approach is often required to determine the appropriate management strategy for each patient.

#### Single Antiplatelet Therapy

A total of 10% of adult surgical candidates receive chronic antiplatelet and/or anticoagulation therapy prior to NCS [57, 58]. Acetylsalicylic acid (ASA) inhibits platelet aggregation by blocking thromboxane synthesis and is widely used to prevent CV events in patients with established CV disease. The prognostic impact of discontinuing ASA prior to NCS is not well understood. In POISE-2, 23% of patients undergoing NCS had CAD and 5.8% of all patients were scheduled for major thoracic surgery. POISE-2 showed that perioperative aspirin use in unselected patients undergoing NCS was not associated with a reduction in death or non-fatal MI, but these patients were at increased risk of major bleeding [59]. This study did not support the routine use of ASA in patients undergoing NCS, but it is unclear whether ASA could be instrumental in reducing postoperative ischemia in patients at higher risk of CV events after surgery.

P2Y12 inhibitors act by inhibiting platelet aggregation in response to ADP and are more potent platelet inhibitors than ASA. Patients at high risk of bleeding who are receiving clopidogrel-based monotherapy as P2Y12 inhibitor monotherapy for chronic coronary syndrome may have their therapy interrupted for a short period of time. The perioperative management of patients on P2Y12 inhibitor monotherapy after an acute coronary event, with or without prior percutaneous revascularization, or for other indications, such as recent stroke, peripheral arterial disease, or aspirin intolerance, requires a multidisciplinary approach [60–63]. Although individualized decisions are required, strategies that may be considered include surgery without interruption of P2Y12 monotherapy, short preoperative interruption, switching to ASA, or perioperative bridging with parenteral P2Y12 or GpIIb/IIIa inhibitors [12].

#### Dual Antiplatelet Therapy

Dual antiplatelet therapy (DAPT) with ASA and a P2Y12 inhibitor (prasugrel, ticagrelor, and clopidogrel) is indicated in patients with a recent percutaneous coronary intervention (PCI) and in patients with a recent acute coronary event. The risk of bleeding and perioperative bleeding complications is further increased in patients treated with DAPT, especially with the potent P2Y12 inhibitors prasugrel and ticagrelor [62]. However, premature discontinuation of DAPT, especially in patients with recent coronary stent implantation, may lead to stent thrombosis and myocardial infarction.

The ACC/AHA recommendations for DAPT therapy for NCS are as follows [13, 14, 64].

1. Elective operations should be deferred for up to 6 months after placement of drug-eluting stents (DES) and for 1 month for bare-metal stents (BMS).
2. In patients treated with DAPT after coronary stent implantation who must undergo surgical procedures that mandate the discontinuation of P2Y12 inhibitor therapy, guidelines recommend continuation of ASA with reinstitution of P2Y12 inhibitors as soon as possible.

3. Elective NCS should not be performed within 30 days after BMS implantation or within 3 months after DES implantation in patients in whom preoperative DAPT discontinuation is required.

The ESC recommendations for antiplatelet therapy for NCS are as follows [12].

- DAPT management recommendation of ESC is primarily to postpone elective NCS until completion of the whole course of DAPT (6 months after elective PCI and 12 months after ACS).
- After elective PCI, it is recommended to delay time-sensitive NCS until a minimum of 1 month of DAPT treatment has been given.
- If interruption of P2Y12 inhibitor is indicated, it is recommended to discontinue clopidogrel for 5 days, ticagrelor for 3–5 days, and prasugrel for 1 week prior to NCS.
- Whenever possible, in patients with an indication for DAPT, surgery should be performed without discontinuation of aspirin.
- Aspirin might be discontinued as a last measure only with very high bleeding risk and a comparably low ischemic risk.
- Although generally not recommended, bridging with an i.v. agent (eptifibatide/tirofiban or cangrelor) might be applicable in rare cases when DAPT cannot be interrupted before NCS (e.g. in patients with very high risk of stent thrombosis, history of recurrent MI, recent PCI).
- If antiplatelet therapy has been interrupted before a surgical procedure, it is recommended to restart therapy as soon as possible (within 48 h) post-surgery, according to interdisciplinary risk assessment.

There is little evidence to suggest that stopping antiplatelet therapy before esophagectomy is safe, although in a small retrospective analysis of 23 patients with prior CAD, there were no differences in ischemic events in patients who stopped antiplatelet therapy 7 days before surgery [55]. Of note, none of the patients in this latter study had recent stent implantation.

In summary, decisions regarding the timing of surgery and whether to continue DAPT after coronary stent implantation are at best individualized. It is recommended to be determined by consensus between the surgeon, anesthesiologist, cardiologist, and patient. The surgical procedure and the risks of delaying the procedure, the risks of ischemia and stent thrombosis, and the risk of bleeding and its consequences should be discussed [12–14, 64].

### 16.7.3 Management of Other Treatments in Coronary Artery Disease

In patients using BB therapy prior to surgery, it is recommended that the medication be continued in the perioperative period. In addition, the use of BBs may also be useful in patients at high CV risk or who have undergone high-risk surgery. Initiation of preoperative BBs prior to high-risk NCS in patients with ≥2 clinical risk factors may be considered to reduce the incidence of perioperative MI [12–14, 64]. The ACC/AHA guidelines recommend the following for perioperative BB therapy [13, 14]:

- Perioperative continuation of BBs is recommended in patients currently receiving this medication.
- BBs may be started in patients in whom preoperative stress testing results are compatible with a moderate to large degree of cardiac ischemia.
- BBs may be initiated in patients with high CV risk.
- BBs should not be started on the day of surgery.
- If BBs are indicated, it should be started 2–7 days before the surgery.

Patients who were taking HMG-CoA inhibitors (also known as statins) prior to surgery or who have an indication for statins should continue statin therapy without interruption in the perioperative and postoperative periods [12, 65]. Routine preoperative initiation of statin therapy in patients without an indication for statins is not recommended. There is some evidence that the use of statins may improve the prognosis of patients with EC by reducing EC-specific mortality and all-cause mortality [66–68]. In contrast, a study from China evaluating the prognostic impact of statins in patients undergoing esophagectomy found no association between statins and improved survival in patients with EC [69].

#### 16.7.3.1 Preoperative Coronary Angiography for Risk Reduction in Coronary Artery Disease

In patients with a past history of CAD, it is imperative to gather information regarding the prior invasive and non-invasive diagnostic tests and therapeutic interventions done for CAD. As aforementioned, routine use of ICA for preoperative evaluation in NCS, including those with known CAD or those with a history of revascularization, is neither recommended nor encouraged. The decision to proceed with ICA should be based on the same indications for ICA in the non-surgical setting for patients with suspected or known CAD [12–14].

#### 16.7.3.2 Perioperative Revascularization in Coronary Artery Disease

Revascularization refers to the alleviation of ischemia by restoring epicardial blood flow by percutaneous intervention or by bypassing the occluded arterial segments by surgery. Coronary artery disease or previous incomplete revascularization is known to be associated with postoperative MACE, but there is no evidence that preoperative revascularization improves outcomes after NCS. In contrast, results from a large randomized controlled trial suggest that percutaneous revascularization is not associated with improved outcomes in patients undergoing high-risk NCS [68]. Percutaneous revascularization requires the use of antiplatelet agents for at least 1 month after percutaneous coronary intervention (PCI), during which time elective procedures are either postponed or performed with a much higher risk of bleeding. Thus, for most patients, revascularization—if indicated—is best performed after EC surgery. Possible exceptions to this rule include acute coronary events prior to elective CABG, high-risk anatomy such as left main disease, or the presence of life-threatening ventricular arrhythmias related to active ischemia [12–14].

## 16.8 Management of Perioperative Myocardial Infarction

The ESC guidelines define perioperative MI as acute cardiomyocyte injury (postoperative hs-cTn T/I release) after surgery. Symptoms, ECG changes or imaging evidence of acute myocardial ischemia may or may not be present [12]. Perioperative MI can be detected with hs-cTn T/I measurements before and serially after surgery (e.g., 24 and 48 h postoperatively) [12]. However, routine monitoring of patients with troponin testing in the absence of myocardial ischemia is not recommended.

Postoperative MI is associated with poor short- and long-term outcomes. Overall, the 1-month mortality in patients who develop perioperative myocardial injury/MI is nearly 10%. Several different pathological mechanisms and clinical phenotypes may contribute to the development of perioperative myocardial injury/MI and troponin elevation, so the etiology is variable and acute atherothrombosis (amenable to treatment with angiography and revascularization) is not the sole cause [12]. Treatment should be determined according to the underlying etiology (Table 16.2).

**Table 16.2** Different diagnosis of clinical conditions associated with elevated postoperative cardiac troponin levels

| | Clinical situations | Mechanism | Treatment |
|---|---|---|---|
| Cardiac cause | Type 1 MI | Atherothrombosis | • ICA<br>• Aspirin<br>• Statin<br>• Monitoring<br>• DAPT after coronary stenting |
| | Type 2 MI | Supply demand mismatch with obvious type 2 trigger (hypotension, anemia) | In case of severe anemia<br>• Immediate transfusion followed by reassessment for ICA |
| | Tachyarrhythmia | Supply demand mismatch | Treat cause |
| | Acute heart failure | Multiple mechanisms | Treat cause |
| | Likely type 2 MI | • Missed type 1 MI<br>• Undocumented hypotension<br>• Mild hypotension | • Aspirin<br>• Statin<br>• Stress imaging/CCTA/ICA<br>• Treat cause |
| Primarily non-cardiac cause | • Severe sepsis<br>• Pulmonary embolism<br>• Stroke | Multiple mechanisms | Treat cause |

*Abbreviations*: *CCTA* coronary computed tomography angiography, *DAPT* dual antiplatelet therapy, *ICA* invasive coronary angiography, *MI* myocardial infarction

## 16.9 Management of Atrial Fibrillation

Perioperative cardiac arrhythmias, especially new-onset atrial fibrillation, are much more common in noncardiac thoracic surgery than in general surgery [70]. The incidence of AF after major thoracic surgery ranges from 9.9% to 19% [70]. New-onset AF occurs in 12–37% of patients who have undergone esophagectomy [71]. The risk of developing AF continues not only during the intraoperative period but also during the first 3 days after surgery in most patients. The mechanism of AF after NCS is complex and its exact pathophysiology remains unclear. The main factors leading to the development of perioperative AF are as follows [70, 71]:

1. Direct trauma to the atrium
2. Infections
3. Ventilation-related oxidative stress
4. Hypo and hypervolemia
5. Anesthesia-induced CV depression
6. Sepsis
7. Release of endogenous catecholamines
8. The presence of preoperatively undetected heart diseases

Independent risk predictors for the occurrence of postoperative AF are male sex, advanced age, preoperative high heart rate, and BNP levels [72]. In addition, AF may be associated with other postoperative complications such as infectious and pulmonary complications, pneumonia, respiratory failure, and anastomotic leakage. The occurrence of postoperative AF is associated with increased length of stay, need for reoperation, and risk of postoperative mortality [71–73].

### 16.9.1 Prevention of Postoperative Atrial Fibrillation

The first step in preventing postoperative AF is to identify patients at risk for AF, optimize hemodynamics, and correct electrolyte imbalances [12–14]. Many agents, including but not limited to BBs, sotalol, colchicine, corticosteroids, amiodarone, statins, and magnesium sulfate, have been used to prevent postoperative AF, but the benefit of these prophylactic measures is not entirely clear [74–80]. Amiodarone has the best evidence for AF prophylaxis, and in a large meta-analysis, preoperative administration of amiodarone was associated with a 60% reduction in postoperative AF [74]. There are also some data suggesting that amiodarone is effective in preventing postoperative AF in patients undergoing esophagectomy [75]. However, amiodarone is associated with frequent side effects that should be considered before using amiodarone as a prophylactic measure.

There is some evidence that statins may be useful in preventing postoperative AF after major thoracic surgery, although the data are insufficient to suggest routine use of status for this purpose [12, 76]. Landiolol, an ultra-short acting BB, prevents perioperative AF after cardiac surgery and is an effective and safe agent in the prevention of AF in patients undergoing major thoracic surgery [12, 78, 79]. Esmolol is a highly selective β1-adrenergic blocker with an ultra-short and fast-acting effect, like landiolol, and can be considered in the prevention and treatment of AF [80]. The potential hemodynamic consequences of using intravenous beta-blockers should be weighed against the perceived benefit of reducing the risk of postoperative AF.

### 16.9.2 Management of Postoperative Atrial Fibrillation and Thromboembolic Complications

Emergency electrical or pharmacological cardioversion is indicated in patients who develop postoperative AF with hemodynamic instability [12–14]. In a randomized controlled trial of patients undergoing cardiac surgery, there was no clear benefit of restoring sinus rhythm over controlling heart rate in hemodynamically stable patients [81]. Therefore, the decision to restore sinus rhythm in patients with postoperative AF should be individualized. However, in stable patients with postoperative AF, it is imperative to ensure optimal ventricular rate control during the arrhythmia, and BBs or dihydropyridine calcium channel blockers could be used for this purpose.

Postoperative AF is associated with thromboembolism and stroke, as are other types of AF, and the available evidence suggests that the association between thromboembolism and postoperative AF is stronger in patients undergoing NCS than in those undergoing cardiac surgery [82]. Postoperative AF was more strongly associated with long-term stroke risk in patients undergoing NCS than in those undergoing cardiac surgery [82]. Therefore, anticoagulation should be considered in all patients with AF. However, the risk of postoperative bleeding should also be considered before initiating anticoagulation, especially in the immediate postoperative period [12].

## 16.10 Management of Oral Anticoagulation in Patients with a Previous Indication for Anticoagulation

There are two main groups of anticoagulants used for long-term anticoagulation: Vitamin K antagonists (VKA) and non-vitamin K antagonist oral anticoagulants (NOAC). Perioperative management of oral anticoagulant (OAC) therapy depends on surgical and patient-related factors, as well as the specific OAC the patient is taking. Anticoagulant therapy is commonly used for several common CV conditions, including stroke, atrial fibrillation, venous thromboembolism, and mechanical valve disease [12].

### 16.10.1 Perioperative Management of Vitamin K Antagonists

Three different compounds are commercially available: warfarin (half-life 36–48 h), acenocoumarol (half-life 12 h), and phenprocoumon (half-life 100 h). Vitamin K antagonists are the mainstay of therapy in patients with mechanical heart valves.

Recommendations for vitamin K antagonists for mechanical heart valves are as follows [12]:

1. In patients with mechanical heart valves, minor surgical procedures, and procedures where bleeding is easily controlled can be performed without VKA interruption.
2. Major surgical procedures that necessitate an INR below 1.5 require VKA interruption and perioperative bridging with heparin should be considered.
3. In patients with mechanical heart valves with a low risk of thromboembolism (e.g. mechanical bileaflet aortic valve in patients with sinus rhythm), bridging may not be needed.
4. In patients with mechanical heart valves with a high risk of thromboembolism (mechanical AVR and any thromboembolic risk factor, an older-generation mechanical AVR, or a mechanical mitral or tricuspid valve replacement), bridging with heparin should be considered during the perioperative time interval when the INR is subtherapeutic.
5. In all conditions, the risks of bleeding should be weighed against the benefits of thromboembolism prevention.
6. Intravenous unfractionated heparin is the only heparin treatment approved for bridging in patients with mechanical heart valves. However, subcutaneous low molecular weight heparins (LMWH) are also used in clinical practice for this purpose.

Because of the availability of NOACs, VKAs are rarely used to prevent thromboembolism in AF patients or to prevent recurrent venous thromboembolism (VTE) in susceptible individuals. Nevertheless, VKAs are still occasionally preferred for some patients. Recommendations for vitamin K antagonists in AF/venous thromboembolism (VTE) are as follows [12–14]:

1. In patients using VKA for AF or VTE, invasive procedures with low bleeding risk can be performed by maintained the INR at the lower level of the therapeutic range without VKA interruption.
2. Bridging therapy may be considered in the following cases with a high thrombotic risk.
   (a) AF with CHA2DS2-VASc score >6.
   (b) Recent cardioembolic stroke <3 months.
   (c) High risk of VTE recurrence.
3. VKAs should be discontinued 3–5 days before procedures with a high risk of bleeding, and routine bridging with heparin is not recommended.

**Table 16.3** Timing of last NOAC dose before NCS according to renal function without bridging

| | Low bleeding risk NCS | High bleeding risk NCS |
|---|---|---|
| Dabigatran | GFR ≥ 80: 24 h<br>GFR 50–79: 36 h<br>GFR 30–49: 48 h<br>GFR15–29: Not indicated<br>GFR < 15: No formal indication for use | GFR ≥ 80: 48 h<br>GFR 50–79:72 h<br>GFR 30–49: 96 h<br>GFR15–29: Not indicated<br>GFR < 15: No formal indication for use |
| Apixaban<br>Rivaroxaban<br>Edoxaban | GFR ≥ 30: 24 h<br>GFR 15–29: 36 h<br>GFR < 15: No formal indication for use | GFR ≥ 15: 48 h<br>GFR < 15: No formal indication for use |

*Abbreviations*: *GFR* glomerular filtration rate, *NCS* non-cardiac surgery

### 16.10.2 Perioperative Management of Management of NOACs

In patients on NOACs (apixaban, dabigatran, edoxaban, and rivaroxaban), perioperative bridging with heparin or LMWH is associated with an increased risk of bleeding without a reduction in thromboembolic events. For NOACs, the optimal timing of preoperative interruption depends on renal function, risk of postoperative bleeding, and the type of agent used. Longer interruption may be required in patients with creatinine clearance <30 mL/min, very low body weight, or advanced age (Table 16.3) [83].

## 16.11 Management of Chronic Heart Failure

Heart failure is a known predictor of perioperative mortality in NCS. The risk of postoperative adverse events associated with HF depends on left ventricular systolic function, hemodynamic status, and the presence of symptoms. On the other hand, patients undergoing NCS may develop acute decompensated HF due to fluid overload and/or comorbidities. In a recently published analysis examining the association between HF and perioperative outcomes in patients undergoing NCS, the presence of HF was associated with an increased rate of in-hospital mortality compared with patients without a diagnosis of HF. Only 4% of the patients included in this study underwent major thoracic surgery (including esophageal surgery), but HF was more common in this subset of patients [84].

To reduce the risk of poor postoperative outcomes, optimal guideline-directed medical therapy is recommended before NCS [12–14]. Fluid balance is one of the most important factors to consider in HF patients. Baseline medical therapy should be continued throughout the perioperative period, but the effects of medications in the perioperative period should also be considered. In patients who are receiving BB treatment prior to surgery, it is recommended that this be continued in the perioperative period [12–14]. Data on the perioperative use of renin-angiotensin-aldosterone system (RAAS) inhibitors are inconclusive. Withdrawal of medications carries the risk of hypertension, whereas continuation of medications carries the risk of hypotension. A study evaluating the effect of RAAS inhibitors in esophagectomy patients with EC showed no difference between those on and those not on RAAS inhibitors in terms of major adverse cardiovascular events, infection rates, overall survival, and disease-free survival. However, in this study, it was not known how many of the cases received RAAS inhibitors for HF [85]. There is no data on the perioperative efficacy of angiotensin receptor-neprilysin inhibitors, which reduce mortality in HF patients, but hypotension is more common than in patients receiving angiotensin-converting enzyme inhibitors [86]. In the perioperative period, a balance between volume status, electrolyte disturbances, and diuretic use should be maintained in patients with HF [12]. Retrospective studies have reported that the risk of acute renal failure may increase with the use of intraoperative diuretics [87]. Sodium-glucose co-transporter 2 inhibitors are recommended as first-line therapy in patients with HF with reduced ejection fraction. Consideration should be given to interrupting sodium-glucose co-transporter-2 inhibitor treatment for at least 3 days prior to high-risk NCS [12]. In cases of postoperative acute HF, the general principles of diagnostic work-up and therapy of acute HF should be applied [12].

## 16.12 Management of Valvular Heart Disease

The presence of valvular heart disease (VHD) should be considered during the preoperative evaluation, as it is associated with an increased risk of perioperative cardiovascular complications following NCS. Patients with suspected VHD should undergo echocardiography to quantify the severity of stenosis or regurgitation. The perioperative risk varies depending on the severity of the VHD and the type of surgery. In patients with severe VHD undergoing NCS, a multidisciplinary approach should be used to evaluate valvular intervention and timing of surgery. The ESC/ESA guidelines prioritize the presence of symptoms as the basis for the decision algorithm for elective NCS [12].

### 16.12.1 Aortic Valve Stenosis and Regurgitation

The perioperative risk associated with aortic stenosis (AS) depends on the severity of symptoms such as angina, dyspnea, and syncope, as well as other determinants such as the presence of comorbidities, left ventricular systolic function, and the presence of concomitant CAD. Perioperative management of high-risk patients scheduled for NCS is important because AS is a predictor of postoperative HF, ACS, and mortality. Aortic valve replacement (AVR) has been associated with reduced in-hospital and 1-month mortality in patients with AS undergoing high-risk NCS. The decision to perform surgical aortic valve replacement or transcatheter aortic valve implantation (TAVI) should be made according to the 2021 ESC/European Association for Cardio-Thoracic Surgery (EACTS) guidelines for the management of VHD [88]. In patients with severe aortic regurgitation (AR), it is recommended that AR be treated prior to high-risk NCS.

The recommendations for the treatment of AS and AR in patients undergoing NCS are as follows [12]:

1. For symptomatic AS patients; AVR (surgical AVR or TAVI) is recommended before elective high-risk surgery.
2. For asymptomatic severe AS; AVR (surgical AVR or TAVI) decision should be considered with the heart team.
3. In patients with symptomatic severe AR or asymptomatic severe AR and left ventricular end-systolic diameter >50 mm or resting left ventricular ejection fraction ≤50%, valve surgery is recommended prior to elective high-risk NCS.

### 16.12.2 Mitral Valve Stenosis and Regurgitation

Noncardiac surgery can be performed with a relatively low risk of complications in patients with mild mitral stenosis (MS) and in asymptomatic patients with moderate to severe MS. In symptomatic patients, percutaneous mitral commissurotomy should be considered before high-risk NCS. In patients with moderate-to-severe MS who are not candidates for percutaneous mitral commissurotomy, NCS should be performed only when indicated [12].

For mitral regurgitation (MR), the cause of MR (primary or secondary) and left ventricular function should be assessed in the perioperative period. Patients with secondary MR due to ischemic etiology are at high risk of CV complications during NCS [89].

The recommendations for the treatment of MS and MR in patients undergoing NCS are as follows [12].

1. In patients with moderate-to-severe rheumatic MS and symptoms or systolic pulmonary artery pressure >50 mmHg, valve intervention is recommended before elective high-risk NCS (Class 1C).
2. Patients with severe symptomatic MR should be evaluated for valve treatment prior to high-risk elective NCS.
3. Valve intervention should be considered prior to NCS in patients with symptomatic severe secondary MR despite guideline-directed medical therapy (Class IIa).
4. In patients with symptomatic severe primary MR or asymptomatic severe primary MR with LV dysfunction (Left ventricular end-systolic diameter ≥40 mm and/or left ventricular ejection fraction ≤60%), valve intervention should be considered before high-risk NCS (Class IIa).

## References

1. Uhlenhopp DJ, Then EO, Sunkara T, Gaduputi V. Epidemiology of esophageal cancer: update in global trends, etiology and risk factors. Clin J Gastroenterol. 2020;13(6):1010–21. https://doi.org/10.1007/s12328-020-01237-x.

2. Huang FL, Yu SJ. Esophageal cancer: risk factors, genetic association, and treatment. Asian J Surg. 2018;41(3):210–5. https://doi.org/10.1016/j.asjsur.2016.10.005.
3. Cunningham D, Allum WH, Stenning SP, Thompson JN, Van de Velde CJ, Nicolson M, et al. Perioperative chemotherapy versus surgery alone for resectable gastroesophageal cancer. N Engl J Med. 2006;355(1):11–20. https://doi.org/10.1056/NEJMoa055531.
4. van Hagen P, Hulshof MC, van Lanschot JJ, Steyerberg EW, van Berge Henegouwen MI, Wijnhoven BP, et al. Preoperative chemoradiotherapy for esophageal or junctional cancer. N Engl J Med. 2012;366(22):2074–84. https://doi.org/10.1056/NEJMoa1112088.
5. Reijneveld EAE, Bor P, Dronkers JJ, Argudo N, Ruurda JP, Veenhof C. Impact of curative treatment on the physical fitness of patients with esophageal cancer: a systematic review and meta-analysis. Eur J Surg Oncol. 2022;48(2):391–402. https://doi.org/10.1016/j.ejso.2021.08.015.
6. Birkmeyer JD, Siewers AE, Finlayson EV, Stukel TA, Lucas FL, Batista I, et al. Hospital volume and surgical mortality in the United States. N Engl J Med. 2002;346(15):1128–37. https://doi.org/10.1056/NEJMsa012337.
7. Bronson NW, Luna RA, Hunter JG. Tailoring esophageal cancer surgery. Semin Thorac Cardiovasc Surg. 2012;24(4):275–87. https://doi.org/10.1053/j.semtcvs.2012.11.001.
8. Siegel R, Naishadham D, Jemal A. Cancer statistics, 2013. CA Cancer J Clin. 2013;63(1):11–30. https://doi.org/10.3322/caac.21166.
9. Theochari CA, Theochari NA, Kokkinidis DG, Dellaportas D, Kosmopoulos M, Triantafyllou T, et al. Myocardial infarction after esophagectomy for esophageal cancer: a systematic review. Eur Surg. 2022;54(1):24–31.
10. Markar S, Gronnier C, Duhamel A, Bigourdan JM, Badic B, du Rieu MC, et al. Pattern of postoperative mortality after esophageal cancer resection according to center volume: results from a large European multicenter study. Ann Surg Oncol. 2015;22(8):2615–23. https://doi.org/10.1245/s10434-014-4310-5.
11. Low DE, Kuppusamy MK, Alderson D, Cecconello I, Chang AC, Darling G, et al. Benchmarking complications associated with esophagectomy. Ann Surg. 2019;269(2):291–8. https://doi.org/10.1097/SLA.0000000000002611.
12. Halvorsen S, Mehilli J, Cassese S, Hall TS, Abdelhamid M, Barbato E, et al. 2022 ESC Guidelines on cardiovascular assessment and management of patients undergoing non-cardiac surgery. Eur Heart J. 2022;43(39):3826–924. https://doi.org/10.1093/eurheartj/ehac270.
13. Fleisher LA, Fleischmann KE, Auerbach AD, Barnason SA, Beckman JA, Bozkurt B, et al. 2014 ACC/AHA guideline on perioperative cardiovascular evaluation and management of patients undergoing noncardiac surgery: a report of the American College of Cardiology/American Heart Association Task Force on Practice Guidelines. Circulation. 2014;130(24):e278–333. https://doi.org/10.1161/CIR.0000000000000106.
14. Fleisher LA, Fleischmann KE, Auerbach AD, Barnason SA, Beckman JA, Bozkurt B, et al. 2014 ACC/AHA guideline on perioperative cardiovascular evaluation and management of patients undergoing noncardiac surgery: executive summary: a report of the American College of Cardiology/American Heart Association Task Force on Practice Guidelines. Circulation. 2014;130(24):2215–45. https://doi.org/10.1161/CIR.0000000000000105.
15. ASA Physical Status Classification System developed by Committee on Economics. Last Amended: 13 Dec 2020 (original approval: 15 Oct 2014). https://www.asahq.org/standards-and-guidelines/asa-physicalstatus-classification-system.
16. Sato S, Nakatani E, Higashizono K, Nagai E, Taki Y, Nishida M, et al. The impact of the American Society of Anesthesiology—physical Status classification system on the treatment and prognosis of patients with esophageal cancer undergoing esophagectomy. Int J Clin Oncol. 2022;27(8):1289–99. https://doi.org/10.1007/s10147-022-02190-0.
17. Onishi S, Tajika M, Tanaka T, Yamada K, Abe T, Higaki E, et al. Prognostic impact of sarcopenic obesity after neoadjuvant chemotherapy followed by surgery in elderly patients with esophageal squamous cell carcinoma. J Clin Med. 2020;9(9):2974. https://doi.org/10.3390/jcm9092974.
18. Kouzu K, Tsujimoto H, Sugasawa H, Ishibashi Y, Hase K, Kishi Y, et al. Modified geriatric nutrition risk index as a prognostic predictor of esophageal cancer. Esophagus. 2021;18(2):278–87. https://doi.org/10.1007/s10388-020-00795-w.

19. Lee TH, Marcantonio ER, Mangione CM, Thomas EJ, Polanczyk CA, Cook EF, et al. Derivation and prospective validation of a simple index for prediction of cardiac risk of major noncardiac surgery. Circulation. 1999;100(10):1043–9. https://doi.org/10.1161/01.cir.100.10.1043.
20. Smilowitz NR, Gupta N, Guo Y, Beckman JA, Bangalore S, Berger JS. Trends in cardiovascular risk factor and disease prevalence in patients undergoing non-cardiac surgery. Heart. 2018;104(14):1180–6. https://doi.org/10.1136/heartjnl-2017-312391.
21. Reeh M, Metze J, Uzunoglu FG, Nentwich M, Ghadban T, Wellner U, et al. The PER (Preoperative Esophagectomy Risk) score: a simple risk score to predict short-term and long-term outcome in patients with surgically treated esophageal cancer. Medicine (Baltimore). 2016;95(7):e2724. https://doi.org/10.1097/MD.0000000000002724.
22. Bilimoria KY, Liu Y, Paruch JL, Zhou L, Kmiecik TE, Ko CY, et al. Development and evaluation of the universal ACS NSQIP surgical risk calculator: a decision aid and informed consent tool for patients and surgeons. J Am Coll Surg. 2013;217(5):833–42.e423. https://doi.org/10.1016/j.jamcollsurg.2013.07.385.
23. Cohen ME, Liu Y, Ko CY, Hall BL. An examination of American College of Surgeons NSQIP surgical risk calculator accuracy. J Am Coll Surg. 2017;224(5):787–795.e1. https://doi.org/10.1016/j.jamcollsurg.2016.12.057.
24. Gergen AK, Halpern AL, Helmkamp L, Torphy RJ, White AM, Mitchell JD, et al. Outcomes after converted minimally invasive to open esophagectomy in patients with esophageal cancer. Ann Thorac Surg. 2021;112(5):1593–9. https://doi.org/10.1016/j.athoracsur.2020.11.025.
25. Steins Bisschop CN, Velthuis MJ, Wittink H, Kuiper K, Takken T, van der Meulen WJ, et al. Cardiopulmonary exercise testing in cancer rehabilitation: a systematic review. Sports Med. 2012;42(5):367–79. https://doi.org/10.2165/11598480-000000000-00000.
26. Moran J, Wilson F, Guinan E, McCormick P, Hussey J, Moriarty J. Role of cardiopulmonary exercise testing as a risk-assessment method in patients undergoing intra-abdominal surgery: a systematic review. Br J Anaesth. 2016;116(2):177–91. https://doi.org/10.1093/bja/aev454.
27. O'Neill L, Moran J, Guinan EM, Reynolds JV, Hussey J. Physical decline and its implications in the management of oesophageal and gastric cancer: a systematic review. J Cancer Surviv. 2018;12(4):601–18. https://doi.org/10.1007/s11764-018-0696-6.
28. Sivakumar J, Sivakumar H, Read M, Sinclair RCF, Snowden CP, Hii MW. The role of cardiopulmonary exercise testing as a risk assessment tool in patients undergoing oesophagectomy: a systematic review and meta-analysis. Ann Surg Oncol. 2020;27(10):3783–96. https://doi.org/10.1245/s10434-020-08638-9.
29. Steffens D, Ismail H, Denehy L, Beckenkamp PR, Solomon M, Koh C, et al. Preoperative cardiopulmonary exercise test associated with postoperative outcomes in patients undergoing cancer surgery: a systematic review and meta-analyses. Ann Surg Oncol. 2021;28(12):7120–46. https://doi.org/10.1245/s10434-021-10251-3.
30. Lam S, Alexandre L, Hardwick G, Hart AR. The association between preoperative cardio pulmonary exercise-test variables and short-term morbidity after esophagectomy: a hospital-based cohort study. Surgery. 2019;166(1):28–33. https://doi.org/10.1016/j.surg.2019.02.001.
31. Sivakumar J, Forshaw MJ, Lam S, Peters CJ, Allum WH, Whibley J, et al. Identifying the limitations of cardiopulmonary exercise testing prior to esophagectomy using a pooled analysis of patient-level data. Dis Esophagus. 2022;35(11):doac005. https://doi.org/10.1093/dote/doac005.
32. Guinan EM, Bennett AE, Doyle SL, O'Neill L, Gannon J, Foley G, et al. Measuring the impact of oesophagectomy on physical functioning and physical activity participation: a prospective study. BMC Cancer. 2019;19(1):682. https://doi.org/10.1186/s12885-019-5888-6.
33. Inoue T, Ito S, Kanda M, Niwa Y, Nagaya M, Nishida Y, et al. Preoperative six-minute walk distance as a predictor of postoperative complication in patients with esophageal cancer. Dis Esophagus. 2020;33(2):doz050. https://doi.org/10.1093/dote/doz050.
34. Kondo S, Inoue T, Yoshida T, Saito T, Inoue S, Nishino T, et al. Impact of preoperative 6-minute walk distance on long-term prognosis after esophagectomy in patients with esophageal cancer. Esophagus. 2022;19(1):95–104. https://doi.org/10.1007/s10388-021-00871-9.

35. Faller JW, Pereira DDN, de Souza S, Nampo FK, Orlandi FS, Matumoto S. Instruments for the detection of frailty syndrome in older adults: a systematic review. PLoS One. 2019;14(4):e0216166. https://doi.org/10.1371/journal.pone.0216166.
36. Park MG, Haro G, Mabeza RM, Sakowitz S, Verma A, Lee C, et al. Association of frailty with clinical and financial outcomes of esophagectomy hospitalizations in the United States. Surg Open Sci. 2022;9:80–5. https://doi.org/10.1016/j.sopen.2022.05.003.
37. Yurttas T, Hidvegi R, Filipovic M. Biomarker-based preoperative risk stratification for patients undergoing non-cardiac surgery. J Clin Med. 2020;9(2):351. https://doi.org/10.3390/jcm9020351.
38. Weber M, Luchner A, Seeberger M, Mueller C, Liebetrau C, Schlitt A, et al. Incremental value of high-sensitive troponin T in addition to the revised cardiac index for peri-operative risk stratification in non-cardiac surgery [published correction appears in Eur Heart J. 2013 Jun;34(24):1853. Manfred, Seeberger [corrected to Seeberger, Manfred]]. Eur Heart J. 2013;34(11):853–62. https://doi.org/10.1093/eurheartj/ehs445.
39. Duceppe E, Patel A, Chan MTV, Berwanger O, Ackland G, Kavsak PA, et al. Preoperative N-terminal pro-B-type natriuretic peptide and cardiovascular events after noncardiac surgery: a cohort study. Ann Intern Med. 2020;172(2):96–104. https://doi.org/10.7326/M19-2501.
40. Rodseth RN, Biccard BM, Le Manach Y, Sessler DI, Lurati Buse GA, Thabane L, et al. The prognostic value of pre-operative and post-operative B-type natriuretic peptides in patients undergoing noncardiac surgery: B-type natriuretic peptide and N-terminal fragment of pro-B-type natriuretic peptide: a systematic review and individual patient data meta-analysis. J Am Coll Cardiol. 2014;63(2):170–80. https://doi.org/10.1016/j.jacc.2013.08.1630.
41. Hou JL, Gao K, Li M, Ma JY, Shi YK, Wang Y, et al. Increased N-terminal pro-brain natriuretic peptide level predicts atrial fibrillation after surgery for esophageal carcinoma. World J Gastroenterol. 2008;14(16):2582–5. https://doi.org/10.3748/wjg.14.2582.
42. Cai GL, Chen J, Hu CB, Yan ML, Xu QH, Yan J. Value of plasma brain natriuretic peptide levels for predicting postoperative atrial fibrillation: a systemic review and meta-analysis. World J Surg. 2014;38(1):51–9. https://doi.org/10.1007/s00268-013-2284-2.
43. Szczeklik W, LeManach Y, Fronczek J, Polok K, Conen D, McAlister FA, et al. Preoperative levels of natriuretic peptides and the incidence of postoperative atrial fibrillation after noncardiac surgery: a prospective cohort study. CMAJ. 2020;192(49):E1715–22. https://doi.org/10.1503/cmaj.200840.
44. Amar D, Zhang H, Shi W, Downey RJ, Bains MS, Park BJ, et al. Brain natriuretic peptide and risk of atrial fibrillation after thoracic surgery. J Thorac Cardiovasc Surg. 2012;144(5):1249–53. https://doi.org/10.1016/j.jtcvs.2012.06.051.
45. Chang HY, Chang WT, Liu YW. Application of transthoracic echocardiography in patients receiving intermediate- or high-risk noncardiac surgery. PLoS One. 2019;14(4):e0215854. https://doi.org/10.1371/journal.pone.0215854.
46. Ai D, Lasala J, Mehran JR, Xu G, Banchs J, Cata JP. Preoperative echocardiographic parameters of diastolic dysfunction did not provide a predictive value for postoperative atrial fibrillation in lung and esophageal cancer surgery. J Cardiothorac Vasc Anesth. 2015;29(5):1127–30. https://doi.org/10.1053/j.jvca.2015.01.012.
47. Nagatsuka Y, Sugimura K, Miyata H, Shinnno N, Asukai K, Hara H, et al. Predictive value of preoperative echocardiographic assessment for postoperative atrial fibrillation after esophagectomy for esophageal cancer. Esophagus. 2021;18(3):496–503. https://doi.org/10.1007/s10388-020-00804-y.
48. Brecher O, Gulati H, Roistacher N, Zhang H, Shi W, Thaler HT, et al. Preoperative echocardiographic indices of diastolic dysfunction and brain natriuretic peptide in predicting postoperative atrial fibrillation after noncardiac surgery. Anesth Analg. 2017;124(4):1099–104. https://doi.org/10.1213/ANE.0000000000001471.
49. Chow CK, Teo KK, Rangarajan S, Islam S, Gupta R, Avezum A, et al. Prevalence, awareness, treatment, and control of hypertension in rural and urban communities in high-, middle-, and low-income countries. JAMA. 2013;310(9):959–68. https://doi.org/10.1001/jama.2013.184182.

50. Futier E, Lefrant JY, Guinot PG, Godet T, Lorne E, Cuvillon P, et al. Effect of individualized vs standard blood pressure management strategies on postoperative organ dysfunction among high-risk patients undergoing major surgery: a randomized clinical trial. JAMA. 2017;318(14):1346–57. https://doi.org/10.1001/jama.2017.14172.
51. Im C, Oh TK, Song IA. Association between use of preoperative antihypertensive medication and 90-Day mortality after noncardiac surgery: a retrospective cohort study. Am J Hypertens. 2020;33(6):534–42. https://doi.org/10.1093/ajh/hpaa012.
52. Liang J, Li G, Xu J, Wang T, Jia Y, Zhai Q, et al. Hypertension predicts a poor prognosis in patients with esophageal squamous cell carcinoma. Oncotarget. 2018;9(18):14068–76. https://doi.org/10.18632/oncotarget.23774.
53. Williams B, Mancia G, Spiering W, Agabiti Rosei E, Azizi M, Burnier M, et al. 2018 ESC/ESH Guidelines for the management of arterial hypertension [published correction appears in Eur Heart J. 2019 Feb 1;40(5):475]. Eur Heart J. 2018;39(33):3021–104. https://doi.org/10.1093/eurheartj/ehy339.
54. Friedell ML, Van Way CW III, Freyberg RW, Almenoff PL. β-Blockade and operative mortality in noncardiac surgery: harmful or helpful? [published correction appears in JAMA Surg. 2015 Aug;150(8):820]. JAMA Surg. 2015;150(7):658–63. https://doi.org/10.1001/jamasurg.2015.86.
55. Schizas D, Theochari NA, Theochari CA, Kokkinidis DG, Domi V, Mpaili E, et al. Perioperative management of antiplatelet therapy in patients with history of coronary artery disease undergoing surgery for esophageal cancer: a single-center experience. In Vivo. 2019;33(2):621–6. https://doi.org/10.21873/invivo.11519.
56. Fujikawa T, Tanaka A, Abe T, Yoshimoto Y, Tada S, Maekawa H. Effect of antiplatelet therapy on patients undergoing gastroenterological surgery: thromboembolic risks versus bleeding risks during its perioperative withdrawal. World J Surg. 2015;39(1):139–49. https://doi.org/10.1007/s00268-014-2760-3.
57. Go AS, Mozaffarian D, Roger VL, Benjamin EJ, Berry JD, Blaha MJ, et al. Heart disease and stroke statistics—2014 update: a report from the American Heart Association. Circulation. 2014;129(3):e28–e292. https://doi.org/10.1161/01.cir.0000441139.02102.80.
58. Hornor MA, Duane TM, Ehlers AP, Jensen EH, Brown PS Jr, Pohl D, et al. American College of Surgeons' guidelines for the perioperative management of antithrombotic medication. J Am Coll Surg. 2018;227(5):521–536.e1. https://doi.org/10.1016/j.jamcollsurg.2018.08.183.
59. Devereaux PJ, Mrkobrada M, Sessler DI, Leslie K, Alonso-Coello P, Kurz A, et al. Aspirin in patients undergoing noncardiac surgery. N Engl J Med. 2014;370(16):1494–503. https://doi.org/10.1056/NEJMoa1401105.
60. Vranckx P, Valgimigli M, Jüni P, Hamm C, Steg PG, Heg D, et al. Ticagrelor plus aspirin for 1 month, followed by ticagrelor monotherapy for 23 months vs aspirin plus clopidogrel or ticagrelor for 12 months, followed by aspirin monotherapy for 12 months after implantation of a drug-eluting stent: a multicentre, open-label, randomised superiority trial. Lancet. 2018;392(10151):940–9. https://doi.org/10.1016/S0140-6736(18)31858-0.
61. Mehran R, Baber U, Sharma SK, Cohen DJ, Angiolillo DJ, Briguori C, et al. Ticagrelor with or without aspirin in high-risk patients after PCI. N Engl J Med. 2019;381(21):2032–42. https://doi.org/10.1056/NEJMoa1908419.
62. Watanabe H, Domei T, Morimoto T, Natsuaki M, Shiomi H, Toyota T, et al. Effect of 1-month dual antiplatelet therapy followed by clopidogrel vs 12-month dual antiplatelet therapy on cardiovascular and bleeding events in patients receiving PCI: the STOPDAPT-2 randomized clinical trial. JAMA. 2019;321(24):2414–27. https://doi.org/10.1001/jama.2019.8145.
63. Aoyama T, Atsumi Y, Hara K, Kazama K, Tamagawa H, Tamagawa A, et al. Postoperative bleeding after esophagectomy for esophageal cancer in patients receiving antiplatelet and anticoagulation treatment. Anticancer Res. 2020;40(4):2359–64. https://doi.org/10.21873/anticanres.14204.
64. Levine GN, Bates ER, Bittl JA, Brindis RG, Fihn SD, Fleisher LA, et al. 2016 ACC/AHA guideline focused update on duration of dual antiplatelet therapy in patients with coronary artery disease: a report of the American College of Cardiology/American Heart Association

Task Force on Clinical Practice Guidelines. J Thorac Cardiovasc Surg. 2016;152(5):1243–75. https://doi.org/10.1016/j.jtcvs.2016.07.044.
65. Visseren FLJ, Mach F, Smulders YM, et al. 2021 ESC Guidelines on cardiovascular disease prevention in clinical practice [published correction appears in Eur Heart J. 2022 Nov 7;43(42):4468]. Eur Heart J. 2021;42(34):3227–337. https://doi.org/10.1093/eurheartj/ehab484.
66. Alexandre L, Clark AB, Bhutta HY, Chan SS, Lewis MP, Hart AR. Association between statin use after diagnosis of esophageal cancer and survival: a population-based cohort study. Gastroenterology. 2016;150(4):854–e17. https://doi.org/10.1053/j.gastro.2015.12.039.
67. Cardwell CR, Spence AD, Hughes CM, Murray LJ. Statin use after esophageal cancer diagnosis and survival: a population based cohort study. Cancer Epidemiol. 2017;48:124–30. https://doi.org/10.1016/j.canep.2017.04.015.
68. McFalls EO, Ward HB, Moritz TE, Goldman S, Krupski WC, Littooy F, Pierpont G, Santilli S, Rapp J, Hattler B, Shunk K, Jaenicke C, Thottapurathu L, Ellis N, Reda DJ, Henderson WG. Coronary-artery revascularization before elective major vascular surgery. N Engl J Med. 2004;351(27):2795–804. https://doi.org/10.1056/NEJMoa041905.
69. Chen Y, Li F, Wu K, Zhao J, Yang Y, Qi Y, et al. Do statins improve the survival time after esophagectomy?—a propensity score matching study. Transl Cancer Res. 2020;9(4):2295–9. https://doi.org/10.21037/tcr.2020.03.51.
70. Xie K, Zhang W, Fang J, Guo Y, Fang M, Ding Z, et al. Prevalence and risk factors of atrial fibrillation during lung and esophageal surgery: a prospective observational study. Medicine (Baltimore). 2018;97(30):e11549. https://doi.org/10.1097/MD.0000000000011549.
71. Seesing MFJ, Borggreve AS, Ruurda JP, van Hillegersberg R. New-onset atrial fibrillation after esophagectomy for cancer. J Thorac Dis. 2019;11(Suppl 5):S831–4. https://doi.org/10.21037/jtd.2019.02.03.
72. Day RW, Jaroszewski D, Chang YH, Ross HJ, Paripati H, Ashman JB, et al. Incidence and impact of postoperative atrial fibrillation after minimally invasive esophagectomy. Dis Esophagus. 2016;29(6):583–8. https://doi.org/10.1111/dote.12355.
73. Seesing MFJ, Scheijmans JCG, Borggreve AS, van Hillegersberg R, Ruurda JP. The predictive value of new-onset atrial fibrillation on postoperative morbidity after esophagectomy. Dis Esophagus. 2018;31(11) https://doi.org/10.1093/dote/doy028.
74. Oesterle A, Weber B, Tung R, Choudhry NK, Singh JP, Upadhyay GA. Preventing postoperative atrial fibrillation after noncardiac surgery: a meta-analysis. Am J Med. 2018;131(7):795–804.e5. https://doi.org/10.1016/j.amjmed.2018.01.032.
75. Tisdale JE, Wroblewski HA, Wall DS, et al. A randomized, controlled study of amiodarone for prevention of atrial fibrillation after transthoracic esophagectomy. J Thorac Cardiovasc Surg. 2010;140(1):45–51. https://doi.org/10.1016/j.jtcvs.2010.01.026.
76. Amar D, Zhang H, Heerdt PM, Park B, Fleisher M, Thaler HT. Statin use is associated with a reduction in atrial fibrillation after noncardiac thoracic surgery independent of C-reactive protein. Chest. 2005;128(5):3421–7. https://doi.org/10.1378/chest.128.5.3421.
77. Saran T, Perkins GD, Javed MA, Annam V, Leong L, Gao F, et al. Does the prophylactic administration of magnesium sulphate to patients undergoing thoracotomy prevent postoperative supraventricular arrhythmias? A randomized controlled trial. Br J Anaesth. 2011;106(6):785–91. https://doi.org/10.1093/bja/aer096.
78. Sakamoto A, Hamasaki T, Kitakaze M. Perioperative landiolol administration reduces atrial fibrillation after cardiac surgery: a meta-analysis of randomized controlled trials. Adv Ther. 2014;31(4):440–50. https://doi.org/10.1007/s12325-014-0116-x.
79. Ojima T, Nakamori M, Nakamura M, et al. Randomized clinical trial of landiolol hydrochloride for the prevention of atrial fibrillation and postoperative complications after oesophagectomy for cancer. Br J Surg. 2017;104(8):1003–9. https://doi.org/10.1002/bjs.10548.
80. Gassanov N, Er F. Ultraschnell wirksame Betablocker Esmolol und Landiolol: Aktuelle Rolle in der Intensiv- und Notfallmedizin [The role of ultrarapid acting betablocker esmolol and landiolol in critically ill patients]. Dtsch Med Wochenschr. 2019;144(18):1280–5. https://doi.org/10.1055/a-0936-3872.

81. Gillinov AM, Bagiella E, Moskowitz AJ, Raiten JM, Groh MA, Bowdish ME, et al. Rate control versus rhythm control for atrial fibrillation after cardiac surgery. N Engl J Med. 2016;374(20):1911–21. https://doi.org/10.1056/NEJMoa1602002.
82. Lin MH, Kamel H, Singer DE, Wu YL, Lee M, Ovbiagele B. Perioperative/postoperative atrial fibrillation and risk of subsequent stroke and/or mortality. Stroke. 2019;50(6):1364–71. https://doi.org/10.1161/STROKEAHA.118.023921.
83. Steffel J, Collins R, Antz M, Cornu P, Desteghe L, Haeusler KG, Oldgren J, Reinecke H, Roldan-Schilling V, Rowell N, Sinnaeve P, Vanassche T, Potpara T, Camm AJ, Heidbüchel H, External reviewers. 2021 European Heart Rhythm Association Practical Guide on the use of non-vitamin K antagonist oral anticoagulants in patients with atrial fibrillation. Europace. 2021;23(10):1612–76. https://doi.org/10.1093/europace/euab065. Erratum in: Europace. 2021 Jun 28.
84. Smilowitz NR, Banco D, Katz SD, Beckman JA, Berger JS. Association between heart failure and perioperative outcomes in patients undergoing non-cardiac surgery. Eur Heart J Qual Care Clin Outcomes. 2021;7(1):68–75. https://doi.org/10.1093/ehjqcco/qcz066.
85. Wang X, Sweigert P, Eguia E, Varsnik MA, Renz CR, Terrasse WA, et al. Impact of angiotensin system inhibitors on esophageal cancer survival. Surg Open Sci. 2020;3:34–8. https://doi.org/10.1016/j.sopen.2020.08.001.
86. McMurray JJ, Packer M, Desai AS, Gong J, Lefkowitz MP, Rizkala AR, et al. Angiotensin-neprilysin inhibition versus enalapril in heart failure. N Engl J Med. 2014;371(11):993–1004. https://doi.org/10.1056/NEJMoa1409077.
87. Tagawa M, Ogata A, Hamano T. Pre- and/or intra-operative prescription of diuretics, but not renin-angiotensin-system inhibitors, is significantly associated with acute kidney injury after non-cardiac surgery: a retrospective cohort study. PLoS One. 2015;10(7):e0132507. https://doi.org/10.1371/journal.pone.0132507.
88. Vahanian A, Beyersdorf F, Praz F, Milojevic M, Baldus S, Bauersachs J, et al. 2021 ESC/EACTS Guidelines for the management of valvular heart disease. Eur Heart J. 2022;43:561–632. https://doi.org/10.1093/eurheartj/ehab395.
89. Bajaj NS, Agarwal S, Rajamanickam A, Parashar A, Poddar KL, Griffin BP, et al. Impact of severe mitral regurgitation on postoperative outcomes after noncardiac surgery. Am J Med. 2013;126:529–35. https://doi.org/10.1016/j.amjmed.2012.12.005.

# Cardio-Oncology: Cancer and Treatment-Related Cardiotoxicity and Imaging Methods for Assessment of Cardiotoxicity

17

Rengin Cetin Guvenc, Emel Celiker Guler, and Tolga Sinan Güvenc

## Abbreviations

| | |
|---|---|
| 2D | Two-dimensional |
| 3D | Three-dimensional |
| CAC | Coronary artery calcium |
| CAD | Coronary artery disease |
| CCTA | Cardiac computed tomography angiography |
| CT | Computed tomography |
| CTRCD | Cancer therapy-related cardiac dysfunction |
| EC | Esophageal cancer |
| ECV | Extracellular volume |
| ESC | European Society of Cardiology |
| FDG | Fluorodeoxyglucose |
| FP | Fluoropyrimidines |
| GLS | Global longitudinal strain |
| HF | Heart failure |
| ICI | Immune checkpoint inhibitor |
| IMRT | Intensity-modulated proton beam therapy |
| irAE | Immune-related adverse effects |
| LGE | Late gadolinium enhancement |

R. C. Guvenc
Cardiology Department, Okan University School of Medicine, Istanbul, Turkey

E. C. Guler
Cardiology Department, Koc University School of Medicine, Istanbul, Turkey

T. S. Güvenc (✉)
Cardiology Department, Istinye University School of Medicine, Istanbul, Turkey
e-mail: tolgasinan.guvenc@istinye.edu.tr


O. Engin (ed.), *Risk Factors and Therapy of Esophagus Cancer*,
https://doi.org/10.1007/978-3-031-47024-0_17

| | |
|---|---|
| LVEF | Left ventricular ejection fraction |
| MHD | Mean heart dose |
| NCCN | National Comprehensive Cancer Network |
| PD-1 | Programmed death receptor 1 |
| PET | Positron emission tomography |
| RT | Radiotherapy |
| SPECT | Single-photon emission computed tomography |
| TTE | Transthoracic echocardiography |
| TTS | Takotsubo syndrome |

## 17.1 Introduction

Cardio-oncology and therapy-related cardiotoxicity are two complementary definitions that come to the fore in the emergence of cardiovascular disease secondary to oncological diseases and their treatment. The term cardio-oncology includes the definition of cardiotoxicity associated with cancer treatments, in addition to the direct or indirect effects of the cancer itself in causing cardiovascular disease [1].

Cancer therapy-induced cardiotoxicity is defined as damage to all cardiac structures affected at different levels by radiotherapy (RT) and chemotherapy that occurs during and after cancer treatment and can lead to long-term adverse outcomes, including cardiac death. 2022 European Society of Cardiology (ESC) guidelines on cardio-oncology, developed in collaboration with the European Hematology Association, the European Society for Therapeutic Radiology and Oncology, and the International Cardio-Oncology Society Committee, define chemotherapy-induced cardiotoxicity for heart failure (HF) as one or more of the following: (1) symptoms or signs associated with heart failure—from mild to severe requiring advanced heart failure management strategies; (2) new reduction in left ventricular ejection fraction (LVEF) <40%; (3) reduction in LVEF ≤10% in the presence of LVEF 40–49% and new relative decrease in global longitudinal strain (GLS) >15% or new increase in cardiac biomarkers, or reduction in LVEF ≥10% in the presence of LVEF 40–49% or LVEF ≥50% and new relative decrease in GLS >15% from baseline and/or new increase in cardiac biomarkers. Other definitions and adverse event grading of cancer therapy-related cardiotoxicity are shown in Table 17.1 [1, 2].

Thoracic malignancies such as lung, esophageal, breast, and Hodgkin's lymphoma cause major cardiovascular events. Unlike most other cancers, esophageal cancer (EC) in advanced stages can spread directly to the pericardium, airways, pulmonary artery, aorta, and heart. In particular, upper EC tends to invade the aorta and carotid arteries due to their location. Both the invasion of nearby structures and the autocrine and paracrine effects of cancers can cause serious cardiovascular complications, such as aorto-esophageal fistula, superior vena cava syndrome, pericarditis, and pericardial effusion, which in the long term can lead to cardiac tamponade or constrictive pericarditis, and thromboembolism due to increased thrombogenicity. Early diagnosis and prompt treatment are essential to improve patient outcomes [1].

**Table 17.1** European Society of Cardiology and National Cancer Institute Definitions for Adverse Events Related to Cancer Treatments

| Category/severity | Subcategories/definitions |
|---|---|
| *European Society of Cardiology Cardio-oncology Study Group definitions* | |
| Heart failure | Symptomatic/asymptomatic |
| Myocarditis (mostly related to immunotherapy) | Fulminant/non-fulminant/steroid refractory |
| Vascular disease | Acute coronary syndrome/main coronary arteries or microvascular disease/other vessel lesion/ cerebrovascular events/vasospastic angina |
| Arterial hypertension | |
| Brady- or tachy-arrhythmias | |
| Pericardial disease | Pericarditis/pericardial effusion/tamponade |
| Venous or arterial thrombosis | |
| *The National Cancer Institute common terminology criteria for adverse events* | |
| Grade 1—mild | Asymptomatic or mild symptoms, clinical or diagnostic observations only, intervention not indicated |
| Grade 2—moderate | Minimal, local or noninvasive intervention indicated |
| Grade 3—severe or medically significant but not immediately life-threatening | Hospitalization or prolongation of hospitalization indicated |
| Grade 4—life-threatening consequences | Urgent intervention indicated |
| Grade 5—death related to adverse event | |

Modified from European Society of Cardiology Guidelines on Cardio-oncology and National Cancer Institute Definitions for Adverse Events [1, 2]

With improvements in EC treatment modalities, as cancer-specific survival increases, the proportion of cancer therapy-induced cardiotoxicity increases, and cardiovascular disease becomes the most common cause of mortality not directly related to neoplasms [3].

## 17.2 Therapy-Related Cardiotoxicity

### 17.2.1 Chemoradiotherapy

Esophageal cancer is a highly aggressive form of cancer, and as a result, its survival rates are lower compared to other types of thoracic malignancies. This low survival rate has made it challenging to determine the frequency of cardiac events related to late toxicity in the long term [4, 5]. However, advancements in modern neoadjuvant chemoradiotherapy (CRT) regimens and techniques for shielding cardiac tissue from radiation have led to a decrease in associated cardiotoxicity. It is important to note that while these improvements have resulted in increased survival rates, they may also increase the risk of treatment-induced late cardiotoxicity [4, 5].

Chemoradiotherapy is the mainstay of definitive treatment for locally advanced EC. Depending on the chemotherapy and RT regimens, cardiotoxicity may occur in the acute (up to 2 weeks), early (within 1 year) and late (1 year after the treatment) phases of treatment [6–9].

### 17.2.2 Radiation Therapy

Radiotherapy, along with chemotherapy, is the primary modality for locoregional EC. While it is a critical component of curative peri/pre/postoperative treatments for locally advanced disease, its use alone is limited to palliative therapy for patients who are ineligible for chemotherapy and/or surgery [6].

It is well known that during RT, the radiation beam travels in different directions and interacts with the human body, affecting both healthy and cancerous tissues (Table 17.2). This radiation can affect blood vessel permeability by causing

**Table 17.2** Mechanisms or radiation-induced cardiac injury, potential outcomes, and management strategies to alleviate or treat radiation-induced cardiac dysfunction

| Exposed area | Mechanisms | Outcomes | Management strategies |
|---|---|---|---|
| Coronary arteries | Increased capillary permeability<br>Endothelial dysfunction<br>Intimal proliferation<br>Progressive fibrosis<br>Luminal narrowing<br>Upstream thrombogenesis<br>Microvascular thrombosis | Ischemia<br>Myocardial infarction<br>Coronary artery disease (particularly ostial lesions and left main or left anterior descending artery stenosis)<br>Sudden cardiac death | Anti ischemic treatment<br>Statins<br>Antiplatelets<br>Coronary revascularization |
| Myocardium | Microvascular dysfunction<br>Ischemia<br>Diffuse interstitial fibrosis | Arrhythmias<br>Diastolic dysfunction<br>Restrictive cardiomyopathy<br>Heart failure | Antiarrhythmic agents<br>Medical treatment for heart failure<br>Device treatment for heart failure<br>Cardiac transplantation |
| Pericardium | Acute and chronic inflammation<br>Fibrosis | Acute or chronic pericarditis<br>Pericardial tamponade<br>Constrictive pericarditis | Pericardiocentesis<br>Medical treatment<br>Surgery |
| Valvular apparatus | Fibrosis<br>Valvular thickening and retraction—calcification | Aortic stenosis or regurgitation/mitral stenosis or regurgitation | Medical treatment<br>Surgical repair or valve replacement<br>Percutaneous repair or valve replacement |
| Conduction system | Fibrosis | Atrioventricular blocks QTc prolongation<br>Supraventricular or ventricular arrhythmias | Antiarrhythmic drugs<br>Pacemaker and/or intracardiac defibrillator (ICD) implantation<br>Percutaneous ablation |

vasodilation and cell damage in target and non-target organs [3, 10, 11]. That can happen directly through its particles and free oxygen radicals, resulting in DNA single and double-strand breaks, RNA helix damage, intracellular protein damage and endothelial basement membrane damage [10–12]. Although most of its potential energy is lost during radiation scattering, it can accumulate in the body over time and trigger inflammation and other mechanisms that cause cardiovascular damage, even if the irradiated area is outside the thorax [10, 13]. The process, which starts with inflammation and ends with fibrosis, affects all structures of the heart, such as the pericardium, endocardium, myocardium, conduction system, coronary arteries and valvular components of the heart, as well as other tissues [3]. Additionally, cardiac structures are at risk due to their proximity to the esophagus, both in terms of the risk of direct cancer invasion and spread, and from radiation scatter during treatment. Although cardiac structures have been shown to be relatively more resistant to RT, the use of higher dose RT regimens and radiation intensity in EC may increase the cardiotoxic effect [11].

The recommended doses are 41.4 Gy, 45 Gy, and 50.4 Gy for preoperative, postoperative, and nonsurgical candidates, respectively, but these maximum doses should not be exceeded per The National Comprehensive Cancer Network (NCCN) guidelines [6]. Apart from the fact that there are no data showing that higher doses are beneficial, further dose escalation is associated with decreased survival [6, 14]. Since the first description of the relationship between radiation and cardiac disease by Hankok et al., many studies have been published showing the strong correlation and linear relationship between mean heart dose (MHD) and cardiac disease and mortality [15–18]. MHD is a measure used in clinical practice to determine radiation exposure to the heart [10]. Studies have used an acceptable threshold of 3–7 Gy for MHD. As there is no safe MHD (1 Gy increase per MHD up to 7.4% risk of cardiovascular disease), radiation dose should be minimized as much as possible [1, 6, 10, 19]. Intensity-modulated RT, proton beam therapy, intensity-modulated proton beam therapy (IMRT), 3D conformal RT, external beam RT are different techniques used in current clinical practice and trials for the treatment of EC [6]. The NCCN currently recommends the use of IMRT for definitive, pre/postoperative treatment of EC because it is feasible with low toxicity and acceptable side effects to the lungs and heart [6]. However, to further reduce cardiotoxicity, simulation of treatment planning should be performed using CT or an immobilization device to prevent respiratory movement to maintain reproducibility and protect the effect of large cardiac volumes [6, 20]. However, besides radiation dose and modality, age, and presence of previous cardiovascular disease and its risk factors such as diabetes and hypertension are important indicators of cardiotoxicity [1]. Therefore, studies have reported two different vulnerable populations for RT. Radiation exposure under 15 years of age was found to be associated with an absolute and relative risk of high mortality [21, 22]. On the other hand, one study showed that being older than 75 years was associated with more than grade 3 cardiotoxicity compared with relatively younger patients with EC (30% vs. 3%) [23]. While the first phenomenon can be explained by the radiation sensitivity of developing myocytes and the longer life expectancy of younger patients, the second situation can be attributed to the abundance of comorbidities in elderly patients. Other risk factors for the development of radiation-induced cardiotoxicity are: (1) large cardiac volume irradiated, (2) organ-sparing effect: anterior/posterior positioning, (3) tumor location, (4) total exposure time, (5) concomitant cardiotoxic chemotherapy (e.g. anthracyclines, 5-fluorouracil) [3, 6].

## 17.2.3 Chemotherapy

The Preoperative Chemoradiotherapy for Esophageal or Junctional Cancer trial demonstrated that preoperative chemoradiation for locoregional EC is associated with reduced survival and local recurrence rates compared to chemotherapy and surgery alone [6, 24, 25]. However, chemotherapeutic agents can be used alone for preoperative treatment, as well as for systemic treatment of locally advanced or metastatic EC. Although various combination therapies are available for chemotherapy in the treatment of esophageal carcinoma, the major drug groups are FLOT (fluorouracil, leucovorin, oxaliplatin, and docetaxel), FOLFOX (leucovorin calcium, fluorouracil, and oxaliplatin) regimes, and immune checkpoint inhibitors. Additionally, drugs such as Trastuzumab (for HER2-overexpressing adenocarcinoma), Ramucirumab, Fam-trastuzumab deruxtecan-nxki, Entrectinib, and Larotrectinib (rarely used in EC) are recommended for special and rare conditions as a part of second-line/subsequent therapy or target therapy [6, 25]. The cardiotoxic effects associated with the major drug groups are provided below.

### 17.2.3.1 FLOT/FOLFOX-Related Cardiotoxicity

Fluoropyrimidines (FP) are one of the main component of treatment for all advanced ECs, whether they are metastatic or not [25]. Capecitabine, an oral prodrug, is designed to inhibit RNA and DNA synthesis by activating within the tumor cell [26]. The main pathophysiology leading to cardiotoxicity is endothelial damage, vasospasm, and thrombus formation, which may cause myocardial ischemia, coronary artery disease, acute coronary syndrome, and arrhythmias [26, 27]. Free oxygen radicals have been shown to increase the risk of endothelial and myocardial damage by triggering vasospasm [26, 28]. The risk of cardiotoxicity is higher in patients with pre-existing cardiac disease, high doses, concomitant use of certain cardiotoxic chemotherapeutics (e.g., cisplatin/leucovorin), and RT [29, 30]. The rate of administration is also a contributing factor, as cardiotoxic side effects are more common after long infusion episodes [29, 31, 32]. The less cardiotoxicity is associated with the short half-life of FPs when administered as a bolus [32].

Unlike other chemotherapeutic agents, fluoropyrimidines have a high potential for silent ischemia, which means that about half of the patients do not have any complaints, and resting angina is more common than exertion-induced angina [1, 26, 33]. Therefore, careful follow-up of the patient is important, and dizziness is among the most common non-cardiac complaints [27]. It may be associated with episodes of bradycardia, tachyarrhythmia, or secondary left ventricular failure in the accompanying ischemic myocardium. Electrocardiographic variabilities, cardiac biomarkers (troponins I-T, creatine kinase myocardial band, and B-type natriuretic peptide), and echocardiographic findings are not highly sensitive for detecting abnormalities due to FP-induced cardiovascular events [34]. However, the presence of symptoms correlates with an increase in biomarker levels and ECG abnormalities [34]. Asymptomatic patients who undergo FP therapy should be carefully evaluated with screening using ECG, Holter-ECG monitoring, and stress tests in selected cases to prevent cardiovascular events [27].

To prevent FP-related cardiotoxicity, it is recommended to avoid combination regimens if possible, use reduced doses, administer the medication for a short time, and combine it with anti-ischemic/antiarrhythmic drugs. And also, stress tests should be part of the diagnosis [1].

#### 17.2.3.2 Platinum-Related Cardiotoxicity

Platinum derivatives have an important role for the perioperative treatment of ECs. They are included in combination therapy as oxaliplatin and cisplatin, but oxaliplatin is recommended due to its lower side effects [6, 25]. The mechanism of action is based on increased mitochondrial oxidative stress, caspase 3 activity in the endoplasmic reticulum, deterioration in mitochondrial structure and function, and subsequent damage to cardiomyocytes and endothelial cells [35, 36]. In addition to cardiac side effects, renal side effects are also prominent, and they can lead to myocardial injury, infarction, and rarely, heart failure, as well as trigger renal tubular necrosis [37]. Fluid replacement is necessary to prevent renal failure, and close monitoring of signs and symptoms, ECG monitoring, and checking cardiac biomarkers are important for early detection of cardiotoxicity development [1].

#### 17.2.3.3 Taxane-Related Cardiotoxicity

Paclitaxel and docetaxel are commonly used to treat esophageal squamous cell carcinoma (SCC) [25]. Cardiac side effects are thought to be mostly related to the conduction system, with reports of bradycardia and atrioventricular blocking effects. However, the general consensus is that cardiac side effects occur mostly when these drugs are used in combination regimens [38] Therefore, routine cardiac monitoring is not recommended in patients without risk factors who are receiving this drug due to their low cardiac side effect profiles. There is currently insufficient evidence to suggest that these drugs have direct cardiotoxic effects [1, 38].

#### 17.2.3.4 Immune Checkpoint Inhibitors-Related Cardiotoxicity

Immunotherapy is a groundbreaking treatment method in cancer treatment that activates the immune system to eliminate neoplastic cells. Since its introduction, it has been increasingly used in the treatment of many cancers, including Hodgkin's lymphoma, non-small cell lung cancer, colorectal cancer, renal cell cancer, severe solid tumors, and esophageal carcinoma (EC). Immune checkpoint inhibitors (ICI), such as Nivolumab and Pembrolizumab, have been shown to significantly improve median overall survival in phase III trials, including ATTRACTION-3, Checkmate-649, KEYNOTE-181, and KEYNOTE-590 in patients with EC [6, 39–42].

ICIs do not suppress immunity but instead activate cytotoxic T lymphocytes and facilitate elimination of neoplastic cells via immune activation. Monoclonal IgG agents bind to checkpoint proteins, including cytotoxic T-lymphocyte antigen 4, programmed death receptor 1 (PD-1), and programmed death-ligand 1 on the surface of cancerous and normal healthy cells, inhibiting them [43, 44]. This inactivation leads to the destruction of cancer cells by cytotoxic T cells. However, as the potential effect of ICIs increases, the side effect profiles secondary to nonspecific immune activation tend to be potent. These adverse effects specific to ICIs are called immune-related adverse effects (irAE) [44]. Myocardial cells express the PD1 receptor and its ligand, which could protect cardiac myocytes against aggressive immune attack [45]. Nivolumab, pembrolizumab, and Dostarlimab-gxly (approved in August 2021 by the FDA) act on PD1 inactivators and block unique negative signaling that prevents immune-related diseases in myocardium [6]. ICI-related cardiotoxicity depends on secondary group effects and specific uses in EC and has been reported with a frequency of around 0.1% [46]. This rate is higher when combination schemes are used and can be dose-dependent for certain agents. The onset of irAEs is usually around 6 weeks after the start of treatment, although the onset of cardiac side effects can vary between 12 and 20 weeks and rarely reported later [1, 47]. Although cardiotoxic side effects are rare, they can be fatal, such as myocarditis and myocarditis-related heart failure.

Symptoms of cardiotoxicity caused by ICIs can be mild and vague at first but can worsen rapidly, leading to clinical progression from benign myocarditis to cardiogenic shock. Therefore, close follow-up of patients receiving ICIs for cardiotoxicity is essential. Clinicians should maintain a low threshold for clinical suspicion in patients who present with symptoms such as chest pain, shortness of breath, palpitations, or fatigue. ECG findings typically demonstrate non-specific ST segment and T wave changes, sinus tachycardia, and occasionally normal patterns, QT prolongation, diffuse T wave inversion, ventricular arrhythmias, and AV conduction defects. Inflammation of the adjacent pericardium can also lead to ECG features of pericarditis. Cardiac biomarker elevation is used as a first-line diagnostic tool and is useful for predicting adverse cardiac events. Troponin level (cTn) >40 ng/L and hs-cTs >14 ng/L on admission are associated with major adverse cardiac events, including developing left ventricular dysfunction and cardiac death [1, 43, 44]. Additionally, BNP and NT-proBNP levels can be used to evaluate volume overload related to left ventricular dysfunction and is useful for ruling out heart failure. For this purpose, BNP <100 pg/mL and NT-proBNP <125 pg/mL threshold could be used [1, 48].

All suspected patients with ICI-related cardiotoxicity should undergo a transthoracic echocardiography (TTE) evaluation. Echocardiography is a useful tool for the comprehensive assessment of cardiac function, as it can not only detect myocarditis and associated ventricular function but also identify other cardiac pathologies, such as pleural and pericardial effusions. While myocardial biopsy is considered the gold standard diagnostic method, in most cases the diagnosis can be established with echocardiography and cardiac magnetic resonance (CMR) without a need for invasive verification [1, 44, 45, 48, 49]. Cardiac biopsy is only recommended for the rare patient that requires a specific diagnosis [49]. For the management of myocarditis secondary to ICIs; hospitalization, close monitoring of hemodynamic parameters, monitoring with cardiac biomarkers, ECG, and echocardiography, and treatment with high-dose steroids (methylprednisolone 500–1000 mg iv. bolus) for at least 3 days is recommended [50]. Transfer of the patient to the intensive care unit in case of any instability and cardiology team evaluation is essential for the treatment of advanced heart failure.

The cardio-oncology consensus recommends resuming ICI therapy after recovery, with careful consideration of any grade +2 cardiac events and life-threatening cardiovascular complications [1, 51, 52]. However, if such complications are present, permanent discontinuation is essential.

In addition to myocarditis and myocarditis-related heart failure, ICIs can also have other cardiotoxic effects, such as non-aggressive pericarditis, pericardial effusion, and non-inflammatory heart failure. As a result, patients treated with ICIs may experience myocardial infarction due to increased thrombogenicity and progressive atherosclerosis, brady/tachyarrhythmias, ischemic stroke, and venous thromboembolism. Therefore, closer follow-up and modification of risk factors are recommended for patients with multiple risk factors [1].

## 17.3 Cardiovascular Imaging Methods for Patients Undergoing Esophageal Cancer Treatment

The descriptive term cancer therapy-related cardiac dysfunction (CTRCD) was introduced in 2022 by the ESC guidelines on cardio-oncology, which encompass the broad spectrum of potential presentations and the etiological link with various cancer therapies, including chemotherapy, targeted agents, immune therapies, and radiation therapy [1]. Although no specific therapy is known for CTRCD, baseline risk assessment and early recognition of functional and structural abnormalities can prevent further damage. Multimodality cardiac imaging is recommended for detecting and screening CTRCD [1, 53]. LVEF is currently recommended, if possible, with three-dimensional TTE or CMR along with global longitudinal strain assessment using speckle-tracking echocardiography as diagnostic tools for cardiotoxicity [1, 53]. Moreover, novel promising imaging techniques such as T1 mapping, T2 mapping, extracellular volume (ECV) quantification, and late gadolinium enhancement by CMR can evaluate myocardial edema, inflammation, and fibrosis. Additionally, coronary artery calcium (CAC) score and cardiac computed tomography angiography (CCTA), as well as nuclear cardiology imaging techniques such as single-photon emission computed tomography (SPECT) and positron emission tomography (PET), play an increasing role in cardio-oncology [53].

### 17.3.1 Echocardiography

Echocardiography is the preferred imaging modality for assessing the risk, screening, and diagnosing of CTRCD. It's widely available, exposes patients to no ionizing radiation, and assesses left and right ventricular function, chamber dilation, left ventricular hypertrophy, regional wall motion abnormalities, diastolic function, valvular heart disease, pulmonary arterial pressure, and pericardial disease [10, 54]. The recommended frequency of echocardiographic screening varies based on the patient's baseline cardiovascular toxicity risk assessment. A baseline comprehensive TTE is recommended for all cancer patients at high and very high risk of cardiovascular toxicity before and during anticancer therapy. High-risk and very high-risk patients should have a TTE every 2 years, while low to moderate-risk patients should undergo TTE screening every 5 years [1].

Current guideline define CTRCD as a reduction of LVEF and/or relative changes in global longitudinal strain (GLS) [1]. In the 2022 ESC guidelines on cardio-oncology, CTRCD is categorized based on LVEF and GLS:

1. Severe (new LVEF reduction to <40%).
2. Moderate (new LVEF reduction by ≥10 percentage points to an LVEF of 40–49% or new LVEF reduction by <10 percentage points to an LVEF of 40–49% and either new relative decline in GLS by >15% from baseline).
3. Mild (LVEF ≥50% and the new relative decline in GLS by >15% from baseline).

Although CTRCD data specific to EC is somewhat limited, available evidence suggests that cardiac dysfunction following treatment can indeed be very common. For example, a retrospective study of 15 patients with esophageal and gastroesophageal junctional cancer demonstrated a significant drop in LVEF in 80% of patients (from 63% to 58%) after chemoradiotherapy [55]. Similarly, Tripp et al. have observed a 5% decrease in mean LVEF after treatment in patients with EC [56]. As such, monitoring for CTRCD is essential to avoid delays in initiating preventive measures that can ameliorate the negative consequences of cardiac dysfunction.

Two-dimensional TTE calculation methods, including the recommended Simpson's biplane method, can be employed to measure left ventricular ejection fraction. However, when available, three-dimensional (3D) TTE is recommended due to its better reproducibility and accuracy [57]. 2D volume calculations have several limitations, such as geometric assumptions, foreshortened views, and high inter- and intra-observer variability. These limitations can cause failure to detect minor variations in systolic and diastolic function, which can result in missed diagnoses of cardiotoxicity [57, 58]. In contrast, 3D TTE can overcome these limitations by eliminating the need for geometric modeling and potential errors caused by foreshortened apical views. It has become more widely accepted in routine cardio-oncology practice, as it offers better accuracy and correlation with the gold standard non-invasive method, CMR measurements [59, 60].

Ultrasound-enhancing contrast agents can improve the delineation of the endocardial border and image quality in poor acoustic windows, which are common in patients with a history of radiation therapy. Left ventricular contrast agents are recommended when two contiguous segments from any apical view are not well observed [53].

The measurement of LVEF is the gold standard for assessing myocardial systolic function. However, it has significant limitations in detecting early subclinical changes. Myocardial deformation measured by 2D speckle-tracking echocardiography can assess early changes in myocardial function before a decrease in LVEF occurs and has a higher prognostic value [61–63].

There are three principal components of strain (radial, circumferential, and longitudinal), but GLS is a widely recognized deformation parameter that evaluates the longitudinal aspect of myocardial contraction. GLS has been shown to be more sensitive than LVEF in detecting subtle myocardial dysfunction [64, 65]. Impaired GLS is associated with mortality, even when LVEF is normal (Fig. 17.1). Therefore, strain imaging is crucial for identifying cardiotoxicity in the early stages.

While modern radiation protocols have significantly reduced the incidence of pericardial disease after chest RT [3, 66], pericardial diseases (pericarditis, effusion, and/or constriction) remain the most common type of cardiotoxicity associated with chest RT administration, with a prevalence of 48% in EC [18]. Pericardial disease may occur in acute (days to months) and chronic phases (months to years) [67], and its clinical presentation can range from asymptomatic to progressive, sometimes resulting in heart failure and death [68]. Echocardiography is the method of choice for the initial evaluation when pericardial disease is suspected due to its high sensitivity in detecting anatomical and hemodynamic changes. It can diagnose pericardial thickening, pericardial effusion, and characteristic hemodynamic features of constrictive pericarditis. Additionally, it can differentiate between constriction and restriction by assessing early diastolic annulus velocity

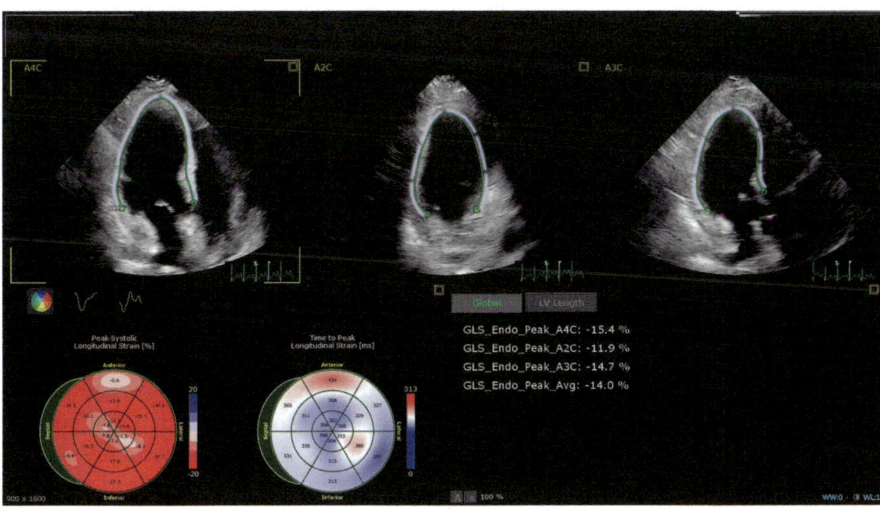


**Fig. 17.1** A 48-year-old female patient with a history of metastatic invasive ductal carcinoma underwent chemotherapy with HER2 inhibitors. Left ventricular strain imaging findings suggest a low global longitudinal strain following the chemotherapy, compatible with subclinical left ventricular dysfunction. Left ventricular ejection fraction was measured as 61.5% during the same study, while a repeat examination showed an ejection fraction of 54.7% 3 months later

and annulus reverse using cardiac tissue Doppler analysis, strain, and strain rate imaging via speckle tracking imaging. However, distinguishing between restriction and constriction is often challenging in patients with a history of chest RT, as reasonably restrictive physiology occurs in these patients due to myocardial fibrosis. Therefore, a multimodality approach is typically required. Evaluating pericardial thickening and calcification with cardiac CT and assessing pericardial gadolinium enhancement and septal shift with cardiac MRI can aid in differentiation.

Chest RT is a major risk factor for the development of valvular heart disease (VHD). The acute effects of radiation on heart valves are usually subtle, and VHD is typically observed 10 or more years after cancer treatment, with reported incidence rates of up to 40% [69], directly related to the RT dose [70, 71]. Echocardiography is the primary imaging modality for the diagnosis and management of VHD. It is suitable for assessing valvular thickening, calcification, regurgitation, and stenosis, and is highly accurate in detecting any degree of valvular disease. However, it should be noted that multimodality imaging with multidetector CT provides critical information regarding the anatomical relationship of various cardiovascular structures to the sternum, as well as the extent of RT-related mediastinal and pulmonary fibrosis and aortic calcification if intervention is required [72].

Echocardiography is a vital imaging tool for screening and diagnosing cardiotoxicity as it offers a comprehensive evaluation of the heart without exposing patients to radiation. Nevertheless, echocardiography has certain limitations in cancer patients, such as inadequate acoustic windows, challenges in breath-holding due to pulmonary fibrosis, and the presence of acoustic shadows caused by tissue calcification [53].

### 17.3.2 Cardiac Magnetic Resonance

CMR is a powerful non-invasive imaging tool in the cardio-oncology field, offering detailed information on the heart's structure and function. Its unique tissue characterization capability enables the evaluation of myocardial inflammation, infiltration, and edema, as well as the detection of valvular and pericardial diseases. Moreover, it allows assessment of myocardial perfusion and provides information regarding extracardiac findings, thus enabling early diagnosis and clinical decision-making in cardiotoxicity [73, 74]. Despite its numerous advantages, CMR has some limitations. The cost of the procedure can be relatively expensive, and it may not be suitable for patients with claustrophobia or metal implants. Additionally, acquiring and analyzing images requires a significant amount of time, which may limit its availability. Furthermore, image quality may be suboptimal in patients with pulmonary fibrosis or acute heart failure who cannot breath-hold repeatedly or have arrhythmias [53].

CMR is considered the gold standard for assessing ventricular volumes and systolic function due to its superior ability to discriminate between endocardial and epicardial borders. It offers high temporal resolution (25–50 ms), spatial resolution (1–2 mm), high signal-to-noise ratio, accuracy, and reproducibility with low intra- and inter-observer variability. The steady-state free precession sequence is preferred for cine imaging, where a series of short-axis slices are analyzed from the base to the apex, and typically acquired in 10–15 min [75]. The left or right ventricular ejection fractions, volumes, and masses can be measured without making any geometric assumptions. Compared to 2D echocardiography, CMR provides a more accurate assessment of LVEF reduction. On the other hand, 3D TTE has an excellent correlation with CMR measurements for LVEF assessment [76]. Therefore, CMR should be considered for evaluating LVEF when echocardiography is not available or non-diagnostic due to its limitations [1].

Advanced imaging techniques such as T1 and T2 mapping are valuable for evaluating myocardial tissue properties, including inflammation, fibrosis, and edema [77, 78]. T1 mapping is a quantitative imaging technique that measures the relaxation time of protons in myocardial tissue. T1 relaxation time is used to assess extracellular volume (ECV) of the myocardium, which quantifies the amount of interstitial space in the myocardium. Changes in ECV can occur in response to myocardial injury, inflammation, or fibrosis, and it is the most sensitive parameter for detecting diffuse myocardial fibrosis. T2-weighted imaging is a valuable non-invasive imaging technique that can detect myocardial edema. T2-weighted images are sensitive to tissue water content and provide information about tissue edema, inflammation, and ischemia. T2 mapping, on the other hand, is a quantitative imaging technique that measures the transverse relaxation time of protons in myocardial tissue. T2 relaxation time can be used to assess myocardial edema, which is an early and reversible feature of myocardial injury. T2-weighted imaging and T2 mapping techniques are primarily used to diagnose myocarditis, a common cause of myocardial edema. They can detect the presence and severity of myocardial edema in patients suspected of having myocarditis, aiding in diagnosis and management. CMR is recommended for all patients with suspected myocarditis, particularly in ICI-associated myocarditis [1]. Although no specific MRI features are described for ICI-induced myocarditis in the literature, modified Lake Louise criteria are recommended for diagnosis. Moreover, CMR can differentiate ICI-associated myocarditis from Takotsubo syndrome (TTS).

Late gadolinium enhancement (LGE) is the gold standard for non-invasive assessment of myocardial scar [76]. Images are typically acquired 10–20 min after injection of a contrast agent, usually gadolinium. Gadolinium accumulates in the scar region, which appears as bright areas due to increased uptake of the contrast agent (Fig. 17.2). The pattern and distribution of LGE allows differentiation of the causes of myocardial dysfunction [77, 79].

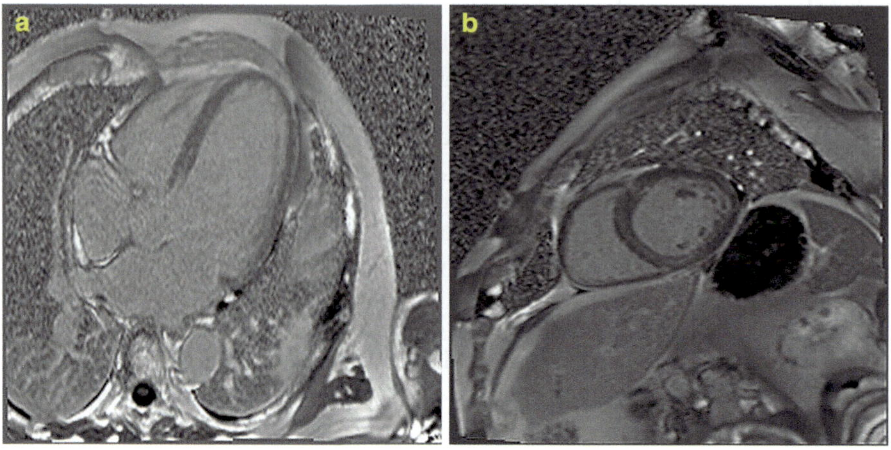


**Fig. 17.2** A 56-year-old patient with renal cell carcinoma underwent treatment with immune checkpoint inhibitors. Mid-myocardial late gadolinium enhancement in the left ventricle on long-axis (**a**) and short-axis (**b**) views is compatible with immune-checkpoint inhibitor-induced myocarditis. The patient had a normal left ventricular ejection fraction before the treatment

### 17.3.3 Cardiac Computed Tomography

Cardiac computed tomography (CCT) has become a valuable diagnostic tool in cardio-oncology due to its ability to detect and assess the significance of coronary artery disease (CAD) by providing functional and structural data of the heart, imaging myocardium, pericardium, valvular and aortic calcifications. It is the only imaging modality that can assess the burden of coronary atherosclerosis [80]. Recent technological advances offer low radiation dose exposure, fast acquisition time, and improved spatial and temporal resolution. However, it still has some disadvantages, such as the need for contrast agents, susceptibility to motion and respiratory artifacts, and ionizing radiation.

ECG-gated non-contrast CT is used to assess coronary artery calcium and screen for CAD (Fig. 17.3). Coronary calcium scanning is an accurate and sensitive method for assessing the progression of coronary artery disease and stratifying cardiovascular risk [81]. The coronary calcium score is usually calculated using the Agatston score, a tool for monitoring subclinical atherosclerosis and identifying patients who may benefit from primary prevention [82, 83]. CAC can also be assessed by non-ECG-gated chest CT, although its diagnostic accuracy is lower than ECG-gated acquisition [84, 85]. It is reasonable to assess coronary calcium burden by non-ECG-gated chest CT for cardiovascular risk stratification and to guide primary prevention therapy, as it is routinely performed for planning chest radiotherapy and cancer staging [81].

Coronary computed tomography angiography is a well-established non-invasive imaging modality for the assessment of coronary artery disease. CCTA has a sensitivity of 100%, specificity of 93%, negative predictive value of 100%, and positive predictive value of 95% on a per-patient basis for excluding CAD with ≥50%

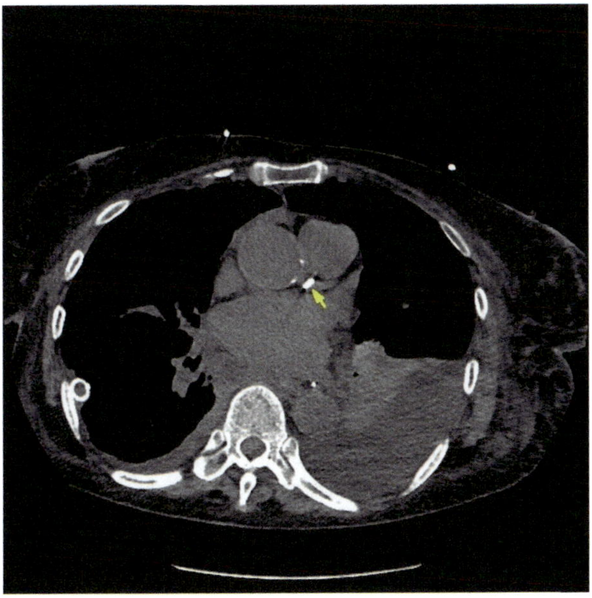

**Fig. 17.3** A 69-year-old female patient with no risk factors for atherosclerosis but with a past medical history of radiotherapy and chemotherapy (with paclitaxel and carboplatin) due to esophageal carcinoma. Non-ECG gated computed tomography shows an osteal left main coronary artery calcification (arrow), compatible with radiotherapy-induced coronary artery disease

luminal stenosis compared with invasive coronary angiography [86]. Thus, CCTA is a robust modality for excluding CAD with high sensitivity. It can be used to assess CAD when coronary angiography is contraindicated due to advanced malignancy and thrombocytopenia [1].

Radiation therapy can accelerate the development of atherosclerosis and plaque rupture, particularly in patients with a history of chest RT who are also at risk for CAD. As a result, individuals receiving radiotherapy should be closely monitored for signs of CAD. According to the 2022 ESC cardio-oncology guidelines, asymptomatic patients who have received more than 15 Gy mean heart dose (≥35 Gy to a volume exposing the heart if mean heart dose is not available) should undergo non-invasive screening for CAD every 5–10 years, beginning 5 years after RT [1]. The screening may involve using CAC scoring, CCTA, or functional stress imaging modalities. However, in the presence of severe calcification, assessing luminal stenosis with CCTA may be suboptimal due to blooming artifacts [53].

Although Takotsubo syndrome (TTS) is not directly related to cancer, there have been some reports of an association between TTS and cancer, most likely due to the malignancy itself, cardiotoxic agents, and intense emotional or physical stressors related to diagnosis, investigation, and treatment are recognized predisposing factors for TTS [87–89]. Therefore, invasive coronary angiography is usually required to exclude acute myocardial infarction in TTS, but CCTA is an alternative in patients with suspected TTS [1].

Cardiac CT is capable of evaluating both left and right ventricular function, volume, and mass. It has been shown to have good diagnostic accuracy and reproducibility when compared to CMR [90]. Additionally, if images are acquired using retrospective ECG gating, it can also assess regional wall motion abnormalities, constrictive physiology, and systolic/diastolic volumes, although this does come with a higher radiation dose. Therefore, cardiac CT is typically only recommended when CMR is contraindicated [53].

### 17.3.4 Nuclear Imaging and Positron Emission Tomography

Nuclear imaging techniques, such as multi-gated radionuclide angiography (MUGA), SPECT, and PET are considered important in assessing cardiac disease in cancer survivors [1, 91]. In a MUGA scan, a small amount of a radioactive substance is injected into the patient, which binds to red blood cells. Then, a gamma camera is used to produce images of the heart, providing accurate and reproducible measurements of cardiac chamber and LVEF [92]. However, due to radiation exposure and limitations in assessing other structural and hemodynamic features, such as valvular disease and pulmonary artery pressure, it is typically considered a third-line modality after echocardiography and CMR [1, 93].

Myocardial perfusion imaging using SPECT and PET is capable of detecting inducible ischemia, wall-motion abnormalities, and myocardial viability. Studies have reported the incidence of resting and stress-induced perfusion defects in patients who received chest RT to be between 14% and 60% [94, 95]. Radionuclide imaging using SPECT and PET is useful in following up patients with a high risk of CAD. PET, despite having several advantages, including improved spatial and temporal resolution and absolute blood flow quantification compared to SPECT, is less preferred in clinical practice due to its high cost and limited availability. Furthermore, PET with 18F-fluorodeoxyglucose (FDG) PET/CT can assess myocarditis by providing metabolic information on inflammation, as evidenced by increased myocardial FDG uptake. However, its limitations include low sensitivity and the requirement of a strict carbohydrate diet. As a result, PET is considered a diagnostic tool only if CMR is not available or is contraindicated [53].

## References

1. Lyon AR, López-Fernández T, Couch LS, Asteggiano R, Aznar MC, Bergler-Klein J, Boriani G, Cardinale D, Cordoba R, Cosyns B, Cutter DJ, de Azambuja E, de Boer RA, Dent SF, Farmakis D, Gevaert SA, Gorog DA, Herrmann J, Lenihan D, Moslehi J, Moura B, Salinger SS, Stephens R, Suter TM, Szmit S, Tamargo J, Thavendiranathan P, Tocchetti CG, van der Meer P, van der Pal HJH, ESC Scientific Document Group. 2022 ESC Guidelines on cardio-oncology developed in collaboration with the European Hematology Association (EHA), the European Society for Therapeutic Radiology and Oncology (ESTRO) and the International Cardio-Oncology Society (IC-OS). Eur Heart J. 2022;43(41):4229–361. https://doi.org/10.1093/eurheartj/ehac244.
2. Common Terminology Criteria for Adverse Events (CTCAE), Version 5.0. U.S. Department of Health and Human Services National Institutes of Health, National Cancer Institute. 2017.
3. Jaworski C, Mariani JA, Wheeler G, Kaye DM. Cardiac complications of thoracic irradiation. J Am Coll Cardiol. 2013;61(23):2319–28. https://doi.org/10.1016/j.jacc.2013.01.090. Epub 2013 Apr 10.

4. Beukema JC, de Groot C, Plukker JTM, Vliegenthart R, Langendijk JA, van Luijk P, van Melle JP, Prakken NHJ, Muijs CT. Late cardiac toxicity of neo-adjuvant chemoradiation in esophageal cancer survivors: a prospective cross-sectional pilot study. Radiother Oncol. 2022;167:72–7. https://doi.org/10.1016/j.radonc.2021.11.029. Epub 2021 Dec 2.
5. Wang X, Palaskas NL, Yusuf SW, Abe JI, Lopez-Mattei J, Banchs J, Gladish GW, Lee P, Liao Z, Deswal A, Lin SH. Incidence and onset of severe cardiac events after radiotherapy for esophageal cancer. J Thorac Oncol. 2020;15(10):1682–90. https://doi.org/10.1016/j.jtho.2020.06.014. Epub 2020 Jun 26.
6. NCCN Clinical Practice Guidelines in Oncology (NCCN Guidelines®) esophageal and esophagogastric junction cancers, Version 5.2022—5 Dec 2022.
7. Florescu M, Cinteza M, Vinereanu D. Chemotherapy-induced cardiotoxicity. Maedica (Bucur). 2013;8(1):59–67.
8. Albini A, Pennesi G, Donatelli F, Cammarota R, De Flora S, Noonan DM. Cardiotoxicity of anticancer drugs: the need for cardio-oncology and cardio-oncological prevention. J Natl Cancer Inst. 2010;102(1):14–25. https://doi.org/10.1093/jnci/djp440.
9. Dolci A, Dominici R, Cardinale D, Sandri MT, Panteghini M. Biochemical markers for prediction of chemotherapy-induced cardiotoxicity: systematic review of the literature and recommendations for use. Am J Clin Pathol. 2008;130(5):688–95. https://doi.org/10.1309/AJCPB66LRIIVMQDR.
10. Bergom C, Bradley JA, Ng AK, Samson P, Robinson C, Lopez-Mattei J, Mitchell JD. Past, present, and future of radiation-induced cardiotoxicity: refinements in targeting, surveillance, and risk stratification. JACC CardioOncol. 2021;3(3):343–59. https://doi.org/10.1016/j.jaccao.2021.06.007.
11. Spetz J, Moslehi J, Sarosiek K. Radiation-induced cardiovascular toxicity: mechanisms, prevention, and treatment. Curr Treat Options Cardiovasc Med. 2018;20(4):31. https://doi.org/10.1007/s11936-018-0627-x.
12. Eriksson D, Stigbrand T. Radiation-induced cell death mechanisms. Tumour Biol. 2010;31(4):363–72. https://doi.org/10.1007/s13277-010-0042-8. Epub 2010 May 20.
13. Haugnes HS, Wethal T, Aass N, et al. Cardiovascular risk factors and morbidity in long-term survivors of testicular cancer: a 20-year followup study. J Clin Oncol. 2010;28:4649–57.
14. Chun SG, Hu C, Choy H, Komaki RU, Timmerman RD, Schild SE, Bogart JA, Dobelbower MC, Bosch W, Galvin JM, Kavadi VS, Narayan S, Iyengar P, Robinson CG, Wynn RB, Raben A, Augspurger ME, MacRae RM, Paulus R, Bradley JD. Impact of intensity-modulated radiation therapy technique for locally advanced non-small-cell lung cancer: a secondary analysis of the NRG oncology RTOG 0617 randomized clinical trial. J Clin Oncol. 2017;35(1):56–62. https://doi.org/10.1200/JCO.2016.69.1378. Epub 2016 Oct 31.
15. Hancock SL, Tucker MA, Hoppe RT. Factors affecting late mortality from heart disease after treatment of Hodgkin's disease. JAMA. 1993;270(16):1949–55.
16. Takeuchi Y, Murakami Y, Kameoka T, Ochi M, Imano N, Takahashi I, Nishibuchi I, Kimura T, Kawahara D, Saito A, Nagata Y. Analysis of cardiac toxicity after definitive chemoradiotherapy for esophageal cancer using a biological dose-volume histogram. J Radiat Res. 2020;61(2):298–306. https://doi.org/10.1093/jrr/rraa001.
17. Tamari K, Isohashi F, Akino Y, Suzuki O, Seo Y, Yoshioka Y, Hayashi Y, Nishida T, Takehara T, Mori M, Doki Y, Ogawa K. Risk factors for pericardial effusion in patients with stage I esophageal cancer treated with chemoradiotherapy. Anticancer Res. 2014;34(12):7389–93.
18. Wei X, Liu HH, Tucker SL, Wang S, Mohan R, Cox JD, Komaki R, Liao Z. Risk factors for pericardial effusion in inoperable esophageal cancer patients treated with definitive chemoradiation therapy. Int J Radiat Oncol Biol Phys. 2008;70(3):707–14. https://doi.org/10.1016/j.ijrobp.2007.10.056. Epub 2008 Jan 11.
19. Beukema JC, Kawaguchi Y, Sijtsema NM, Zhai TT, Langendijk JA, van Dijk LV, van Luijk P, Teshima T, Muijs CT. Can we safely reduce the radiation dose to the heart while compromising the dose to the lungs in oesophageal cancer patients? Radiother Oncol. 2020;149:222–7. https://doi.org/10.1016/j.radonc.2020.05.033. Epub 2020 May 21.

20. Scarsbrook A, Ward G, Murray P, et al. Respiratory-gated (4D) contrast-enhanced FDG PET-CT for radiotherapy planning of lower oesophageal carcinoma: feasibility and impact on planning target volume. BMC Cancer. 2017;17:671.
21. Tukenova M, Guibout C, Oberlin O, et al. Role of cancer treatment inlong-term overall and cardiovascular mortality after childhood cancer. J Clin Oncol. 2010;28:1308–15.
22. Totterman K, Pesonene E, Siltanen P. Radiation related chronic heartdisease. Chest. 1983;6:875–8.
23. Morota M, Gomi K, Kozuka T, Chin K, Matsuura M, Oguchi M, Ito H, Yamashita T. Late toxicity after definitive concurrent chemoradiotherapy for thoracic esophageal carcinoma. Int J Radiat Oncol Biol Phys. 2009;75(1):122–8. https://doi.org/10.1016/j.ijrobp.2008.10.075. Epub 2009 Mar 26.
24. Noordman BJ, Verdam MGE, Lagarde SM, et al. Effect of neoadjuvant chemoradiotherapy on health-related quality of life in esophageal or junctional cancer: results from the randomized CROSS trial. J Clin Oncol. 2018;36:268–75.
25. Obermannová R, Alsina M, Cervantes A, Leong T, Lordick F, Nilsson M, van Grieken NCT, Vogel A, Smyth EC, ESMO Guidelines Committee. Oesophageal cancer: ESMO Clinical Practice Guideline for diagnosis, treatment and follow-up. Ann Oncol. 2022;33(10):992–1004. https://doi.org/10.1016/j.annonc.2022.07.003. Epub 2022 Jul 29.
26. Shiga T, Hiraide M. Cardiotoxicities of 5-fluorouracil and other fluoropyrimidines. Curr Treat Options in Oncol. 2020;21(4):27. https://doi.org/10.1007/s11864-020-0719-1.
27. Cucciniello L, Bidoli E, Viel E, Canale ML, Gerratana L, Lestuzzi C. The puzzling clinical presentation of fluoropyrimidines cardiotoxicity. Front Cardiovasc Med. 2022;9:960240. https://doi.org/10.3389/fcvm.2022.960240.
28. Pinedo HM, Peters GF. Fluorouracil: biochemistry and pharmacology. J Clin Oncol. 1988;6(10):1653–64. https://doi.org/10.1200/JCO.1988.6.10.1653.
29. Kosmas C, Kallistratos MS, Kopterides P, Syrios J, Skopelitis H, Mylonakis N, Karabelis A, Tsavaris N. Cardiotoxicity of fluoropyrimidines in different schedules of administration: a prospective study. J Cancer Res Clin Oncol. 2008;134(1):75–82. https://doi.org/10.1007/s00432-007-0250-9.
30. Jensen SA, Sorensen JB. Risk factors and prevention of cardiotoxicity induced by 5-fluorouracil or capecitabine. Cancer Chemother Pharmacol. 2006;58(4):487–93. https://doi.org/10.1007/s00280-005-0178-1.
31. Meydan N, Kundak I, Yavuzsen T, Oztop I, Barutca S, Yilmaz U, Alakavuklar MN. Cardiotoxicity of de Gramont's regimen: incidence, clinical characteristics and long-term follow-up. Jpn J Clin Oncol. 2005;35(5):265–70. https://doi.org/10.1093/jjco/hyi071. Epub 2005 Apr 26.
32. Labianca R, Beretta G, Clerici M, Fraschini P, Luporini G. Cardiac toxicity of 5-fluorouracil: a study on 1083 patients. Tumori. 1982;68(6):505–10. https://doi.org/10.1177/030089168206800609.
33. Lestuzzi C, Vaccher E, Talamini R, Lleshi A, Meneguzzo N, Viel E, Scalone S, Tartuferi L, Buonadonna A, Ejiofor L, Schmoll HJ. Effort myocardial ischemia during chemotherapy with 5-fluorouracil: an underestimated risk. Ann Oncol. 2014;25(5):1059–64. https://doi.org/10.1093/annonc/mdu055.
34. Fontanella C, Aita M, Cinausero M, Aprile G, Baldin MG, Dusi V, Lestuzzi C, Fasola G, Puglisi F. Capecitabine-induced cardiotoxicity: more evidence or clinical approaches to protect the patients' heart? Onco Targets Ther. 2014;7:1783–91. https://doi.org/10.2147/OTT.S65653.
35. Ma W, Wei S, Zhang B, Li W. Molecular mechanisms of cardiomyocyte death in drug-induced cardiotoxicity. Front Cell Dev Biol. 2020;8:434. https://doi.org/10.3389/fcell.2020.00434.
36. Varga ZV, Ferdinandy P, Liaudet L, Pacher P. Drug-induced mitochondrial dysfunction and cardiotoxicity. Am J Physiol Heart Circ Physiol. 2015;309(9):H1453–67. https://doi.org/10.1152/ajpheart.00554.2015. Epub 2015 Sep 18.
37. Zsengeller ZK, Ellezian L, Brown D, Horvath B, Mukhopadhyay P, Kalyanaraman B, Parikh SM, Karumanchi SA, Stillman IE, Pacher P. Cisplatin nephrotoxicity involves mitochondrial injury with impaired tubular mitochondrial enzyme activity. J Histochem Cytochem. 2012;60:521–9.

38. Salvatorelli E, Menna P, Cascegna S, Liberi G, Calafiore AM, Gianni L, Minotti G. Paclitaxel and docetaxel stimulation of doxorubicinol formation in the human heart: implications for cardiotoxicity of doxorubicin-taxane chemotherapies. J Pharmacol Exp Ther. 2006;318(1):424–33. https://doi.org/10.1124/jpet.106.103846. Epub 2006 Apr 13.
39. Sun JM, Shen L, Shah MA, et al. Pembrolizumab plus chemotherapy versus chemotherapy alone for first-line treatment of advanced oesophageal cancer (KEYNOTE-590): a randomised, placebo-controlled, phase 3 study. Lancet. 2021;398:759–71.
40. Janjigian YY, Shitara K, Moehler M, et al. First-line nivolumab plus chemotherapy versus chemotherapy alone for advanced gastric, gastrooesophageal junction, and oesophageal adenocarcinoma (CheckMate 649): a randomised, open-label, phase 3 trial. Lancet. 2021;398:27–40.
41. Kato K, Cho BC, Takahashi M, et al. Nivolumab versus chemotherapy in patients with advanced oesophageal squamous cell carcinoma refractory or intolerant to previous chemotherapy (ATTRACTION-3): a multicentre, randomised, open-label, phase 3 trial. Lancet Oncol. 2019;20:1506–17.
42. Kojima T, Muro K, Francois E, et al. Pembrolizumab versus chemotherapy as second-line therapy for advanced esophageal cancer: phase III KEYNOTE-181 study. J Clin Oncol. 2019;37:2.
43. Zhou YW, Zhu YJ, Wang MN, Xie Y, Chen CY, Zhang T, Xia F, Ding ZY, Liu JY. Immune checkpoint inhibitor-associated cardiotoxicity: current understanding on its mechanism, diagnosis and management. Front Pharmacol. 2019;10:1350. https://doi.org/10.3389/fphar.2019.01350.
44. Chhabra N, Kennedy J. A review of cancer immunotherapy toxicity: immune checkpoint inhibitors. J Med Toxicol. 2021;17(4):411–24. https://doi.org/10.1007/s13181-021-00833-8. Epub 2021 Apr 7.
45. Varricchi G, Marone G, Mercurio V, Galdiero MR, Bonaduce D, Tocchetti CG. Immune checkpoint inhibitors and cardiac toxicity: an emerging issue. Curr Med Chem. 2018;25(11):1327–39. https://doi.org/10.2174/0929867324666170407125017.
46. Yang S, Asnani A. Cardiotoxicities associated with immune checkpoint inhibitors. Curr Probl Cancer. 2018;42:422–32. https://doi.org/10.1016/j.currproblcancer.2018.07.002.
47. Wang DY, Okoye GD, Neilan TG, Johnson DB, Moslehi JJ. Cardiovascular toxicities associated with cancer immunotherapies. Curr Cardiol Rep. 2017;19(3):21. https://doi.org/10.1007/s11886-017-0835-0.
48. McDonagh TA, Metra M, Adamo M, Gardner RS, Baumbach A, Böhm M, Burri H, Butler J, Čelutkienė J, Chioncel O, Cleland JGF, Coats AJS, Crespo-Leiro MG, Farmakis D, Gilard M, Heymans S, Hoes AW, Jaarsma T, Jankowska EA, Lainscak M, Lam CSP, Lyon AR, McMurray JJV, Mebazaa A, Mindham R, Muneretto C, Francesco Piepoli M, Price S, Rosano GMC, Ruschitzka F, Kathrine Skibelund A, ESC Scientific Document Group. 2021 ESC Guidelines for the diagnosis and treatment of acute and chronic heart failure. Eur Heart J. 2021;42(36):3599–726. https://doi.org/10.1093/eurheartj/ehab368. Erratum in: Eur Heart J. 2021 Oct 14.
49. Kindermann I, Barth C, Mahfoud F, Ukena C, Lenski M, Yilmaz A, Klingel K, Kandolf R, Sechtem U, Cooper LT, Böhm M. Update on myocarditis. J Am Coll Cardiol. 2012;59(9):779–92. https://doi.org/10.1016/j.jacc.2011.09.074.
50. Zhang L, Zlotoff DA, Awadalla M, Mahmood SS, Nohria A, Hassan MZO, et al. Major adverse cardiovascular events and the timing and dose of corticosteroids in immune checkpoint inhibitor-associated myocarditis. Circulation. 2020;141:2031–4.
51. Brahmer JR, Lacchetti C, Schneider BJ, Atkins MB, Brassil KJ, Caterino JM, Chau I, Ernstoff MS, Gardner JM, Ginex P, Hallmeyer S, Holter Chakrabarty J, Leighl NB, Mammen JS, McDermott DF, Naing A, Nastoupil LJ, Phillips T, Porter LD, Puzanov I, Reichner CA, Santomasso BD, Seigel C, Spira A, Suarez-Almazor ME, Wang Y, Weber JS, Wolchok JD, Thompson JA, in collaboration with the National Comprehensive Cancer Network. Management of immune-related adverse events in patients treated with immune checkpoint inhibitor therapy: American Society of Clinical Oncology Clinical Practice Guideline. J Clin Oncol. 2018;36:1714–68. https://doi.org/10.1200/JCO.2017.77.6385.

52. Zarifa A, Albittar A, Kim PY, Hassan S, Palaskas N, Iliescu C, Durand JB, Lopez-Mattei J. Cardiac toxicities of anticancer treatments: chemotherapy, targeted therapy and immunotherapy. Curr Opin Cardiol. 2019;34:441–50. https://doi.org/10.1097/HCO.0000000000000641.
53. Čelutkienė J, Pudil R, López-Fernández T, et al. Role of cardiovascular imaging in cancer patients receiving cardiotoxic therapies: a position statement on behalf of the Heart Failure Association (HFA), the European Association of Cardiovascular Imaging (EACVI) and the Cardio-Oncology Council of the European Society of Cardiology (ESC) [published correction appears in Eur J Heart Fail. 2021 Feb;23(2):345]. Eur J Heart Fail. 2020;22(9):1504–24. https://doi.org/10.1002/ejhf.1957.
54. Plana JC, Thavendiranathan P, Bucciarelli-Ducci C, Lancellotti P. Multi-modality imaging in the assessment of cardiovascular toxicity in the cancer patient. JACC Cardiovasc Imaging. 2018;11:1173–86.
55. Mukherjee S, Aston D, Minett M, Brewster A, Crosby TD. The significance of cardiac doses received during chemoradiation of oesophageal and gastrooesophageal junctional cancers. Clin Oncol. 2003;15(3):115–20.
56. Tripp P, Malhotra HK, Javle M, Shaukat A, Russo R, De Boer S, Podgorsak M, Nava H, Yang GY. Cardiac function after chemoradiation for esophageal cancer: comparison of heart dose-volume histogram parameters to multiple gated acquisition scan changes. Dis Esophagus. 2005;18(6):400–5. https://doi.org/10.1111/j.1442-2050.2005.00523.x.
57. Lambert J, Lamacie M, Thampinathan B, Altaha MA, Esmaeilzadeh M, Nolan M, et al. Variability in echocardiography and MRI for detection of cancer therapy cardiotoxicity. Heart. 2020;106:817–23. https://doi.org/10.1136/heartjnl-2019-316297.
58. Chuang ML, Hibberd MG, Salton CJ, Beaudin RA, Riley MF, Parker RA, et al. Importance of imaging method over imaging modality in noninvasive determination of left ventricular volumes and ejection fraction: assessment by two- and three-dimensional echocardiography and magnetic resonance imaging. J Am Coll Cardiol. 2000;35:477–84. https://doi.org/10.1016/s0735-1097(99)00551-3.
59. Jenkins C, Chan J, Hanekom L, Marwick TH. Accuracy and feasibility of online 3-dimensional echocardiography for measurement of left ventricular parameters. J Am Soc Echocardiogr. 2006;19(9):1119–28. https://doi.org/10.1016/j.echo.2006.04.002.
60. Jenkins C, Moir S, Chan J, Rakhit D, Haluska B, Marwick TH. Left ventricular volume measurement with echocardiography: a comparison of left ventricular opacification, three-dimensional echocardiography, or both with magnetic resonance imaging. Eur Heart J. 2009;30(1):98–106. https://doi.org/10.1093/eurheartj/ehn484.
61. Sawaya H, Sebag IA, Plana JC, Januzzi JL, Ky B, Tan TC, Cohen V, Banchs J, Carver JR, Wiegers SE, Martin RP, Picard MH, Gerszten RE, Halpern EF, Passeri J, Kuter I, Scherrer-Crosbie M. Assessment of echocardiography and biomarkers for the extended prediction of cardiotoxicity in patients treated with anthracyclines, taxanes, and trastuzumab. Circ Cardiovasc Imaging. 2012;5(5):596–603. https://doi.org/10.1161/CIRCIMAGING.112.973321. Epub 2012 Jun 28.
62. Trivedi SJ, Tang S, Byth K, Stefani L, Lo Q, Otton J, Jameson M, Tran D, Batumalai V, Holloway L, Delaney GP, Koh ES, Thomas L. Segmental cardiac radiation dose determines magnitude of regional cardiac dysfunction. J Am Heart Assoc. 2021;10(7):e019476. https://doi.org/10.1161/JAHA.120.019476. Epub 2021 Mar 20.
63. Mignot A, Donal E, Zaroui A, Reant P, Salem A, Hamon C, Monzy S, Roudaut R, Habib G, Lafitte S. Global longitudinal strain as a major predictor of cardiac events in patients with depressed left ventricular function: a multicenter study. J Am Soc Echocardiogr. 2010;23(10):1019–24. https://doi.org/10.1016/j.echo.2010.07.019. Epub 2010 Sep 1.
64. Walker V, Lairez O, Fondard O, Pathak A, Pinel B, Chevelle C, et al. Early detection of subclinical left ventricular dysfunction after breast cancer radiation therapy using speckle-tracking echocardiography: association between cardiac exposure and longitudinal strain reduction (BACCARAT study). Radiat Oncol. 2019;14:204. https://doi.org/10.1186/s13014-019-1408-8.

65. Trivedi SJ, Choudhary P, Lo Q, Sritharan HP, Iyer A, Batumalai V, et al. Persistent reduction in global longitudinal strain in the longer term after radiation therapy in patients with breast cancer. Radiother Oncol. 2019;132:148–54. https://doi.org/10.1016/j.radonc.2018.10.023.
66. Filopei J, Frishman W. Radiation-induced heart disease. Cardiol Rev. 2012;20(4):184–8. https://doi.org/10.1097/CRD.0b013e3182431c23.
67. Bovelli D, Plataniotis G, Roila F, ESMO Guidelines Working Group. Cardiotoxicity of chemotherapeutic agents and radiotherapy-related heart disease: ESMO clinical practice guidelines. Ann Oncol. 2010;21(Suppl 5):v277–82.
68. Beukema JC, van Luijk P, Widder J, Langendijk JA, Muijs CT. Is cardiac toxicity a relevant issue in the radiation treatment of esophageal cancer? Radiother Oncol. 2015;114(1):85–90.
69. Lancellotti P, Nkomo VT, Badano LP, Bergler J, Bogaert J, Davin L, et al. Expert Consensus for multi-modality imaging evaluation of cardiovascular complications of radiotherapy in adults: a report from the European Association of Cardiovascular Imaging and the American Society of Echocardiography. J Am Soc Echocardiogr. 2013;26:1013–32.
70. Cutter DJ, Schaapveld M, Darby SC, Hauptmann M, van Nimwegen FA, Krol AD, Janus CP, van Leeuwen FE, Aleman BM. Risk of valvular heart disease after treatment for Hodgkin lymphoma. J Natl Cancer Inst. 2015;107(4):djv008. https://doi.org/10.1093/jnci/djv008.
71. Hull MC, Morris CG, Pepine CJ, Mendenhall NP. Valvular dysfunction and carotid, subclavian, and coronary artery disease in survivors of hodgkin lymphoma treated with radiation therapy. JAMA. 2003;290(21):2831–7. https://doi.org/10.1001/jama.290.21.2831.
72. Kamdar AR, Meadows TA, Roselli EE, et al. Multidetector computed tomographic angiography in planning of reoperative cardiothoracic surgery. Ann Thorac Surg. 2008;85(4):1239–45. https://doi.org/10.1016/J.ATHORACSUR.2007.11.075.
73. Drafts BC, Twomley KM, D'Agostino R, Lawrence J, Avis N, Ellis LR, et al. Low to moderate dose anthracycline-based chemotherapy is associated with early noninvasive imaging evidence of subclinical cardiovascular disease. JACC Cardiovasc Imaging. 2013;6:877–85.
74. Giusca S, Korosoglou G, Montenbruck M, Geršak B, Schwarz AK, Esch S, et al. Multiparametric early detection and prediction of cardiotoxicity using myocardial strain, T1 and T2 mapping, and biochemical markers: a longitudinal cardiac resonance imaging study during 2 years of follow-up. Circ Cardiovasc Imaging. 2021;14:e012459.
75. Kramer CM, Barkhausen J, Bucciarelli-Ducci C, Flamm SD, Kim RJ, Nagel E. Standardized cardiovascular magnetic resonance imaging (CMR) protocols: 2020 update. J Cardiovasc Magn Reson. 2020;22:17. https://doi.org/10.1186/s12968-020-00607-1.
76. Walker J, Bhullar N, Fallah-Rad N, Lytwyn M, Golian M, Fang T, et al. Role of three-dimensional echocardiography in breast cancer: comparison with two-dimensional echocardiography, multiple-gated acquisition scans, and cardiac magnetic resonance imaging. J Clin Oncol. 2010;28(21):3429–36. https://doi.org/10.1200/jco.2009.26.7294.
77. Podlesnikar T, Delgado V, Bax JJ. Cardiovascular magnetic resonance imaging to assess myocardial fibrosis in valvular heart disease. Int J Cardiovasc Imaging. 2018;34:97–112. https://doi.org/10.1007/s10554-017-1195-y.
78. Messroghli DR, Moon JC, Ferreira VM, Grosse-Wortmann L, He T, Kellman P, et al. Clinical recommendations for cardiovascular magnetic resonance mapping of T1, T2, T2 and extracellular volume: a consensus statement by the Society for Cardiovascular Magnetic Resonance (SCMR) endorsed by the European Association for Cardiovascular Imaging (EACVI). J Cardiovasc Magn Reson. 2017;19:75. https://doi.org/10.1186/s12968-017-0389-8.
79. Mahrholdt H, Wagner A, Judd RM, Sechtem U, Kim RJ. Delayed enhancement cardiovascular magnetic resonance assessment of nonischaemic cardiomyopathies. Eur Heart J. 2005;26:1461–74. https://doi.org/10.1093/eurheartj/ehi258.
80. Carrabba N, Berteotti M, Taborchi G, Ciatti F, Acquafresca M, Moroni M, Migliorini A, Miele V, Marchionni N, Valenti R. Integration of CTA in the diagnostic workup of new onset chest pain in clinical practice. Biomed Res Int. 2019;2019:2647079. https://doi.org/10.1155/2019/2647079.
81. Hecht HS. Coronary artery calcium scanning: past, present, and future. JACC Cardiovasc Imaging. 2015;8:579–96.

82. Grundy SM, Stone NJ, Bailey AL, Beam C, Birtcher KK, Blumenthal RS, et al. 2018 AHA/ACC/AACVPR/AAPA/ABC/ACPM/ADA/AGS/APhA/ASPC/NLA/PCNA Guideline on the management of blood cholesterol: a report of the American college of Cardiology/American Heart Association Task Force on clinical practice guidelines. Circulation. 2019;139:e1082–143. https://doi.org/10.1161/cir.0000000000000625.
83. Roos CTG, van den Bogaard VAB, Greuter MJW, Vliegenthart R, Schuit E, Langendijk JA, et al. Is the coronary artery calcium score associated with acute coronary events in breast cancer patients treated with radiotherapy? Radiother Oncol. 2018;126:170–6. https://doi.org/10.1016/j.radonc.2017.10.009.
84. Phillips WJ, Johnson C, Law A, Turek M, Small AR, Dent S, et al. Comparison of Framingham risk score and chest-CT identified coronary artery calcification in breast cancer patients to predict cardiovascular events. Int J Cardiol. 2019;289:138–43. https://doi.org/10.1016/j.ijcard.2019.01.056.
85. Xie X, Zhao Y, de Bock GH, de Jong PA, Mali WP, Oudkerk M, Vliegenthart R. Validation and prognosis of coronary artery calcium scoring in nontriggered thoracic computed tomography: systematic review and meta-analysis. Circ Cardiovasc Imaging. 2013;6(4):514–21. https://doi.org/10.1161/CIRCIMAGING.113.000092. Epub 2013 Jun 11.
86. Stolzmann P, Goetti R, Baumueller S, et al. Prospective and retrospective ECG-gating for CT coronary angiography perform similarly accurate at low heart rates. Eur J Radiol. 2011;7:85.
87. Desai R, Desai A, Abbas SA, Patel U, Bansod S, Damarlapally N, et al. National prevalence, trends and outcomes of Takotsubo syndrome in hospitalizations with prior history of mediastinal/intrathoracic cancer and radiation therapy. Int J Cardiol. 2020;309:14–8.
88. Sattler K, El-Battrawy I, Lang S, Zhou X, Schramm K, Tülümen E, et al. Prevalence of cancer in Takotsubo cardiomyopathy: short and long-term outcome. Int J Cardiol. 2017;238:159–65.
89. Omerovic E, Citro R, Bossone E, Redfors B, Backs J, Bruns B, et al. Pathophysiology of Takotsubo syndrome—a joint scientific statement from the HFA TTS and Myocardial Function Working Group of the ESC—Part 2: vascular pathophysiology, gender and sex hormones, genetics, chronic cardiovascular problems and clinical implications. Eur J Heart Fail. 2022;24:274–86.
90. Raman SV, Shah M, McCarthy B, Garcia A, Ferketich AK. Multi-detector row cardiac computed tomography accurately quantifies right and left ventricular size and function compared with cardiac magnetic resonance. Am Heart J. 2006;151:736–44. https://doi.org/10.1016/j.ahj.2005.04.029.
91. Kelly JM, Babich JWPET. Tracers for imaging cardiac function in cardiooncology. Curr Cardiol Rep. 2022;24:247–60. https://doi.org/10.1007/s11886-022-0164.
92. Gottdiener JS, Mathisen DJ, Borer JS, Bonow RO, Myers CE, Barr LH, Schwartz DE, Bacharach SL, Green MV, Rosenberg SA. Doxorubicin cardiotoxicity: assessment of late left ventricular dysfunction by radionuclide cineangiography. Ann Intern Med. 1981;94(4 pt 1):430–5. https://doi.org/10.7326/0003-4819-94-4-430.
93. Dhir V, Yan AT, Nisenbaum R, Sloninko J, Connelly KA, Barfett J, et al. Assessment of left ventricular function by CMR versus MUGA scans in breast cancer patients receiving trastuzumab: a prospective observational study. Int J Cardiovasc Imaging. 2019;35:2085–93.
94. Heidenreich PA, Schnittger I, Strauss HW, Vagelos RH, Lee BK, Mariscal CS, et al. Screening for coronary artery disease after mediastinal irradiation for Hodgkin's disease. J Clin Oncol. 2007;25:43–9. https://doi.org/10.1200/jco.2006.07.0805.
95. Gayed IW, Liu HH, Yusuf SW, Komaki R, Wei X, Wang X, et al. The prevalence of myocardial ischemia after concurrent chemoradiation therapy as detected by gated myocardial perfusion imaging in patients with esophageal cancer. J Nucl Med. 2006;47:1756–62.

# 18 Acid-Base Balance, Fluid Electrolyte Balance in Patients with Esophageal Cancer

Ufuk Uylas, Nurhilal Kiziltoprak, Ramazan Gundogdu, Mert Ercan, and Erdinc Kamer

Fluids and electrolytes are continuously exchanged between various body compartments and between the body and the external environment. Proper physiological function includes the preservation of the volume and composition of the body's fluids. Further, fluid volume maintenance requires that fluid intake and excretion be balanced. Failure to achieve fluid and electrolyte balance can result in severe and fatal complications in multiple organ systems.

Changes in fluid volume and content can occur before, after, and during surgery. In addition, changes in the amount of fluid and ionic content may occur in trauma and sepsis, depending on the body's response and the event itself. Liquid and ion control of the postoperative patient is essential to preventing problems.

The most common fluid and electrolyte problems arise due to the deterioration in the control systems that provide fluid-electrolyte balance. This review supplies a background on body water balance, including sources of water loss. Next, it discusses the fluid compartments of the body. It then describes fluid balance disorders, including hyponatremia and hypernatremia. The following section details normal and abnormal electrolyte functions. The disease states associated with elevated or deficient sodium, potassium, calcium, phosphorus, and magnesium are described.

U. Uylas
Gastroenterological Surgery Clinic, Gaziantep City Hospital, Gaziantep, Turkey

N. Kiziltoprak
Department of General Surgery, Sultan 2. Abdulhamid Khan Training and Research Hospital, University of Health Sciences, Istanbul, Turkey

R. Gundogdu
Dr. Turgut Noyan Training and Research Hospital General Surgery Clinic, Başkent University, Ankara, Turkey

M. Ercan · E. Kamer (✉)
Department of General Surgery, Izmir City Hospital, University of Health Sciences, Izmir, Turkey



O. Engin (ed.), *Risk Factors and Therapy of Esophagus Cancer*,
https://doi.org/10.1007/978-3-031-47024-0_18

The final topic is acid-base balance, including respiratory and metabolic contributors to disease and control. Throughout, this review focuses on control systems that ensure fluid and electrolyte balance, including buffering systems and drivers of exchange and transport.

## 18.1 Daily Water Intake

Water intake is affected by environment, personal habits, and physical activity. The same person may consume different amounts on different days. Human metabolism provides its water in two ways. First, approximately 2100 mL/day is consumed orally in liquid form. Second, approximately 200 mL/day of water is synthesized during carbohydrate oxidation. In total, approximately 2300 mL of water is required per day [1].

## 18.2 Body Fluids

### 18.2.1 Total Body Water

For every 10 units of total body weight; It consists of 5 units of water in an adult female and 6 units of water in a male individual [2]. For a 70 kg male individual, approximately 42 kg, or 6/10 of it, consists of total body water (TBW). Body morphology manifests itself with a decrease in TBW of 1–2 in 10 units in obese. The group that should be regulated by increasing TBW by 10% is the population with nutritional deficiency. The highest TBW in the human body is in the postnatal period, consisting of 8 units of TBW per 10 weights. This rate decreases to 6.5 at the age of 1 and reaches the adulthood stage by decreasing over the years.

Average body fluid varies depending on age, sex, and body fat percentage. More water is present in lean tissues than in fat and bone, which include muscular tissue and organs that are solid. Muscular people have a higher percent TBW than obese people. In later years of age human body fluid gets down amount of total. Young people contain higher amounts of water relative to their body weight than older people. In advanced ages, the percentage of fat tissue in body weight increases, this is the main mechanism in the decrease in water percentage. The isotope dilution method, bioelectrical impedance analysis, skinfold thickness measurement, and resonance cavity perturbation are commonly used to measure the water composition of the human body [3].

## 18.2.2 Body Water Loss per Daily

### 18.2.2.1 Imperceptible Loss of Water

Fluid lost through the respiratory tract, skin, perspiration, and feces is called insensible water loss. It may not be fully balanced with intake because it is continuous and unpredictable (Table 18.1).

#### Water Loss from the Skin

Even those without congenital sweat glands can experience insensible losses of water through their skin, which happens independently of sweating. About 300–400 mL/day of water is lost by diffusion through the skin. The cornified skin layer rich in cholesterol forms a layer that prevents the high loss to occur by diffusion. After severe skin burns, this area can become bare, causing the evaporation rate to increase ten times to 3–5 L/day. For extensive burns, it may be necessary to administer intravenous fluids to maintain the fluid balance [4].

#### Water Loss from the Lungs

Imperceptible loss of water from inhalation is about 300–400 mL/day. Before being evacuated, air that enters the respiratory system is moistened up to a steam pressure of approx. 47 mmHg. Water is continuously lost from the lungs because the pressure of the vapors of the air that is inhaled is typically less than 47 mmHg. In cold conditions (at below-zero temperatures), the atmospheric vapor pressure drops to almost 0 mmHg, worsening water loss from the lungs as the temperature drops. In cold conditions (at below-zero temperatures), the atmospheric vapor pressure drops to almost 0 mmHg, worsening water loss every dropping temperature. In respiratory system, this mechanism clarifies why it feels dried when it's chilly outside [5].

#### Loss of Water by Sweat

Normal human sweat volume is about 100 mL/day. Water loss through sweating may increase to 1–2 L/s according to the external ambient temperature and the increase in motor movements [6].

**Table 18.1** Daily loss of body water

| | Normal condition (mL/day) |
|---|---|
| 1. Insensible water loss | |
| • Skin | 300–400 |
| • Lungs | 300–400 |
| • Sweat | 100 |
| • Feces | 100 |
| 2. Water loss from kidneys | 500–1500 |

#### Water Loss from Feces

The amount of water lost in feces in normal individuals is about 100 mL/day. In exceptional cases such as diarrhea, the daily loss can reach a few liters [7].

#### Water Loss from Kidneys

Many mechanisms control the urinary excretion rate. In kidneys managing the evacuation rate of these chemicals is the most crucial step in maintaining a balance between the human being's intake and outflow of water as well as the ingestion and release of the majority of electrolytes. For example, urine output may decrease to 0.5 L/day in thirst, or it may increase to 20 L/day in a person who drinks a lot of water. Intake of sodium can range from 20 to 300 to 500 mEq/day. The water and mineral balance are adjusted precisely by parenchymal mechanisms in kidney by changing uptake and secretion in addition to making up for the too much fluid and electrolyte losses that happen in some illness situations [8].

## 18.3 Liquid Chambers in Body

TBW is made by three main functional liquid chambers in body includes the intracellular fluid (ICF), the extracellular interstitial fluid, and plasma (Table 18.2). TBW can also be distributed based on two compartments, extracellular fluid (ECF) and ICF because extracellular fluid consists of both plasma and the fluid of interstitial part. Synovium, peritoneum, pericardium, ocular and cerebrospinal spaces include some liquids named transcellular fluid. Transcellular fluid is usually considered a special type of ECF, but its composition can be different in both plasma and interstitial space liquids. Transcellular fluid volume in the body is approximately 1–2 L [9].

### 18.3.1 Intracellular Fluid Compartment

About 28 of 42 L of fluid in humans are distributed in approximately 100 trillion cells in the intracellular fluid compartment. ICF accounts for approximately 66% of the TBW, representing 40% of the total weight. It's mainly found in muscle of skeletal. Even in diverse creatures, from the most basic microbes to humans, the fluid inside of every single cell includes its own unique blend of various components. As a result, the ICF of every type of cell is viewed as a single sizable fluid compartment. ICF can be calculated indirectly by deducting TBW from the ECF volume [10].

**Table 18.2** Fluid compartments

| Intracellular fluid | Extracellular fluid | Transcellular fluid |
|---|---|---|
| | Plasma<br>Interstitial fluid | Cerebrospinal synovial peritoneal pericardial intraocular fluid |

### 18.3.2 Extracellular Fluid Compartment

ECF includes all other liquids outside of cells. ECF accounts for one-third of TBW and 20% of total body weight. A normal 70-pound man has about 14 L of ECF. Plasma constitutes 5% of ECF weight, and interstitial fluid constitutes 15%. The non-cellular component of blood is called plasma. Through the pores of capillary membranes, the plasma and interstitial fluid are constantly exchanging chemicals. With the exception of proteins, those pores are extremely transparent to practically all ECF solutes. ECFs are constantly varied, so plasma and interstitial fluids (which have a higher concentration in plasma) have approximately the same contents, except for proteins. ECF can be measured using indicator dilution methods. Sodium-bromide (NaBr) and radioactive sulfate distribution volumes have been used to measure ECF in clinical trials [11].

## 18.4 Blood Volume

Blood is composed of 40% red blood cells and 60% plasma, though the ratios might vary from person to person depending on sex, weight, and other factors. Blood makes up 7% of the adult body weight and is about 5 L. Since blood is in its own space, the circulatory system, blood is considered a separate fluid compartment [12].

### 18.4.1 Composition of Fluid Compartments, Components of Extracellular, and Intracellular Fluids

Plasma and interstitial fluid ion compositions are similar. ECF also contains large amounts of bicarbonate ($HCO_3^-$), chloride ($Cl^-$), sodium ($Na^+$), and few levels of potassium ($K^+$), calcium ($Ca^{2+}$), magnesium ($Mg^{2+}$), phosphate ($PO_4^{3-}$), and organic acids. In ECF, there is a balance between the main cation, sodium, and the main anions, chloride, and bicarbonate. In ICF, the main cations are, and the main anions are sulfate, phosphate, potassium and magnesium, and proteins [13].

The cation attentiveness is slightly higher in plasma than in the interstitial fluid (approximately 2% more) due to the Donnan effect. The presence of high protein in the results of plasma in a higher plasma cation content in the plasma than in the interstitial fluid. However, for practical purposes, the ion concentration in the interstitial fluid and plasma is considered to be approximately equal. Proteins increase plasma osmolarity and stabilize the forces that provide capillary endothelial permeability. Sodium-containing fluids increase as we increase the osmotic pressure and draw fluid into the environment, the volume of both intravascular and interstitial cavities [14].

#### 18.4.1.1 Intracellular Fluid Components

The ICF is apart from the ECF with the cell membrane. This membrane is highly conductive to water and selective to most electrolytes. Unlike ECF, ICF contains little sodium and chloride and almost no calcium. It contains plenty of potassium-phosphate ions and moderate amounts of Mg-sulfate ions. The ICF protein content is also almost four times that of plasma.

#### 18.4.1.2 Osmotic Pressure

The movement of water through the cell membrane is mainly associated with osmosis. The water passes through the semipermeable membrane until it reaches osmotic equality, equalizing its concentration on both sides. This transition is associated with solute concentrations on both sides of the cell membrane. Sodium, glucose, and blood urea nitrogen (BUN) are the main determinants of osmolality. The ICF and ECF osmolalities are kept between 290 and 310 mOsm, and the balance is achieved with the increase and decrease of fluid in the ECF area [15, 16].

## 18.5 Changes in Body Fluid

### 18.5.1 Normal Fluid and Electrolyte Exchange

Daily salt intake is 3–5 g/day. The kidneys provide sodium balance. In cases of hypovolemia or hyponatremia, excretion of sodium can be deductible by 1 mEq/day. In cases of hypernatremia, excretion can be increased up to 5000 mEq/day [17].

### 18.5.2 Fluid Balance Disorders

ECF loss is common in surgical patients. The loss of gastrointestinal fluids (widespread reason of depletion bulk of fluids in surgery-diseased individuals) due to nasogastric aspiration, diarrhea, vomiting, or enterocutaneous fistula. Besides, intra-abdominal conditions such as soft tissue injuries, burns, peritonitis, and obstruction or prolonged surgical procedures can cause massive volume losses. Acute volume losses present with cardiovascular and central nervous system findings. Additional tissue findings, such as decreased skin turgor and sunken eyes, are observed in chronic ECF losses. An increased BUN level may occur if a serious loss reduces glomerular filtration. Sodium of Urine will typically be low grade, at 20 mEq/L, and urine osmolality will typically be greater than serum osmolality. When fluid is lost, blood sodium levels may be high, normal, or low since the level of sodium in the blood does not always represent volume status [18].

### 18.5.3 Concentration Changes

Plasma sodium concentration measurement is the most practical method to evaluate a patient's fluid status since it gives results close to plasma osmolality. The normal plasma sodium value is 135–145 mEq/L. Low plasma sodium is hyponatremia, and elevated is hypernatremia [19].

#### 18.5.3.1 Hyponatremia

The most prevalent electrolyte problem, hyponatremia, is found in 15–25% of hospitalized patients. ESS volume may be high, normal, or low in hyponatremia. Sodium depletion or a dilutional sodium deficiency is frequently observed [20]. Possible causes should be carefully considered. Hyperosmolar causes such as hyperglycemia or mannitol infusion should be identified. Consumption or dilution conditions should then be evaluated. In the absence of kidney disease, hyponatremia may be tied to increased fluid consumption and a low urinary sodium level (<20 mEq/L) [21].

Dilutional hyponatremia is often due to increased extracellular water. This may be caused by excessive oral water intake or intravenous fluid therapy. In postoperative patients, dilutional hyponatremia may develop after free water absorption from the kidneys due to increased antidiuretic hormone (ADH) release. Especially in older individuals, various drugs (tricyclic antidepressants, antipsychotics, angiotensin-converting enzyme inhibitors) may cause dilutional hyponatremia by causing water retention. Fluid overload does not usually present physical examination findings, but hemodilution can be detected in laboratory examination [22].

Hypovolemic hyponatremia occurs due to loss of sodium-containing fluids or decreased intake. The main causes are a low-sodium diet, vomiting, diarrhea, gastrointestinal losses, nasogastric drainage, and losses due to primary renal disease or diuretics [23].

Normovolemic hyponatremia develops in cases where particles increase compared to water with hyperglycemia or mannitol-like drugs. Glucose increases the passage of water into the ESS, and hyponatremia may occur when the osmotic pressure is normal or high. If plasma lipid and protein levels are high, there is no any real extracellular sodium decreased compared to normal water, which may cause pseudohyponatremia. In the case of normovolemic hyponatremia, the presence of water intoxication and inappropriate ADH syndrome should be investigated [24].

##### Consequences of Hyponatremia

Neurological symptoms (seizure, headache, nausea, lethargy, disorientation) may be seen in rapid decreases in plasma sodium levels. The rapid decrease of sodium levels below 115–120 mmol/L may cause brain edema, cerebral herniation, seizure, coma, permanent brain damage, and death [25].

The brain and other tissues react to hyponatremia by transferring organic solutes like sodium, chloride, potassium, and glutamate outside the cells and into the extracellular chamber over the course of a few days. This lessens tissue edema and osmotic water influx into cells [26].

There is a risk of osmotic neuron damage from demyelination (loss of the myelin sheath of nerves) during the correction of chronic hyponatremia. By reducing hypertonic solutions below 180–216 mg/dL (10–12 mmol/L) in 1 day time zone and below 324 mg/dL (18 mmol/L) in 2 day time zone demyelination can be prevented [27].

### 18.5.3.2 Hypernatremia

Hypernatremia causes increased osmolality. It may develop due to water loss from the ECF (which concentrates sodium ions) or excess sodium in the ECF. Like hyponatremia, ECF may be increased, normal, or decreased in hypernatremia [28]. Hypernatremia may be hypervolemic, normovolemic, or hypovolemic.

Hypervolemic hypernatremia can be caused by administering fluids containing high amounts of sodium bicarbonate. It may also be caused by hyperaldosteronism in Cushing's syndrome due to increased mineralocorticoid levels. Concentration of urine sodium is >20 mEq/L, and osmolarity is >300 mOsm/L [29].

Renal or non-renal water losses are the reasons for normovolemic hypernatremia. Dehydration from this hypernatremia occurs when the ECF loses primary water. The inability to secrete ADH, which is necessary for the kidneys to retain water, may be the cause of normovolemic hypernatremia. The condition known as "diabetes insipidus" is caused by an ADH shortage, which causes the kidneys to secrete high volumes of diluted urine. Dehydration and an elevated sodium chloride concentration are brought on by this secretion in the ECF. A form of nephrogenic diabetes insipidus results from the kidneys' inability to respond to ADHs in certain types of renal disease [30].

Dehydration from less water intake than water loss, which can occur through sweating during continuous severe activity, is a more frequent cause of hypernatremia linked with a drop in ECF volume [31]. Hypovolemic hypernatremia may be caused by water loss. Renal losses may occur with diabetes insipidus and diuretic use. Non-renal losses consist of the gastrointestinal and cutaneous systems. In hypovolemic hypernatremia, the urinary concentration of sodium is <20 mEq/L, and its osmolality is <300–400 mOsm/L [32].

Compared to hyponatremia, hypernatremia is far less common. Severe symptoms often only appear when plasma sodium concentrations rapidly and significantly rise over 158–160 mmol/L. One explanation is that hypernatremia encourages acute thirst, which serves as protection against significant rises in plasma and ECF sodium levels. Water consumption rises in hypernatremia as a result of thirst. Only in patients with thirst disorder or fluid restriction due to other causes does symptomatic hypernatremia emerge. There are little symptoms until the sodium level of serum exceeds 160 mEq/L, however, these symptoms have a high mortality and morbidity rate. Hyperosmolarity is the cause of the symptoms, which can include seizures, coma, and death in addition to nervous system restlessness. The water movement from the intracellular area into the hyperosmolar extracellular environment might lead to cellular dehydration. In this situation, the straining of the brain arteries may lead to subarachnoid hemorrhage. In hypovolemic hypernatremia, tachycardia, hypotension, and dry and sticky mucosa are all common [33].

With an excessive input of sodium chloride to the ECF, hypernatremia is also a possibility. Hypernatremia typically occurs from an over-hydrated state because an excess of extracellular sodium chloride is frequently linked to more than some water retained in the kidneys. For instance, increased release of the hormone aldosterone, which retains sodium, might result in mild hypernatremia and overhydration. In these circumstances, hypernatremia is not severe since the kidneys are reabsorbing more sodium and water due to increased aldosterone release [34].

Clinicians must first analyze irregularities in plasma sodium before deciding whether the abnormality is caused by primary sodium loss or gain or primary water loss or gain. Hypernatremia can be treated by giving hypoosmotic sodium chloride or dextrose solutions. However, it is wise to gradually treat hypernatremia in patients whose plasma sodium content has been rising for a while. As a result, the cell is protected from volume changes by defense mechanisms that hypernatremia also activates. These defense mechanisms, which are the opposite of those that occur in hyponatremia, include those that raise the amounts of intracellular sodium and other solutes [35].

#### 18.5.3.3 Potassium Disorders

Humans consume an average of 50–100 mEq potassium daily. The amount of extracellular potassium is kept inside a narrow limit through renal excretion. The renal excretion of potassium is 10–700 mEq/day. Although the amount in the extracellular compartment is only 2% of all potassium, it is critical for cardiac and neuromuscular function. A slight change in potassium can have a severe cardiac effect. Intracellular and extracellular distribution of potassium may change in catabolic conditions such as injury, acidosis, surgical stress, and tissue catabolism [36].

##### Hyperkalemia

Normal serum potassium is between 3.5 and 5.5 mEq/L, and a value above 5.5 mEq/L is called hyperkalemia. Hyperkalemia may develop because of excessive potassium intake from oral or intravenous fluids, lysis of red cells after transfusion, excessive potassium transfer from cells to ECF, or impaired renal excretion of potassium. Rhabdomyolysis, hemolysis, and crush injuries may disrupt the cell membrane, causing intracellular potassium to pass inside ECF. Potassium transfer from the intracellular space to the ECF can also increase due to a rapid increase in ECF osmolarity. Acidosis, hyperglycemia, and IV mannitol administration may cause this situation [37]. Since almost all of the potassium in the body (98%) is in the intracellular space, even a small amount passing into the ECF can cause a significant increase in ESS potassium. Some medications, like NSAIDs (non-steroidal anti-inflammatory drugs), ACE inhibitors (inhibitors of angiotensin converting enzyme) and diuretics the potassium-sparing ones, can cause hyperkalemia, especially if there is kidney failure. Aldosterone plays a role in potassium excretion, and drugs that inhibit aldosterone (spironolactone and angiotensin-converting enzyme inhibitors) may cause hyperkalemia. Since potassium excretion occurs in the kidneys, hyperkalemia occurs in acute and chronic renal failure [38].

Hyperkalemia affects the gastrointestinal, neuromuscular, and cardiovascular systems. Nausea, diarrhea, intestinal colic, and vomiting are gastrointestinal symptoms. Neurovascular symptoms can range because of weakness (starting from the hand and foot) to ascending paralysis and respiratory failure. Findings on the cardiovascular system first manifest themselves on the electrocardiogram (ECG) and then progress to arrhythmia and cardiac arrest. The ECG may show elongated PR interval, an enlarged QRS complex, flat downed P wave, pointed T waves, and as hyperkalemia deepens, even ventricular fibrillation [39].

#### Hypokalemia

Hypokalemia is more widespread than hyperkalemia in surgical patients. Potassium can be lost from pathological gastrointestinal secretions, inadequate potassium intake, increased renal excretion, diarrhea, fistula, vomiting, and high nasogastric drainage. Alternatively, excess potassium transfer into the intracellular space may occur due to insulin therapy. Metabolic alkalosis can also cause hypokalemia; every 0.1 increase in hydrogen potential (pH) in alkalosis causes a 0.3 mEq/L decrease in potassium. Decreased magnesium can also result in potassium loss from the kidneys. This effect is also seen in magnesium-reducing drugs (amphotericin, aminoglycosides, cisplatin, and ifosfamide) [40, 41]. In this case, it is difficult to correct the potassium value unless the magnesium value is brought to the normal range [42, 43].

Hypokalemia has effects on the muscular system. Patients may develop contractility disorder of the smooth muscle of the gastrointestinal tract, skeletal muscles, and heart muscle. Findings can contain weakness, constipation, ileus, fatigue, decreased paralysis, tendon reflexes, and cardiac arrest. U waves, flattening of the T wave, ST segment changes, and arrhythmias can be seen on the ECG [44].

### 18.5.3.4 Calcium Disorders

Most calcium is in the bone matrix, so less than 1% is in ECF. This calcium is present in three forms: 40% protein-bound, 10% as complexes with anions such as phospate, and 50% in ionized form. The measurable form is the ionized form, which provides neuromuscular stability. Total serum calcium is influenced by albumin; each 1 g/dL reduce in albumin decreases serum calcium by 0.8 mg/dL. Changes in pH also change the concentration of ionized calcium. In acidosis, the protein binding ratio of calcium decreases, so the ionized calcium fraction increases [45].

Most calcium is excreted through the intestines, but urinary excretion occurs. Calcium balance is under hormonal control and is not urgent in acute surgery as symptoms develop over time. However, ionized calcium is critical in neuromuscular function [46].

#### Hypercalcemia

The normal value range for calcium is 8.5–10.5 mEq/L, while ionized calcium is between 4.2 and 4.8 mg/dL. Above these values is hypercalcemia. Hypercalcemia develops in primary hyperparathyroidism, and these patients are seen on an outpatient basis. Hypercalcemia can also occur in bone metastasis or parathyroid-associated protein-secreting malignancy patients, which are inpatient groups [47]. Symptoms of hypercalcemia vary according to severity. Gastrointestinal symptoms (nausea, vomiting, and abdominal pain), neurological disorders, musculoskeletal weakness, pain, and impaired renal function can be observed. ECG findings may contain Decrement of QT interval, prolongation of PR and QRS intervals, increase of QRS voltage, atrioventricular block, expansion of T wave, complete block, flattening, and cardiac arrest. Cardiac symptoms may manifest as hypertension, cardiac arrhythmia, and increased digitalis toxicity [48].

#### Hypocalcemia

Hypocalcemia is a calcium level drops below of 8.5 mEq/L (4.2 mg/dL for ionized calcium). Hypocalcemia can be caused by extensive infections of soft tissue, pancreatitis, hypoparathyroidism, renal failure, pancreatic and small intestine fistulas, necrotizing fasciitis, tumor lysis syndrome, and hypomagnesemia. Parathyroid adenomas cause chronic hypercalcemia. Transient hypocalcemia is common after surgery because of atrophy of other glands and increased remineralization of bone (hunger bone syndrome). In this case, high-dose calcium supplementation may be required [49]. In breast and prostate cancer, bone formation increases due to increased osteoblastic activity, which may cause hypocalcemia [50]. During tumor lysis and rhabdomyolysis, hyperphosphatemia can cause hypocalcemia because calcium precipitates with organic anions. Hypocalcemia can also result from the chelation of calcium with fatty acids in pancreatitis or binding with citrate in blood transfusion. Hypocalcemia rarely develops due to low oral intake since calcium stores in the bone compensate for a long time [51].

Although calcium is low in hypoproteinemia, symptoms do not develop. Conversely, in alkalosis, hypocalcemia symptoms may develop despite normal calcium values. Cardiac and neuromuscular symptoms are not observed until ionized calcium decreases up to 2.5 mg/dL. Hypocalcemia symptoms contain paresthesia of the face and extremities, carpopedal spasm, stridor, muscle cramps, tetany, and seizure. Patients develop hyperreflexia. Spasm development may be seen when tapping on the facial nerve (Chvostek's sign) and in the hand when pressure is applied to the upper extremity with a sphygmomanometer (Trousseau's sign). Hypocalcemia can cause decreased cardiac contractility and heart failure. ECG may find QT interval elongation, heart block, T wave reversal, and fibrillation of ventricles [52].

### 18.5.3.5 Phosphorus Abnormalities

An internal divalent anion called phosphorus is primarily present in metabolically active cells. Phosphorus is a component of high-energy phosphate products like adenosine triphosphate (ATP) and contributes to the energy production process during glycolysis. Renal excretion exerts tight control over serum phosphate levels [53].

#### Hyperphosphatemia

Higher oral consumption, decreased urine phosphorus excretion, or higher conversion to endogenous phosphate can all lead to hyperphosphatemia. Most occurrences of hyperphosphatemia are caused by patients' reduced excretion due to renal failure. By lowering urine excretion, hypoparathyroidism and hyperthyroidism can cause hyperphosphatemia. Endogenous phosphorus release rises and results in hyperphosphatemia in conditions such as rhabdomyolysis, hemolysis, tumor lysis syndrome, sepsis, profound malignant hyperthermia, and hypothermia. Although hyperphosphatemia frequently has no symptoms, it can result in the buildup of calcium-phosphate complexes in soft tissue [54, 55].

#### Hypophosphatemia

Hypophosphataemia develops due to decreased phosphorus intake, transfer of phosphorus to the intracellular region, or increased phosphorus excretion. Chronic hypophosphatemia may be caused by decreased gastrointestinal absorption in malabsorption, decreased intake of phosphate binders, and decreased dietary intake. In respiratory alkalosis, insulin therapy, hungry bone syndrome, and refeeding syndrome acute hypophosphatemia may develop due to the transfer of phosphorus to the intracellular region. Clinical findings usually do not occur unless hypophosphatemia is severe. Symptoms include muscle weakness or cardiac dysfunction [56].

### 18.5.3.6 Abnormalities of Magnesium

Like potassium, magnesium is mostly found intracellularly and is the fourth most prevalent element in the body. The bones are where the body stores half of its 2000 mEq of magnesium. Serum albumin has a third of the extracellular magnesium bound to it. As a result, not all bodily stores of magnesium may be reflected in plasma during hypoalbuminemia. The top limit of the normal range should be the only site where magnesium substitution is allowed. About 20 mEq of magnesium should be consumed each day with a typical diet; this quantity is eliminated in both urine and feces. Magnesium is excreted by the kidneys with magnesium insufficiency at a rate of less than 1 mEq/day [57].

#### Hypermagnesemia

Hypermagnesemia parallels changes in potassium excretion in severe renal failure. As such, magnesium-containing antacids and laxatives must be limited in the renal failure patients to prevent toxic levels. Symptomatic hypermagnesemia may be caused by intravenous overdose with total parenteral nutrition, thermal injury, massive trauma, and severe acidosis. Symptoms can include nausea, vomiting, weakness, neuromuscular dysfunction, lethargy, hyporeflexia, and impaired cardiac activity that can progress to hypotension and arrest. ECG findings are the same as hyperkalemia, with widened QRS complex, increased PR interval, and pointed T waves [58].

#### Hypomagnesemia

Magnesium loss is typical in hospitalized patients, especially those who are seriously unwell [59]. The calcium/magnesium receptors in the kidney regulate magnesium balance [60]. Hypomagnesemia may be brought on by decreased oral or intravenous magnesium intake, increased renal excretion, or extrarenal pathological losses. Starvation, drunkenness, extended IV fluid treatment, and complete parenteral nutrition with inadequate magnesium are some causes of decreased intake. Losses can result from gastrointestinal problems such as diarrhea, malabsorption, and acute pancreatitis as well as renal excretion brought on by excessive alcohol consumption, the use of diuretics, amphotericin B treatment, primary aldosteronism, and other factors.

Many enzymes depend on the magnesium ion to function properly. Hyperactive reflexes, positive presence of Chvostek's and Trousseau's symptom of sign, tetany, and muscular tremors are symptoms that are comparable to calcium shortage. Seizures and delirium can result from severe insufficiency. Long QT and PR intervals, torsades de pointes, P wave flattening or inversion, ST segment depression, and arrhythmias can all be seen on the ECG. In addition to having negative effects on the neurological system, hypomagnesemia can also lead to hypocalcemia and refractory hypokalemia. Hypomagnesemia makes it challenging to maintain potassium and calcium hemostasis when hypokalemia and hypocalcemia are both present. Consequently, these individuals should get intensive magnesium replacement [61, 62].

## 18.6 Acid-Base Balance

A large amount of acid is produced in our body, and the pH can be kept within normal ranges by buffering with kidney production of $HCO_3^-$. This buffering is necessary for organs to function normally. The normal value range of pH is between 7.35 and 7.45. Values less than 7.35 are called acidemia, and this disorder is called acidosis. On the other hand, values greater than 7.45 are alkalemia, and this condition is called alkalosis. Acid-base homeostasis is achieved by the lungs, kidneys, and a complex buffering system [63].

Our body operates buffering systems to correct metabolic acidosis, including intracellular buffers and extracellular bicarbonate in muscle and bone. Proteins and phosphates in the intracellular area and the bicarbonate-carbonic acid system in the extracellular area are among the important buffers. Other buffering systems include ventilation (Kussmaul's respiration) and increased reabsorption and production of bicarbonate in the kidneys. The kidney furthermore increases hydrogen excretion, which increases the excretion of $NH_4^+$ ($H^+ + NH_3^+ = NH_4^+$) in the urine [64].

Blood $pCO_2$ is firmly controlled by ventilation of alveolar cells through respiratory centers located in the pons and medulla oblongata [65]. In acid-base metabolism disorders, respiratory disorders are compensated by metabolic compensation and metabolic disorders are compensated by respiratory compensation. Henderson-Hasselbalch's equation demonstrates how metabolic and respiratory parameters regulate pH (Table 18.3). As shown, pH is determined by the ratio of the bicarbonate ($HCO_3$) concentration to the arterial partial pressure of carbon dioxide ($pCO_2$) [66, 67].

Correction of metabolic disorders is achieved by ventilation changes in response to hydrogen-sensitive receptors in the carotid and brain stem. When the receptors

**Table 18.3** The Henderson-Hasselbalch's equation, anion gap (AG), and corrected AG formula

| | Formula |
|---|---|
| AG | $Na^+ - (Cl^- + HCO_3^-)$ |
| Corrected AG | Actual AG − [2.5(4.5 − albumin)] |
| The Henderson-Hasselbalch's equation | $pH = pK + \log [HCO_3^-] / [0.03 \times (pCO_2)]$ |

*pK* equilibrium constant

are stimulated, ventilation increases. While the stimulation of these receptors increases acidosis, it decreases alkalosis. The kidneys increase or reducing bicarbonate reabsorption in response to respiratory alkalosis or acidosis to compensate for respiratory abnormalities. While compensatory changes in ventilation are rapid, the compensatory response of the kidney is slow. Compensation may begin after the first 6 h and may take days. For this reason, acid-base disorders are called acute if they occur before the compensation of the kidneys starts and chronic if they continue after renal compensation [68].

Interstitial and intracellular acid-base balance is mixed and differs in each tissue. Since blood is part of the extracellular compartment, blood is used to detect acid-base imbalance. ECF is important on determining tissue pH because blood is easy to access. Normal blood gas ranges are an arterial blood pH of 7.40 (7.35–7.45); partial pressure of $O_2$ ($pO_2$) >70 mmHg; oxygen saturation >90%; $pCO_2$ 35–45 mmHg; $HCO_3^-$ 24–30 mEq/L and deficit of base +2.3 to −2.4 mEq/L. In venous blood, normal pH is 7.36 (7.31–7.41), $pCO_2$ 42–55 mmHg, $pO_2$ 30–50 mmHg, $HCO_3^-$ 24–28 mEq/L, deficit of base +2.3 to −2.4 mEq/L, and oxygen saturation 60–85% [69].

The capacity of the respiratory system to supply oxygen to the blood is shown by arterial blood gas, whereas tissue oxygenation is shown by venous blood gas. If $pO_2$ is less than 60 mmHg, the reduction in hemoglobin saturation will compromise oxygen transport to tissues and hemoglobin saturation must stay above 90% [70]. Studies have shown that lactate and ECF pH play significant roles in the immune system, T cell activation, extracellular matrix production, and angiogenesis [71]. The smooth continuance of activities like protein synthesis, cell development, and reproduction is ensured by maintaining the ICF pH in balance. The pH is diverse throughout the subcellular compartments, which makes a scientific assessment of ICF acid-base balance challenging even though there are several publications on control mechanisms [72]. It is hard to adequately portray the health of all other organs using blood alone since each organ controls its pH to a different extent. Our knowledge of and ability to treat human acid-base problems will be improved by determining cell pH in diverse organs under varied situations and by developing technologies [73].

As mentioned, two-thirds of the total body fluid is ICF, and one-third is ECF. In addition, ECF is divided into interstitial fluid (ISF), intravascular plasma volume, and transcellular fluid. The transcellular space is covered with epithelium, such as the renal-urinary system epithelium, gastrointestinal cavity tract, and ducts of sweat glands. Since the contents of these fields are open to the outside perimeter, they change at different rates from the rest of the body in illness and health. Areas that do not open to the outside perimeter, such as cerebrospinal fluid, pleural, and peritoneal cavities, may reflect the acid-base state instead of determining HDS [74].

Regulation of ECF acid-base disorders can have unexpected damaging effects on ICF. For instance, when ICF in the central nervous system is acidified due to intracranial hemorrhage, it signals the brain's respiratory center for hyperventilation. However, hyperventilation that inhibits neuronal acidity also causes peripheral respiratory alkalosis. Correction of this hyperventilation may interfere with the regulation of brain pH [75].

## 18.7 Metabolic Disorders

### 18.7.1 Metabolic Acidosis

Metabolic acidosis is caused by increased acid intake and production or increased bicarbonate loss. In the body, the quantity of the negatively charged (anions) and positively charged (cations) ions in all balanced. Some anions (like as negatively charged pyruvate, sulfate, and lactate or serum proteins) cannot be measured in clinical laboratories, so there are less unmeasured cations than anions. This results in a positive anion gap (AG). AG should be calculated in any patient presenting by metabolic acidosis. The normal AG range is 3–11 mEq/L [76]. AG is mainly dependent on the albumin level, so the AG value should be corrected for the albumin value (hypoalbuminemia lowers AG) [69, 77] (Table 18.3).

Metabolic acidosis associated with increased AG can occur with the intake of exogenous acids such as salicylates, ethylene glycol, or methanol. It also occurs with increased production of endogenous acids in ketoacidosis (β-Hydroxybuturate and acetoacetate), lactic acidosis (lactate), and kidney failure (organic acids) [78].

In surgical patients, severe metabolic acidosis is frequently caused by lactic acidosis. In circulatory shock, inadequate tissue perfusion results in subsequent hypoxia and lactate generation. Exogenous bicarbonate administration should be substituted with volume replacement in the course of treatment to restore circulation. The pH returns to normal with sufficient perfusion and lactic acid is quickly digested in the liver. Bicarbonate therapy did not lower morbidity and mortality or restore cellular functioning in investigations of lactic acidosis and ketoacidosis that were conducted in humans [79].

The release of oxygen at the tissue level is prevented by excessive bicarbonate administration, which moves the oxyhemoglobin dissolution curve to the left and results in arrhythmias that are challenging to cure. Furthermore, intracellular acidosis is exacerbated by sodium bicarbonate. The exogenous bicarbonate forms carbonic acid when it mixes with additional hydrogen ions, and this carbonic acid subsequently breaks down into $CO_2$ and water, raising the $pCO_2$. Patients who have an existing acute respiratory distress syndrome may experience worsening breathing anomalies as a result of this hypercarbia. CO may enter cells, whereas bicarbonate stays outside of cells and exacerbates intracellular acidosis. Although lactate levels during resuscitation may not be a reliable indicator of clinical condition, they can be fairly high in critically damaged individuals who have passed away [80].

External acid supply ($HCl^-$ or $NH_4^+$), diarrhea, bicarbonate loss as a result of gastrointestinal conditions (fistula, ureterosigmoidostomy), or renal losses can all cause metabolic acidosis with normal AG. Since the loss of bicarbonate is followed by a gain in Cl in these situations, the AG is unaffected. To determine if a renal source of the bicarbonate loss exists, $[NH_4^+]$ can be tested in the urine. A renal tubular acidosis study should be carried out if there is a low urine [$NH_4^+$] in hyperchloremic acidosis, which suggests that kidney is the location of loss. Distal renal tubular acidosis results from reduced acid secretion, whereas proximal renal tubular acidosis is caused by reduced tubular reabsorption of $HCO_3^-$. The carbonic anhydrase inhibitor acetazolamide also results in the kidneys losing bicarbonate [81].

### 18.7.2 Metabolic Alkalosis

Normal acid-base hemostasis prevents metabolic alkalosis except there is increased bicarbonate production and renal excretion of bicarbonate is impaired. The loss of stable acids or increased bicarbonate can cause metabolic alkalosis, which becomes more profound with potassium loss. Most patients also have hypokalemia for extracellular potassium ions are replaced by intracellular hydrogen ions, thereby buffering the hydrogen ions from the increased $HCO_3^-$ [82].

Duodenal disease in the adult or pyloric stenosis in the child results in loss of gastric-type fluid can produce hypochloremic and hypokalemic metabolic alkalosis. Briefly, when vomiting in the presence of an open pylorus, there is also loss of stomach contents and pancreatic, biliary, and intestinal secretions; however, when vomiting in the presence of an obstructed pylorus, only gastric juice rich in chlorine and hydrogen is lost, resulting in hypochloremic alkalosis [83].

Urinary bicarbonate is initially elevated to counteract alkalosis. In addition, potassium ion excretion results in hydrogen ion reabsorption. Aldosterone-induced sodium reabsorption elevates the evacuation of potassium in response to the fluid imbalance found with metabolic alkalosis. Hypokalemia as a result results in paradoxical aciduria, which is the expulsion of hydrogen ions under alkalosis circumstances. After providing enough urine volume, the potassium deficiency is addressed by replacing the fluid shortfall with isotonic fluids [84, 85].

### 18.7.3 Respiratory Disorders

#### 18.7.3.1 Respiratory Acidosis

Respiratory acidosis occurs with $CO_2$ retention due to a decrease in alveolar ventilation. The response to respiratory acidosis develops late, as compensation is mainly through renal mechanisms. The underlying cause of acute respiratory acidosis is targeted during treatment. To guarantee proper ventilation, certain steps are done. To boost minute ventilation during these operations, volume expansion may be necessary utilizing non-invasive positive airway pressure or endotracheal intubation. While arterial $pCO_2$ remains high in chronic respiratory acidosis, bicarbonate concentration gradually increases as renal compensation improves [86, 87].

#### 18.7.3.2 Respiratory Alkalosis

The most severe case of respiratory alkalosis occurs in surgical patients and results from alveolar hyperventilation. Pain, anxiety, neurological conditions (including injury to the central nervous system), and mechanical breathing assistance are some of the causes. Some medications, such as salicylates, are examples of other causes; thyrotoxicosis, gram-negative bacteremia, hypoxemia, and fever are among the other causes. The rapid development of hypocapnia supports the structuring of free calcium together with circulating albumin and introduces potassium and phosphate into the cell, resulting in symptomatic hypokalemia, hypophosphatemia, and hypocalcemia with arrhythmia, paresthesia, muscular cramps, and convulsions. The underlying reason should be treated first, but hyperventilation should be treated with regulated ventilation [88].

### 18.7.4 Acid-Base External Balance

Acid-base balance from a metabolic point of view means of the tuning of stable acids (such as protein, nucleic acid, and phospholipids) produced from the diet. Sodium, potassium, or calcium salts of an organic anion species that can be metabolized to $CO_2$ and $OH^-$ can essentially become $HCO_3^-$ salts. Organic chlorinated salt cations, including basic charged amino acids and positively charged inorganic ions ($Na^+$, $K^+$, $Ca^{2+}$) in the emergence of net acid charge; contribute to the net acid load. Net alkalinity can be produced in some vegetarian diets. The provision of external balance occurs when the sum of the acids taken directly from the outside and produced by the body as a result of metabolism is equal to the acids that can be excreted in the urine [89].

Acids or alkalis stabilized by ATP consumption are transported to ECF by the plasma membrane transport mechanism. The cell has self-protective solutions from high acid content, including the Na-driven $Cl/HCO_3$ exchanger, Na-H exchanger, Na-$HCO_3$ cotransporter, and $H^+$ ATPase channels. The energy required for the movement of $H^+$ to the ECF can be derived directly from ATP or indirectly from ATP hydrolysis. Acid loads accumulated in ECF are transported to the kidney through the circulation and excreted from there [90].

In cellular alkalization, carrier mechanisms that throw the chemical and electrical charge from the inside out due to the $HCO_3$ gradient difference are located in the plasma membrane and take part in the correction of the cell pH. Mechanisms preventing excessive cell alkalinization include the $Cl/HCO_3^-$ exchanger and $NaHCO_3$ cotransport (1:3 stoichiometry) channels [91].

In the process of elimination of acid or alkaline loads from cells in the urine, the balanced excretion process of net acid and net alkaline loads; that is, acid phosphate salts or $HCO_3^-$ salts, $NH_4^+$ (ammonium) balance, and various mechanisms; that is, $HCO_3^-$ reabsorption and filtration, $H^+$ secretion are involved. One mEq $H^+$ of fixed acid is created per kilogram of body weight each day. On the other hand, the lungs clear around 20 mol/day of volatile acid as $CO_2$. When the body's acid load rises, the kidneys produce more ammonia, which raises net acid excretion [73].

### 18.7.5 Acid-Base Internal Balance

Most body cells have plasma membrane ion transporters that regulate intracellular pH [92]. Cell alkalizing carriers protect cells against over-acidification and acidify the ECF in response to acid loading. When ECF alkalinization occurs as a result of HCl release into the stomach lumen (which is referred to as the alkaline tide), these transporters also function to alkalize cells. The $NaHCO_3$ cotransporter (2 or 3 $HCO_3^-$ response 1 $Na^+$) and the neutral-loaded $Cl^-$–$HCO_3^-$ exchanger are additional transporters on cell membranes that shield the cell from excessive alkalinization [93].

Plasma levels of [$HCO_3^-$] and [$H^+$] are what provide the body its substantial buffering power. Numerous cells containing carbonic anhydrase enzymes may play a role in participation into acid-base homeostasis, according to this theory. The carbonic anhydrase in the red blood cell has a very high enzyme activity. Another significant source of overall buffering capability is the hydroxyapatite crystals found in the bone matrix ($Ca_{10}(PO_4)_6(OH)_2$). Even if the cost will be a loss of bone mineral mass, the $H^+$-ATPases of osteoclasts in chronic acidosis can maintain a nearly constant level of plasma bicarbonate [94]. Finally, intracellular and extracellular pH are also regulated by cellular acid or base absorption. All body cells load acid charges and base residues into the ECF for excretion because buffered surplus acid and base removed in urine from the HDS. This creates an internal-external equilibrium [95].

In homeostasis of acid-base main role of the lung is arrange the $pCO_2$ level in artery, which has a normal value range of 35–45 mmHg. Air entering and leaving the lungs at different rates and depths affects how much carbon dioxide is eliminated. In 1 min generally the average individual breathes between 14 and 18 times, and tidal volume is the breathing amount of air by each time. Adjustments in pH of patient's, arterial $pO_2$, and $pCO_2$ might cause chemoreceptors which based in medulla and arteries to boost or reduce breathing. While respiratory alkalosis can result from a drop in $pCO_2$ during hyperventilation, hypoventilation raises $pCO_2$ and causes respiratory acidosis [96].

Red blood cells, which carry $CO_2$ to the lungs, promote cell and plasma interactions in acid-base balance. The red blood cells that are in circulation subsequently disperse the $CO_2$ that was created in the body cells by cellular respiration to the nearby ICF. Red blood cells' deoxyhemoglobin absorbs $CO_2$ as a result of the Haldane effect. In the presence of carbonic anhydrase, this $CO_2$ reacts with $H_2O$ to produce $H^+$ and $HCO_3^-$. The Bohr effect states that $H^+$ binds to hemoglobin when the acidity is high. The next step is that the anion exchangers, which make up 3/10 of the plasma membrane structure, enable the replacement of $HCO_3^-$ with $Cl^-$. As a result, the bicarbonate in venous plasma rises and blood [$Cl^-$] falls. Tissue $CO_2$ is thus mostly supplied to the lungs through venous plasma as $HCO_3^-$. The procedure is reversed at the lungs. The pulmonary ICF releases $CO_2$ into the alveolar airways. Next, the $Cl^-/HCO_3^-$ exchanger is reversed to lower the $CO_2$ in plasma and red blood cells [97].

It seems doubtful that red blood cell anion exchanges function as a mechanism to counteract metabolic alkalosis. This is due to the inhibition of transporting $CO_2$

and worsening of respiratory acidosis of tissue caused by low rate of plasma $Cl^-$ and high $HCO_3^-$ in alkalosis; in other words, anion exchanges raise $pCO_2$ and $HCO_3^-$ independently. Thus, until the purge of $CO_2$ enables the $CO_2$ removal ratio to equal the $CO_2$ generation ratio and a recent steady-state blood $pCO_2$ grade is attained, systemic respiratory acidosis will deteriorate [98].

## References


1. Armstrong LE, Johnson EC. Water intake, water balance, and the elusive daily water requirement. Nutrients. 2018;10(12):1928. https://doi.org/10.3390/nu10121928.
2. Aloia JF, Vaswani A, Flaster E, Ma R. Relationship of body water compartments to age, race, and fat-free mass. J Lab Clin Med. 1998;132(6):483–90. https://doi.org/10.1016/s0022-2143(98)90126-3.
3. Zhou SG, Chen W. Human body water composition measurement: methods and clinical application. Zhongguo Yi Xue Ke Xue Yuan Xue Bao. 2018;40(5):603–9. Chinese. Abstract English. https://doi.org/10.3881/j.issn.1000-503X.10661.
4. Alrefai H, Mathis SL, Hicks SM, Pivovarova AI, MacGregor GG. Salt and water balance after sweat loss: a study of Bikram yoga. Physiol Rep. 2020;8(22):e14647. https://doi.org/10.14814/phy2.14647.
5. Ferrus L, Guenard H, Vardon G, Varene P. Respiratory water loss. Respir Physiol. 1980;39(3):367–81. https://doi.org/10.1016/0034-5687(80)90067-5.
6. Bettley FR, Grice K. Transepidermal water loss. Br Med J. 1968;1(5590):514. https://doi.org/10.1136/bmj.1.5590.514-a.
7. Dmitrieva NI, Burg MB. Increased insensible water loss contributes to aging related dehydration. PLoS One. 2011;6(5):e20691. https://doi.org/10.1371/journal.pone.0020691. Epub 2011 May 31.
8. Lu HA. Diabetes insipidus. Adv Exp Med Biol. 2017;969:213–25. https://doi.org/10.1007/978-94-024-1057-0_14.
9. Pain RW. Body fluid compartments. Anaesth Intensive Care. 1977;5(4):284–94. https://doi.org/10.1177/0310057X7700500403.
10. Marken Lichtenbelt WD, Fogelholm M. Increased extracellular water compartment, relative to intracellular water compartment, after weight reduction. J Appl Physiol (1985). 1999;87(1):294–8. https://doi.org/10.1152/jappl.1999.87.1.294.
11. Holliday MA. Extracellular fluid and its proteins: dehydration, shock, and recovery. Pediatr Nephrol. 1999;13(9):989–95. https://doi.org/10.1007/s004670050741.
12. Gómez Perales JL. Blood volume analysis by radioisotopic dilution techniques: state of the art. Appl Radiat Isot. 2015;96:71–82. https://doi.org/10.1016/j.apradiso.2014.11.014. Epub 2014 Nov 20.
13. Bedard C, Piette C, Venance L, Destexhe A. Extracellular and intracellular components of the impedance of neural tissue. Biophys J. 2022;121(6):869–85. https://doi.org/10.1016/j.bpj.2022.02.022.
14. Kurbel S. Are extracellular osmolality and sodium concentration determined by Donnan effects of intracellular protein charges and of pumped sodium? J Theor Biol. 2008;252(4):769–72. https://doi.org/10.1016/j.jtbi.2008.02.022. Epub 2008 Feb 23.
15. Keren K, Yam PT, Kinkhabwala A, Mogilner A, Theriot JA. Intracellular fluid flow in rapidly moving cells. Nat Cell Biol. 2009;11(10):1219–24. https://doi.org/10.1038/ncb1965. Epub 2009 Sep 20.
16. Drummond JC. Colloid osmotic pressure and the formation of posttraumatic cerebral edema. Anesthesiology. 2010;112(5):1079–81. https://doi.org/10.1097/ALN.0b013e3181d94e53.
17. Ball SG. Hyponatraemia. J R Coll Physicians Edinb. 2010;40(3):240–5. https://doi.org/10.4997/JRCPE.2010.312.

18. Gross P. Treatment of hyponatremia. Intern Med. 2008;47(10):885–91. https://doi.org/10.2169/internalmedicine.47.0918. Epub 2008 May 15.
19. Vantyghem MC, Balavoine AS, Wémeau JL, Douillard C. Hyponatremia and antidiuresis syndrome. Ann Endocrinol (Paris). 2011;72(6):500–12. https://doi.org/10.1016/j.ando.2011.10.001.
20. Miller M. Syndromes of excess antidiuretic hormone release. Crit Care Clin. 2001;17(1):11–23, v. https://doi.org/10.1016/s0749-0704(05)70149-4.
21. Marco Martínez J. Hiponatremia: clasificación y diagnóstico diferencial [Hyponatremia: classification and differential diagnosis]. Endocrinol Nutr. 2010;57(Suppl 2):2–9. Spanish. https://doi.org/10.1016/S1575-0922(10)70016-4.
22. Hix JK, Silver S, Sterns RH. Diuretic-associated hyponatremia. Semin Nephrol. 2011;31(6):553–66. https://doi.org/10.1016/j.semnephrol.2011.09.010.
23. Mohottige D, Lehrich RW, Greenberg A. Hypovolemic hyponatremia. Front Horm Res. 2019;52:93–103. https://doi.org/10.1159/000493240.
24. Spasovski G, Vanholder R, Allolio B, Annane D, Ball S, Bichet D, Decaux G, Fenske W, Hoorn EJ, Ichai C, Joannidis M, Soupart A, Zietse R, Haller M, van der Veer S, Van Biesen W, Nagler E, Hyponatraemia Guideline Development Group. Clinical practice guideline on diagnosis and treatment of hyponatraemia. Eur J Endocrinol. 2014;170(3):G1–47. https://doi.org/10.1530/EJE-13-1020. Erratum in: Eur J Endocrinol. 2014 Jul;171(1):X1.
25. Corona G, Giuliani C, Verbalis JG, Forti G, Maggi M, Peri A. Hyponatremia improvement is associated with a reduced risk of mortality: evidence from a meta-analysis. PLoS One. 2015;10(4):e0124105. https://doi.org/10.1371/journal.pone.0124105.
26. Rangan GK, Dorani N, Zhang MM, Abu-Zarour L, Lau HC, Munt A, Chandra AN, Saravanabavan S, Rangan A, Zhang JQJ, Howell M, Wong AT. Clinical characteristics and outcomes of hyponatraemia associated with oral water intake in adults: a systematic review. BMJ Open. 2021;11(12):e046539. https://doi.org/10.1136/bmjopen-2020-046539.
27. Tzamaloukas AH, Shapiro JI, Raj DS, Murata GH, Glew RH, Malhotra D. Management of severe hyponatremia: infusion of hypertonic saline and desmopressin or infusion of vasopressin inhibitors? Am J Med Sci. 2014;348(5):432–9. https://doi.org/10.1097/MAJ.0000000000000331.
28. Conley SB. Hypernatremia. Pediatr Clin N Am. 1990;37(2):365–72. https://doi.org/10.1016/s0031-3955(16)36874-2.
29. Ilardi A. Diagnostic and therapeutic approach to hypernatremia. Diagnosis (Berl). 2022;9(4):403–10. https://doi.org/10.1515/dx-2022-0034.
30. Muhsin SA, Mount DB. Diagnosis and treatment of hypernatremia. Best Pract Res Clin Endocrinol Metab. 2016;30(2):189–203. https://doi.org/10.1016/j.beem.2016.02.014. Epub 2016 Mar 4.
31. Seay NW, Lehrich RW, Greenberg A. Diagnosis and management of disorders of body tonicity-hyponatremia and hypernatremia: core curriculum 2020. Am J Kidney Dis. 2020;75(2):272–86. https://doi.org/10.1053/j.ajkd.2019.07.014. Epub 2019 Oct 10.
32. Chand R, Chand R, Goldfarb DS. Hypernatremia in the intensive care unit. Curr Opin Nephrol Hypertens. 2022;31(2):199–204. https://doi.org/10.1097/MNH.0000000000000773.
33. Qian Q. Hypernatremia. Clin J Am Soc Nephrol. 2019;14(3):432–4. https://doi.org/10.2215/CJN.12141018. Epub 2019 Feb 6.
34. Lindner G, Funk GC. Hypernatremia in critically ill patients. J Crit Care. 2013;28(2):216.e11–20. https://doi.org/10.1016/j.jcrc.2012.05.001. Epub 2012 Jul 2.
35. Yun G, Baek SH, Kim S. Evaluation and management of hypernatremia in adults: clinical perspectives. Korean J Intern Med. 2023;38(3):290–302. https://doi.org/10.3904/kjim.2022.346.
36. Lim S. Approach to hypokalemia. Acta Med Indones. 2007;39(1):56–64.
37. Adrogué HJ, Lederer ED, Suki WN, Eknoyan G. Determinants of plasma potassium levels in diabetic ketoacidosis. Medicine (Baltimore). 1986;65(3):163–72. https://doi.org/10.1097/00005792-198605000-00004.
38. Palmer BF, Clegg DJ. Diagnosis and treatment of hyperkalemia. Cleve Clin J Med. 2017;84(12):934–42. https://doi.org/10.3949/ccjm.84a.17056.

39. Sarwar CM, Papadimitriou L, Pitt B, Piña I, Zannad F, Anker SD, Gheorghiade M, Butler J. Hyperkalemia in heart failure. J Am Coll Cardiol. 2016;68(14):1575–89. https://doi.org/10.1016/j.jacc.2016.06.060.
40. Zietse R, Zoutendijk R, Hoorn EJ. Fluid, electrolyte and acid-base disorders associated with antibiotic therapy. Nat Rev Nephrol. 2009;5(4):193–202. https://doi.org/10.1038/nrneph.2009.17.
41. Gennari FJ. Hypokalemia. N Engl J Med. 1998;339(7):451–8. https://doi.org/10.1056/NEJM199808133390707.
42. Unwin RJ, Luft FC, Shirley DG. Pathophysiology and management of hypokalemia: a clinical perspective. Nat Rev Nephrol. 2011;7(2):75–84. https://doi.org/10.1038/nrneph.2010.175.
43. Baker LW, Trautman C. Refractory hypokalemia: a quiz. Am J Kidney Dis. 2022;79(1):A15–7. https://doi.org/10.1053/j.ajkd.2021.06.032.
44. Mandal AK. Hypokalemia and hyperkalemia. Med Clin North Am. 1997;81(3):611–39. https://doi.org/10.1016/s0025-7125(05)70536-8.
45. Pepe J, Colangelo L, Biamonte F, Sonato C, Danese VC, Cecchetti V, Occhiuto M, Piazzolla V, De Martino V, Ferrone F, Minisola S, Cipriani C. Diagnosis and management of hypocalcemia. Endocrine. 2020;69(3):485–95. https://doi.org/10.1007/s12020-020-02324-2. Epub 2020 May 4.
46. Helmeste DM, Tang SW. The role of calcium in the etiology of the affective disorders. Jpn J Pharmacol. 1998;77(2):107–16. https://doi.org/10.1254/jjp.77.107.
47. French S, Subauste J, Geraci S. Calcium abnormalities in hospitalized patients. South Med J. 2012;105(4):231–7. https://doi.org/10.1097/SMJ.0b013e31824e1737.
48. Minisola S, Pepe J, Piemonte S, Cipriani C. The diagnosis and management of hypercalcaemia. BMJ. 2015;350:h2723. https://doi.org/10.1136/bmj.h2723.
49. Cooper MS, Gittoes NJ. Diagnosis and management of hypocalcaemia. BMJ. 2008;336(7656):1298–302. https://doi.org/10.1136/bmj.39582.589433.BE. Erratum in: BMJ. 2008 Jun 28;336(7659).
50. Hakami Y, Khan A. Hypoparathyroidism. Front Horm Res. 2019;51:109–26. https://doi.org/10.1159/000491042. Epub 2018 Nov 19.
51. Nadar R, Shaw N. Investigation and management of hypocalcaemia. Arch Dis Child. 2020;105(4):399–405. https://doi.org/10.1136/archdischild-2019-317482. Epub 2020 Jan 3.
52. Compston JE. Investigation of hypocalcaemia. Clin Endocrinol. 1995;42(2):195–8. https://doi.org/10.1111/j.1365-2265.1995.tb01862.x.
53. Vervloet MG, van Ballegooijen AJ. Prevention and treatment of hyperphosphatemia in chronic kidney disease. Kidney Int. 2018;93(5):1060–72. https://doi.org/10.1016/j.kint.2017.11.036.
54. Barbar T, Jaffer Sathick I. Tumor lysis syndrome. Adv Chronic Kidney Dis. 2021;28(5):438–446.e1. https://doi.org/10.1053/j.ackd.2021.09.007.
55. Rastogi A, Bhatt N, Rossetti S, Beto J. Management of hyperphosphatemia in end-stage renal disease: a new paradigm. J Ren Nutr. 2021;31(1):21–34. https://doi.org/10.1053/j.jrn.2020.02.003.
56. Felsenfeld AJ, Levine BS. Approach to treatment of hypophosphatemia. Am J Kidney Dis. 2012;60(4):655–61. https://doi.org/10.1053/j.ajkd.2012.03.024.
57. Van Laecke S. Hypomagnesemia and hypermagnesemia. Acta Clin Belg. 2019;74(1):41–7. https://doi.org/10.1080/17843286.2018.1516173.
58. Krendel DA. Hypermagnesemia and neuromuscular transmission. Semin Neurol. 1990;10(1):42–5. https://doi.org/10.1055/s-2008-1041252.
59. Pham PC, Pham PA, Pham SV, Pham PT, Pham PM, Pham PT. Hypomagnesemia: a clinical perspective. Int J Nephrol Renovasc Dis. 2014;7:219–30. https://doi.org/10.2147/IJNRD.S42054.
60. Ayuk J, Gittoes NJ. Treatment of hypomagnesemia. Am J Kidney Dis. 2014;63(4):691–5. https://doi.org/10.1053/j.ajkd.2013.07.025.
61. Tseng MH, Konrad M, Ding JJ, Lin SH. Clinical and genetic approach to renal hypomagnesemia. Biom J. 2022;45(1):74–87. https://doi.org/10.1016/j.bj.2021.11.002. Epub 2021 Nov 10.

62. Rosner MH, Ha N, Palmer BF, Perazella MA. Acquired disorders of hypomagnesemia. Mayo Clin Proc. 2023;98(4):581–96. https://doi.org/10.1016/j.mayocp.2022.12.002. Epub 2023 Mar 3.
63. Quade BN, Parker MD, Occhipinti R. The therapeutic importance of acid-base balance. Biochem Pharmacol. 2021;183:114278. https://doi.org/10.1016/j.bcp.2020.114278.
64. Swenson ER. Metabolic acidosis. Respir Care. 2001;46(4):342–53.
65. Chand R, Swenson ER, Goldfarb DS. Sodium bicarbonate therapy for acute respiratory acidosis. Curr Opin Nephrol Hypertens. 2021;30(2):223–30. https://doi.org/10.1097/MNH.0000000000000687.
66. Ayers P, Warrington L. Diagnosis and treatment of simple acid-base disorders. Nutr Clin Pract. 2008;23(2):122–7. https://doi.org/10.1177/0884533608314534.
67. Harrison RA. Acid-base balance. Respir Care Clin N Am. 1995;1(1):7–21.
68. Gomez H, Kellum JA. Understanding acid base disorders. Crit Care Clin. 2015;31(4):849–60. https://doi.org/10.1016/j.ccc.2015.06.016.
69. Seifter JL. Body fluid compartments, cell membrane ion transport, electrolyte concentrations, and acid-base balance. Semin Nephrol. 2019;39(4):368–79. https://doi.org/10.1016/j.semnephrol.2019.04.006.
70. Wagner CA, Imenez Silva PH, Bourgeois S. Molecular pathophysiology of acid-base disorders. Semin Nephrol. 2019;39(4):340–52. https://doi.org/10.1016/j.semnephrol.2019.04.004.
71. Frangiosa A, De Santo LS, Anastasio P, De Santo NG. Acid-base balance in heart failure. J Nephrol. 2006;19(Suppl 9):S115–20.
72. Settergren G, Gårdebäck M. Acid-base balance. J Cardiothorac Vasc Anesth. 1996;10(4):566–7. https://doi.org/10.1016/s1053-0770(05)80040-0.
73. Brewer ED. Disorders of acid-base balance. Pediatr Clin N Am. 1990;37(2):429–47. https://doi.org/10.1016/s0031-3955(16)36878-x.
74. Schoeller DA, van Santen E, Peterson DW, Dietz W, Jaspan J, Klein PD. Total body water measurement in humans with 18O and 2H labeled water. Am J Clin Nutr. 1980;33:2686–93.
75. Leblanc M. Acid-base balance in acute renal failure and renal replacement therapy. Best Pract Res Clin Anaesthesiol. 2004;18(1):113–27. https://doi.org/10.1016/j.bpa.2003.08.001.
76. Kraut JA, Madias NE. Metabolic acidosis: pathophysiology, diagnosis and management. Nat Rev Nephrol. 2010;6(5):274–85. https://doi.org/10.1038/nrneph.2010.33.
77. Lim S. Metabolic acidosis. Acta Med Indones. 2007;39(3):145–50.
78. Raphael KL. Metabolic acidosis and subclinical metabolic acidosis in CKD. J Am Soc Nephrol. 2018;29(2):376–82. https://doi.org/10.1681/ASN.2017040422.
79. Matyukhin I, Patschan S, Ritter O, Patschan D. Etiology and management of acute metabolic acidosis: an update. Kidney Blood Press Res. 2020;45(4):523–31. https://doi.org/10.1159/000507813.
80. Fenves AZ, Emmett M. Approach to patients with high anion gap metabolic acidosis: core curriculum 2021. Am J Kidney Dis. 2021;78(4):590–600. https://doi.org/10.1053/j.ajkd.2021.02.341.
81. Adeva-Andany MM, Fernández-Fernández C, Mouriño-Bayolo D, Castro-Quintela E, Domínguez-Montero A. Sodium bicarbonate therapy in patients with metabolic acidosis. ScientificWorldJournal. 2014;2014:627673. https://doi.org/10.1155/2014/627673.
82. Palmer BF, Alpern RJ. Metabolic alkalosis. J Am Soc Nephrol. 1997;8(9):1462–9. https://doi.org/10.1681/ASN.V891462.
83. Khanna A, Kurtzman NA. Metabolic alkalosis. J Nephrol. 2006;19(Suppl 9):S86–96.
84. Emmett M. Metabolic alkalosis: a brief pathophysiologic review. Clin J Am Soc Nephrol. 2020;15(12):1848–56. https://doi.org/10.2215/CJN.16041219.
85. Do C, Vasquez PC, Soleimani M. Metabolic alkalosis pathogenesis, diagnosis, and treatment: core curriculum 2022. Am J Kidney Dis. 2022;80(4):536–51. https://doi.org/10.1053/j.ajkd.2021.12.016.
86. Wall RE. Respiratory acid-base disorders. Vet Clin North Am Small Anim Pract. 2001;31(6):1355–67, viii. https://doi.org/10.1016/s0195-5616(01)50106-0.
87. Epstein SK, Singh N. Respiratory acidosis. Respir Care. 2001;46(4):366–83.

88. Foster GT, Vaziri ND, Sassoon CS. Respiratory alkalosis. Respir Care. 2001;46(4):384–91.
89. Oh MS. New perspectives on acid-base balance. Semin Dial. 2000;13(4):212–9. https://doi.org/10.1046/j.1525-139x.2000.00061.x.
90. Sławuta P, Noszczyk-Nowak A, Nowakowski H. Acid-base balance parameters and a value of anion gap of arterial and venous blood in Małopolski horses. Pol J Vet Sci. 2010;13(4):581–5.
91. Oh MS. Inevitability of balance restoration. Electrolyte Blood Press. 2010;8(1):18–24. https://doi.org/10.5049/EBP.2010.8.1.18.
92. Laski ME, Kurtzman NA. Acid-base disorders in medicine. Dis Mon. 1996;42(2):51–125. https://doi.org/10.1016/s0011-5029(96)90004-8.
93. Claiborne JB, Edwards SL, Morrison-Shetlar AI. Acid-base regulation in fishes: cellular and molecular mechanisms. J Exp Zool. 2002;293(3):302–19. https://doi.org/10.1002/jez.10125.
94. Bobulescu IA, Moe OW. $Na^+/H^+$ exchangers in renal regulation of acid-base balance. Semin Nephrol. 2006;26(5):334–44. https://doi.org/10.1016/j.semnephrol.2006.07.001.
95. Story DA. Bench-to-bedside review: a brief history of clinical acid-base. Crit Care. 2004;8(4):253–8. https://doi.org/10.1186/cc2861.
96. Stickland MK, Lindinger MI, Olfert IM, Heigenhauser GJ, Hopkins SR. Pulmonary gas exchange and acid-base balance during exercise. Compr Physiol. 2013;3(2):693–739. https://doi.org/10.1002/cphy.c110048.
97. Nakamura M, Shirai A, Yamazaki O, Satoh N, Suzuki M, Horita S, Yamada H, Seki G. Roles of renal proximal tubule transport in acid/base balance and blood pressure regulation. Biomed Res Int. 2014;2014:504808. https://doi.org/10.1155/2014/504808.
98. Bertini A, Milani GP, Simonetti GD, Fossali EF, Faré PB, Bianchetti MG, Lava SA. Na(+), K(+), Cl(−), acid-base or $H_2O$ homeostasis in children with urinary tract infections: a narrative review. Pediatr Nephrol. 2016;31(9):1403–9. https://doi.org/10.1007/s00467-015-3273-5.

# Esophageal Ca Staging and Management According to Current Guidelines

19

Levent Kaptanoglu and Yalcin Burak Kara

## 19.1 Incidence and Epidemiology

Oesophageal cancer remains a major health problem globally and is the seventh most common cancer worldwide. Approximately 604,000 new cases were diagnosed in 2020. In addition, it is the sixth most common cause of cancer-related mortality, with an estimated 544,000 deaths in 2020 [1]. Male dominance reflects the diagnosis, there is a twofold to threefold difference in incidence and mortality rates between the sexes. Esophageal cancer cases can be seen much more in developing versus developed countries for men, but are comparable for women [2]. Eastern Asia, Southern Africa, Eastern Africa, Northern Europe, and South-Central Asia are most common parts of the world for esophageal malignancies [1]. Older age (<50 years) represents high incidence, but young age tends to be diagnosed in more advanced stages [3].

Two subtypes of esophageal cancer can be randomized: esophageal squamous-cell carcinoma (SCC) and esophageal adenocarcinoma (AC). SCC remains as most common type. However, the incidence of AC is rising in several regions of Europe and North America. Dietary changes were blamed for this. Heavy alcohol consumption and smoking are the major risk factors for esophageal SCC in Western populations [4]. In developing countries nutritional deficiencies and nitrosamines were held responsible [5]. Hot temperature of food and beverages consumption in Turkey and pickled vegetables consumption in China can be example for this condition.

Obesity, gastroesophageal reflux disease, esophageal intestinal metaplasia, and decreasing incidence of chronic *Helicobacter pylori* (*H. pylori*) infection remain major risk factors for AC [4, 6–9].

L. Kaptanoglu (✉) · Y. B. Kara
Department of General Surgery, VM Medical Park Pendik Hospital, Bahcesehir University, Istanbul, Turkey



O. Engin (ed.), *Risk Factors and Therapy of Esophagus Cancer*,
https://doi.org/10.1007/978-3-031-47024-0_19

## 19.2 Diagnosis, Pathology and Molecular Biology

### 19.2.1 Diagnosis

The guidelines of the American College of Gastroenterology should be followed, for screening of precursor lesions (oesophageal intestinal metaplasia) in high-risk patients, surveillance, and endoscopic ablation of precursor lesions [10, 11].

The algorithm of diagnose and staging can be seen in Table 19.1. History and physical examination remain major start-up point for all patients. All patient should be questioned for symptoms of appetite, dysphagia, gastrointestinal bleeding, recurrent aspiration, or emesis. And also, weight loss should be calculated carefully. Upper intestinal endoscopy is the gold standard diagnostic tool for physicians. Distal esophagus is favorite area for AC, whereas SCC is mostly seen in the proximal to middle esophagus [12]. All suspicious lesions should be biopsied, at least 6–8 representative biopsies should be taken.

### 19.2.2 Pathology

Diagnosis should be based on the histological tumor type classified according to the World Health Organization (WHO) criteria [13]. The prognostic and therapeutic relevance are main outcomes for differentiation of esophageal SCC and AC. Immunohistochemical (IHC) staining should be handy and also other less frequently occurring tumor types, such as neuroendocrine tumors/carcinomas,

**Table 19.1** Diagnostic and staging investigations in esophageal cancer

| Procedure | Purpose |
|---|---|
| FBC | Assess for iron-deficiency anemia |
| Renal and liver function | Assess renal and liver function to determine appropriate therapeutic options |
| Endoscopy and biopsy | Obtain tissue for diagnosis, histological classification and molecular biomarkers, e.g. PD-L1 and HER2 status (AC) |
| EUS | Accurate assessment of T and N stage in potentially resectable tumors |
| Bronchoscopy | Assess tumor growth towards central airways; complementary to EUS, especially when tumor stricture precludes EUS |
| CT thorax abdomen | Staging of tumor to detect local/distant lymphadenopathy and metastatic disease |
| PET-CT | Staging of tumor to detect local/distant lymphadenopathy and metastatic disease |
| Laparoscopy | Exclude occult metastatic disease involving peritoneum/diaphragm, especially in locally advanced (T3/T4) ACs of the OGJ infiltrating the anatomical cardia |

*AC* adenocarcinoma, *CT* computed tomography, *EUS* endoscopic ultrasound, *FBC* full blood count, *HER2* human epidermal growth factor receptor 2, *N* node, *OGJ* esophagogastric junction, *PD-L1* programmed death-ligand 1, *PET* positron emission tomography, *T* tumor lymphomas, mesenchymal tumors, melanomas or secondary tumor. They must be differentiated from SCC and AC.

### 19.2.3 Recommendations

- An upper intestinal endoscopy should be performed for the patients with new dysphagia and gastrointestinal bleeding. Other symptoms can be classified as recurrent aspiration or emesis and weight loss and/or loss of appetite [III, A]. Diagnosis should be made by histopathological assessment of multiple (_6) endoscopic biopsies to guarantee an adequate representation of the tumor [I, B].
- Histological diagnosis should be reported according to the WHO criteria [IV, A].
- Sometimes SCC and AC cannot be differentiated by using morphological features. IHC staining is recommended to differentiate for poorly differentiated and undifferentiated cancers [V, B] [14–17].

## 19.3 Staging and Risk Assessment

Staging paves, the road for successful treatment of esophageal cancer. Complete clinical examination, endoscopy, and computed tomography (CT) or positron emission tomography (PET) with [18F]2-fluoro-2-deoxy-D-glucose (FDG) remains as gold standard diagnostic tools. Staging of tumor and node is succeeded by Endoscopic ultrasound (EUS). Endoscopic resection offers more precise staging in addition to therapeutic benefit [18, 19].

EUS may reveal T4b status with invasion towards the airways, pericardium, or aorta and also give chance for lymph node biopsies. Because of tumoral strictures not give usage of EUS bronchoscopy with endobronchial ultrasonography can be proper choice.

FDGePET (typically carried out as PETeCT) is helpful in diagnosing undetected distant metastases. It should be performed for surgical candidates. However, the availability of PETeCT differs between countries and centers [20–23].

Our current practice recommends diagnostic laparoscopy, especially for (T3/T4) ACs of the OGJ infiltrating the anatomical cardia [24, 25], to detect peritoneal metastases.

Esophageal cancer should be staged according to the American Joint Committee on Cancer AJCC/UICC TNM (tumor-node-metastasis) 8th edition staging system [26].

To decide medical risk assessment, blood count, liver, pulmonary, cardiac, and renal function tests are needed. Nutritional status and history of weight loss should be assessed according to the European Society for Clinical Nutrition and Metabolism (ESPEN) guidelines [27]. More than half of patients lose >5% of their body weight before surgery and this is an increased operative risk, worsens a patient's quality of life (QoL) and is associated with poor survival in advanced disease. Nutrition remains as major part of successful therapy and should be pursued according to

ESPEN guidelines [28]. Physical activity remains as supporting factor for successful surgeries [29, 30]. An exercise program may improve of QoL [31]. Literature review gives us clues for perioperative exercise regimen to neoadjuvant chemotherapy (ChT) improves outcomes [32, 33].

### 19.3.1 Recommendations

- Initial staging and risk assessment should include physical examination, endoscopy and contrast-enhanced CT or FDG-PET-CT scan of the thorax, abdomen—pelvis. EUS is very helpful in T and N evaluation [III, A].
- FDG-PET should be carried out in candidates for esophagectomy [III, B].
- Patients with (T3/T4), including cardia invasion deserves laparoscopy [IV, B].
- Final TNM stage should follow AJCC/UICC guidelines and staging manual [IV, A].
- According to ESPEN guidelines nutritional support can be designed [26–33].

## 19.4 Management of Local and Locoregional Diseases

Treatment plan should be organized very carefully. Histological type of tumor, TNM stage, tumor location, and the patient's status (performance status and comorbidities) play major role in planning. Patients suffering from malnutrition should be evaluated and undergo corrections for their status. In most of the cases, enteral feeding is necessary, either via feeding jejunostomy or via nasogastric tube. Most experienced surgeons do not prefer stent application [34]. Figure 19.1 reflects treatment options of localized esophageal and OGJ cancer.

### 19.4.1 Early Disease (cT1 N0 M0)

Endoscopic en bloc resection, using either endoscopic mucosal resection (EMR) or endoscopic submucosal dissection (ESD), is the treatment of choice for lesions with intraepithelial high-grade dysplasia and most T1 tumors [35, 36]. Lack of the deep resection margin and lymph node metastases remain major obstacle for successful resection as definitive treatment [35, 36].

Risk factors for lymph node metastasis are depth of invasion, lymphovascular invasion, low differentiation grade, ulceration, and large tumor size [37, 38].

For esophageal AC, endoscopic resection can usually be considered curative in all T1a cancers and, in the absence of other risk factors for lymph node metastasis, also in the most superficial submucosally involved T1b cancers (sm1, invasion depth <500 mm, no ulceration) [35]. For AC there is no evidence favoring either EMR or ESD, but EMR should normally be preferred in small lesions, while ESD should be considered in lesions >15 mm, poorly lifting tumors and tumors at risk of submucosal invasion [37].

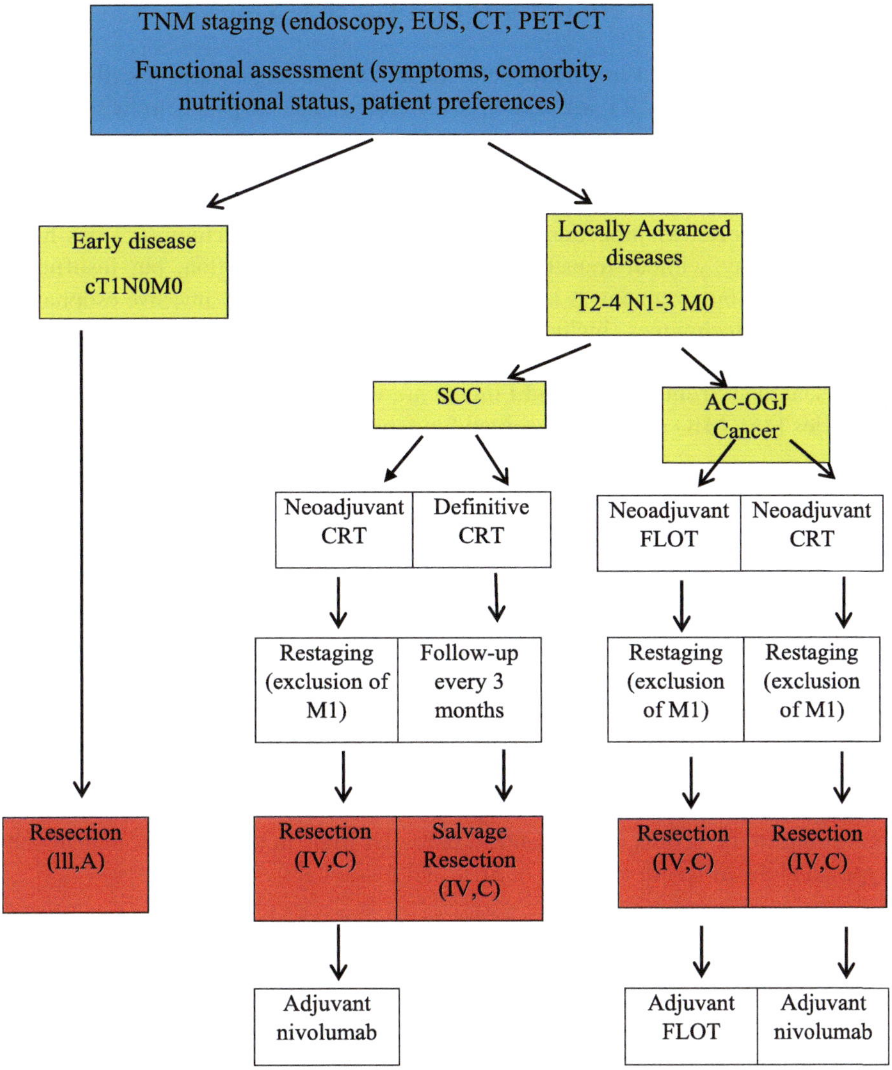


**Fig. 19.1** Treatment algorithm for local/locoregional resectable esophageal and OGJ cancer

For both histological subtypes, T2 N1 patients should be offered resective surgery with appropriate lymphadenectomy. Chemoradiotherapy (CRT) is another treatment modality [38, 39].

## 19.4.2 Patients Suffering from cT2–T4 or cN1–3 M0

Surgery remains as first-line therapeutic method in this stage. There is still an ongoing debate, definitive CRT with surveillance and salvage esophagectomy is as good as surgery.

Transthoracic esophagectomy with en bloc two-field lymphadenectomy is preferred method in our current practice. We perform Ivor Lewis procedure for distal tumors and McKeown procedure for mid and upper esophageal tumors. Trans-hiatal esophagectomy without transthoracic Access is another option, but insufficient lymphadenectomy remains as an obstacle [40, 41]. Minimally invasive esophagectomy (MIO) techniques, including robotics are handy for us recently. Literature review reveals comparable results MIO with open surgeries [42–45].

Researchers from Sweden and Finland are in favor for MIO compared to open surgeries [46]. MIO should be reserved for experienced centers.

## 19.4.3 Pre- and Perioperative Treatment

Chemotherapy and chemoradiotherapy still remain as a treatment choice prior to surgery. Literature reveals increased resection rates with no tumor at the margin (R0) and survival rates in esophageal cancer and should be considered in all patients with locally advanced resectable disease [47–53].

A randomized phase III trial in stage I–II esophageal cancer showed that preoperative CRT did not improve R0 resection rate or survival but increased postoperative mortality [54–56].

The treatment paradigms for esophageal SCC versus esophageal AC differs according to the results of randomized phase III trials in the two histological subtypes, and the differing response of SCC and AC to CRT.

### 19.4.3.1 SCC

Based on the results of the Chemoradiotherapy for Esophageal Cancer Followed by Surgery Study (CROSS), preoperative CRT can be recommended as a standard of care for SCC of the esophagus [50]. Weekly carboplatin-paclitaxel combined with radiation followed by esophagectomy showed improved survival compared with surgery alone for both SCC and AC. Survival rates are increased for SCC with the help of this trimodal therapy. SCC may show high response rates CRT [50], therefore can be applied in selected cases [57–59].

Current practice offers modern and better RT techniques, therefore 3-year OS rate of 47.8% and median OS of 35.9 months in patients with esophageal SCC could be reached [60]. Definitive CRT is recommended for cervically localized tumors where surgery would entail a laryngectomy.

### 19.4.3.2 AC

CROSS, study revealed importance of preoperative CRT. Even after complete clinical tumor response to preoperative CRT or ChT, patients with resectable oesophageal AC should proceed to surgery, as data for a watch-and-wait strategy following complete clinical remission are currently limited [50]. If the patients with oesophageal SCC or AC are not suitable for surgery, the recommendation is definitive chemoradiotherapy [57–60]. Four cycle of cisplatine with/without capecitabine is first choice for CRT regimen. Standard dose of RT is 50.4 Gy in 28 fractions or 50 Gy in 25 fractions.

### 19.4.4 Recommendations

- Multidisciplinary assessment and planning before any treatment is mandatory [IV, A].
- MIO should be performed in surgical centers including experienced staff [II, A].
- Most T1 tumors or lesions which is high-grade dysplasia can be resected by endoscopically by either EMR or ESD [III, A].
- Resective surgery with appropriate lymphadenectomy should be recommended for patients with involved deep endoscopic resection margins or significant risk factors for lymph node metastases [III, A].
- Pre- and perioperative ChT or CRT should be considered in all patients with locally advanced resectable disease [I, A].
- Locally advanced esophageal SCC should be treated with CRT followed by surgery [I, A] or definitive CRT with close surveillance and salvage surgery for local tumor persistence or progression [II, B]. Definitive CRT could be used for cervical tumors requires a laryngectomy [III, B].
- Patients with resectable, locally advanced esophageal AC or OGJ cancer should be treated with neoadjuvant CRT based on the CROSS regimen or perioperative ChT (FLOT) followed by surgery [I, A; ESMO-MCBS v1.1 score: A].
- Complete clinical tumor response to preoperative CRT or ChT does not support final treatment. Surgery still remains first choice of therapy [IV, C].
- When esophageal SCC or AC is unresectable or locally advanced tumors, the recommended treatment option is definitive CRT [I, A] [50, 53, 57, 60].

## 19.5 Management of Advanced and Metastatic Disease

Conditions such as metastatic disease, unresectable tumors or cannot be treated with CRT show poor prognosis and estimated survival time is less than 1 year [61, 62].

A proposed algorithm for the treatment of advanced esophageal SCC is shown in Fig. 19.2.

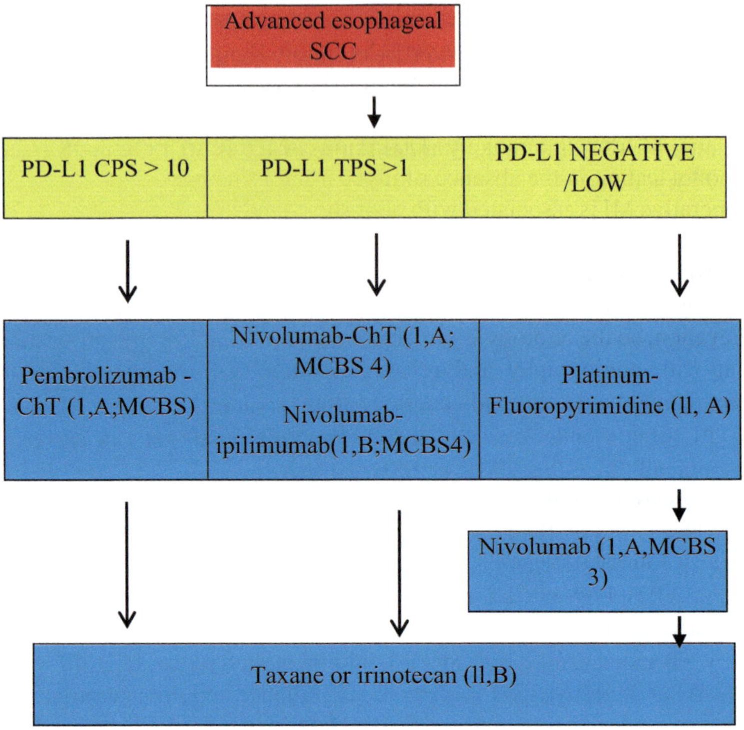


**Fig. 19.2** Treatment algorithm for advanced esophageal SCC. Red and yellow: general categories or stratification; blue: systemic anticancer therapy. *AC* adenocarcinoma, *ChT* chemotherapy, *CPG* Clinical Practice Guideline, *CPS* combined positive score, *EMA* European Medicines Agency, *FDA* Food and Drug Administration, *MCBS* Magnitude of Clinical Benefit Score, *OGJ* esophago-gastric junction, *PDL1* programmed death-ligand 1, *SCC* squamous-cell carcinoma, *TPS* tumor proportion score. (a) For treatment of esophageal AC and OGJ cancer, see the ESMO CPG for gastric cancer. (b) EMA approval is for tumors with PD-L1 CPS 10, FDA approval is irrespective of PD-L1 expression. (c) ESMO-MCBS v1.191 was used to calculate scores for therapies/indications approved by the EMA or FDA

## 19.5.1 First-Line ChT for Esophageal SCC

Standard first-line ChT for esophageal SCC is a platinum fluoropyrimidine doublet [62–65]. The phase III GO2 trial recruited patients with advanced gastroesophageal cancer, including esophageal SCC, who were unsuitable for full dose ChT due to advanced age or frailty and demonstrated equivalent outcomes and reduced toxicity with dose-reduced oxaliplatin capecitabine [66].

### 19.5.2 Other Treatment Options for Esophageal SCC

For patients with esophageal SCC, second-line nivolumab monotherapy is an option based on the results of the phase III ATTRACTION-3 trial.

Taxane or irinotecan chemotherapy regimen should be used as second-line treatment option for esophageal SCC [67–70].

#### 19.5.2.1 Recommendations

A platinum and fluoropyrimidine chemotherapy regimen is first choice and standard treatment for advanced esophageal SCC [II, A]. Secondary choice is Dose-reduced oxaliplatin capecitabine for patients who are not tolerated with full-dose ChT [I, A].

- Pembrolizumab ChT is recommended for advanced, untreated esophageal SCC. The greatest benefit is seen in patients with a PD-L1 CPS_10 [I, A; ESMO-MCBS v1.1 score: 4; European Medicines Agency (EMA) approval is for tumors with PD-L1 CPS_10, Food and Drug Administration (FDA) approval is irrespective of PD-L1 expression].
- Nivolumab is recommended in patients with tumors expressing PD-L1 with a TPS_1% [I, A; ESMOMCBS v1.1 score: 4]. Nivolumab ipilimumab can be given, but a lower radiological response rate and increased risk of early progression and death in patients treated without ChT needs to be considered [I, B; ESMOMCBS v1.1 score: 4] [62–65].

### 19.5.3 Other Treatment Choices for Advanced Esophageal SCC

- Nivolumab is recommended for esophageal SCC previously treated with platinum fluoropyrimidine ChT [I, A; ESMO-MCBS v1.1 score: 3].
- Where approved, pembrolizumab may be an option for patients with previously treated SCC who have not received first-line treatment with ICIs and have a PD-L1 CPS_10 [I, A; ESMO-MCBS v1.1 score: 3; FDA approved, not EMA approved].
- ChT with a taxane or irinotecan can be considered in fit patients who have been previously treated with platinum fluoropyrimidine and/or nivolumab or pembrolizumab [II, B] [62–65].

### 19.5.4 Supportive Care and Nutrition

- Patients with advanced esophageal cancer need early palliative care referral. They also need nutritional support [I, A].

### 19.5.5 Follow-Up, Long-Term Implications and Survivorship

For esophageal and OGJ cancers have different surveillance strategies. Although the majority (nearly 90%) of relapses occur within the first 2 years after completion of local therapy, potentially treatable relapses have been reported >5 years after local therapy [71, 72]. Metachronous malignancies should also be considered in long-term survivors.

Patient symptoms, nutritional status, and psychological support play major role in pursuing these cases. A physician should be responsible for future visits. Absence of the esophagus, side effects of CRT and psychological problems still remain as major obstacles. A multidisciplinary team including dietician, radiologist, gastroenterologist, psychologist and social worker should be handy all the time. Even complete response to definitive CRT does not complete the whole therapy. After 3 months, gastroscopy with biopsies if needed, and CT scan should be performed, in order to detect early recurrence. Salvage surgery may be required [73].

#### 19.5.5.1 Recommendations

- The majority (w90%) of relapses occur within the first 2 years after completion of local therapy. History, physical examination, patient complaints, and general appearance are main points in follow-up [V, A].
- After complete response, 3 months interval follow-up should be recommended. Endoscopy with biopsy, CT scan can be used for early detection [IV, B] [71–73].

## References

1. Sung H, Ferlay J, Siegel RL, et al. Global Cancer Statistics 2020: GLOBOCAN estimates of incidence and mortality worldwide for 36 cancers in 185 countries. CA Cancer J Clin. 2021;71(3):209–49.
2. Arnold M, Abnet CC, Neale RE, et al. Global burden of 5 major types of gastrointestinal cancer. Gastroenterology. 2020;159(1):335–49.
3. Codipilly DC, Sawas T, Dhaliwal L, et al. Epidemiology and outcomes of young-onset esophageal adenocarcinoma: an analysis from a population-based database. Cancer Epidemiol Biomarkers Prev. 2021;30(1):142–9.
4. Thun M, Linet MS, Cerhan JR, et al. Cancer epidemiology and prevention. 4th ed. New York: Oxford University Press; 2018.
5. McCormack VA, Menya D, Munishi MO, et al. Informing etiologic research priorities for squamous cell esophageal cancer in Africa: a review of setting-specific exposures to known and putative risk factors. Int J Cancer. 2017;140(2):259–71.
6. El-Serag HB, Hashmi A, Garcia J, et al. Visceral abdominal obesity measured by CT scan is associated with an increased risk of Barrett's oesophagus: a case-control study. Gut. 2014;63(2):220–9.
7. O'Doherty MG, Freedman ND, Hollenbeck AR, et al. A prospective cohort studyofobesity and riskofoesophageal and gastric denocarcinoma in the NIH-AARP Diet and Health Study. Gut. 2012;61(9):1261–8.
8. Parsonnet J, Friedman GD, Vandersteen DP, et al. Helicobacter pylori infection and the risk of gastric carcinoma. N Engl J Med. 1991;325(16):1127–31.

9. Arnold M, Laversanne M, Brown LM, et al. Predicting the future burden of esophageal cancer by histological subtype: international trends in incidence up to 2030. Am J Gastroenterol. 2017;112(8):1247–55.
10. Parfitt JR, Miladinovic Z, Driman DK. Increasing incidence of adenocarcinoma of the gastroesophageal junction and distal stomach in Canada—an epidemiological study from 1964–2002. Can J Gastroenterol. 2006;20(4):271–6.
11. Shaheen NJ, Falk GW, Iyer PG, et al. ACG clinical guideline: diagnosis and management of Barrett's esophagus. Am J Gastroenterol. 2016;111(1):30–50.
12. Rustgi AK, El-Serag HB. Esophageal carcinoma. N Engl J Med. 2014;371(26):2499–509.
13. Nagtegaal ID, Odze RD, Klimstra D, et al. The 2019 WHO classification of tumours of the digestive system. Histopathology. 2020;76(2):182–8.
14. Shen L, Kato K, Kim SB, et al. Tislelizumab versus chemotherapy as second-line treatment for advanced or metastatic esophageal squamous cell carcinoma (RATIONALE-302): a randomized phase III study. J Clin Oncol. 2022;40(26):3065–76.
15. Prince EA, Sanzari JK, Pandya D, et al. Analytical concordance of PD-L1 assays utilizing antibodies from FDA-approved diagnostics in advanced cancers: a systematic literature review. JCO Precis Oncol. 2021;5:953–973, 1002.
16. Yeong J, Lum HYJ, Teo CB, et al. Choice of PD-L1 immunohistochemistry assay influences clinical eligibility for gastric cancer immunotherapy. Gastric Cancer. 2022;25:741–50.
17. Lordick F, Carneiro F, Cascinu S, et al. Gastric cancer: ESMO Clinical Practice Guideline for diagnosis, treatment and follow-up. Ann Oncol. 2022; https://doi.org/10.1016/j.annonc.2022.07.004.
18. Catalano MF, Van Dam J, Sivak MV. Malignant esophageal strictures: staging accuracy of endoscopic ultrasonography. Gastrointest Endosc. 1995;41(6):535–9.
19. Krill T, Baliss M, Roark R, et al. Accuracy of endoscopic ultrasound in esophageal cancer staging. J Thorac Dis. 2019;11(suppl 12):s1602–9.
20. van Vliet EPM, Heijenbrok-Kal MH, Hunink MGM, et al. Staging investigations for oesophageal cancer: a meta-analysis. Br J Cancer. 2008;98(3):547–57.
21. Flamen P, Lerut A, Van Cutsem E, et al. Utility of positron emission tomography for the staging of patients with potentially operable esophageal carcinoma. J Clin Oncol. 2000;18(18):3202–10.
22. Heeren PAM, Jager PL, Bongaerts F, et al. Detection of distant metastases in esophageal cancer with 18F-FDG PET. J Nucl Med. 2004;45(6):980–7.
23. Findlay JM, Bradley KM, Maile EJ, et al. Pragmatic staging of oesophageal cancer using decision theory involving selective endoscopic ultrasonography, PET and laparoscopy. Br J Surg. 2015;102(12):1488–99.
24. van de Ven S, Bugter O, Hardillo JA, et al. Screening for head and neck second primary tumors in patients with esophageal squamous cell cancer: a systematic review and meta-analysis. United European Gastroenterol J. 2019;7(10):1304–11.
25. Gertsen EC, Brenkman HJF, van Hillegersberg R, et al. 18F-fludeoxyglucose-positron emission tomography/computed tomography and laparoscopy for staging of locally advanced gastric cancer: a multicenter prospective Dutch cohort study (PLASTIC). JAMA Surg. 2021;156(12):e215340.
26. Rice TW, Ishwaran H, Blackstone EH, et al. Recommendations for clinical staging (cTNM) of cancer of the esophagus and esophagogastric junction for the 8th edition AJCC/UICC staging manuals. Dis Esophagus. 2016;29(8):913–9.
27. Cederholm T, Barazzoni R, Austin P, et al. ESPEN guidelines on definitions and terminology of clinical nutrition. Clin Nutr. 2017;36(1):49–64.
28. Bischoff SC, Austin P, Boeykens K, et al. ESPEN guideline on home enteral nutrition. Clin Nutr. 2020;39(1):5–22.
29. Sinclair R, Navidi M, Griffin SM, et al. The impact of neoadjuvant chemotherapy on cardiopulmonary physical fitness in gastrooesophageal adenocarcinoma. Ann R Coll Surg Engl. 2016;98(6):396–400.

30. Whibley J, Peters CJ, Halliday LJ, et al. Poor performance in incremental shuttle walk and cardiopulmonary exercise testing predicts poor overall survival for patients undergoing esophagogastric resection. Eur J Surg Oncol. 2018;44(5):594–9.
31. van Vulpen JK, Hiensch AE, van Hillegersberg R, et al. Supervised exercise after oesophageal cancer surgery: the PERFECT multicentre randomized clinical trial. Br J Surg. 2021;108(7):786–96.
32. Tully R, Loughney L, Bolger J, et al. The effect of a pre- and postoperative exercise programme versus standard care on physical fitness of patients with oesophageal and gastric cancer undergoing neoadjuvant treatment prior to surgery (The PERIOP-OG Trial): study protocol for a randomised controlled trial. Trials. 2020;21(1):638.
33. Kotzerke D, Moritz F, Mantovani L, et al. The performance of three oncogeriatric screening tools—G8, optimised G8 and CARG—in predicting chemotherapy-related toxicity in older patients with cancer. A prospective clinical study. J Geriatr Oncol. 2019;10(6):937–43.
34. Mariette C, Gronnier C, Duhamel A, et al. Self-expanding covered metallic stent as a bridge to surgery in esophageal cancer: impact on oncologic outcomes. J Am Coll Surg. 2015;220(3):287–96.
35. di Pietro M, Canto MI, Fitzgerald RC. Endoscopic management of early adenocarcinoma and squamous cell carcinoma of the esophagus: screening, diagnosis, and therapy. Gastroenterology. 2018;154(2):421–36.
36. Weusten B, Bisschops R, Coron E, et al. Endoscopic management of Barrett's esophagus: European Society of Gastrointestinal Endoscopy (ESGE) Position Statement. Endoscopy. 2017;49(2):191–8.
37. Pimentel-Nunes P, Dinis-Ribeiro M, Ponchon T, et al. Endoscopic submucosal dissection: European Society of Gastrointestinal Endoscopy (ESGE) Guideline. Endoscopy. 2015;47(9):829–54.
38. Yamashina T, Ishihara R, Nagai K, et al. Long-term outcome and metastatic risk after endoscopic resection of superficial esophageal squamous cell carcinoma. Am J Gastroenterol. 2013;108(4):544–51.
39. Cao Y, Liao C, Tan A, et al. Meta-analysis of endoscopic submucosal dissection versus endoscopic mucosal resection for tumors of the gastrointestinal tract. Endoscopy. 2009;41(9):751–7.
40. Kato K, Ito Y, Nozaki I, et al. Parallel-group controlled trial of surgery versus chemoradiotherapy in patients with stage I esophageal squamous cell carcinoma. Gastroenterology. 2021;161(6):1878–86.
41. Hulscher JBF, van Sandick JW, de Boer AGEM, et al. Extended transthoracic resection compared with limited transhiatal resection for adenocarcinoma of the esophagus. N Engl J Med. 2002;347(21):1662–9.
42. Biere SSAY, van Berge Henegouwen MI, Maas KW, et al. Minimally invasive versus open oesophagectomy for patients with oesophageal cancer: a multicentre, open-label, randomised controlled trial. Lancet. 2012;379(9829):1887–92.
43. Maas KW, Cuesta MA, van Berge Henegouwen MI, et al. Quality of life and late complications after minimally invasive compared to open esophagectomy: results of a randomized trial. World J Surg. 2015;39(8):1986–93.
44. Mariette C, Markar SR, Dabakuyo-Yonli TS, et al. Hybrid minimally invasive esophagectomy for esophageal cancer. N Engl J Med. 2019;380(2):152–62.
45. van der Sluis PC, van der Horst S, May AM, et al. Robot-assisted minimally invasive thoracolaparoscopic esophagectomy versus open transthoracic esophagectomy for resectable esophageal cancer: a randomized controlled trial. Ann Surg. 2019;269(4):621–30.
46. Gottlieb-Vedi E, Kauppila JH, Mattsson F, et al. Long-term survival in esophageal cancer after minimally invasive esophagectomy compared to open esophagectomy. Ann Surg. 2021; https://doi.org/10.1097/SLA.0000000000004645.
47. Sjoquist KM, Burmeister BH, Smithers BM, et al. Survival after neoadjuvant chemotherapy or chemoradiotherapy for resectable oesophageal carcinoma: an updated meta-analysis. Lancet Oncol. 2011;12(7):681–92.

48. Ronellenfitsch U, Schwarzbach M, Hofheinz R, et al. Preoperative chemo(radio)therapy versus primary surgery for gastroesophageal adenocarcinoma: systematic review with meta-analysis combining individual patient and aggregate data. Eur J Cancer. 2013;49(15):3149–58.
49. Allum WH, Stenning SP, Bancewicz J, et al. Long-term results of a randomized trial of surgery with or without preoperative chemotherapy in esophageal cancer. J Clin Oncol. 2009;27(30):5062–7.
50. van Hagen P, Hulshof MCCM, van Lanschot JJB, et al. Preoperative chemoradiotherapy for esophageal or junctional cancer. N Engl J Med. 2012;366(22):2074–84.
51. Cunningham D, Allum WH, Stenning SP, et al. Perioperative chemotherapy versus surgery alone for resectable gastroesophageal cancer. N Engl J Med. 2006;355(1):11–20.
52. Ychou M, Boige V, Pignon JP, et al. Perioperative chemotherapy compared with surgery alone for resectable gastroesophageal adenocarcinoma: an FNCLCC and FFCD multicenter phase III trial. J Clin Oncol. 2011;29(13):1715–21.
53. Al-Batran SE, Homann N, Pauligk C, et al. Perioperative chemotherapy with fluorouracil plus leucovorin, oxaliplatin, and docetaxel versus fluorouracil or capecitabine plus cisplatin and epirubicin for locally advanced, resectable gastric or gastro-oesophageal junction adenocarcinoma (FLOT4): a randomised, phase 2/3 trial. Lancet. 2019;393(10184):1948–57.
54. Markar SR, Gronnier C, Pasquer A, et al. Role of neoadjuvant treatment in clinical T2N0M0 oesophageal cancer: results from a retrospective multi-center European study. Eur J Cancer. 2016;56:59–68.
55. Goense L, Visser E, Haj Mohammad N, et al. Role of neoadjuvant chemoradiotherapy in clinical T2N0M0 esophageal cancer: a population-based cohort study. Eur J Surg Oncol. 2018;44(5):620–5.
56. Mariette C, Dahan L, Mornex F, et al. Surgery alone versus chemoradiotherapy followed by surgery for stage I and II esophageal cancer: final analysis of randomized controlled phase III trial FFCD 9901. J Clin Oncol. 2014;32(23):2416–22.
57. Herskovic A, Martz K, al-Sarraf M, et al. Combined chemotherapy and radiotherapy compared with radiotherapy alone in patients with cancer of the esophagus. N Engl J Med. 1992;326(24):1593–8.
58. Markar S, Gronnier C, Duhamel A, et al. Salvage surgery after chemoradiotherapy in the management of esophageal cancer: is it a viable therapeutic option? J Clin Oncol. 2015;33(33):3866–73.
59. Vincent J, Mariette C, Pezet D, et al. Early surgery for failure after chemoradiation in operable thoracic oesophageal cancer. Analysis of the non-randomised patients in FFCD 9102 phase III trial: chemoradiation followed by surgery versus chemoradiation alone. Eur J Cancer. 2015;51(13):1683–93.
60. Crosby T, Hurt CN, Falk S, et al. Long-term results and recurrence patterns from SCOPE-1: a phase II/III randomised trial of definitive chemoradiotherapy +/− cetuximab in oesophageal cancer. Br J Cancer. 2017;116(6):709–16.
61. Moehler M, Maderer A, Thuss-Patience PC, et al. Cisplatin and 5-fluorouracil with or without epidermal growth factor receptor inhibition panitumumab for patients with non-resectable, advanced or metastatic oesophageal squamous cell cancer: a prospective, openlabel, randomised phase III AIO/EORTC trial (POWER). Ann Oncol. 2020;31(2):228–35.
62. Chau I, Ayers D, Goring S, et al. Comparative effectiveness of nivolumab versus clinical practice for advanced gastric or gastroesophageal junction cancer. J Comp Eff Res. 2020;9(2):103–14.
63. Hayashi K, Ando N, Watanabe H, et al. Phase II evaluation of protracted infusion of cisplatin and 5-fluorouracil in advanced squamous cell carcinoma of the esophagus: a Japan Esophageal Oncology Group (JEOG) Trial (JCOG9407). Jpn J Clin Oncol. 2001;31(9):419–23.
64. Bleiberg H, Conroy T, Paillot B, et al. Randomised phase II study of cisplatin and 5-fluorouracil (5-FU) versus cisplatin alone in advanced squamous cell oesophageal cancer. Eur J Cancer. 1997;33(8):1216–20.
65. Lorenzen S, Schuster T, Porschen R, et al. Cetuximab plus cisplatin-5-fluorouracil versus cisplatin-5-fluorouracil alone in first-line metastatic squamous cell carcinoma of the

esophagus: a randomized phase II study of the Arbeitsgemeinschaft Internistische Onkologie. Ann Oncol. 2009;20(10):1667–73.
66. Hall PS, Swinson D, Cairns DA, et al. Efficacy of reduced-intensity chemotherapy with oxaliplatin and capecitabine on quality of life and cancer control among older and frail patients with advanced gastroesophageal cancer: the GO2 phase 3 randomized clinical trial. JAMA Oncol. 2021;7(6):869–77.
67. Shitara K, Özgüroğlu M, Bang YJ, et al. Pembrolizumab versus paclitaxel for previously treated, advanced gastric or gastro-oesophageal junction cancer (KEYNOTE-061): a randomised, open-label, controlled, phase 3 trial. Lancet. 2018;392(10142):123–33.
68. Kato K, Tahara M, Hironaka S, et al. A phase II study of paclitaxel by weekly 1-h infusion for advanced or recurrent esophageal cancer in patients who had previously received platinum-based chemotherapy. Cancer Chemother Pharmacol. 2011;67(6):1265–72.
69. Muro K, Hamaguchi T, Ohtsu A, et al. A phase II study of single-agent docetaxel in patients with metastatic esophageal cancer. Ann Oncol. 2004;15(6):955–9.
70. Burkart C, Bokemeyer C, Klump B, et al. A phase II trial of weekly irinotecan in cisplatin-refractory esophageal cancer. Anticancer Res. 2007;27(4c):2845–8.
71. Rodríguez-Camacho E, Pita-Fernández S, Pértega-Díaz S, et al. Characteristics and pattern of recurrence after curative surgery in oesophageal cancer. Rev Esp Enferm Dig. 2015;107(9):539–46.
72. Ni W, Yang J, Deng W, et al. Patterns of recurrence after surgery and efficacy of salvage therapy after recurrence in patients with thoracic esophageal squamous cell carcinoma. BMC Cancer. 2020;20(1):144.
73. Conroy T, Galais MP, Raoul JL, et al. Definitive chemoradiotherapy with FOLFOX versus fluorouracil and cisplatin in patients with oesophageal cancer (PRODIGE5/ACCORD17): final results of a randomised, phase 2/3 trial. Lancet Oncol. 2014;15(3):305–14.

# Endoscopic Treatment in Esophagus Cancer: Endoscopic Mucosal Resection and Endoscopic Submucosal Dissection

# 20

Fevzi Cengiz

## Abbreviations

| | |
|---|---|
| AJCC | American Joint Committee on Cancer |
| EMR | Endoscopic mucosal resection |
| EMR-P | Precut EMR |
| ER | Endoscopic resection |
| ESD | Endoscopic submucosal dissection |
| EUS | Endoscopic ultrasonography |
| FDG | Fluorodeoxyglucose |
| HGD | High-grade dysplasia |
| HPMC | Hydroxypropyl methylcellulose |
| JSGE | Japanese Society of Gastroenterological Endoscopy |
| LVI | Lymphovascular invasion |
| NCCN | National Comprehensive Cancer Network |
| NCDB | National Cancer Database |
| PET/CT | Integrated positron emission tomography/computerized tomography |
| RFA | Radiofrequency ablation |
| SCC | Squamous cell carcinoma |

## 20.1 Introduction

Endoscopic resection is an alternative to surgical resection of mucosal and submucosal neoplastic lesions [1]. The epidemiology of esophageal cancer has evolved over the past two decades. The most obvious change is a reversal in the rate of

F. Cengiz (✉)
Surgery Department, Medicine Faculty, Izmir Kâtip Celebi University, Izmir, Turkey



O. Engin (ed.), *Risk Factors and Therapy of Esophagus Cancer*,
https://doi.org/10.1007/978-3-031-47024-0_20

adenocarcinoma of squamous cell cancers and a shift in the stage distribution [2]. The incidence of superficial esophageal cancer (*no deeper than the submucosa*) is increasing, particularly in Asian countries where screening for upper gastrointestinal tract cancers is common [3]. A similar trend has been seen in the United States, where routine endoscopic surveillance for malignancy and high-grade dysplasia (*HGD*) has been recommended in patients with Barrett's esophagus, a complication of long-standing gastroesophageal reflux disease [4].

Endoscopic resection offers a chance for both accurate diagnosis and treatment. Endoscopic resections are performed with endoscopic instruments developed for Endoscopic Mucosal Resection (*EMR*) or Endoscopic Submucosal Dissection (*ESD*) using a snare endoscopically. In this way, they are ideal methods for the curative treatment of lesions limited to the superficial layers of the mucosa and submucosa. However, it should be noted that these techniques are only suitable for patients with a very low risk of lymph node metastasis or at risk for esophageal surgery [5].

## 20.2 Detection and Evaluation of Superficial Esophageal Cancer

Accurately assessing the extent of disease is a crucial aspect of determining the appropriate treatment strategy for superficial esophageal cancer. The depth of tumor invasion, particularly the presence or absence of submucosal involvement, is a significant prognostic factor for early esophageal cancers. When cancer cells penetrate beyond the mucosal layer and invade the submucosa, it signifies a higher risk of metastasis and disease progression. Lymphatic vessels are predominantly present in the submucosal layer of the esophagus, and their involvement facilitates the spread of cancer cells to nearby lymph nodes. If submucosal invasion is detected, it indicates a greater likelihood of lymph node metastasis, which can impact treatment decisions and prognosis. Therefore, an accurate assessment of tumor size is required to guide treatment [6].

Early esophageal cancers are classified as Tis (*non-invasive neoplasia called carcinoma in situ or high-grade dysplasia* [*HGD*]) and T1 tumors, which are divided into T1a and T1b, depending on the depth of invasion [7]. In a series of 3963 patients surgically treated for localized esophageal cancer from the National Cancer Database (*NCDB*), the risk of nodal metastases for T1a and T1b tumors was 5% versus 16.6% [8].

## 20.3 T-Stage Classification of Superficial Esophageal Cancer and Prognostic Pathological Factors

A more comprehensive subclassification for early esophageal cancers has been proposed by Japanese researchers to determine prognosis and tailor treatment (Fig. 20.1) [9]. According to this classification, mucosal tumors are divided into three types according to the depth of invasion: M1—limited to the epithelial layer,

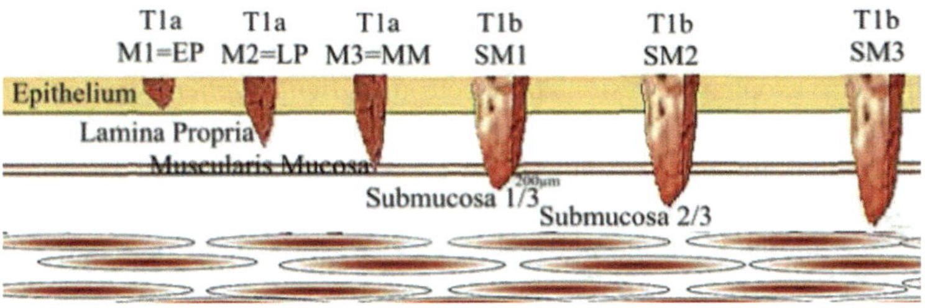


**Fig. 20.1** Subclassification for superficial cancer

M2—limited to the lamina propria, and M3—refers to tumors limited to the muscularis mucosa. M1 tumors correspond to Tis stage in the American Joint Committee on Cancer (*AJCC*) stage definition, while M2 and M3 tumors are considered T1a lesions. Tumors invading the submucosa are subclassified as follows: SM1—Invades the shallowest third of the submucosa, SM2—Invades the intermediate third of the submucosa, SM3—Invades the lower third of the submucosa [9]. All of these subcategories, regardless of histology, are considered T1b disease according to the AJCC stage definitions.

The lymph node metastasis rate of superficial adenocarcinomas is not higher than that of squamous cell carcinomas (*SCCs*) [5]. Since M1 and M2 tumors do not have the possibility of lymph node metastasis, they are very suitable for endoscopic treatment. The risk of lymph node metastasis in M3 tumors is *0–12%* [10]. In the evaluation of nodal involvement, the second important factor other than the depth of invasion is pathological factors. In M3 tumors, lymphovascular invasion, one of the pathological factors, should be considered [11]. In addition to the depth of tumor (*T*) invasion, other tumor characteristics that may affect the risk of lymph node metastasis; the morphological features of the lesion (*flat-type* versus *non-flat* [*elevated*], *depressed, or ulcerated*), tumor size, presence of lymphovascular invasion, and degree of histological differentiation [12, 13].

ER should be avoided because of the risk of lymph node metastasis of esophageal tumors extending to the T1b submucosa and the risk of local and distant metastases [14]. While SM1 in Japanese clinical practice and publications accepts the treatment of esophageal tumors with limited (*defined as ≤200 µm depth*) and good prognostic features (*macroscopically polypoid or flat, well or moderately differentiated, without lymphovascular invasion*) with ESD, regardless of histology in the guidelines, esophagectomy with lymphadenectomy is recommended for T1b tumors.

## 20.4 Morphological Classification of Superficial Esophageal Cancer

In staging superficial esophageal cancer, it is necessary first to detect and predict the depth of invasion. Endoscopy is the main and even the only method for detecting superficial esophageal cancer. The classification system of the Japanese Society of

Gastroenterological Endoscopy (*JSGE*) based on morphological features, which can also be applied to epithelial cancers in other parts of the gastrointestinal tract, is also applied to esophageal lesions by electronic (*digital-optical*) and chromoendoscopic evaluation after lesion detection (Table 20.1).

The depth of invasion of superficial esophageal cancer can be predicted by observing the changes in the esophageal microvascular structure with magnified endoscopic examination after morphological evaluation [15] (Fig. 20.2).

## 20.5 Endoscopic Ultrasonography (*EUS*)

Endoscopic evaluation and endoscopic ultrasonography (*EUS*) have been the main techniques used to diagnose the depth of cancer invasion. EUS after endoscopic evaluation does not contribute significantly to diagnostic accuracy, and the accuracy of EUS for T staging is highly dependent on operator experience and technique. EUS evaluation of superficial esophageal neoplasms has been found to be interpreted as more deeply invasive than the true T stage [16, 17]. A more advanced diagnosis than it is may lead to more invasive treatments, such as esophagectomy and chemoradiotherapy for cancers that can be treated with ER. As a result, if ER is possible after endoscopic examination, EUS may not be necessary afterward. However, the use of EUS can be planned in cases in between.

## 20.6 Positron Emission Tomography/Computerized Tomography Using Fluorodeoxyglucose (*PET/CT—FDG*)

For patients with suspected locally advanced disease, FDG-PET/CT should ideally be performed prior to ER when it may affect treatment outcomes. There is no consensus on the role of integrated FDG-PET/CT scanning in the evaluation of patients with superficial esophageal cancer. National Comprehensive Cancer Network (*NCCN*) guidelines recommend obtaining FDG-PET/CT for all patients with esophageal cancer, but there are no specific guidelines for superficial cancers [18].

**Table 20.1** Morphological classification system of superficial gastrointestinal lesions

| | | |
|---|---|---|
| Type 0—I; polypoid or protuberant lesions | 0—Ip | Pedunculated |
| | 0—Is | Sessile |
| Type 0—II; flat lesions | 0—IIa | Slightly elevated type |
| | 0—IIb | Flat type |
| | 0—IIc | Slightly depressed type |
| Type 0—III; excavated type | 0—III | Superficial and excavated type |

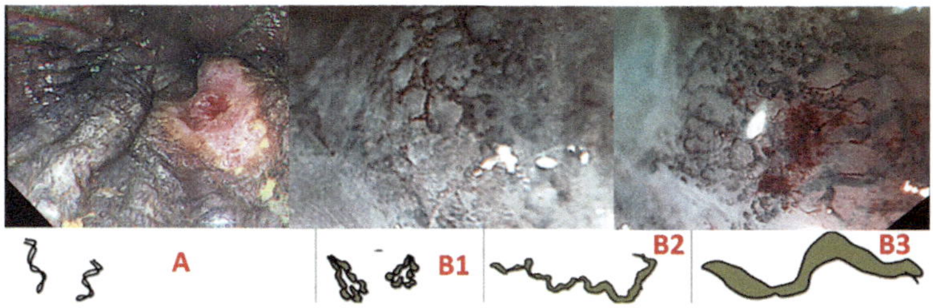


**Fig. 20.2** Magnifying endoscopy classification of image

## 20.7 Superficial Esophageal Cancer Treatment

Endoscopic treatment; ER is recommended instead of surgical resection in elderly patients interested in an esophageal-sparing approach for their intramucosal tumors (*M1, M2, M3 without lymphovascular invasion*) or with multiple comorbidities and high surgical risk [19]. There are limited studies due to the lack of randomized studies comparing ER with esophagectomy and long-term follow-up results after ER. Nevertheless, ER is a viable option for patients in treating mucosal-confined superficial cancers based on esophageal preservation and the morbidity and mortality of esophagectomy [17].

There are two procedures used for ER. The first is endoscopic mucosal resection (*EMR*), which includes snare resection of the dysplastic lesion. The second is endoscopic submucosal dissection (*ESD*), and therapeutic gastroscope and apparatus and blades developed for dissection are used to dissection the lesion from the submucosa.

EMR techniques can be broadly divided into aspiration (*suction and cut*) and non-aspiration (*lift and cut*) techniques. Submucosal injection is often used to create a cushion or space between the lesion and the deeper muscularis propria layer during various resection procedures, in ER, allowing for easier dissection and removal of the lesion while minimizing the risk of complications. Wrinkling or non-raising of the lesion during injection is also suggestive of invasion of the muscularis propria [12].

Saline can be used but is rapidly absorbed. To overcome this limitation, hypertonic saline, 50% dextrose, 10% glycerol, 5% fructose, fibrinogen blend, sodium hyaluronate, and hydroxypropyl methylcellulose (*HPMC*), 6% hydroxyethyl starch were used [18, 20, 21]. Its preferred solution is HPMC because it is widely available, less expensive than sodium hyaluronate, and as effective as sodium hyaluronate [22]. For an effective submucosal fluid cushion, at least 10–40 mL of solution should be injected [23].

In the aspiration method, if desired, the lesion is removed from the muscularis propria after submucosal injection; it is sucked and resected [24]. This technique is most commonly performed with a transparent cap attached to the end of the endoscope, if desired, preceded by a rubber band (*known as EMR-C and EMR-L*) [25]. This cap is placed on the lesion, and suction is applied by pulling the lesion into the cap. The lesion is then resected through the endoscope with a snear inserted into the cap. There are commercial EMR kits designed for this technique.

The non-aspiration method describes resection with a snear after grasping the lesion with a grasper to remove it from the muscularis propria. This technique was the first for EMR and is very difficult to implement. Today, classical EMR, submucosal injection followed by snear resection technique, is mainly applied. However, resectioning lesions larger than 2 cm with EMR is very difficult. In large lesions, it is impossible to obtain a solid surgical margin after partial resection with EMR and to reach a definite conclusion that the entire lesion has been removed. ESD allows larger lesions to be excised with an intact surgical margin [26]. While the en bloc resection rate is 100% in patients with esophageal squamous cell cancer who underwent ESD resection, this rate declines to 53% in patients who underwent EMR, with local recurrence rates of 1% versus 10%, respectively [27].

ESD is a specialized ER technique that uses an ESD blade to excise the lesion by cutting through the submucosa. It can remove mucosal and submucosal tumors, regardless of lesion size. ESD requires several steps to perform. First, electronic chromoendoscopy or true chromoendoscopy is applied to detect the lesion and its border. Then, the lesion's periphery is marked from a solid border of 3–5 mm, a submucosal injection is made under the marks. A circumferential incision is made with the marked area ESD blade, providing access for a mucosal flap and submucosal dissection. The submucosal solution intermittently is injected under the mucosal flap and is completed by dissection with the ESD knife until the entire lesion is separated from the submucosal area. Submucosal dissection is the most difficult step of the ESD procedure, usually managing the vessels in the submucosal area and continuously keeping the endoscope in the submucosal plane. Dissection must be completed without breaking the pathological lesion superficially or damaging the muscularis propria by going deep. During ESD, various electrocautery settings are used for incision, dissection, and coagulation. A clear cap attached to the tip of the endoscope provides better control of the dissection step. Various ESD blades are available, and blade selection largely depends on the endoscopist's experience and preference [28]. Adverse events related to the ESD procedure are safe in experienced hands. However, immediate side effects were observed in 13% of the procedures, including 3% perforation and 10% bleeding in the early period [12]. In the late period, ulcer-related bleeding in the esophageal structure or scar tissue can be observed at a rate of 7%.

Precut EMR (*EMR-P*) is a hybrid technique. It is a modification of the standard ESD technique, and although the first two stages are the same as ESD, it is called EMR and not submucosal dissection. It is a simplified hybrid approach in which a snare excises the lesion by submucosal injection, circumferential incision, and EMR. EMR-P is not significantly different from ESD regarding the complete and en bloc resection rates for flat lesions of 20–30 mm [29]. This method minimizes the submucosal dissection, which tends to be the most challenging and time-consuming part of the procedure.

## 20.8 Surgical Treatment

Although randomized studies are not available, retrospective study results suggest that ER and surgical outcomes are similar for patients with superficial tumors confined to the mucosa [30, 31]. In data-based studies, different population results have been reached in ER versus surgery. Although ER results are advantageous in terms of mortality, they did not show a significant difference in survival among T1a patients. In contrast, better survival rates were achieved with esophagectomy for T1b patients [32–35]. Patients treated with ER had higher 30-day survival rates than those treated surgically. However, 5-year survival was lower in the ER group than in the surgery group, attributed to the ER outcomes of patients with T1b tumors [5]. In meta-analysis studies, however, patients who underwent ER had significantly fewer adverse events, a lower procedure-related mortality rate, and similar stricture rates [36]. However, ER has a higher recurrence rate, lower complete (*R0*) resection rate, and moderate but significantly worse long-term survival rates [36].

In long-term results, it has been shown that a cure can be achieved in the follow-up of ER despite surgery—5-year survival rates after ER range from 76% to 100%. However, survival is lower for multicentric lesions or circumferentially or invade beyond the lamina propria. Relapses occur in 3–32% of patients and can often be treated with local therapy [4, 37, 38]. Additional radiofrequency ablation (*RFA*) to endoscopic therapy may allow the treatment of larger lesions with a lower recurrence rate [7, 39, 40].

If there is a local recurrence after endoscopic resection, esophagectomy, radiotherapy, or chemoradiotherapy is usually selected as the appropriate treatment. Most patients should be restaged with PET/CT [41–43].

## References


1. Technology status report evaluation. Endoscopic mucosal resection. Gastrointest Endosc. 2000;52:860–3.
2. Devesa SS, Blot WJ, Fraumeni JF Jr. Changing patterns in the incidence of esophageal and gastric carcinoma in the United States. Cancer. 1998;83:2049–53.
3. The Paris endoscopic classification of superficial neoplastic lesions: esophagus, stomach, and colon: November 30 to December 1, 2002. Gastrointest Endosc. 2003;58:S3–43. https://doi.org/10.1016/s0016-5107(03)02159-x.
4. Endo M, Takeshita K, Inoue H. Endoscopic mucosal resection of esophageal cancer. Gan To Kagaku Ryoho. 1995;22:192–5.
5. Merkow RP, Bilimoria KY, Keswani RN, Chung J, Sherman KL, Knab LM, Posner MC, Bentrem DJ. Treatment trends, risk of lymph node metastasis, and outcomes for localized esophageal cancer. J Natl Cancer Inst. 2014;106:dju133. https://doi.org/10.1093/jnci/dju133.
6. Ning B, Abdelfatah MM, Othman MO. Endoscopic submucosal dissection and endoscopic mucosal resection for early stage esophageal cancer. Ann Cardiothorac Surg. 2017;6:88–98. https://doi.org/10.21037/acs.2017.03.15.
7. Pacifico RJ, Wang KK, Wongkeesong LM, Buttar SN, Lutzke LS. Combined endoscopic mucosal resection and photodynamic therapy versus esophagectomy for management of early adenocarcinoma in Barrett's esophagus. Clin Gastroenterol Hepatol. 2003;1:252–7.

8. Suzuki H, Masuda K, Fujisaki J, Okuwaki S. Endoscopic treatment of gastrointestinal cancers—indication and limitation. Nihon Rinsho. 1996;54:1699–704.
9. Tanabe S, Koizumi W, Higuchi K, Sasaki T, Nakatani K, Hanaoka N, Ae T, Ishido K, Mitomi H, Saigenji K. Clinical outcomes of endoscopic oblique aspiration mucosectomy for superficial esophageal cancer. Gastrointest Endosc. 2008;67:814–20. https://doi.org/10.1016/j.gie.2007.11.034.
10. Białek A, Wiechowska-Kozłowska A, Pertkiewicz J, Polkowski M, Milkiewicz P, Karpińska K, Ławniczak M, Starzyńska T. Endoscopic submucosal dissection for treatment of gastric subepithelial tumors (with video). Gastrointest Endosc. 2012;75:276–86. https://doi.org/10.1016/j.gie.2011.08.029.
11. Kim GH, Choi KD, Gong CS, Lee IS, Park YS, Han M, Na HK, Ahn JY, Lee JH, Jung KW, Kim DH, Song HJ, Lee GH, Jung HY. Comparison of the treatment outcomes of endoscopic and surgical resection of GI stromal tumors in the stomach: a propensity score-matched case-control study. Gastrointest Endosc. 2020;91:527–36. https://doi.org/10.1016/j.gie.2019.10.020.
12. Conio M, Rajan E, Sorbi D, Norton I, Herman L, Filiberti R, Gostout CJ. Comparative performance in the porcine esophagus of different solutions used for submucosal injection. Gastrointest Endosc. 2002;56:513–6. https://doi.org/10.1067/mge.2002.128107.
13. Fujishiro M, Yahagi N, Kashimura K, Mizushima Y, Oka M, Matsuura T, Enomoto S, Kakushima N, Imagawa A, Kobayashi K, Hashimoto T, Iguchi M, Shimizu Y, Ichinose M, Omata M. Different mixtures of sodium hyaluronate and their ability to create submucosal fluid cushions for endoscopic mucosal resection. Endoscopy. 2004;36:584–9. https://doi.org/10.1055/s-2004-814524.
14. Yokota T, Sugihara K, Yoshida S. Endoscopic mucosal resection for colorectal neoplastic lesions. Dis Colon Rectum. 1994;37:1108–11. https://doi.org/10.1007/BF02049812.
15. Pimentel-Nunes P, Libânio D, Bastiaansen BAJ, Bhandari P, Bisschops R, Bourke MJ, Esposito G, Lemmers A, Maselli R, Messmann H, Pech O, Pioche M, Vieth M, Weusten BLAM, van Hooft JE, Deprez PH, Dinis-Ribeiro M. Endoscopic submucosal dissection for superficial gastrointestinal lesions: European Society of Gastrointestinal Endoscopy (ESGE) Guideline—update 2022. Endoscopy. 2022;54:591–622. https://doi.org/10.1055/a-1811-7025.
16. Oyama T. Endoscopic diagnosis and treatment of superficial Barrett's esophageal adenocarcinoma: Japanese perspective. Dig Endosc. 2022;2:27–30. https://doi.org/10.1111/den.14147.
17. Ishihara R. Endoscopic diagnosis and treatment of superficial esophageal squamous cell cancer: present status and future perspectives. Curr Oncol. 2022;29:534–43. https://doi.org/10.3390/curroncol29020048.
18. Fasoulas K, Lazaraki G, Chatzimavroudis G, Paroutoglou G, Katsinelos T, Dimou E, Geros C, Zavos C, Kountouras J, Katsinelos P. Endoscopic mucosal resection of giant laterally spreading tumors with submucosal injection of hydroxyethyl starch: comparative study with normal saline solution. Surg Laparosc Endosc Percutan Tech. 2012;22:272–8. https://doi.org/10.1097/SLE.0b013e318251553c.
19. Sumiyama K, Tajiri H, Gostout CJ, Kawamura M, Imazu H, Ohya TR, Ikeda K, Goda K, Saito S, Kato T. Chemically assisted submucosal injection facilitates endoscopic submucosal dissection of gastric neoplasms. Endoscopy. 2010;42:627–32. https://doi.org/10.1055/s-0029-1244223.
20. Fujishiro M, Yahagi N, Kashimura K, Mizushima Y, Oka M, Enomoto S, Kakushima N, Kobayashi K, Hashimoto T, Iguchi M, Shimizu Y, Ichinose M, Omata M. Comparison of various submucosal injection solutions for maintaining mucosal elevation during endoscopic mucosal resection. Endoscopy. 2004;36:579.
21. Lee SH, Park JH, Park DH, Chung IK, Kim HS, Park SH, Kim SJ, Cho HD. Clinical efficacy of EMR with submucosal injection of a fibrinogen mixture: a prospective randomized trial. Gastrointest Endosc. 2006;64:691.
22. Polymeros D, Kotsalidis G, Triantafyllou K, Karamanolis G, Panagiotides JG, Ladas SD. Comparative performance of novel solutions for submucosal injection in porcine stomachs: an ex vivo study. Dig Liver Dis. 2010;42:226.

23. Narahara H, Iishi H, Tatsuta M, Uedo N, Sakai N, Yano H, Otani T. Effectiveness of endoscopic mucosal resection with submucosal saline injection technique for superficial squamous carcinomas of the esophagus. Gastrointest Endosc. 2000;52:730.
24. Poppers DM, News GB. Endoscopic mucosal resection of colonic lesions: current applications and future prospects. Med Clin North Am. 2008;92:687.
25. Fleischer DE, Wang GQ, Dawsey S, Tio TL, Newsome J, Kidwell J, Prifti S. Tissue band ligation followed by snare resection (band and snare): a new technique for tissue acquisition in the esophagus. Gastrointest Endosc. 1996;44:68.
26. Berger A, Rahmi G, Perrod G, Pioche M, Canard JM, Cesbron-Métivier E, Boursier J, Samaha E, Vienne A, Lépilliez V, Cellier C. Long-term follow-up after endoscopic resection for superficial esophageal squamous cell carcinoma: a multicenter Western study. Endoscopy. 2019;51:298–306. https://doi.org/10.1055/a-0732-5317.
27. Takahashi H, Arimura Y, Masao H, Okahara S, Tanuma T, Kodaira J, Kagaya H, Shimizu Y, Hokari K, Tsukagoshi H, Shinomura Y, Fujita M. Endoscopic submucosal dissection is superior to conventional endoscopic resection as a curative treatment for early squamous cell carcinoma of the esophagus (with video). Gastrointest Endosc. 2010;72:255–64. https://doi.org/10.1016/j.gie.2010.02.040.
28. Bhatt A, Abe S, Kumaravel A, Vargo J, Saito Y. Indications and techniques for endoscopic submucosal dissection. Am J Gastroenterol. 2015;110:784–91. https://doi.org/10.1038/ajg.2014.425. Epub 2015 Jan 27.
29. Toyonaga T, Man-I M, Morita Y, Azuma T. Endoscopic submucosal dissection (ESD) versus simplified/hybrid ESD. Gastrointest Endosc Clin N Am. 2014;24:191–9. https://doi.org/10.1016/j.giec.2013.11.004.
30. Yuan B, Liu L, Huang H, Li D, Shen Y, Wu B, Liu J, Yang M, Wang Z, Lu H, Liu Y, Liao L, Wang F. Comparison of the short-term and long-term outcomes of surgical treatment versus endoscopic treatment for early esophageal squamous cell neoplasia larger than 2 cm: a retrospective study. Surg Endosc. 2019;33:2304–12. https://doi.org/10.1007/s00464-018-6524-2.
31. Huang B, Xu MC, Pennathur A, Li Z, Liu Z, Wu Q, Wang J, Luo K, Bai J, Wei Z, Xiang J, Fang W, Zhang J. Endoscopic resection with adjuvant treatment versus esophagectomy for early-stage esophageal cancer. Surg Endosc. 2022;36:1868.
32. Lee SH, Cho WY, Kim HJ, Kim HJ, Kim HJ, Kim YH, Chung IK, Kim HS, Park SH, Kim SJ. A new method of EMR: submucosal injection of a fibrinogen mixture. Gastrointest Endosc. 2004;59:220.
33. Yamamoto H, Koiwai H, Yube T, Yamamoto H, Koiwai H, Yube T, Isoda N, Sato Y, Sekine Y, Higashizawa T, Utsunomiya K, Ido K, Sugano K. A successful single-step endoscopic resection of a 40 millimeter flat-elevated tumor in the rectum: endoscopic mucosal resection using sodium hyaluronate. Gastrointest Endosc. 1999;50:701.
34. Das A, Singh V, Fleischer DE, Sharma VK. A comparison of endoscopic treatment and surgery in early esophageal cancer: an analysis of surveillance epidemiology and end results data. Am J Gastroenterol. 2008;103:1340–5. https://doi.org/10.1111/j.1572-0241.2008.01889.x.
35. Semenkovich TR, Hudson JL, Subramanian M, Mullady DK, Meyers BF, Puri V, Kozower BD. Trends in treatment of T1N0 esophageal cancer. Ann Surg. 2019;270:434–43. https://doi.org/10.1097/SLA.0000000000003466.
36. Kume K. Endoscopic mucosal resection and endoscopic submucosal dissection for early gastric cancer: current and original devices. World J Gastrointest Endosc. 2009;1:21.
37. Nakagawa K, Koike T, Iijima K, Shinkai H, Hatta W, Endo H, Ara N, Uno K, Asano N, Imatani A, Shimosegawa T. Comparison of the long-term outcomes of endoscopic resection for superficial squamous cell carcinoma and adenocarcinoma of the esophagus in Japan. Am J Gastroenterol. 2014;109:348.
38. Pech O, Behrens A, May A, Nachbar L, Gossner L, Rabenstein T, Manner H, Guenter E, Huijsmans J, Vieth M, Stolte M, Ell C. Long-term results and risk factor analysis for recurrence after curative endoscopic therapy in 349 patients with high-grade intraepithelial neoplasia and mucosal adenocarcinoma in Barrett's oesophagus. Gout. 2008;57:1200.

39. Gray NA, Odze RD, Spechler SJ. Buried metaplasia after endoscopic ablation of Barrett's esophagus: a systematic review. Am J Gastroenterol. 2011;106:1899.
40. Manner H, Pech O, Heldmann Y, May A, Pohl J, Behrens A, Gossner L, Stolte M, Vieth M, Ell C. Efficacy, safety, and long-term results of endoscopic treatment for early stage adenocarcinoma of the esophagus with low-risk sm1 invasion. Clin Gastroenterol Hepatol. 2013;11:630.
41. Rajan E, Gostout CJ. Future developments of EMR, techniques and devices. Tech Gastrointest Endosc. 2002;4:51.
42. Ono H. Endoscopic submucosal dissection for early gastric cancer. Chin J Dig Dis. 2005;6:119.
43. Gotoda T. A large endoscopic resection by endoscopic submucosal dissection procedure for early gastric cancer. Clin Gastroenterol Hepatol. 2005;3:S71.

# 21 Management of Cervical Esophageal Cancer

Muhammer Ergenç and Tevfik Kıvılcım Uprak

## 21.1 Surgical Anatomy of Cervical Esophagus

The esophagus is formed by the surrounding structures, while the thoracic part of the esophagus is more spherical, owed to negative intrathoracic pressure. It flattens again in the abdomen as an impact of positive intra-abdominal pressure. Three anatomical constrictions are found in the esophagus. Cricopharyngeal constriction at the upper sphincter (1.5 cm) is the narrowest part. In the upper mediastinum, aortic arch, left atrium, and left bronchus constrict the esophagus anterolaterally to the left, approximately at 22 cm. The third narrowing area is the lower sphincter. It is important to know these areas because ingested foreign materials are often lodged in these areas [1–6].

The cricopharyngeal muscle and up to 2 cm of the cervical esophagus are mostly formed of striated muscle. There is a transformation from striated to smooth muscle, and this transition is present only in the upper 40% of the esophagus [1–6].

The cervical esophagus expands from the cricoid cartilage at the C6 vertebrae superiorly to the suprasternal notch and inferiorly to the T1–T2 interspace. The cervical esophagus is reached with a left neck incision as the cervical esophagus changes its route to the left. There is loose fibroareolar tissue all around the esophagus. The pretracheal fascia, the prevertebral fascia, and the carotid sheaths combine to produce two cervical compartments, the paraesophageal space anteriorly and the retroesophageal space posteriorly. Pretracheal fascia links the pericardium and the diaphragm, respectively, whereas the prevertebral fascia connects the neck and rib cage. Mediastinum infections can swiftly progress to necrotizing mediastinitis, which can be lethal. Most iatrogenic perforations that result in posterior pharyngeal perforation occur above the region of the cricopharyngeal muscle contraction [1–6].

M. Ergenç · T. K. Uprak (✉)
Department of General Surgery, Marmara University School of Medicine, Istanbul, Turkey
e-mail: muhammerergenc@gmail.com; kuprak@gmail.com


O. Engin (ed.), *Risk Factors and Therapy of Esophagus Cancer*,
https://doi.org/10.1007/978-3-031-47024-0_21

The cervical esophagus receives its blood supply from the superior and inferior thyroid arteries on the right and left sides, with smaller branches from the common carotid and subclavian arteries. Venous drainage is via the inferior thyroid vein. Innervation of the cervical esophagus is provided by the recurrent laryngeal nerves and sympathetic chains [7, 8].

### 21.1.1 Recurrent Laryngeal Nerves

The vagus nerve gives off a branch called the right and left recurrent laryngeal nerve. Although the left nerve circles the aortic arch, the right nerve goes posteriorly around the right subclavian artery. The tracheoesophageal groove is where both recurrent nerves continue, although the left nerve travels closer to the esophagus due to the leftward tilt of the cervical esophagus, while the right nerve recurs more laterally along the subclavian. The cricopharyngeal muscle and cervical esophagus are likewise innervated by the recurrent laryngeal nerves. The left recurrent laryngeal nerve must be protected when the cervical esophagus is dissected during surgery. In addition to hoarseness, injury to the recurrent laryngeal nerve also affects the cervical esophagus mobility and the cricopharyngeal muscle, affecting swallowing. Bilateral vocal cord paralysis with airway obstruction and the requirement for a tracheostomy can result from injury to both recurrent nerves [3, 6, 7, 9].

## 21.2 Epidemiology and Risk Factors

According to the Global Cancer Statistics, esophageal cancer (EC) ranked seventh in incidence and sixth in death in 2020. About 70% of cases were diagnosed in men. The incidence and mortality rates differ two- to threefold between males and females. East Asia has the highest regional incidence rates for both genders. Cervical esophageal cancer (CEC) represents less than 10% of all esophageal cancers. Overall, the survival percentage for CEC that is not identified at an early stage is low [10–15].

There are two main subtypes of esophageal cancer: esophageal squamous cell carcinoma (SCC) and esophageal adenocarcinoma (AC). SCC accounts for 90% of esophageal cancer cases worldwide; however, the incidence of AC is increasing [16–18].

The main risk factors for esophageal SCC in Western populations are excessive alcohol consumption, smoking, and their synergistic effects. In low-income countries, including parts of Asia and sub-Saharan Africa, potential dietary components, including nutritional deficiencies and nitrosamines, have been identified; however, the main risk factors for esophageal SCC have yet to be clarified. These risk factors, such as tobacco smoke, alcohol consumption, and betel nut chewing, are also similar in head and neck SCC etiology. Esophageal adenocarcinoma accounts for approximately two-thirds of esophageal cancer cases in high-income countries, and major risk factors include excess body weight, gastroesophageal reflux disease, and esophageal intestinal metaplasia [16–19]. There are studies suggesting that Human papillomavirus infection may be a risk factor for EC [20–22].

## 21.3 Presentation

Dysphagia, like other esophageal cancers, is the most common cause of presentation in cervical esophageal cancer patients. CEC is usually detected at presentation as advanced to the hypopharynx or thoracic esophagus. CECs usually show local invasion into the larynx, thyroid gland, trachea, and upper mediastinal structures because the cervical esophagus is closely associated with these structures. The following symptoms may also be present among the presenting symptoms: weight loss, anemia, neck pain, neck mass, and vocal cord paralysis. On physical examination, cachexia may be observed, and enlarged lymph nodes in the neck or supraclavicular region may be detected. Upper intestinal endoscopy should be performed in patients with new-onset dysphagia, gastrointestinal bleeding, recurrent aspiration or vomiting, and weight loss and/or loss of appetite. CEC is usually detected in an advanced stage by symptoms. However, the widespread use of image-assisted endoscopies, such as narrow-band imaging and blue laser imaging in recent years, has made it possible to detect CEC early [16, 17, 23–26].

## 21.4 Diagnosis and Staging

The clinical diagnosis of esophageal cancer is based on history, physical examination, imaging methods, and biopsy. A patient with cervical squamous cell carcinoma is usually from a low socioeconomic class and has a history of dysphagia, weight loss, heavy smoking, and alcohol use. Flexible endoscopy is used in the evaluation of dysphagia and clinical diagnosis of esophageal cancer. A tissue biopsy is required for the clinical diagnosis of esophageal cancer. Pathologic analysis of these specimens gives both the histologic type and grade of esophageal cancer. Upper intestinal endoscopy should be performed in all patients with new dysphagia, gastrointestinal bleeding, recurrent aspiration or emesis, and weight loss and/or loss of appetite. Biopsies should be taken from all suspicious sites [16, 27, 28].

American Joint Committee on Cancer (AJCC) is the internationally accepted standard for esophageal cancer staging (Fig. 21.1). Eighth Edition of the AJCC Cancer Staging Manual staging of esophageal and esophagogastric epithelial cancers includes clinical staging (cTNM), pathologic staging (pTNM), and post neoadjuvant pathologic staging (ypTNM) stage groups. The tumor grade (G) is important for early-stage cancer staging (pTNM) in patients undergoing resection without neoadjuvant treatment [29].

In Japan Esophageal Society guidelines, mucosal invasion (T1a) depth is evaluated in three layers; M1 points to the involvement of the epithelium, M2 is the invasion of the lamina propria, and M3 is the invasion of muscularis mucosa. Submucosal invasion depth (T1b) is also evaluated in three layers; SM1 describes the

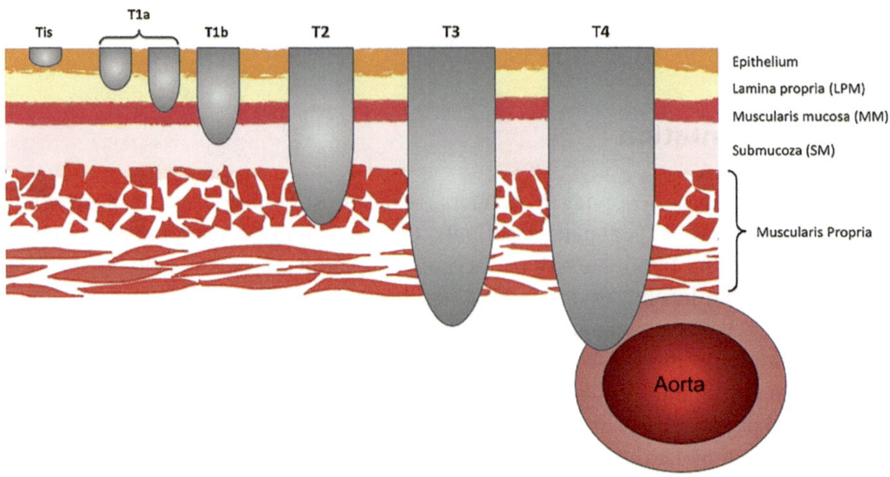


**Fig. 21.1** The Eighth Edition AJCC Cancer Manual TNM Categories. Tis: High-grade dysplasia, T1a: Tumor invades the lamina propria or muscularis mucosae, T1b: Tumor invades the submucosa, T2: Tumor invades the muscularis propria, T3: Tumor invades the adventitia, T4a: Tumor invades adjacent structures such as the pleura, pericardium, azygos vein, diaphragm, or peritoneum and T4b: Tumor invades the major adjacent structures, such as the aorta, vertebral body, or trachea

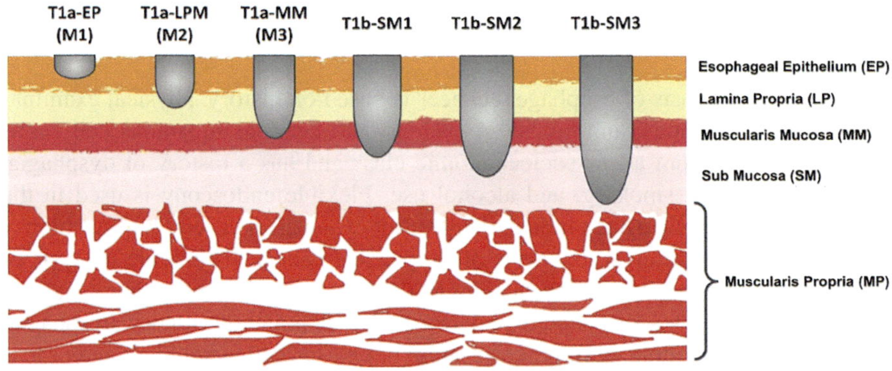


**Fig. 21.2** Japanese Classification of Esophageal Cancer 11th Edition Subclassification for Superficial Cancer. T1a-EP(M1): Carcinoma in-situ (Tis), T1a-LPM(M2): Tumor invades the lamina propria mucosa, T1a-MM(M3): Tumor invades the muscularis mucosa, T1b-SM1: Tumor invades the upper third of the submucosa, T1b-SM2: Tumor invades the middle third of the submucosa and T1b-SM3: Tumor invades the lower third of the submucosa

involvement of the upper third of the submucosa, SM2 is the involvement of the middle third of the submucosa, and SM3 is the involvement of the lower third of the submucosa (Fig. 21.2) [30].

The clinical investigation, endoscopy, and computed tomography (CT) or positron emission tomography (PET) with $^{18}$F-fluoro-2-deoxy-D-glucose (FDG) should be included in staging. Tumors and nodes may be staged using endoscopic ultrasound (EUS). For T1 tumors, it is less accurate; in these cases, endoscopic resection offers more exact staging in addition to therapeutic benefits. In addition to checking the T4b status in invasion to the airways, pericardium, or aorta, EUS can be utilized to locate and biopsy likely lymph node metastases outside the conventional radiation region or outside the targeted resection boundaries. Advanced disorders may not be able to use EUS because of tumor stenosis. Especially when tumor stenosis prevents the use of EUS, endobronchial ultrasonography is a helpful substitute for EUS in assessing tumor development into the central airways [16, 27, 28, 31, 32].

FDG-PET is useful for identifying distant metastases. Cervical SCCs of the esophagus can often be accompanied by head and neck second primary tumors (HNSPTs). Patients with cervical esophageal SCC should undergo a qualified clinical examination of the head and neck region to exclude HNSPTs that have worse prognoses [31, 33, 34].

## 21.5 Management

Multidisciplinary evaluation and treatment planning are essential to adequately evaluate patients and tumors and determine the most appropriate treatment option.

European Society for Medical Oncology (ESMO) guidelines state that neoadjuvant chemoradiotherapy (CRT) followed by surgery and definitive CRT are equally effective for overall survival. Therefore, the ESMO guideline recommends definitive CRT for localized cervical tumors where the surgery will require a laryngectomy. According to National Comprehensive Cancer Network (NCCN) guidelines, cervical or cervicothoracic esophageal cancers closer than 5 cm from the cricopharyngeus should be treated with definitive CRT. Palliative esophagectomy may also be considered in patients with cervical esophageal cancer who develop localized resectable recurrence or incurable stricture after definitive chemoradiotherapy unless there is a distant recurrence. Three treatment modalities are used in Japan: additional therapy following surgery, chemotherapy followed by surgery or CRT depending on the effect of chemotherapy, and preoperative or definitive CRT [13, 16, 28].

The most usual surgical procedure for CEC is total pharyngolaryngoesophagectomy (PLE), but patients' quality of life is severely impaired in the postoperative period because the larynx is resected. A meta-analysis showed that conservative primary surgery is a useful option for managing CEC. Notably, laryngeal sparing surgery showed a pooled 5-year overall survival rate of 35.1%, comparable to definitive CRT. Moreover, the 5-year overall survival rate for surgery without larynx sparing was 14.6%, which may reflect the higher T-classification of these tumors [11, 13].

Percutaneous gastrostomy tube placement may be considered for patients with cervical esophageal tumors receiving definitive chemoradiotherapy or with marginally resectable tumors. It should be evaluated multidisciplinary before the percutaneous gastrostomy tube placement [28].

### 21.5.1 Endoscopic Therapy

Endoscopic resection can be performed as following indications: high-grade intraepithelial neoplasia or mucosal carcinoma (adenocarcinoma: m1–m3, squamous cell carcinoma: m1–m2), without lymph or vascular invasion (histological L0/V0 status), without ulcerations, and G1/G2 grading. Endoscopic resection is also possible in the case of superficial infiltration of adenocarcinoma into the submucosa (sm1) without the risk factor and less than 20 mm [16, 27, 35].

Endoscopic mucosal resection (EMR) and endoscopic submucosal dissection (ESD) are effective endoscopic resection methods for superficial esophageal cancer. EMR and ESD can perform comparable treatment rates with surgical resection in specialized centers. It has been reported that ESD is superior to EMR regarding the en bloc resection rate, R0 en bloc resection rate, and recurrence [36–38].

The upper sphincter muscle usually contracts the cervical esophagus region. Therefore, it is difficult to observe and detect CEC at an early stage. CECs are generally locally extended at diagnosis, invade surrounding structures, and often present with lymph node metastases. The detection rate of superficial esophageal cancer has increased with the use of advanced endoscopy methods such as magnified endoscopy with narrow-band imaging (NBI) and a scope attachment. ESD performed for the cervical esophagus lesions can be technically challenging, and perioperative complications may happen more often than in other parts of the esophagus [39–42].

In the study in which 45 patients with superficial cancer of the cervical esophagus were compared with 375 patients with superficial cancer in the middle thoracic esophagus, ESD has been shown to provide local control safely. However, esophageal stricture was more common after ESD for the cervical esophagus. A study of 26 patients with superficial esophageal neoplasms extending to the cervical esophagus showed ESD involving the cervical esophagus is technically possible. However, circumferential resection may cause refractory postoperative stricture or perforation after endoscopic balloon dilation, so it should be avoided whenever possible [39, 40].

A study of 43 CEC and 282 thoracic esophageal cancer lesions showed that more CEC group patients than the thoracic esophageal cancer group received prophylactic steroid therapy. It has been reported that the stenosis rate of CEC after endoscopic submucosal dissection was found to be higher than thoracic esophageal cancer, and more intensive prophylactic measures can be required for CEC than thoracic esophageal cancer after endoscopic submucosal dissection stenosis [26].

### 21.5.2 Surgery

Despite advances in surgical technique and perioperative care, esophageal cancer remains one of the most challenging conditions facing the surgeon. The principles of esophageal cancer surgery are to achieve complete resection of the tumor and surrounding lymph nodes and to perform reconstruction with optimal functional outcomes and minimal morbidity and mortality. While radical treatment for esophageal adenocarcinoma is multidisciplinary, surgery remains the primary form of treatment. The outcome is highly stage dependent. Esophagectomy should be performed in cases where curative resection can be achieved. The intramural lymphovascular invasion should be considered when evaluated in terms of the surgical margin. An initial surgical margin of at least 5 cm should be targeted. Radical en bloc circumferential resection is among the goals. However, the case may vary according to histopathology and neoadjuvant therapy [43].

#### 21.5.2.1 Lymphadenectomy

Lymph node involvement is one of the most significant prognostic variables. There may be confusing information about lymph node resection areas in the literature. If we divide radical lymphadenectomy into three-field area lymphadenectomy, one-field lymphadenectomy includes only diaphragmatic, right, and left paracardial, lesser curvature, left gastric artery, and common hepatic and splenic vessels. In two-field lymphadenectomy, in addition to the one field, lymph nodes around the para-aortic, right, and left pulmonary hilar, subcarinal, and paratracheal should be included. In three-field lymphadenectomy, in addition to two fields, brachiocephalic, deep lateral, and external cervical nodes, and lymph nodes around the left recurrent nerve are included in the specimen with neck dissection (Fig. 21.3) [44–47].

Radical lymphadenectomy is thought to increase disease-free survival. The literature has shown that when transthoracic esophagectomy is compared with transhiatal resection, more lymph node resection is performed, and better survival is achieved with transthoracic resection [48].

The most used area is the posterior mediastinal space. It is known as the shortest route between the abdomen and the neck. The retrosternal space can be created by blunt dissection behind the sternum or laparoscopic dissection. This route may be preferred after mediastinal sepsis or unsuccessful use of the posterior mediastinal route. The head of the clavicle may be removed due to angulation in the thoracic inlet. The presternal route is preferred when the previous two routes are unavailable. It is approximately 2 cm longer [49].

A gastric tube is commonly used after esophagectomy. It is generally preferred because it requires a single anastomosis and is easy to prepare. It is recommended to prepare an initial conduit of approximately 5 cm by preserving the right gastroepiploic arcade. Preservation of the right gastric artery is important in terms of preserving the intramural vascular arcade and preparing a well-blooded conduit. Pyloroplasty and pyloromyotomy can provide gastric drainage. Kocher maneuver is especially necessary for the presence of a long conduit [50, 51].

#### 21.5.2.2 Colonic Reconstruction

It is preferred, especially in cases where the esophagus and stomach are to be resected or when the stomach cannot be used due to previous surgeries. It is generally less preferred due to more anastomosis needed, and long-term durability is less than a gastric conduit. Isoperistaltic anastomoses are preferred. The vascular

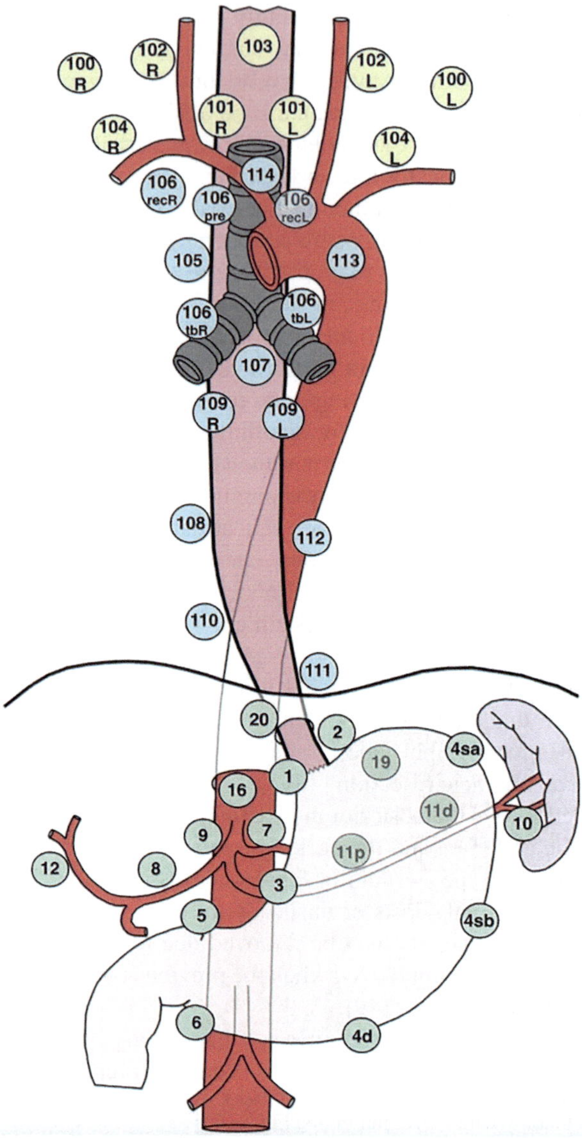


**Fig. 21.3** Japanese Classification of Esophageal Cancer 11th Edition, station number of regional lymph nodes. Cervical lymph nodes are classified as 100: Superficial lymph nodes of neck, 101: Cervical paraesophageal lymph nodes, 102: Deep cervical lymph nodes; 103: Peripharyngeal lymph nodes, 104: Supraclavicular lymph nodes. Thoracic lymph nodes are classified as; 105: Upper thoracic paraesophageal lymph nodes, 106: Thoracic paratracheal lymph nodes, 107: Subcarinal lymph nodes, 108: Middle thoracic paraesophageal lymph nodes, 109: Main bronchus lymph nodes, 110: Lower thoracic paraesophageal lymph nodes, 111: Supradiaphragmatic lymph nodes, 112: Posterior mediastinal lymph nodes, 113: Ligamentum arteriosum lymph nodes, 114: Anterior mediastinal lymph nodes. Abdominal lymph nodes are classified as; 1: Right paracardiac lymph nodes, 2: Left paracardiac lymph nodes, 3: Lesser curvature lymph nodes, 4: Greater curvature lymph nodes, 5: Suprapyloric lymph nodes, 6:Infrapyloric lymph nodes, 7: Left gastric artery lymph nodes, 8: Common hepatic artery lymph nodes, 9: Celiac trunk lymph nodes, 10: Splenic hilum lymph nodes, 11: Splenic artery lymph nodes, 12: Hepatoduodenal ligament lymph nodes, 16: Paraaortic lymph nodes, 19: Infradiaphragmatic lymph nodes, 20: Esophageal hiatus of the diaphragm lymph nodes

structure must be well determined. Generally, the transverse colon, in which the ascending branch of the left colic is protected, or the right colon, in which based the middle colic artery is used. After preoperative bowel cleansing, the whole colon should be mobilized, and variations should be paid attention to. After the colon to be used is selected, its proximal should be cut, and it should be extended towards the chest and neck, and it should be seen that it comes without tension [52].

Microvascular-free pedunculated jejunal transfer can be used in the cervical area, especially in cases of laryngeal and pharyngeal resection. In this method, a jejunum flap of approximately 20 cm with preserved vascular structures is prepared and anastomoses to the esophagus in the cervical area with a pedicle [53].

#### 21.5.2.3 Mc-Keown Esophagectomy Procedure

##### Thoracic Phase

The patient is placed in the left lateral decubitus position. The operating table is flexed to widen the intercostal space. It is performed through the fourth or fifth intercostal space via a right posterolateral thoracotomy. The operation can also be performed using minimally invasive surgery. The operation is started by dividing the arch of the azygos vein. The descending aorta and the adventitia fascia of the esophagus are separated by a pleural incision. The thoracic duct is identified at the level of the azygos vein and can be dissected from the aorta. Para-aortic lymph nodes and thoracic duct are mobilized, and the aortic branches connected to the esophagus are tied. The anterior plane of the dissection is along the pericardium, allowing suspension of the esophagus. The dissection continues caudally to the right pulmonary hilum, and the right bronchial, subcarinal, and left bronchial nodes are dissected. Care is taken in this area to avoid membranous injury of the tracheobronchial tree. The mediastinal pleura is dissected along the right vagus nerve towards the brachiocephalic and subclavian arteries. The right recurrent laryngeal nerve is preserved, and the adjacent lymph node chain is dissected. The pleura is incised along the border of the superior vena cava, and the right paratracheal lymph nodes between the trachea and vena cava are dissected. Dissection should be carried out along the left recurrent laryngeal nerve to the thoracic inlet [54–56].

##### Abdominal Phase

The abdominal phase is started with a laparotomy or laparoscopy to exclude the presence of distant metastases. The stomach is dissected over the right gastroepiploic and right gastric arches, preserving the gastroepiploic arch. Complete freeing is achieved by the division of all posterior attachments of the stomach and duodenocolic ligament. The previously mentioned lymph node stations are dissected [54–56].

During hiatal dissection, it is important to provide adequate space for the passage of the gastric conduit. The stomach is then stapled to form a conduit at the level of the right gastric artery from small curvature using surgical staplers (Fig. 21.4). The remaining stomach can be sutured to the esophagus, or it can be left to be pulled into the cervical area without a complete stapled incision. A gastric tube is created by resecting the specimen after the esophagus is separated along its length, and the stomach and esophagus are transported to the abdomen on a band. A laparoscopic camera bag is typically used to extend the gastric tube into the neck through the rear of a foley catheter for anastomosis [55, 57].

A feeding jejunostomy is routinely placed for postoperative feeding. The omentum close to the transverse colon may be sutured to the abdominal wall to prevent postoperative diaphragmatic herniation [55, 58, 59].

The patient is placed in the supine position for standard stomach mobilization during the second part of the procedure. This can be done in tandem with a cervical dissection on the left side (third stage). The left neck's exposed esophagus makes it easy to perform an anastomosis. In cases where a patient has a mediastinal high nodal disease, it permits a formal nodal dissection of the neck [55, 60].

Although anastomotic leakage is more common in the neck, mortality and morbidity rates are not high. After dissection in the neck, the esophagus is cut with a negative surgical margin, and the pre-prepared gastric or colonic canal is drawn to this area. The anterior opening can be closed with a hand-stitched anastomosis or with a stapler after a posterior side-to-side stapler anastomosis. 2/0 (non-absorbable or long-term absorbable) suture with a single layer, the hand-sewn anastomosis may also be an option (Fig. 21.5) [55, 56, 61–63].

Many studies have been conducted to select the method to be used for reconstruction after esophagectomy. In a meta-analysis of 868 cervical esophageal cancer patients treated primarily with surgery, 57.1% underwent total PLE, and reconstruction was performed using gastric pull-up ($n$ = 287/329, 88.2%), colon interposition ($n$ = 22/329, 6.2%), or jejunal free flap ($n$ = 20/329, 5.6%). Partial PLE was performed in 372 (42.9%) patients and reconstructed with jejunal free flap ($n$ = 256/335, 76.4%), pectoralis major flap ($n$ = 59/335, 17.6%), primary end-to-end anastomosis ($n$ = 17/335, 5.1%), and radial forearm free flap ($n$ = 3/335, 0.9%). Laryngeal protection was achieved in 347 (40%) patients [11].

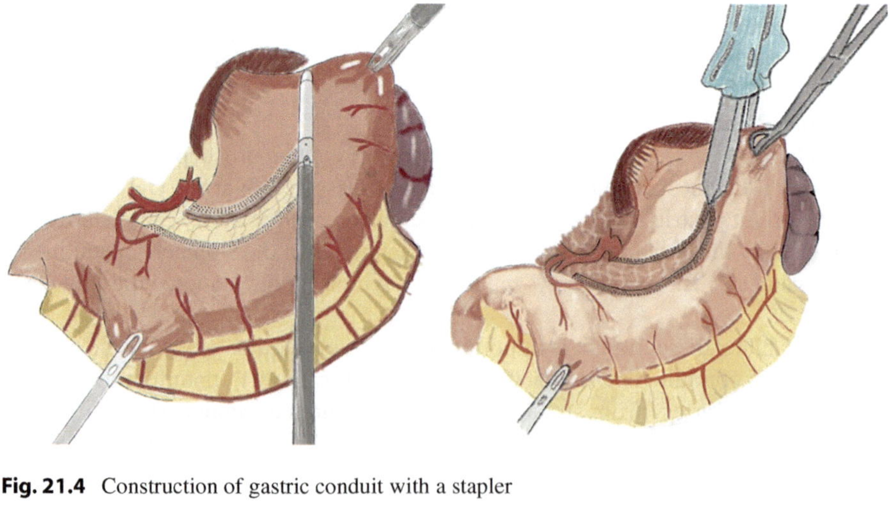

**Fig. 21.4** Construction of gastric conduit with a stapler

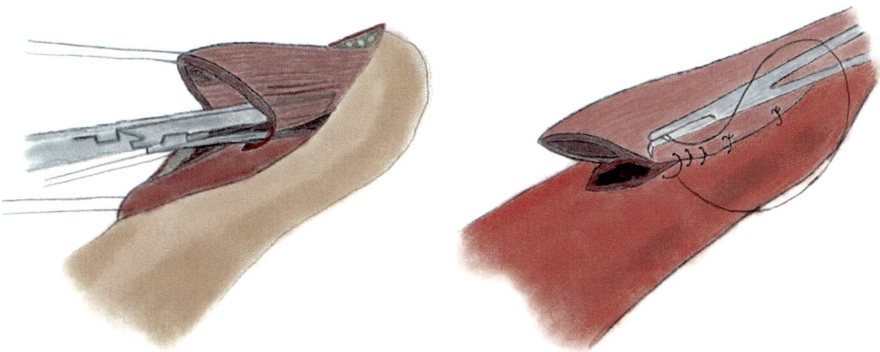

**Fig. 21.5** Anastomosis with a linear stapler

In a study in which 55 cervical esophagectomies and 19 total esophagectomies were performed, reconstruction with free jejunal transfer or gastric pull-up after surgical resection for cervical esophageal carcinoma was found to be equally successful and effective. Larynx-preserving surgery was performed on 24 patients. It has been reported that the choice of the reconstruction method depends on the extent of tumor spread [12].

A study from Italy states that cervical esophageal cancer should be treated with definitive chemotherapy with concomitant radiotherapy (RT). Surgery should be considered only in patients who do not respond completely. Their surgical methods were: three-incision esophagectomy or pharyngo-laryngo-esophagectomy, using either a gastric or colon conduit and pharyngo-laryngectomy with partial esophageal resection and reconstruction with a jejunal free flap [64].

A study evaluating 2159 patients with proximal Esophageal Squamous Cell Carcinoma through the American National Cancer Database shows that surgery should stay a treatment option in carefully selected patients with residual disease or local recurrence after definitive chemoradiotherapy. It emphasizes that the perioperative results of surgery are acceptable [65].

A simple gastric tube ($n = 56$, 37.1%) was commonly used for reconstruction in a multicenter study from Japan in which the results of 151 patients undergoing total PLE were reported. This was followed by a gastric tube with free graft transfer ($n = 53$, 35.1%), sleeve gastrectomy with microvascular anastomosis ($n = 34$, 22.5%), and other procedures ($n = 8$, 5.3%). Reconstruction of 91.4% of the patients was performed with the posterior mediastinal approach. It has been reported that the addition of FGT helps prevent end-gastric complications, while intraoperative evaluation of microcirculation can effectively improve outcomes [66].

### 21.5.3 Chemotherapy

A meta-analysis evaluating 1222 patients showed that definitive chemoradiotherapy is a beneficial first-line therapy for treating cervical esophageal squamous cell carcinoma [15]. In a study evaluating 55 patients with cervical esophageal cancer, concomitant chemoradiotherapy was reported to offer an acceptable chance of long-term survival for locally advanced, unresectable carcinomas of the cervical esophagus [67]. Several chemotherapeutic regimens are used for CEC based on information from treatments for lower esophageal SCC and head and neck squamous cell carcinoma [68].

The recommended agents for definitive chemotherapy, according to the NCCN guideline as follows: (Infusional fluorouracil can be changed with capecitabine) Preferred Regimens: Paclitaxel and carboplatin, Fluorouracil and oxaliplatin, Fluorouracil and cisplatin. Other Recommended Regimens: Cisplatin with docetaxel or paclitaxel, Irinotecan and cisplatin, Paclitaxel and fluoropyrimidine (fluorouracil or capecitabine) [28].

### 21.5.4 Radiotherapy

The treatment guideline for esophageal cancer patients receiving definitive chemoradiation with curative intent is 50–50.4 Gy (total 25–28 fractions) with concomitant chemotherapy. Patients with cT1b-2N+ or cT3-4aN0/N+ cervical esophageal SCC have radical chemoradiotherapy/radiotherapy indications [25, 28, 68].

Applying a sufficient RT dose to the tumor is usually difficult because it is close to critical structures such as the spinal cord and lungs. Current RT techniques, such as intensity-modulated radiation therapy (IMRT) and simultaneous integrated boost (SIB), where the density of radiation can be changed during treatment, allow a dose to a higher dose to the lesion and a reduced dose to adjacent structures. These techniques may be helpful in the treatment of CEC. Regarding elective lymph node irradiation, no clear consensus has not yet been achieved [68–70].

### 21.5.5 Other Treatments

According to guidelines, systemic therapy is recommended as first-line therapy in patients with locally advanced or metastatic esophageal cancer [16, 28]. The choice of regimens for the second line and subsequent therapy is conditional upon initial therapy and performance status. Nivolumab is recommended for second-line or subsequent treatment for esophageal SCC. According to the current NCCN guideline, some targeted therapeutic agents, trastuzumab, pembrolizumab, nivolumab, and entrectinib/larotrectinib have been approved by the FDA for use in advanced esophageal and EGJ cancers [16, 28]. According to a review, cetuximab is not recommended for CEC [68]. Some studies have shown that for loco-regional-advanced CEC, nimotuzumab, in combination with CRT, is effective [71, 72].

Patients with advanced esophageal cancer should be provided with early palliative care and nutritional support [16].

## 21.6 Conclusions

Since cervical esophageal cancer is rare compared to other regions, there is a lack of high-level evidence for its treatment. Management of CEC is complicated because it is usually detected to have progressed to adjacent vital organs from the time of diagnosis. Increasing our knowledge and awareness about cervical esophageal cancer constitutes the first step of studies to enable us to reach more precise results.

**Acknowledgments** Thank you, M. İkbal Akın, MD, and Ahmet Akmercan, MD, for their support regarding medical illustrations.

## References

1. Force SD, Symbas PN, Symbas NP. Esophagus and diaphragm. In: Wood WC, Staley CA, Skandalakis JE, editors. Anatomic basis of tumor surgery. Berlin, Springer; 2010. p. 265–97.
2. Skandalakis JE, Ellis H. Embryologic and anatomic basis of esophageal surgery. Surg Clin North Am. 2000;80(1):85–155. https://doi.org/10.1016/S0039-6109(05)70399-6.
3. Lin J. Chapter 4—Relevant anatomic relations of the esophagus. In: Yeo CJ, editor. Shackelford's surgery of the alimentary tract, 2 Volume Set. 8th ed. Philadelphia: Elsevier; 2019. p. 31–43.
4. Liebermann-Meffert D. Anatomy and embryology of the esophagus. In: Tilanus HW, Attwood SEA, editors. Barrett's esophagus. Dordrecht: Springer Netherlands; 2001. p. 17–30.
5. Jaffe BM. Surgery of the esophagus. In: Orlando RC, editor. Atlas of esophageal diseases. London: Current Medicine Group; 2002. p. 221–42.
6. Deslauriers J, Meyerson S, Patterson A, Cooper J. Pearson's thoracic and esophageal surgery. 3rd ed. Philadelphia: Churchill Livingstone; 2008.
7. Skandalakis JE, Colborn GL, Weidman TA. Skandalakis' surgical anatomy: the embryologic and anatomic basis of modern surgery. Athens, Greece: Paschalidis Medical Publications; 2004.
8. Ugalde PA, Pereira ST, Araujo C. Correlative anatomy for the esophagus. Thorac Surg Clin. 2011;21(2):307–17. https://doi.org/10.1016/j.thorsurg.2010.12.007.
9. Netter FH. Atlas of human anatomy. 6th ed. Philadelphia: Saunders/Elsevier; 2006.
10. Sung H, Ferlay J, Siegel RL, Laversanne M, Soerjomataram I, Jemal A, et al. Global Cancer Statistics 2020: GLOBOCAN estimates of incidence and mortality worldwide for 36 cancers in 185 countries. CA Cancer J Clin. 2021;71(3):209–49. https://doi.org/10.3322/caac.21660.
11. De Virgilio A, Costantino A, Festa BM, Mercante G, Franceschini D, Franzese C, et al. Oncological outcomes of cervical esophageal cancer treated primarily with surgery: a systematic review and meta-analysis. Eur Arch Otorrinolaringol. 2023;280(1):373–90. https://doi.org/10.1007/s00405-022-07589-z.
12. Daiko H, Hayashi R, Saikawa M, Sakuraba M, Yamazaki M, Miyazaki M, et al. Surgical management of carcinoma of the cervical esophagus. J Surg Oncol. 2007;96(2):166–72. https://doi.org/10.1002/jso.20795.
13. Ohno K, Nasu M, Matsui H, Baba Y, Yasuda T, Sakuma J, et al. Real-world treatment patterns and outcomes in Japanese patients with cervical esophageal cancer. Esophagus. 2022;19(4):576–85. https://doi.org/10.1007/s10388-022-00921-w.
14. Du XX, Yu R, Wang ZF, Du DC, Liu QY, Wang RM, et al. Outcomes and prognostic factors for patients with cervical esophageal cancer undergoing definitive radiotherapy or chemoradiotherapy. Bosn J Basic Med Sci. 2019;19(2):186–94. https://doi.org/10.17305/bjbms.2019.3873.
15. De Virgilio A, Costantino A, Festa BM, Mercante G, Franceschini D, Franzese C, et al. Oncological outcomes of squamous cell carcinoma of the cervical esophagus treated with

definitive (chemo-)radiotherapy: a systematic review and meta-analysis. J Cancer Res Clin Oncol. 2022;149:1029. https://doi.org/10.1007/s00432-022-03965-8.
16. Obermannová R, Alsina M, Cervantes A, Leong T, Lordick F, Nilsson M, et al. Oesophageal cancer: ESMO Clinical Practice Guideline for diagnosis, treatment and follow-up. Ann Oncol. 2022;33(10):992–1004. https://doi.org/10.1016/j.annonc.2022.07.003.
17. Salama JK, Palta M, Torok JA. The multidisciplinary management of early stage cervical esophageal cancer. In: Saba NF, El-Rayes BF, editors. Esophageal cancer: prevention, diagnosis and therapy. Cham: Springer International Publishing; 2015. p. 173–85.
18. Domper Arnal MJ, Ferrández Arenas Á, Lanas Arbeloa Á. Esophageal cancer: risk factors, screening and endoscopic treatment in Western and Eastern countries. World J Gastroenterol. 2015;21(26):7933–43. https://doi.org/10.3748/wjg.v21.i26.7933.
19. Huang FL, Yu SJ. Esophageal cancer: risk factors, genetic association, and treatment. Asian J Surg. 2018;41(3):210–5. https://doi.org/10.1016/j.asjsur.2016.10.005.
20. Li X, Gao C, Yang Y, Zhou F, Li M, Jin Q, et al. Systematic review with meta-analysis: the association between human papillomavirus infection and oesophageal cancer. Aliment Pharmacol Ther. 2014;39(3):270–81. https://doi.org/10.1111/apt.12574.
21. Petrick JL, Wyss AB, Butler AM, Cummings C, Sun X, Poole C, et al. Prevalence of human papillomavirus among oesophageal squamous cell carcinoma cases: systematic review and meta-analysis. Br J Cancer. 2014;110(9):2369–77. https://doi.org/10.1038/bjc.2014.96.
22. Yuan W, Li S, Jia J, Wang L, Huang Y, Wang M, et al. Human papillomavirus is an important risk factor for esophageal carcinoma in a Chinese population. J Cancer Res Clin Oncol. 2022;149:5241. https://doi.org/10.1007/s00432-022-04322-5.
23. Buckstein M, Liu J. Cervical esophageal cancers: challenges and opportunities. Curr Oncol Rep. 2019;21(5):46. https://doi.org/10.1007/s11912-019-0801-7.
24. Walker RC, Underwood TJ. Oesophageal cancer. Surgery (Oxford). 2017;35(11):627–34. https://doi.org/10.1016/j.mpsur.2017.09.010.
25. Gong H, Li B. Guidelines for radiotherapy of esophageal carcinoma (2020 edition). Precis Radiat Oncol. 2021;5(2):54–72. https://doi.org/10.1002/pro6.1119.
26. Muroi K, Kakushima N, Furukawa K, Furune S, Ito N, Hirose T, et al. Effects of steroid use for stenosis prevention after endoscopic submucosal dissection for cervical esophageal cancer. Int J Clin Oncol. 2022;27(5):940–7. https://doi.org/10.1007/s10147-022-02139-3.
27. Kuwano H, Nishimura Y, Oyama T, Kato H, Kitagawa Y, Kusano M, et al. Guidelines for diagnosis and treatment of carcinoma of the esophagus April 2012 edited by the Japan Esophageal Society. Esophagus. 2015;12(1):1–30. https://doi.org/10.1007/s10388-014-0465-1.
28. Ajani JA, D'Amico TA, Bentrem DJ, Chao J, Corvera C, Das P, et al. Esophageal and esophagogastric junction cancers, Version 2.2019, NCCN Clinical Practice Guidelines in Oncology. J Natl Compr Cancer Netw. 2019;17(7):855–83. https://doi.org/10.6004/jnccn.2019.0033.
29. Amin MB, Greene FL, Edge SB, Compton CC, Gershenwald JE, Brookland RK, et al. The Eighth Edition AJCC Cancer Staging Manual: continuing to build a bridge from a population-based to a more "personalized" approach to cancer staging. CA Cancer J Clin. 2017;67(2):93–9. https://doi.org/10.3322/caac.21388.
30. Japan Esophageal Society. Japanese classification of esophageal cancer, 11th edition: Part I. Esophagus. 2017;14(1):1–36.
31. van Vliet EP, Heijenbrok-Kal MH, Hunink MG, Kuipers EJ, Siersema PD. Staging investigations for oesophageal cancer: a meta-analysis. Br J Cancer. 2008;98(3):547–57. https://doi.org/10.1038/sj.bjc.6604200.
32. Thakkar S, Kaul V. Endoscopic ultrasound stagingof esophageal cancer. Gastroenterol Hepatol (N Y). 2020;16(1):14–20.
33. Flamen P, Lerut A, Van Cutsem E, De Wever W, Peeters M, Stroobants S, et al. Utility of positron emission tomography for the staging of patients with potentially operable esophageal carcinoma. J Clin Oncol. 2000;18(18):3202–10. https://doi.org/10.1200/jco.2000.18.18.3202.
34. Heeren PA, Jager PL, Bongaerts F, van Dullemen H, Sluiter W, Plukker JT. Detection of distant metastases in esophageal cancer with (18)F-FDG PET. J Nucl Med. 2004;45(6):980–7.

35. Mönig S, Chevallay M, Niclauss N, Zilli T, Fang W, Bansal A, et al. Early esophageal cancer: the significance of surgery, endoscopy, and chemoradiation. Ann N Y Acad Sci. 2018;1434(1):115–23. https://doi.org/10.1111/nyas.13955.
36. Lu JX, Liu DL, Tan YY. Clinical outcomes of endoscopic submucosal tunnel dissection compared with conventional endoscopic submucosal dissection for superficial esophageal cancer: a systematic review and meta-analysis. J Gastrointest Oncol. 2019;10(5):935–43. https://doi.org/10.21037/jgo.2019.06.09.
37. Cao Y, Liao C, Tan A, Gao Y, Mo Z, Gao F. Meta-analysis of endoscopic submucosal dissection versus endoscopic mucosal resection for tumors of the gastrointestinal tract. Endoscopy. 2009;41(9):751–7. https://doi.org/10.1055/s-0029-1215053.
38. Wang HY, Zeng X, Bai SY, Pu K, Zheng Y, Ji R, et al. The safety and efficacy of endoscopic submucosal dissection for treating early oesophageal carcinoma: a meta-analysis. Ann R Coll Surg Engl. 2020;102(9):702–11. https://doi.org/10.1308/rcsann.2020.0177.
39. Iizuka T, Kikuchi D, Hoteya S, Kajiyama Y, Kaise M. Efficacy and safety of endoscopic submucosal dissection for superficial cancer of the cervical esophagus. Endosc Int Open. 2017;5(8):E736–E41. https://doi.org/10.1055/s-0043-112493.
40. Ariyoshi R, Toyonaga T, Tanaka S, Abe H, Ohara Y, Kawara F, et al. Clinical outcomes of endoscopic submucosal dissection for superficial esophageal neoplasms extending to the cervical esophagus. Endoscopy. 2018;50(6):613–7. https://doi.org/10.1055/s-0043-123761.
41. Inoue T, Shichijo S, Cho H, Shoji A, Waki K, Fujii T, et al. Laryngeal elevation for endoscopic submucosal dissection in cervical superficial esophageal cancer at esophageal entrance. Endoscopy. 2021;53(2):E65–E6. https://doi.org/10.1055/a-1187-0826.
42. Tanaka K, Kido K, Sawai S, Ikenoyama Y, Yukimoto H, Hamada Y, et al. Endoscopic submucosal dissection with a novel traction wire for esophageal cancer in the cervical esophagus. Endoscopy. 2022;54(S02):E1055–E6. https://doi.org/10.1055/a-1889-5606.
43. Chan DS, Reid TD, Howell I, Lewis WG. Systematic review and meta-analysis of the influence of circumferential resection margin involvement on survival in patients with operable oesophageal cancer. Br J Surg. 2013;100(4):456–64. https://doi.org/10.1002/bjs.9015.
44. Akiyama H. Surgery for carcinoma of the esophagus. Curr Probl Surg. 1980;17(2):53–120.
45. Akiyama H, Tsurumaru M, Udagawa H, Kajiyama Y. Esophageal cancer. Curr Probl Surg. 1997;34(10):765–834.
46. Jamieson GG, Lamb PJ, Thompson SK. The role of lymphadenectomy in esophageal cancer. Ann Surg. 2009;250(2):206–9. https://doi.org/10.1097/SLA.0b013e3181b16cd1.
47. Akiyama H, Tsurumaru M, Ono Y, Udagawa H, Kajiyama Y. Background of lymph node dissection for squamous cell carcinoma of the esophagus. In: Sato T, Iizuka T, editors. Color atlas of surgical anatomy for esophageal cancer. Tokyo: Springer Japan; 1992. p. 9–24.
48. Hulscher JB, van Sandick JW, de Boer AG, Wijnhoven BP, Tijssen JG, Fockens P, et al. Extended transthoracic resection compared with limited transhiatal resection for adenocarcinoma of the esophagus. N Engl J Med. 2002;347(21):1662–9. https://doi.org/10.1056/NEJMoa022343.
49. Bartels H, Thorban S, Siewert JR. Anterior versus posterior reconstruction after transhiatal oesophagectomy: a randomized controlled trial. Br J Surg. 1993;80(9):1141–4. https://doi.org/10.1002/bjs.1800800924.
50. Arya S, Markar SR, Karthikesalingam A, Hanna GB. The impact of pyloric drainage on clinical outcome following esophagectomy: a systematic review. Dis Esophagus. 2015;28(4):326–35. https://doi.org/10.1111/dote.12191.
51. Akiyama H, Miyazono H, Tsurumaru M, Hashimoto C, Kawamura T. Use of the stomach as an esophageal substitute. Ann Surg. 1978;188(5):606–10. https://doi.org/10.1097/00000658-197811000-00004.
52. DeMeester TR, Johansson KE, Franze I, Eypasch E, Lu CT, McGill JE, et al. Indications, surgical technique, and long-term functional results of colon interposition or bypass. Ann Surg. 1988;208(4):460–74. https://doi.org/10.1097/00000658-198810000-00008.

53. Sasaki TM, Baker HW, McConnell DB, Vetto RM. Free jejunal graft reconstruction after extensive head and neck surgery. Am J Surg. 1980;139(5):650–3. https://doi.org/10.1016/0002-9610(80)90355-4.
54. Acosta MA, Cuesta MA, Bruna M. Atlas of minimally invasive techniques in upper gastrointestinal surgery. Springer; 2021.
55. Wong I, Law S. McKeown esophagectomy. In: Schlottmann F, Molena D, Patti MG, editors. Esophageal cancer: diagnosis and treatment. Cham: Springer International Publishing; 2018. p. 99–107.
56. DeMeester SR. En bloc esophagectomy. In: Schlottmann F, Molena D, Patti MG, editors. Esophageal cancer: diagnosis and treatment. Cham: Springer International Publishing; 2018. p. 109–16.
57. Griffin SM, Raimes SA, Shenfine J. Oesophagogastric surgery E-book: companion to specialist surgical practice. Elsevier Health Sciences; 2013.
58. Watson M, Trufan S, Benbow JH, Gower NL, Hill J, Salo JC. Jejunostomy at the time of esophagectomy is associated with improved short-term perioperative outcomes: analysis of the NSQIP database. J Gastrointest Oncol. 2020;11(2):421.
59. Yoshida N, Eto K, Matsumoto T, Kosumi K, Imamura Y, Iwatsuki M, et al. Omental flap wrapping around the esophagogastric anastomosis and association with anastomotic leak in esophagectomy for esophageal cancer: a propensity score-matching analysis. J Am Coll Surg. 2023;236(1):189–97.
60. Akiyama Y, Iwaya T, Endo F, Shioi Y, Chiba T, Takahara T, et al. Stability of cervical esophagogastrostomy via hand-sewn anastomosis after esophagectomy for esophageal cancer. Dis Esophagus. 2017;30(5):1.
61. Egberts JH, Schniewind B, Bestmann B, Schafmayer C, Egberts F, Faendrich F, et al. Impact of the site of anastomosis after oncologic esophagectomy on quality of life—a prospective, longitudinal outcome study. Ann Surg Oncol. 2008;15(2):566–75. https://doi.org/10.1245/s10434-007-9615-1.
62. Lerut T, Coosemans W, Decker G, De Leyn P, Nafteux P, van Raemdonck D. Anastomotic complications after esophagectomy. Dig Surg. 2002;19(2):92–8. https://doi.org/10.1159/000052018.
63. Orringer MB, Marshall B, Iannettoni MD. Eliminating the cervical esophagogastric anastomotic leak with a side-to-side stapled anastomosis. J Thorac Cardiovasc Surg. 2000;119(2):277–88. https://doi.org/10.1016/s0022-5223(00)70183-8.
64. Valmasoni M, Pierobon ES, Zanchettin G, Briscolini D, Moletta L, Ruol A, et al. Cervical esophageal cancer treatment strategies: a cohort study appraising the debated role of surgery. Ann Surg Oncol. 2018;25(9):2747–55. https://doi.org/10.1245/s10434-018-6648-6.
65. Patel DC, Yang CJ, Liou DZ, Berry MF. Treatment and outcomes of proximal esophageal squamous cell carcinoma. Ann Surg Oncol. 2023;30(2):818–27. https://doi.org/10.1245/s10434-022-12683-x.
66. Okamura A, Watanabe M, Mukoyama N, Ota Y, Shiraishi O, Shimbashi W, et al. A nationwide survey on digestive reconstruction following pharyngolaryngectomy with total esophagectomy: a multicenter retrospective study in Japan. Ann Gastroenterol Surg. 2022;6(1):54–62. https://doi.org/10.1002/ags3.12509.
67. Gkika E, Gauler T, Eberhardt W, Stahl M, Stuschke M, Pöttgen C. Long-term results of definitive radiochemotherapy in locally advanced cancers of the cervical esophagus. Dis Esophagus. 2014;27(7):678–84. https://doi.org/10.1111/dote.12146.
68. Hoeben A, Polak J, Van De Voorde L, Hoebers F, Grabsch HI, de Vos-Geelen J. Cervical esophageal cancer: a gap in cancer knowledge. Ann Oncol. 2016;27(9):1664–74. https://doi.org/10.1093/annonc/mdw183.
69. Ishida Y, Sakanaka K, Fujii K, Itasaka S, Mizowaki T. Intensity-modulated radiotherapy for cervical esophageal squamous cell carcinoma without hypopharyngeal invasion: dose distribution and clinical outcome. J Radiat Res (Tokyo). 2019;60(4):517–26. https://doi.org/10.1093/jrr/rrz019.

70. Li Q, Zhu S, Li S, Deng W. Elective nodal irradiation provides a superior therapeutic modality for lymph node positivity esophageal squamous cell carcinoma patients receiving definitive radiotherapy versus involved-field irradiation. Medicine (Baltimore). 2019;98(3):e14080. https://doi.org/10.1097/md.0000000000014080.
71. Lai X, Gu Q, Zheng X, Liu G, Feng W, Lin X, et al. Combined nimotuzumab with chemoradiotherapy in patients with locally advanced or metastatic esophageal squamous cell carcinoma: a retrospective study. J Cancer Res Ther. 2016;12(Suppl):89–95. https://doi.org/10.4103/0973-1482.191612.
72. Hu J, Chen Z, Lv J, Zheng Z, Bei Y, Chen X, et al. The application of nimotuzumab combined with definitive chemoradiotherapy toward the treatment of locally advanced cervical esophageal carcinoma: a retrospective study. Front Oncol. 2022;12:905422. https://doi.org/10.3389/fonc.2022.905422.

# Robotic Esophagectomy for Esophageal Cancer

# 22

Evangelos Tagkalos and Peter P. Grimminger

## 22.1 Introduction

Updated worldwide collected data from 2020, present esophageal cancer as the ninth most common cancer with more than 600,000 new cases [1]. Furthermore, esophageal cancer is the sixth leading cancer cause of death with almost 550,000 deaths every year worldwide opposed to the 400,000 deaths calculated for year 2012 [1–3]. For the ascending prevalence both most common types of esophageal carcinoma, the squamous cell carcinoma (SCC) and the adenocarcinoma (AC) are responsible. Whereas SCC is still the most prevalent type of esophageal cancer worldwide, western countries face a decline of this type but a significant rise if adenocarcinoma including the adenocarcinoma of the esophagogastric junction (AEG) [1, 2].

Obesity, gastroesophageal reflux disease and Barrett's metaplasia are found to be factors of high risk for the occurrence of AC [4]. Although AC is related with a better 5-year overall survival compared to SCC, it is still a cancer with high mortality rates in studies from the both the western and eastern hemisphere as it is characterized by early metastasis [5, 6]. AC tends to occur in the distal third of the esophagus or as AEG [2]. Curative therapy strategies for esophageal AC and AEG mainly

E. Tagkalos (✉)
Department of General, Visceral and Transplant Surgery, University Medical Center Mainz, Mainz, Germany

UGIRA-Fellow 2022–2023 in Chang Gung Memorial Hospital, Taoyuan, Taiwan
e-mail: evangelos.tagkalos@unimedizin-mainz.de

P. P. Grimminger
Minimally Invasive Surgery and Robotics, Case Observation Center for Robotic Esophageal Surgery, Department of General, Visceral and Transplant Surgery, University Medical Center Mainz, Mainz, Germany
e-mail: peter.grimminger@unimedizin-mainz.de


O. Engin (ed.), *Risk Factors and Therapy of Esophagus Cancer*,
https://doi.org/10.1007/978-3-031-47024-0_22

include transthoracic esophagectomy with abdominal and thoracic lymph node dissection after chemotherapy or chemoradiation in case of locally advanced disease.

Esophagectomy is a technically demanding operation and produces substantial trauma for the patient. The open procedure (OP), which has been the only relevant approach for many decades, was associated with high morbidity and mortality rates exceeding 20% in small-volume centers [7]. The shift from open surgery to minimally invasive approaches resulted in reduced morbidity and mortality rates as low as 0.9% [8]. Mainly three different approaches have been established for the use of minimally invasive surgery in esophagectomy: The hybrid esophagectomy (HE) including a laparoscopic gastric mobilization and lymphadenectomy and open thoracic esophagectomy and reconstruction, the totally minimally invasive esophagectomy (MIE) with the use of laparoscopy and thoracoscopy and the robot-assisted esophagectomy (RAMIE) with robotic or laparoscopic abdominal part and robot-assisted thoracic part [8, 9].

The surgical approaches are critically evaluated for their safety. The question of the anastomotic technique is in the focus as well as the location of the anastomosis, intrathoracic or cervical, and if it is performed intracorporeally. Regarding the extent of lymphadenectomy, recent studies aim to deliver a rational for each tumor entity, AC and SCC, as well as for the exact location, esophagus or esophagogastric junction [9].

## 22.2 RAMIE

In 2003, RAMIE was developed to overcome the technical limitations of MIE. The use of the robotic assistant leads to a very stable three-dimensional, enlarged view. The articulated instruments enable precise preparation with 7 degrees of freedom of movement in very confined spaces such as the posterior mediastinum where the conventional laparoscopy is limited [10]. The first cohort study was published from Utrecht University in 2006. Van Hillegersberg et al. performed 21 consecutive RAMIEs in patients with esophageal carcinoma. In summary, a precise lymph node dissection in the mediastinum was possible with the robotic assistant. Furthermore, this approach provided the potential to reduce postoperative complications with optimal surgical en bloc dissection of the tumor and the periesophageal tissue. A standardized RAMIE procedure was described in the study. The authors came to the conclusion that the RAMIE is a good and feasible minimally invasive technique alternative to OP [11]. The first review of the literature for RAMIE came in 2011 from Clark et al. enclosing nine studies with only 130 patients. The study had a suboptimal level of evidence showing that there was a great need for prospective studies and randomized control trials (RCTs) [12]. Following the latter study, van der Sluis et al. organized and carried out the first and last RCT comparing OP to RAMIE until today, the ROBOT Trial [13].

In this prospective single center RCT 54 patients underwent OP and 55 patients RAMIE. OP consisted of an open three-stage transthoracic esophagectomy through a right posterolateral thoracotomy followed by a laparotomy and ended with the creation of the esophagogastric handsewn end-to-side cervical anastomosis. Likewise, RAMIE consisted of a robotic-assisted thoracoscopy followed by a laparoscopic abdominal phase and the creation of a handsewn cervical esophagogastric anastomosis. Primary endpoint was the rate of postoperative complications as classified by the modified Dindo-Clavien classification (MCDC) [14]. A total of 59% of the RAMIE group presented MCDC surgery-related complications of grade 2 or higher in comparison with 80% of the OP group ($p = 0.02$). Pulmonary complications occurred in 32% of the RAMIE and 58% of the OP group ($p = 0.005$). Cardiac complications were also significantly lower in the RAMIE group (22% vs. 47%; $p = 0.006$). Functional recovery 2 weeks postoperatively was significantly better for RAMIE (70% vs. 50% of the group-patients; $p = 0.04$). Blood loss was significantly lower for thoracic part of the operation in favor of RAMIE with 120 mL (200 mL for OP; $p < 0.001$). The mean postoperative pain as noted in a VAS daily for the first 2 week postoperatively revealed a statistically significant difference in favor of RAMIE ($p = 0.001$). Short-term quality of life ($p = 0.02$ and $p = 0.03$) and physical functioning ($p = 0.03$ and $p = 0.049$) at discharge and 6 weeks after the operation revealed statistically better results for RAMIE as well. On the other hand, RAMIE procedures took significantly more time to complete (349 min vs. 296 min for the OP; $p < 0.001$) with the thoracic part playing the biggest role in this delay (170 min for RAMIE vs. 134 min for the OP; $p < 0.001$). R0 resections, lymph node harvesting, and survival rates did not differ statistically between the two groups [15].

The first evaluations of the learning curve of RAMIE were published by Hernandez et al. and Sarkaria et al. which concluded that the learn effect was noted after 20 and 30–45 cases respectively. A clear cut-off point for the completion of the learning curves is not stated in the latter studies [16, 17]. Van der Sluis et al. assessed the learning curve of RAMIE using the cumulative sum method (CUSUM) for a proctor and a novice to the method surgeon undergoing proctoring in a number of 312 cases. The proctor needed 70 procedures and a time frame of 55 months in order to achieve proficiency of the method, whereas the proctored novice surgeon completed the learning phase after 15 supervised and 9 unsupervised/independent cases (24 cases). The authors conclude that proctoring can crucially reduce the cases need to complete the learning curve [18]. In many centers RAMIE is a procedure with a standardized setting.

## 22.3 HE vs. MIE vs. RAMIE

Very few studies with a little number of patients compared the three minimally invasive techniques. Pneumonia and wound infections were less common in MIE and RAMIE when compared with HE. HE on the other hand, was the technique with the significantly less cumulative ($p < 0.001$; HE: 314 ± 43 min; MIE 339 ± 52 min; RAMIE 410 ± 70 min) and thoracic operative time ($p < 0.001$; HE: 177 ± 26 min; MIE 217 ± 37 min; RAMIE 250 ± 56 min) [19].

Up to date there is not a prospective RCT comparing HE to RAMIE or all minimally invasive techniques (HE, MIE and RAMIE).

## 22.4 MIE vs. RAMIE

Little evidence is provided concerning the possible superiority of one minimally invasive method to the other as no RCT controlling the two methods is finished up to date.

There is currently one multicenter prospective RCT, the ROBOT2-trial (ClinicalTrials.gov Identifier: NCT04306458)—which started recruiting in the beginning of 2021—that controls MIE to RAMIE for adenocarcinoma of the distal esophagus or AEG. Primary endpoint is the extent of lymph node dissection and this study is the first to compare MIE and RAMIE in the western world [20]. Simultaneously there are two Asian multicenter randomized controlled trials finished recruiting esophageal squamous cell carcinoma patients comparing RAMIE to conventional MIE: the REVATE trial (ClinicalTrials.gov Identifier: NCT03713749) [21]. and the RAMIE Trial (ClinicalTrials.gov Identifier: NCT03094351) [22].

Long-term results for these trials are awaited with great interest and might answer the question whether RAMIE is superior to MIE for patients suffering from esophageal cancer.

## 22.5 Basic Principles of Reconstruction Following Esophagectomy

Depending strictly on the anatomical course of the esophagus, an ideal surgical approach will have to follow a left cervical, right thoracic, and median abdominal path. After resection of the esophagus, the stomach, a segment of the small intestine or a segment of the colon can alternatively be used for reconstruction of the continuity of the upper gastrointestinal tract. The stomach represents the most often used organ to replace the esophagus by means of a gastric pull-up after conduit construction, which requires a singular anastomosis (esophagogastrostomy), although the acid and bile reflux are small disadvantages of the method [23]. Although the small intestine has very good blood circulation which facilitates good anastomotic healing, due to its location and dependance on the *A. mesenterica* superior it is only suitable for pulling up into the lower mediastinum, as in the Merendino operation, the limited radical resection of the lower esophagus. The microvascular transfer of free segments of the small intestine to bridge defects after cervical esophageal carcinoma resections plays a dwindling role today due to radiation therapy as a very good treatment alternative [23, 24]. Such cases are mostly reported from big Asian centers where cervical esophageal cancer has a higher prevalence. The colon as a replacement organ is seldom used today as the first choice of reconstruction. The operative burden would be further increased as in the case of isoperistaltic interposition of the transverse colon or the right hemicolon, a total of three high-risk anastomoses must be created (the esophago-colostomy, the colo-gastrostomy, and the colo-colostomy). Diverticula, colitis and also—not uncommon in the age range of 60–70 years—adenomas or colon carcinomas must be ruled out beforehand. The advantages of a primer colonic interposition are the relative good function of colonic tissue, the big achievable lengths enabling an easy cervical placement (the biggest length of all three interposition variants can be achieved through colonic interposition) and the chance of preserving the stomach with all the positive aspects that this includes [25, 26]. The use of colon can still be necessary today in the case of very large tumors at the esophagogastric junction requiring an esophagogastrectomy, in unexpected problematic situations intraoperatively where the stomach can no longer be used as a replacement organ, or in the case of a gastrectomy or partial gastric resection in the patient's history. Another special situation is the secondary loss of the stomach after gastric pull-up due to ischemia of the conduit. Although seldom, such a situation requires an emergency discontinuity-resection. The following reconstruction in 6 months is basically only possible with a colonic segment [27, 28].

## 22.6 Special Aspects of the Esophageal Operation

### 22.6.1 Lymphadenectomy

The lymph node yield is of pivotal importance in surgical treatment of esophageal cancer. Rizk et al. investigated in 2010 a collective of 4627 patients who underwent esophagectomy for esophageal cancer in order to find an association between extend of lymphadenectomy and survival. Extended lymph node harvesting was found to correlate with increased survival for all cancer patients except from patients with well-differentiated pN0M0 or TisN0M0 cancers or patients with 7 or more positive for cancer lymph nodes. After further analysis the study group defined the optimum lymphadenectomy in order to achieve maximum 5-year survival, according to the T stadium as follows: 10 lymph nodes for pT1, 20 for pT2, and 30 or more for stadium pT3/T4. The study was limited from the fact that no uniform protocol for the dissection of the lymph nodes or the pathological examination of the specimen was followed, with the latter resulting in undervaluation of the real numbers [29]. Visser et al. in a meta-analysis of 26 studies evaluated the effect of lymphadenectomy in overall survival (OS) and disease-free survival (DFS). They concluded that increased number of resected lymph nodes was associated with significantly improved OS for both western and eastern studies [(HR = 0.86; 95% CI = 0.77–0.96; $p < 0.01$) and (HR = 0.71; 95% CI = 0.61–0.84; $p < 0.01$) respectively]. Furthermore, DFS was statistically significantly prolonged for the operations with the higher number of resected lymph nodes (HR = 0.72; 95% CI = 0.62–0.84; $p < 0.01$). In most of the controlled studies a minimum of 15–23 lymph nodes should be resected for an optimal staging. The authors also concluded that final lymph node yield depends on many factors such as variety in lymphadenectomy between surgeons, variety in specimen submission and variety of retrieval methods of the pathologists [30].

Regarding the anatomical correlation of the lymphadenectomy, Kurokawa et al. managed to accurately identify the distribution of lymph node metastasis from AEG tumors and evaluated the extent of the needed lymph node dissection in a prospective Japanese national-wide multicenter study. One limitation of this study is that the cohort has been treated by gastrectomy or esophagectomy, according to the length of esophageal tumor infiltration. In case of wide esophageal infiltration however, only esophagectomy was performed and those cases are clinically more considered as esophageal cancer. The exact lymph node stations to be resected were aimed to be identified prior to the operation according to the extent of the tumor invasion of the esophagus. Key outcome of the study is the strong recommendation that upper mediastinal lymph nodes (as the station 106recR lymph nodes) should be dissected in cases with esophageal involvement of more than 4 cm [31]. Retrospective studies show that RAMIE can facilitate safe dissections in upper mediastinum, where absolute precision is demanded as trauma of the underlining vital structures increase morbidity and mortality. The utilization of the robotic assistant is such cases should be further evaluated and might prove to be of great importance [32].

The TIGER multicenter prospective observation trial, which is currently ongoing, tries to achieve a uniform staging system of lymph node metastasis of esophageal carcinoma parallel to the work of Kurokawa et al. In this cohort study, only cases of esophagectomy are included, so a homogeneous set of harvested lymph nodes is expected. The surgeons of the 50 participating centers must separate all resected lymph node stations and the pathologists must examine each station individually, thus delivering homogenous data. Through this very detailed lymph node mapping and evaluation, the study hopes to facilitate a better understanding of the tumor biology and thus facilitate a more precise treatment of patients with esophageal cancer [33].

### 22.6.2 Anastomosis

Up to date there is no consensus for a textbook anastomosis following esophagectomy. Scientific evidence for a general recommendation is still limited. The lack of standardization combined with the numerous anastomotic techniques used for the anastomotic creation following esophagectomy result to an input of heterogeneous information. The latter bias is added upon the fact that no uniform assessment and reporting system of complications existed for many decades, making results of the evaluation of such data trivial. Anastomotic leakage, which is the predominant surgical complication after esophagectomy, is a case with multiple given definitions until the esophagectomy complications consensus group (ECCG) reached to a definition widely accepted in 2015 [34]. Following the suggested system Schröder et al. presented in 2019 substantial data between anastomotic techniques and associated morbidity in 966 patients. The five anastomotic techniques identified were the intrathoracic end-to-side circular-stapled technique (double-stapling or purse-string), the intrathoracic side-to-side linear-stapled technique, the cervical side-to-sided linear-stapled one and lastly the cervical end-to-side handsewn anastomosis. The leakage rates did not differ statistically between the two anastomotic sites ($p = 0.601$) with 15.9% incidence for the intrathoracic anastomosis and 17.2% for the cervical one. On the other hand, intrathoracic anastomosis was associated with statistically fewer overall complications ($p = 0.09$). Furthermore, end-to-side handsewn anastomosis showed the higher leakage rate with 25.1% followed by end-to-side double-stapled intrathoracic anastomosis with 23.3%. The side-to-side linear stapled-anastomosis in thorax provided a leakage rate of 15.6% and 11.8% respectively, whereas the purse-string circular-stapled intrathoracic anastomosis showed a leakage rate of 13.9%. The multivariate analysis confirmed that the anastomotic technique is an independent predictor of leakage [35].

Kuppusamy et al. using the ECCG definitions and the EsoBenchmark database assessed contemporary international outcomes. The collected data from 6022 patients registered between 2015 and 2018 were evaluated. Most patients received a minimally invasive esophagectomy (52.8%) and an intrathoracic anastomosis (63.7%). Anastomotic leakage rates were 11.7% and 13.1% for years 2015–2016 and 2017–2018, respectively. The study shows the trend to minimally invasive approaches. None the less, anastomotic leakage rates above 10% are detected. On the other hand, the 90-day mortality is found to be as little as 4.5% [36].

Franzen et al. further evaluated the impact of such anastomotic leakages in long-term survival of patients who underwent MIE for esophageal cancer. In this international multicenter cohort study, the occurrence of anastomotic leakages was 14.8%. The occurrence alone of such a complication is associated with a significantly deteriorating long-term survival [hazard ratio (HR) 1.68, 95% confidence interval (CI) 1.25–2.24]. Moreover, the severity of the complication showed an inverse relation to the long-term survival of the patient [37].

The Oesophago-Gastric Anastomosis Audit (OGAA), in a prospective, multicenter cohort study, assessed postoperative outcomes from 2247 patients in 41 countries. Particularly, the anastomotic complications and their influence were analyzed. Anastomotic leakage rate was 14.2%. The leakage rate of cervical anastomosis was 20.1% in comparison to the 12.2% of leakage rate of intrathoracic anastomosis. The difference was statistically significant between the anastomotic sites ($p < 0.001$). Contrarily the severity of the intrathoracic anastomotic leakage and the necessity for a reoperation were statistically significant higher compared to that of the cervical leakage ($p < 0.001$ and $p = 0.004$, respectively). Further, the 90-day mortality rate differed statistically between the severity types of the complication (ECCG definition). Type III leakages (localized defect requiring surgical treatment) showed mortality rates of 24.7% whereas Type I leakages (local defect requiring no change in therapy, or treated medically or with dietary modification) only 3.2% [38].

The currently running MIVATE—RCT is comparing the linear stapled intrathoracic anastomosis with the open circular stapled intrathoracic anastomosis (MIE vs. OP) and will try to further differentiate if there benefits when using each method [39]. Furthermore, the diameter of the circular stapler (25 mm vs. 28 mm) is to be evaluated as latest data form retrospective studies indicate no differences between the two, as far anastomotic leakages and strictures are concerned, data that differ to older studies [40, 41]. A clear consensus upon the latter is not reached up to date.

## 22.7 Robotic Esophagectomy Procedures for Cancer

Taking into account the basic aspects described and in combination with today's knowledge for oncological radicality two basic resection and reconstruction procedures and their modifications for the surgical treatment of esophageal carcinoma come into question. The Ivor-Lewis and the McKeown esophageal procedures. A new technique that bypasses the neuralgic step of the transthoracic resection which requires a single lung ventilation will be also described as a very promising alternative that can be carried out robotically (RACE procedure).

### 22.7.1 Ivor Lewis Procedure (Transabdominal, Transthoracic Esophagectomy)

The described robotic-assisted minimally invasive transabdominal and transthoracic esophagectomy with gastric conduit reconstruction and D2 lymph node harvesting consists of two phases: an abdominal and a thoracic. In both phases, the "one surgeon—one assistant" principal will be demonstrated. For the latter, the use of four robotic arms and an assistant port is required. For the anastomotic creation we will describe in detail an end-to-side esophagogastric intrathoracic circular stapled anastomosis.

This procedure is according to the 2022 ESMO guidelines acceptable for the resection of tumors situated in the middle and distal esophagus as well as the gastroesophageal junction (Siewert I and II) [42].

#### 22.7.1.1 Abdominal Phase

The patient is placed in a normal supine position with a 15° reverse Trendelenburg. The da Vinci® Xi patients' cart will be positioned in the right side of the patient and the surgical assistant to the left. The trocar placement in robotic surgery is a very important step in order to facilitate maximum use of space without collisions between the robotic arms. The patient's anatomy plays a major role and should be taken into account prior to the operation. To further elaborate the latter, the CT scan is used to show the position of the stomach and its distance from the umbilicus. The camera will be placed in the midline in such a position that will enable an unproblematic view of the stomach and the transverse colon without maximum extension of the robotic arm in the upward position (like a flip-up action). After inserting a Verres needle 2–4 cm above the umbilicus and 2–4 cm on the left of the midline in the left upper quadrant, the pneumoperitoneum will be applied. The Verres needle will be removed and exchanged with an 8 mm trocar (robotic Arm#4; *t-4*). Through this trocar a dissection device will be inserted (vessel sealer or hook). As mentioned above, the camera trocar (robotic Arm#3; *t-3*) will be placed in the midline above the umbilicus in a position that will facilitate both the preparation of the gastroesophageal junction as well as the pylorus and the right gastroepiploic vessels. The next trocar to be placed is a 12 mm (robotic Arm#2; *t-2*) one on the right upper quadrant in a mirroring position of the robotic Arm#3 in contrast to the midline, where the fenestrated bipolar forceps and the robotic 12 mm stapler can be exchanged. (*In case that a robotic stapler is not applicable, then an 8 mm trocar should be placed for the Arm#2 in order to use the fenestrated bipolar forceps and then, according to the angulation of the stomach, the t-2 or t-3 trocar should be exchanged with a 13 mm trocar so that a hand-held stapler device can be inserted at the final steps of the abdominal phase for creating the gastric conduit*). The next trocar to be placed is an 8 mm-one (robotic Arm#1; *t-1*) in the right lateral subcostal area at least 6 cm (and at least two centimeters under the tenth pleura) to the right of the *t-2*. Through *t-1* a fenestrated tip-up grasper will be inserted. The last trocar to be placed is the assistant 12 mm trocar (*t-5*) in the left lateral subcostal region (Fig. 22.1).

After docking of the robotic patients' cart and inserting the camera (*t-3*), the vessel sealer will be inserted through *t-4* and the fenestrated bipolar forceps through *t-2*. Through *t-1 the tip-up* grasper will lift-up the left upper lobe so that—as a first step—the lesser omentum can be divided. After opening the pars flaccida of the hepatogastric ligament, the dissection will be expanded towards the right diaphragmatic crus. The assistant should provide adequate but gentle contra-traction of the pericardial fatty tissue by retracting the tissue to the patients' left. This facilitates a good surgical plane and enables a better visualization of the lesser omentum.

The following step is to completely mobilize the right side of distal esophagus and the gastroesophageal junction from the diaphragm. The station 1 lymph nodes are prepared so that they can be retrieved later with the final specimen. The next step is to prepare the greater curvature of the stomach. After identifying the gastroepiploic arcade, the greater omentum is dissected caudally. The assistant will hold the omentum to the left side of the patient and the surgeon to the right with respect to the gastroepiploic artery and the spleen. The correct traction and contra-traction between surgeon and assistant are of great importance to avoid unnecessary dissection, especially in obese patients and not "loose" the correct surgical plane. (*Tip: Avoid grasping of the gastroepiploic arcade at all costs. Try changing the position of both grasping instruments (surgeon and assistant) before dissecting the omentum which is held and sealed by the vessel sealer so that adequate traction is always applied in the divided tissue thus facilitating better visualization and control of the*

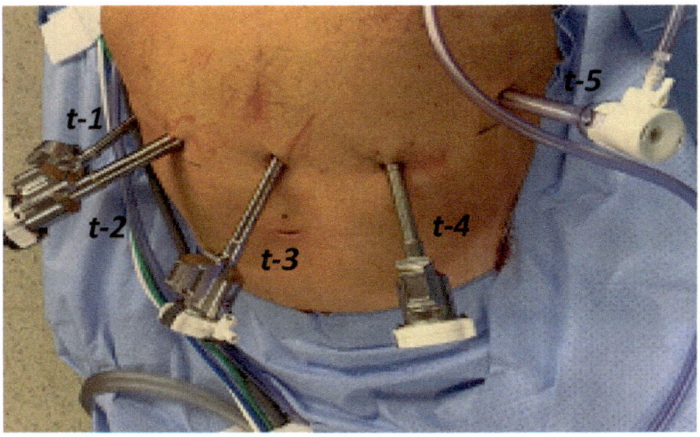


**Fig. 22.1** Trocar placement for the abdominal phase of the Ivor-Lewis procedure

*surgical plane*). After completing a partial omentectomy towards the spleen along the greater curvature of the stomach, the procedure continues with the dissection of the short gastric vessels. At this point, the left gastroepiploic vessels will be sealed and dissected (*Tip: the dissection should be not close to the stomach so that the intramural vascular net of the gastroepiploic arteries is not destroyed*). At this point, the *4sa-* and *4sb*-station lymph nodes are prepared so that they can be retrieved *en bloc* with the specimen. To facilitate an easier dissection the tip-up grasper from *t-1* should retract the stomach to the right of the patient. The assistant (*t-5*) will provide contra-traction by gently retracting the fat pad towards the left shoulder of the patient. The step is finished with the complete mobilization of the gastric fundus. The fundus can then be retracted to enable the preparation along the left diaphragmatic crus. The left side of the abdominal esophagus and the gastroesophageal junction will then be completely mobilized. At this step, the station 2 lymph nodes are prepared so that they can be retrieved later *en bloc* with the specimen. At this point, the left dissection plane will be fused to the right dissection plane which has been developed in the first steps of the operation. (*Tip: The assistant can retract the diaphragmatic tissue with an instrument bluntly at this point. This avoids destruction of the parietal peritoneum of the diaphragm and thus any unnecessary bleeding from the muscle layer*). After freeing of the esophagus from the diaphragmatic attachments, the assistant will gently grasp the posterior wall of the stomach and with an upward traction will facilitate the dissection of the adhesions between the pancreas and the stomach. Furthermore, adhesions to the mesocolon can be now dissected. The tip-up grasper can be of further assistance in the fine dissection (traction at the sixth hour and caudally). The dissection plane evolves then to the pylorus. At this point, the visualization of the right gastroepiploic vessels is mandatory as they should be spared for the vascularization of the conduit. Proceed with great caution when preparing the posterior gastric wall from the transverse mesocolon. The most secure way in our opinion is to lift-up the antrum by lifting up the posterior gastric wall with the fenestrated bipolar forceps (*t-2*) so that the gastroepiploic vessels are in a 90°-angle to your view-axis and always to your left. The tip-up grasper (*t-1*) or the assistant (*t-5*) can provide smooth traction of the mesocolic fatty tissue at the sixth hour of your screen (*Tip: The good visualization is the key to a fine dissection. At this point try to avoid complicated maneuvers and use the least number of instruments needed for a good visualization to avoid unnecessary uncontrolled movements that can lead to a traumatization of the gastroepiploic vessels. The tip-up or even the assistant traction are seldom needed in this step*). The visualization of the duodenum (*Pars I*), after mobilizing of the stomach towards the gallbladder, is the next step. After the mobilization of the stomach in this region, the gastric conduit can be prepared. The tip-up grasper (*t-1*) will lift the left upper liver lobe. The right and the left gastric arteries do both provide vascularization of an intramural plexus and thus the first branches should be preserved (this step does not interfere with the lymphadenectomy of the lesser curvature and the hepatoduodenal ligament). The fatty tissue of the lesser curvature is then dissected to create a fatty-free gastric front for the application of the first stapler (*t-2*). The robotic stapler (SureForm™ Stapler, Intuitive, Sunnyvale, California, USA) is then inserted at the point mentioned above (sparing the first branches of the right gastric artery) at the distal third of the lesser curvature. The conduit should not be too narrow, in order to reduce the risks of a possible ischemia [43]. After using three to four 60 mm staplers the conduit is constructed. At this point a 4–5 cm tissue connection to the fundus should be sparred, a step which is crucial for the anastomotic technique later described in the thoracic part. The stapler is exchanged with the fenestrated bipolar forceps (*t-2*) and the lymph node dissection can be now facilitated by cranially lifting the partially dissected lesser curvature. At this point a monopolar hook (permanent cautery hook) is inserted through *t-4* to enable a finer dissection. Alternatively, a monopolar scissor can be used. We start the dissection medially to the right gastric artery and following this vessel we then land to the proper hepatic artery. The identification of the gastroduodenal artery arising from the proper hepatic artery can then follow and the station 12 lymph nodes can then be finely prepared and remain connected to the specimen's side. The retrieval of the station 8 lymph nodes is then completed after dissecting the anterior and posteromedial side of the common hepatic artery. The next step is to assess the region of the celiac trunk. The pancreatic cranial border lies in close proximity to the vessels and thus fine dissection is required to avoid any pancreatic injuries at this point. The proximal splenic artery is identified at this step. To retrieve the 7, 9 and 11p station lymph nodes, the lesser curvature should be lifted up cranially (*t-2*) enabling visualization to the left gastric vein which can then be divided, followed by the transection of the left gastric artery at its origin [this step could be carried out via a Hem-o-lok (Telefex Medical, Weck Drive, NC) clip applied through *t-4*]. During this procedure the tissue surrounding the celiac trunk the left gastric artery and vein as well as the splenic artery are lifted anteriorly. The left diaphragmatic crura is then reached. After complete mobilization of the abdominal esophagus and the gastroesophageal junction the aortal plane and both pleurae must be clearly visible. The abdominal phase ends with the undocking of the da Vinci® Xi patients' cart and the removal of all the trocars.

#### 22.7.1.2 Thoracic Phase

The patient is placed in a semi-prone position (45° tilt from the left lateral position). The ventilation of the right lung will be obstructed through a double-lumen endotracheal tube or an endotracheal block. In our clinic for the Ivor Lewis procedure, we prefer the double-lumen endotracheal tube as it tends to dislocate less frequently than the endotracheal block. The da Vinci® Xi patients' cart will be positioned at the right side of the operating table and the assistant to left side.

Firstly, the assistant 12 mm trocar (*t-4*) is inserted through the fifth intercostal space along the anterior axillary line. The pneumoperitoneum with an 8 mmHg pressure is then established in the thoracic cavity after visualization of ta correct intrathoracic trocar placement. An 8 mm trocar (robotic Arm#3; *t-3*) will be placed 2–3 cm left and 1–2 cm above the *t-4* at the sixth intercostal space closely to the anterior axillary line. This is the camera trocar. Another 8 mm trocar (robotic Arm#5; *t-5*) is then placed on the fourth intercostal space at least 6 cm distant to *t-3* and 1–2 cm higher that the latter (along the posterior axillary line). The dissection devices will be inserted through *t-5* (*Tip: Always try to insert the trocar in the thoracic cavity under a 90°-angle and in the middle of the intercostal space. This can be troublesome in obese and small patients and the use of a syringe filled with 0.9% NaCl and a 21 G needle can be used to evaluate the best position for the trocar placement prior to trocar insertion*). A 12 mm trocar (robotic Arm#2; *t-2*) is then inserted through the eighth intercostal space at the posterior axillary line with its center 1–2 cm above *t-3* and at least 6 m distal to the latter (to avoid collisions). The last trocar to be placed is an 8 mm trocar (robotic Arm#1; *t-1*) at the tenth intercostal space at least 6 m distal to *t-2* and 1 cm above the posterior axillary line. Positioning trocars above the line that connects the scapula tip and the pelvis should be avoided (Fig. 22.2).

The standard setup is a hook (or vessel sealer) through *t-5*, a fenestrated bipolar forceps through *t-2* and a tip-up grasper through *t-1*.

The dissection of the parietal pleura starts at the end of the abdominal plane, at the region of the inferior pulmonary ligament and the pericardium, where the anterior side of the esophagus is identified. The dissection of the pleura continues gradually above the subcarinal lymph nodes to the azygos arch and expand above the azygos vein, parallel and medially to the right vagus nerve. The use of the *t-1* is seldom needed in this step and the assistant provides contra-traction by retracting the tissue at a sixth hour position of our screen. The right paratracheal lymph nodes will be retrieved separately at this point. The posterior and anterior parts of the azygos vein are then freed from the surround tissue so that an adequate space is created for the application of distal and proximal Hem-o-lok (Telefex Medical, Weck Drive, NC) clips through *t-2*. The vessel sealer is used to hold the azygos vein during the clip application and will then dissect the vein after sealing. The small bronchial artery that is located in close proximity to the posterior wall of the azygos vein cranially and to the patients' right, should be carefully identified and transected. The pleura is then dissected caudally parallel to the azygos vein and is expanded to the aortal layer. The paraesophageal lymph nodes are then dissected. The thoracic duct can be respected or taken down. To avoid a chyle-leakage we clip the thoracic duct in the lower mediastinum with the use of a Hem-o-lok (Telefex Medical, Weck Drive, NC) clip. The esophagus is then completely mobilized from the pericardial layer with respect to the left and right pulmonary veins followed by mobilization

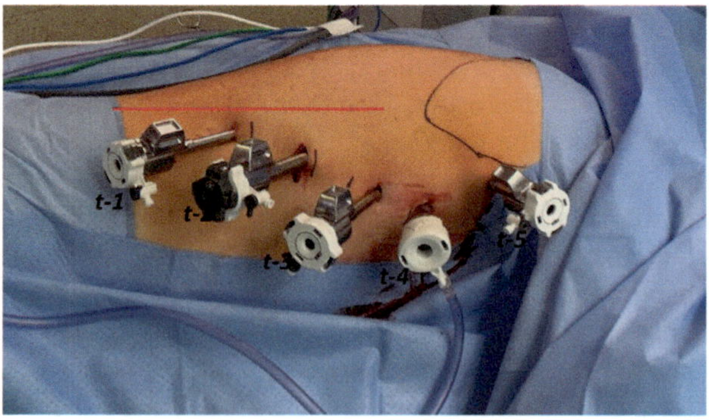


**Fig. 22.2** Trocar placement for the thoracic phase of the Ivor-Lewis procedure. The red interrupted line shows the upper level that a trocar should be placed

form the left and right bronchus as well as the trachea. The left and right bronchus lymph nodes will not be separated but prepared so that they can be retrieved *en bloc* with the specimen (*Tip 1: Extra caution should be taken during these steps to avoid thermal damage to the airway system. The use of a bipolar instrument facilitates a more controlled thermal injury to the tissue when compared to a monopolar one; the power level of the applied energy can also be modified/reduced in such steps; Tip 2: The left bronchus is easier to identify as it is fully expanded through the use of the left lung whereas the right bronchus is collapsed*). The vagus nerve should be transected with respect to the bronchial branches if possible. The tip-up grasper is used to retract the esophagus anteriorly (12th hour of are view) and thus facilitate a better traction and visualization of the right surgical plane. The assistant is responsible for the sixth hour contra-traction of the tissue. When retrieving the subcarinal lymph nodes the assistant will have to gently press the bronchial system with a closed forceps (bluntly) to avoid any tissue damage from grasping. After this step the esophagus is fully mobilized above the diaphragm and any connection to the diaphragmatic crura should now be taken down. The posterior mediastinal as well as the supradiaphragmatic lymph nodes will be retrieved *en bloc* with the specimen as well as the subcarinal ones (*Tip: Bulky lymph nodes that are not easy to dissect en bloc with the specimen can be dissected separately. Never compromise the security of an airway or other important mediastinal structures in order to achieve an en bloc resections of such lymph node stations*). Now the mobilization of the esophagus is complete and the monopolar hook is used to dissect the esophagus above the level of the transected azygos vein (*Tip 1: The nasogastric tube should be retrieved many centimeters before the opening of the esophagus through the anesthesiologist, so that is situated cranially to our proximal dissection margin; Tip 2: The use of an esophageal bougie can facilitate an easier dissection of the stretched mucosal layer*). Through the assistant trocar a monofilament suture is inserted and a purse-string of the proximal esophageal end is made robotically. The both ends of the suture are then externalized through *t-4*. Through *t-4* a grasper will secure the distal esophageal resected end. Prior to the latter the conduit should be brough to the thoracic cavity under gentle traction of the fatty tissue of the greater curvature (*Tip: The right angulation of the conduit is of vital importance in order to avoid any strangulation. The lesser curvature stapler line is situated opposite to the aorta*). The da Vinci Xi® patients' cart is undocked. The *t-4* is removed and a mini thoracotomy is performed by extending the trocar incision 2–3 cm anteriorly and 1–2 cm posteriorly (fifth intercostal space). A wound protector—in our case the Alexis protector (Alexis™ Laparoscopic System, Applied Medical)—is inserted through the mini thoracotomy. The grasper which is still holding the transected esophagus through the mini thoracotomy will be later retrieved to externalize the specimen and partially the gastric conduit. Prior to externalization of the specimen the head of the circular stapler—25 or 28 mm (CEEATM, Covidien, Mansfield, MA, USA)—will be internalized through the mini thoracotomy. The head will be inserted in the proximal esophageal end and secured through the purse-string. A hand-held 5 mm grasper through *t-5* and—in this step—the hand-held robotic camera through *t-1*, are needed for the completion of this step. After that the specimen is partially externalized, a small incision is made at the end of the lesser curvature at the stapler line and the stapler-saft is inserted through the incision and brought in the thoracic cavity. The shaft pin of the stapler is exteriorized cranially near the greater curvature of the gastric conduit. The shaft and the head are connected and approximated under continuous visualization. At this point a hand-held grasper (through *t-2* or *t-4*) is used to remove the fatty tissue of the greater omentum from the anastomotic fronts to avoid simultaneous stapling of such tissue in the anastomosis. The end-to-side circular anastomosis is created (Fig. 22.3). The specimen is then divided from the gastric conduit via a linear stapler inserted from the mini thoracotomy (Endo-GIATM, Covidien, Mansfield, MA, USA) (*Tip: The bougie used for an easier dissection of the esophagus can be used after the anastomotic creation and before the use of the linear stapler to dissect the specimen from the gastric conduit in order to avoid narrowing of the conduit below the anastomosis*). Single interrupted monofilament sutures can be used to secure the anastomosis (alternatively a continuous running barbed reabsorbable suture can be used). A pleural tent and the use of a 180–270° omental-flap can be further created to reinforce the anastomosis. A nasogastric tube will be placed as well as a thoracic tube via the *t-1* after its removal. The

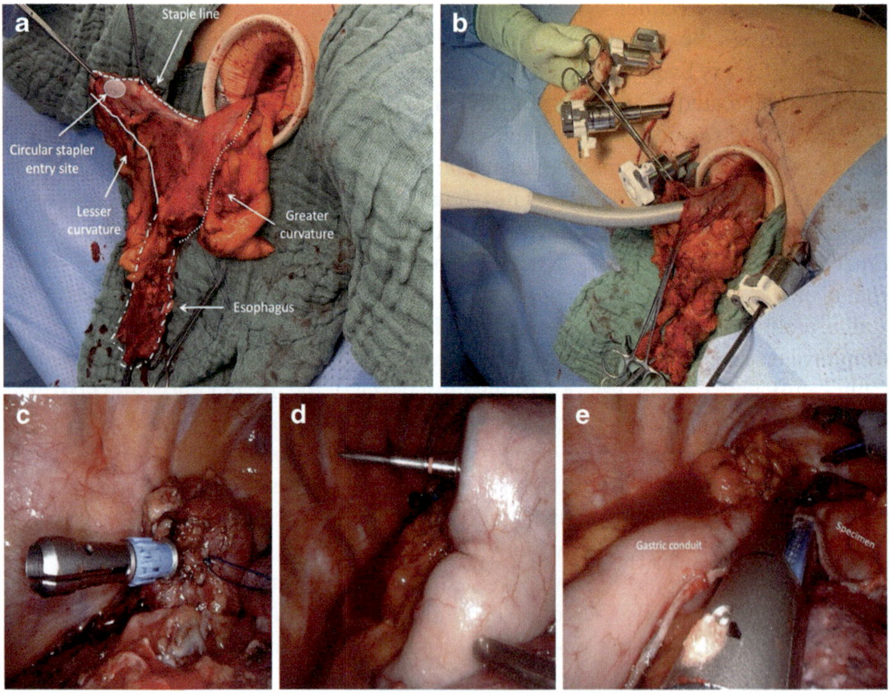


**Fig. 22.3** (**a**) The partial externalization of the specimen and the insertion point of the stapler; (**b**) The specimen is brought back to the thoracic cavity to create the anastomosis; (**c**) The head of the circular stapler is inserted and tightened through a purse string; (**d**) The shaft pin is exteriorized at the cranially; (**e**) After creation of the anastomosis, the specimen is divided from the conduit through a linear stapler

trocars are removed as well as the Alexis protector and the wounds are closed. Prior to closing the wound the right lung will be fully expanded under visualization.

### 22.7.2 McKeown Procedure (Transthoracic, Transabdominal and Cervical Esophagectomy)

The described robotic-assisted minimally invasive transthoracic, transabdominal and cervical esophagectomy with gastric conduit reconstruction and D2 lymph node harvesting consists of three phases: a thoracic, an abdominal, and a cervical. In all phases, the "one surgeon—one assistant" principal will be demonstrated. For the latter, the use of four robotic arms and an assistant port is required. For the anastomotic creation, we will describe in detail an end-to-side cervical esophagogastric circular stapled anastomosis.

#### 22.7.2.1 Thoracic Phase

The thoracic phase of the McKeown procedure shares many steps of the thoracic phase of the Ivor-Lewis procedure. The patient is placed in a semi-prone position (45° tilt from the left lateral position). The ventilation of the right lung will be obstructed through a double-lumen endotracheal tube or an endotracheal block (*Tip: To facilitate an easier traction of the trachea that will enable a better plane for the left recurrent laryngeal nerve lymphadenectomy, an endotracheal block should be used instead of the bigger double-lumen endotracheal tube if possible*). The da Vinci® Xi patients' cart will be positioned at the right side of the operating table and the assistant to left side. The trocar position can be altered to a higher intercostal space for each trocar. That means that *t-1* (robotic Arm#1) will be placed in the ninth intercostal space, *t-2* (robotic Arm#2) in the seventh intercostal space, *t-3* (robotic Arm#3) which is the camera trocar in the fifth intercostal space and *t-5* (robotic Arm#4) in the third intercostal space. All robotic trocars are 8 mm. The assistant 12 mm trocar can be placed in the in the fourth intercostal space. The dissection of the parietal pleura starts at the end of the abdominal plane, at the region of the inferior pulmonary ligament and the pericardium where the anterior side of the esophagus is identified. The dissection of the pleura continues gradually above the subcarinal lymph nodes to the azygos arch and expand above the azygos vein parallel and medially to the right vagus nerve. The right paratracheal lymph nodes will be retrieved separately at this point. The posterior and anterior parts of the azygos vein is then freed from the surround tissue so that adequate space is created for the application of a distal and a proximal Hem-o-lok (Telefex Medical, Weck Drive, NC) clip through *t-2*. The vessel sealer is used to hold the azygos vein during the clip application and will then dissect the vein after sealing. The small bronchial artery that is located in close proximity to the posterior wall of the azygos vein cranially and to the patients right should be carefully identified and transected. The pleura is then dissected caudally parallel to the azygos vein and is expanded to the aortal layer. The paraesophageal lymph nodes are then dissected. The thoracic duct can be respected or taken down. To avoid a chyle-leakage, we clip the thoracic duct in the lower mediastinum with the use of a Hem-o-lok (Telefex Medical, Weck Drive, NC) clip. The esophagus is then completely mobilized from the pericardial layer with respect to the left and right pulmonary veins followed by mobilization form the left and right bronchus as well as the trachea. The left and right bronchus lymph nodes will be not separated but prepared so that they can be retrieved *en bloc* with the specimen. The vagus nerve should be transected with respect to the bronchial branches if possible. After this step the esophagus is fully mobilized above the diaphragm and below the azygos vein and any connection to the diaphragmatic crura should now be taken down. The posterior mediastinal as well as the supradiaphragmatic lymph nodes will be retrieved en-bloc with the specimen as well as the subcarinal ones. For the next step that will take place in the upper mediastinum we suggest that the instruments are exchanged as follows: tip-up grasper through *t-5*, monopolar hook or monopolar scissors through *t-3*, camera through *t-2* (remember to redo the targeting) and fenestrated bipolar forceps (or bipolar forceps) through *t-1*. This alternative setting can facilitate a controlled dissection of the upper mediastinum. Firstly, the lymph nodes of the right recurrent laryngeal nerve (RLN) will be retrieved. The parietal pleura should be incised parallel to the right vagus nerve and up to the right subclavian artery that is easily identifiable. Key is to find the recurring point of the right RLN caudally to the subclavian artery. After that retrieving the right RLN lymph nodes can be done separately from the specimen. The following step of the lymphadenectomy of the left RLN requires traction of the trachea in a clockwise manner. That means that the trachea should be rotated with the help of the assistant through pressure on the tracheal cartilage. Great caution of the membranous part of the trachea should be given (*Tip: The use of a gauze between the assistant's instrument and the trachea can minimize the risk of perforation*). The tip-up grasper through *t-1* is used to retract the esophagus dorsally and the assistant will gently rotate the trachea medially as described above. The instrument of the assistant should be at the sixth hour of our screen. The soft tissue of the left paratracheal space will be carefully dissected leaving the left RLN untouched. The ventral lymph nodes are dissected firstly followed by the dorsal ones. After that the esophagus is further mobilized as cranially as possible. The thoracic phase ends after the placement of a thoracic tube through *t-1* and the full expansion of the right lung under visualization.

#### 22.7.2.2 Abdominal Phase

The abdominal phase of the McKeown procedure follows the same steps as the Ivor Lewis procedure. To enable a smoother passage of the specimen and the conduit through the posterior mediastinum to the neck, the specimen can be divided from the gastric conduit and reattached to it with interrupted sutures at the tip of the gastric conduit as in the RACE procedure (see below). The abdominal phase ends after the anastomotic creation in the neck with the gentle retrieval of a few centimeters of the gastric conduit in the abdomen. The pyloric region should be near the esophageal hiatus.

#### 22.7.2.3 Cervical Phase

The cervical phase should start before the end of the abdominal phase. A second surgical team can carry out this phase. The patient is still placed in supine position and the head is tilted to the right of the patient and the neck is stretched through the positioning of a small pillow under it. The anatomical landmarks such as the jugulum and the medial side of the left sternocleidomastoid (SCM) muscle are used to place the correct skin incision which should be 3–4 cm in length. The incision is extended just above the jugulum and along the medial side of the left SCM muscle (Fig. 22.4). The platysma is dissected and the soft tissue is opened layer by layer to the thoracic inlet. The cervical esophagus is identified and with finger blunt dissection is encircled with a loop to facilitate easier traction of the organ. Through the very high mobilization of the thoracic esophagus, this step can be easily performed. The specimen is then retracted from the neck and the adjacent conduit will appear in the thoracic inlet. The esophagus is then dissected, the specimen is freed and given to further histopathological examination, a purse string is placed in the proximal end of the cervical esophagus and head of the circular stapler (preferably 25 mm; CEEATM, Covidien, Mansfield, MA, USA) is inserted and tightened (with the purse-string). Through the tip of the gastric conduit, and after controlling the correct positioning to avoid an organoaxial malrotation, a small incision via electrocautery will enable the insertion of the stapler shaft. The stapler should be positioned so that the posterior surface of the conduit will be involved in the anastomosis. The shaft pin of the stapler is exteriorized cranially at the posterior gastric wall of the gastric conduit. The shaft and the head are connected and approximated. The end-to-side circular stapled anastomosis is created. The stapler is retrieved and the proximal and distal tissue "donuts" are controlled. A nasogastric tube is then placed under digital control in the conduit and the remaining blind sack of the proximal conduit where the stapler was inserted is resected via a linear stapler (GIA™, Covidien, Mansfield, MA, USA). The anastomosis can be further secured with interrupted absorbable monofilament sutures. A small soft drainage is put posteriorly to the anastomosis and the wounds are closed with interrupted sutures (platysma and skin). The cervical phase is completed.

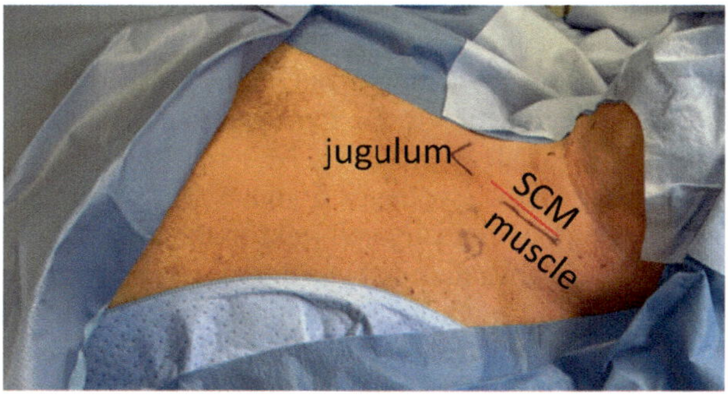


**Fig. 22.4** The jugulum and the medial border of the left sternocleidomastoid muscle are marked with blue. The interrupted red line demonstrates the skin incision

### 22.7.3 Robotic Assisted Transhiatal and Transcervical Esophagectomy (RACE Procedure)

Although fully minimally invasive techniques such as MIE and RAMIE do minimize the substantial trauma of an esophagectomy, both require a single lung ventilation through the thoracic phase. Patients suffering from impaired pulmonary function or who have undergone thoracic operations may not be able to be operated transthoracic. On the other hand, there is evidence that the transhiatal approach (alternative to the transthoracic approach without the opening of the thoracic cavity) can be associated with a poorer lymph node yield. The latter may have an impact in the overall survival as well as the disease-free survival of patients treated with a transhiatal approach although not strictly proven up to date from the literature. The RACE procedure is developed as an intention to maximize the radicality of the transhiatal approach, and thus not jeopardize the oncological aspect of the operation, while combining the advantages of bypassing the neuralgic transthoracic step. To succeed this, a technically demanding transcervical procedure is added to the transhiatal approach. The later technique is described in cadaveric operations as well as case series [44–46]. In this chapter, we will demonstrate our experience with the use of the da Vinci Xi® system in our case series.

#### 22.7.3.1 Transhiatal Phase

The transhiatal phase consists of the same steps using the same instruments as the abdominal phase of the Ivor-Lewis procedure described above. After the dissection of the left gastric vein and artery and completion of the abdominal lymphadenectomy, the dissection plane is extended cranially with respect to the right pleura that should not be opened. The pericardium is situated anteriorly, the right pleura is the right border of our dissection-plane and the esophagus creates the posterior border. The plane between the esophagus and the pericardium is avascular and the paraoesophageal lymph nodes can be prepared so that they can be retrieved *en bloc* with the specimen. The tip-up grasper, the vessel sealer and the fenestrated bipolar forceps are used in this step and traction from the assistant is seldom needed. The left border of the dissection is the aortic layer. The mesoesophagus is carefully dissected. After developing the dissection plane 3–5 cm above the esophageal hiatus the thoracic duct can be visualized to the right and can respected or clipped and dissected. For the dissection the tip-up grasper should carefully provide a small elevation of the pericardium and the fenestrated forceps should gently provide the posterolateral traction to the right, without opening the right pleura. A Hem-o-lok (Telefex Medical, Weck Drive, NC) can be then applied through *t-4*. After completely freeing the esophagus from the pericardium the subcarinal lymph nodes are assessed further cranially and right to the left pulmonary vein. The carina and the main bronchi are situated above the subcarinal lymph nodes and will be confronted after mobilizing of the latter lymph node packet. The main bronchi lymph nodes can be then mobilized and left connected to the periesophageal tissue so that they can be retrieved with the specimen. Alternatively, they can be removed separately. Advancing the dissection plane cranially, the mobilization of the esophagus from the membranous part of the trachea (pars membranacea) can be achieved. The dissection is finished at the level of the azygos vein. The vein dissection should not be conducted as an uncontrolled bleeding at this point is very difficult to handle. At this point, we return to the abdominal cavity and finalize the gastric conduit with the division of the specimen at the gastric fundus (in the Ivor Lewis procedure the specimen remains attached to the conduit). Therefore, the specimen should be connected to the gastric conduit via interrupted sutures in an end-to-end fashion in order to provide the narrowest diameter for the later pull-through maneuver through the posterior mediastinum that follows in the *cervical phase* without compromising the diameter of the conduit and thus its vascularization [*Tip: The anterior part of the conduit is marked with a continuous blue line (tip of a blue sterile marker) to provide evidence for a safe conduit positioning and to prevent a catastrophic kinking afterwards*]. The transhiatal phase is ended.

#### 22.7.3.2 Transcervical Phase

The patient is placed in supine position. The head is tilted to the right of the patient and the neck can be stretched through the positioning of a small pillow under it. The anatomical landmarks such as the jugulum and the median side of the left sternocleidomastoid (SCM) muscle are used to place the correct skin incision which should be 3–4 cm in length (Fig. 22.4). The incision is extended just above the jugulum and along the medial side of the left SCM muscle. The platysma is dissected and the soft tissue is opened layer by layer as in the McKeown procedure to the thoracic inlet. The cervical esophagus is identified with finger blunt dissection. A small Alexis wound protector (Applied Medical, Rancho Santa Margarita, California, United States) is then applied. A GelPOINT Mini (Applied Medical, Rancho Santa Margarita, California, United States) was used in our cases. Alternatively, a plain normal sterile glove can be used and secured in the Alexis wound protector and the trocars can be placed by opening the tip of the fingers and securing them with a tie (any suture). Key point is to create a closed system with at least 5 mmHg pressure. The da Vinci® Xi patients' cart is situated at the patients right and the arms are docked outside of the body (at the GelPOINT Mini). The robotic Arm#2 (fenestrated bipolar forceps; *t-1*), Arm#3 (camera trocar; *t-2*) and Arm#4 (vessel sealer or synchro seal; *t-3*) are placed with 8 mm trocars in a triangle formation whereas a 5 mm (*t-4*) assistant trocar is placed opposite to the camera trocar as in a rhombus (Fig. 22.5). The thoracic inlet is approached and the dissection is continued along the left recurrent laryngeal nerve (LRN). The left LRN lymph nodes can be freed from the nerve and dissected separately. The membranous part of the trachea that was partially mobilized from the esophagus caudally through the transhiatal phase is now completely mobilized through blunt dissection or the use of a bipolar instrument. Extra caution is suggested to avoid tracheal lesions at this point (*Tip: If such a lesion occurs, concern on choosing the retrosternal route for the reconstruction. In such a case the abdominal cavity will be reopened*). The right subclavian artery is then meet at the right anterolateral side of the esophagus (left upper part of our view) and should be carefully detached from the esophagus with extra caution given on the right LRN. Under the pars membranacea and the

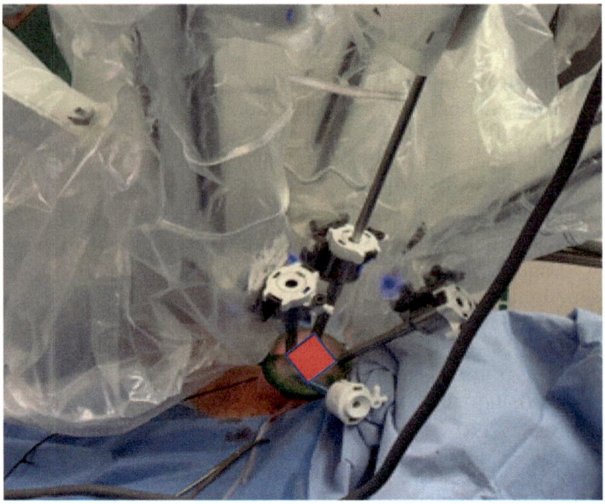

**Fig. 22.5** Trocar placement for the transcervical phase of the RACE procedure. The instruments are placed in each tip of a rhombus (red)

subclavian artery the two surgical planes (the transhiatal and transcervical) are met and connected. At this point, the azygos arch is clearly seen. The azygos is lateralized and preserved. Bleeding at this point will be (as in the transhiatal phase) difficult to handle and so the vein is sparred. The esophagus is now totally mobile. The da Vinci® Xi patients' cart is undocked and the trocars are removed together with the GelPOINT Mini. The esophagus is then dissected, a purse string is placed in the proximal end and head of the circular stapler (preferably 25 mm; CEEATM, Covidien, Mansfield, MA, USA) is inserted and tightened (purse-string). The specimen is retrieved through gentle traction. At the end of the specimen the connected gastric conduit will appear. The steps that follow are the same to the anastomotic creation of the McKeown procedure described above (McKeown; cervical phase).

## 22.8 General Complications Following Esophagectomy

The comparative high risk of surgery, especially of the transthoracic esophagectomy (risk of surgery = risk of anesthesia + risk of surgery) is based on several factors. Esophageal cancer patients very often suffer from relevant comorbidities such as COPD (chronic obstructive pulmonary disease) cardiac diseases. A number of such patients are obese and at the same time malnourished or are underweight to the point of cachexia [47, 48]. The esophagectomy is a radical intervention that takes place in spaces with anatomical proximity to sensitive vascular (aorta, celiac trunk, pulmonary veins, azygos vein), bronchopulmonary (pars membranacea of the trachea, right main bronchus), cardiac (pericardium, left atrium), nervous (vagus nerves, recurrent nerves) and other structures (thoracic duct). These structures can be damaged primarily directly or indirectly (e.g. thermally) during the operation, or they can be digested secondarily in the early postoperative course through the escape of aggressive gastric acid, bile acid or pancreatic enzymes or through inflammatory processes [49, 50].

Typical complications of the transthoracic esophagectomy with gastric pull-up reconstruction include:

- Overall Morbidity and Mortality. A large international multi-center study with 30 participating centers and 2944 included patients showed a major complication rate (type III–V according to MCDC) after transthoracic esophagectomy of 49%. The 30-day mortality was 5% and in-hospital mortality was 7.3% [51].
- Pulmonary complications ranging from mild Pneumonia to ARDS (adult respiratory distress syndrome) are the most common complications and rates of more than 30% are described in large studies [51].
- Cardiac complications with atrial fibrillation being the most common cardiac one, are reported in rates of 15–25% [52].
- Leakage of the anastomosis ranging from self-limiting situation that request no reintervention other than the null to mouth and the insertion of a nasogastric tube up to total conduit necrosis requiring immediate reoperation with externalization of the cervical esophagus (esophagostoma) with disruption of the continuity of the upper gastrointestinal tract. Still rates over 10% are reported even when minimally invasive techniques are used [36].
- Chylothorax is described with an incidence between 0.4% and 4% in large studies and occur after injury to the thoracic duct. Most cases are easily treated with dietary alterations whereas the treatment of persistent chylothorax remains controversial until today and has a major negative impact—when uncontrolled—in the postoperative course of the patients [53].
- Recurrent laryngeal nerve injuries with vocal cord palsy is reported in a latest randomized control trial controlling RAMIE to MIE with up to 32.6% for the robotic operation (vs. 27.1% for MIE; $p = 0.258$). In both operations the right and left RLN lymph nodes are resected and the reported rats are the initial rates of palsy (a substantial proportion of this injuries is expected to heal over time) [54].
- Fistulas between the airway and the conduit are rarely reported. In a large retrospective study of 1204 Ivor-Lewis procedures, only 1.1% of trachea-bronchial fistulas occurred postoperatively the management of whom was trivial and 38.5% of the involved patients died through sepsis [55]. Although rare this complication requires immediate action to minimize further deterioration of the patients' general condition.
- Late complications such us delayed gastric emptying, herniation through the esophageal hiatus (paraconduit hernia), anastomotic strictures, redundancy of colonic- or even gastric segments as well as bile or acid reflux and dumping are reported. Many of the latter cases are revealed through a good follow-up and early diagnosis of minor symptoms can lead to a better handling of such cases [50].

## 22.9 Complications During Robotic Procedures

If a major life-threatening complication occurs, then the minimally invasive aspect of the operation is not to be respected. The latter means that emergency conversion and use of all possible recourses to stabilize the patient is mandatory. We should not forget that the minimally invasive techniques are used to provide further benefit for the patient and lower the perioperative risks of an open procedure. Nonetheless, with the implementation of robotic esophageal surgery especially in the thoracic cavity where the esophagus is in close proximity to major vessels and the airway, extra caution and maximum alert from the whole surgical team during the process should be the case. Major intraoperative complications are not often reported after robotic esophageal surgery [56, 57].

A big retrospective study using data maintained from the FDA's (U.S. Food and Drug Administration) MAUDE (Manufacturer and User Facility Device Experience) database which included robotic procedures over a period of 14 years (2000–2013), showed 13.1% significant patient injuries in 10.624 cases. Mortality of 1.4% was described. The study showed that inadequate training in emergencies was the major contributor to disastrous events [57].

An emergency conversion for a major intrathoracic bleeding is a nightmare scenario for every member of the robotic team (console surgeon, bedside assistant surgeon, scrub nurse, circulating nurse and anesthesiologist). The fact that time from the undocking of the robot until the opening of the human cavity and the manual compression/control of a bleeding consist of several seconds or minutes, even among the most prepared teams, can result to an *exitus in tabula*. In order to minimize the chaos that can arise from such stressful situations the robotic team should simulate such scenarios routinely. Each member of the team should have a clear priorly given role and the simulation should be timed. The needed surgical instrument sets for such a conversion, as well as multiple suction-devices should be at reach and always standing by for immediate use (for example: thoracotomy set, vascular set). An emergency patients' cart roll-out (emergency undocking) should be easily manageable from all the members of the robotic team—nurses and doctors. Such a simulation of an emergency roll-out can even take place after the end of any elective robotic surgical procedure [56].

In case of bleeding that cannot be controlled robotically but can be compressed, a robotic arm can be used to provide constant pressure to the bleeding point. Simultaneously, all the other arms, including the camera can be removed and the thoracotomy can take place. This is the so-called *front arm flip-up method* and when it can be used, provides more time to the team. Alternatively, the bedside assistant surgeon can compress a bleeding and the robotic system can be fully undocked [56].

The da Vinci platform facilitates a highly magnified view thus facilitates fine tissue dissection but at the same time the operating field is narrowed. The robotic instruments should always be on screen and should be never moved in positions outside the screen margins. The same rule applies for the instruments inserted through the assistant trocar. Moreover, the lack of *tactile sense* of the robotic arms (no feedback to the surgeon) can produce severe injuries when in areas outside the screen view without the surgeon even noticing of the latter [56, 57].

Another not common but tragical mistake is the removal of the wrong arm instrument from the assistant. Even in stressful situations the console surgeon and the assistant should **clarify the number of the robotic arm and the instrument to take out or exchange**. *For example: a grasper that is compressing a bleeding vessel cannot be "accidentally" removed due to misunderstanding and create a major complication from a minor one* [56].

*Good cooperation of the robotic team* is mandatory to minimize the stress in extreme situations and thus facilitate quicker and better control of each emergency. The clear role of every team member in such condition remains the cornerstone for successful management.

## References


1. Jacques F, Murielle C, Isabelle S, Donald MP, Marion P, Ariana Z, Freddie B. Cancer statistics for the year 2020: an overview. Int J Cancer. 2021; https://doi.org/10.1002/ijc.33588.
2. Gupta B, Kumar N. Worldwide incidence, mortality and time trends for cancer of the oesophagus. Eur J Cancer Prev. 2017;26(02):107–18.
3. Ferlay J, Soerjomataram I, Dikshit R, et al. Cancer incidence and mortality worldwide: sources, methods and major patterns in GLOBOCAN 2012. Int J Cancer. 2015;136(05):E359–86.
4. Uhlenhopp DJ, Then EO, Sunkara T, Gaduputi V. Epidemiology of esophageal cancer: update in global trends, etiology and risk factors. Clin J Gastroenterol. 2020;13(6):1010–21.
5. Njei B, McCarty TR, Birk JW. Trends in esophageal cancer survival in United States adults from 1973 to 2009: a SEER database analysis. J Gastroenterol Hepatol. 2016;31:1141–6.
6. Hou H, Meng Z, Zhao X, et al. Survival of esophageal cancer in China: a pooled analysis on hospital-based studies from 2000 to 2018. Front Oncol. 2019;9:548.
7. Birkmeyer JD, Siewers AE, Finlayson EV, et al. Hospital volume and surgical mortality in the United States. N Engl J Med. 2002;346(15):1128–37.
8. Luketich JD, Pennathur A, Awais O, et al. Outcomes after minimally invasive esophagectomy: review of over 1000 patients. Ann Surg. 2012;256(01):95–103.
9. Haverkamp L, Seesing MFJ, Ruurda JP, Boone J, van Hillegersberg R. Worldwide trends in surgical techniques in the treatment of esophageal and gastroesophageal junction cancer. Dis Esophagus. 2017;30:1–7.
10. Ruurda JP, van Vroonhoven TJ, Broeders IA. Robot-assisted surgical systems: a new era in laparoscopic surgery. Ann R Coll Surg Engl. 2002;84:223–6.
11. Van Hillegersberg R, Boone J, Draaisma WA, Broeders IAMJ, Giezeman MJMM, Rinkes IHMB. First experience with robot-assisted thoracoscopic esophagolymphadenectomy for esophageal cancer. Surg Endosc. 2006;20(9):1435–9.
12. Clark J, Sodergren MH, Purkayastha S, Mayer EK, James D, Athanasiou T, et al. The role of robotic assisted laparoscopy for oesophagogastric oncological resection; an appraisal of the literature. Dis Esophagus. 2011;24(4):240–50.
13. Van der Sluis PC, Ruurda JP, van der Horst S, Verhage RJJ, Besselink MGH, Prins JDM. Robot-assisted minimally invasive thoraco-laparoscopic esophagectomy versus open transthoracic esophagectomy for resectable esophageal cancer, a randomized con-trolled trial (ROBOT trial). Trials. 2012;13(230):1–9.
14. Clavien PA, Barkun J, de Oliveira ML, Vauthey JN, Dindo D, Schulick RD, de Santibañes E, Pekolj J, Slankamenac K, Bassi C, Graf R, Vonlanthen R, Padbury R, Cameron JL, Makuuchi

M. The Clavien-Dindo classification of surgical complications: five-year experience. Ann Surg. 2009;250(2):187–96.
15. Van der Sluis PC, van der Horst S, May AM, Schippers C, Brosens LAA, Joore HCA, et al. Robot-assisted minimally invasive thoracolaparoscopic esophagectomy versus open transthoracic esophagectomy for resectable esophageal cancer. A randomized controlled trial. Ann Surg. 2019;269(4):621–30.
16. Hernandez JM, Dimou F, Weber J, Almhanna K, Hoffe S, Shridhar R, Karl R, Meredith K. Defining the learning curve for robotic-assisted esophagogastrectomy. J Gastrointest Surg. 2013;17(8):1346–51.
17. Sarkaria IS, Rizk NP, Grosser R, Goldman D, Finley DJ, Ghanie A, Sima CS, Bains MS, Adusumilli PS, Rusch VW, Jones DR. Attaining proficiency in robotic-assisted minimally invasive esophagectomy while maximizing safety during procedure development. Innovations (Phila). 2016;11:268–73.
18. Van der Sluis PC, Ruurda JP, van der Horst S, Goense L, van Hillegersberg R. Learning curve for robot-assisted minimally invasive thoracoscopic esophagectomy: results from 312 cases. Ann Thorac Surg. 2019;106(1):264–71.
19. Grimminger PP, Tagkalos E, Hadzijusufovic E, Corvinus F, Babic B, Lang H. Change from hybrid to fully minimally invasive and robotic esophagectomy is possible without compromises. Thorac Cardiovasc Surg. 2019;67(7):589–96.
20. Tagkalos E, van der Sluis PC, Berlth F, Poplawski A, Hadzijusufovic E, Lang H, van Berge Henegouwen MI, Gisbertz SS, Müller-Stich BP, Ruurda JP, Schiesser M, Schneider PM, van Hillegersberg R, Grimminger PP. Robot-assisted minimally invasive thoraco-laparoscopic esophagectomy versus minimally invasive esophagectomy for resectable esophageal adenocarcinoma, a randomized controlled trial (ROBOT-2 trial). BMC Cancer. 2021;21(1):1060. https://doi.org/10.1186/s12885-021-08780-x.
21. Chao YK, Li ZG, Wen YW, Kim DJ, Park SY, Chang YL, van der Sluis PC, Ruurda JP, van Hillegersberg R. Robotic-assisted esophagectomy vs video-assisted thoracoscopic esophagectomy (REVATE): study protocol for a randomized controlled trial. Trials. 2019;20:346.
22. Yang Y, Zhang X, Li B, Li Z, Sun Y, Mao T, Hua R, Yang Y, Guo X, He Y, Li H, Chen H, Tan L. Robot-assisted esophagectomy (RAE) versus conventional minimally invasive esophagectomy (MIE) for resectable esophageal squamous cell carcinoma: protocol for a multicenter prospective randomized controlled trial (RAMIE trial, robot-assisted minimally invasive Esophagectomy). BMC Cancer. 2019;19:60.
23. Hung PC, Chen HY, Tu YK, Kao YS. A comparison of different types of esophageal reconstructions: a systematic review and network meta-analysis. J Clin Med. 2022;11(17):5025.
24. Norberg ST. New phosphate langbeinites, $K_2MTi(PO_4)_3$ (M = Er, Yb or Y), and an alternative description of the langbeinite framework. Acta Crystallogr B. 2002;58(Pt 5):743–9.
25. de Delva PE, Morse CR, Austen WG Jr, Gaissert HA, Lanuti M, Wain JC, et al. Surgical management of failed colon interposition. Eur J Cardiothorac Surg. 2008;34(2):432–7; discussion 7.
26. Bakshi A, Sugarbaker DJ, Burt BM. Alternative conduits for esophageal replacement. Ann Cardiothorac Surg. 2017;6(2):137–43.
27. Barkley C, Orringer MB, Iannettoni MD, Yee J. Challenges in reversing esophageal discontinuity operations. Ann Thorac Surg. 2003;76(4):989–94; discussion 95.
28. Orringer MB. Reversing esophageal discontinuity. Semin Thorac Cardiovasc Surg. 2007;19(1):47–55.
29. Rizk NP, Ishwaran H, Rice TW, Chen LQ, Schipper PH, Kesler KA, Law S, Lerut TE, Reed CE, Salo JA, Scott WJ, Hofstetter WL, Watson TJ, Allen MS, Rusch VW, Blackstone EH. Optimum lymphadenectomy for esophageal cancer. Ann Surg. 2010;251(1):46–50.
30. Visser E, Markar SR, Ruurda JP, Hanna GB, van Hillegersberg R. Prognostic value of lymph node yield on overall survival in esophageal cancer patients: a systematic review and meta-analysis. Ann Surg. 2017;269(2):261–8.
31. Kurokawa Y, Takeuchi H, Doki Y, Mine S, Terashima M, Yasuda T, Yoshida K, Daiko H, Sakuramoto S, Yoshikawa T, Kunisaki C, Seto Y, Tamura S, Shimokawa T, Sano T, Kitagawa

Y. Mapping of lymph node metastasis from esophagogastric junction tumors: a prospective nationwide multicenter study. Ann Surg. 2021;274(1):120–7.
32. van der Horst S, de Maat MFG, van der Sluis PC, Ruurda JP, van Hillegersberg R. Extended thoracic lymph node dissection in robotic-assisted minimal invasive esophagectomy (RAMIE) for patients with superior mediastinal lymph node metastasis. Ann Cardiothorac Surg. 2019;8(2):218–25.
33. Hagens ERC, van Berge Henegouwen MI, van Sandick JW, Cuesta MA, van der Peet DL, Heisterkamp J, Nieuwenhuijzen GAP, Rosman C, Scheepers JJG, Sosef MN, van Hillegersberg R, Lagarde SM, Nilsson M, Räsänen J, Nafteux P, Pattyn P, Hölscher AH, Schröder W, Schneider PM, Mariette C, Castoro C, Bonavina L, Rosati R, de Manzoni G, Mattioli S, Garcia JR, Pera M, Griffin M, Wilkerson P, Chaudry MA, Sgromo B, Tucker O, Cheong E, Moorthy K, Walsh TN, Reynolds J, Tachimori Y, Inoue H, Matsubara H, Kosugi SI, Chen H, Law SYK, Pramesh CS, Puntambekar SP, Murthy S, Linden P, Hofstetter WL, Kuppusamy MK, Shen KR, Darling GE, Sabino FD, Grimminger PP, Meijer SL, Bergman JJGHM, Hulshof MCCM, van Laarhoven HWM, Mearadji B, Bennink RJ, Annema JT, Dijkgraaf MGW, Gisbertz SS. Distribution of lymph node metastases in esophageal carcinoma [TIGER study]: study protocol of a multinational observational study. BMC Cancer. 2019;19:662.
34. Low DE, Alderson D, Cecconello I, Chang AC, Darling GE, D'Journo XB, Griffin SM, Hölscher AH, Hofstetter WL, Jobe BA, Kitagawa Y, Kucharczuk JC, Law SY, Lerut TE, Maynard N, Pera M, Peters JH, Pramesh CS, Reynolds JV, Smithers BM, van Lanschot JJ. International consensus on standardization of data collection for complications associated with esophagectomy: Esophagectomy Complications Consensus Group (ECCG). Ann Surg. 2015;262(2):286–94.
35. Schröder W, Raptis DA, Schmidt HM, Gisbertz SS, Moons J, Asti E, Luyer MDP, Hölscher AH, Schneider PM, van Berge Henegouwen MI, Nafteux P, Nilsson M, Räsanen J, Palazzo F, Mercer S, Bonavina L, Nieuwenhuijzen GAP, Wijjnhoven BPL, Pattyn P, Grimminger PP, Bruns CJ, Gutschow CA. Anastomotic techniques and associated morbidity in total minimally invasive transthoracic esophagectomy: results from the EsoBenchmark Database. Ann Surg. 2019;270(5):820–6.
36. Kuppusamy MK, Low DE, International Esodata Study Group (IESG). Evaluation of international contemporary operative outcomes and management trends associated with esophagectomy: a 4-year study of >6000 patients using ECCG definitions and the online Esodata Database. Ann Surg. 2022;275(3):515–25.
37. Fransen LFC, Berkelmans GHK, Asti E, van Berge Henegouwen MI, Berlth F, Bonavina L, Brown A, Bruns C, van Daele E, Gisbertz SS, Grimminger PP, Gutschow CA, Hannink G, Hölscher AH, Kauppi J, Lagarde SM, Mercer S, Moons J, Nafteux P, Nilsson M, Palazzo F, Pattyn P, Raptis DA, Räsanen J, Rosato EL, Rouvelas I, Schmidt HM, Schneider PM, Schröder W, van der Sluis PC, Wijnhoven BPL, Nieuwenhuijzen GAP, Luyer MDP, EsoBenchmark Collaborative. The effect of postoperative complications after minimally invasive esophagectomy on long-term survival: an international multicenter cohort study. Ann Surg. 2020;274(6):e1129–37.
38. Griffiths EA, Oesophago-Gastric Anastomosis Study Group on behalf of the West Midlands Research Collaborative. Rates of anastomotic complications and their management following esophagectomy: results of the Oesophago-Gastric Anastomosis Audit (OGAA). Ann Surg. 2021;275:e382–91.
39. Nickel F, Probst P, Studier-Fischer A, Nienhüser H, Pauly J, Kowalewski KF, Weiterer S, Knebel P, Diener MK, Weigand MA, Büchler MW, Schmidt T, Müller-Stich BP. Minimally Invasive Versus open AbdominoThoracic Esophagectomy for esophageal carcinoma (MIVATE)—study protocol for a randomized controlled trial DRKS00016773. Trials. 2021;22(1):41.
40. Tagkalos E, van der Sluis PC, Uzun E, Berlth F, Staubitz J, Gockel I, van Hillegersberg R, Lang H, Grimminger PP. The circular stapled esophagogastric anastomosis in esophagectomy: no differences in anastomotic insufficiency and stricture rates between the 25 mm and 28 mm circular stapler. J Gastrointest Surg. 2021;25:2242.

41. Allen W, Wells CI, Greenslade M, Bissett IP, O'Grady G. Association between circular stapler diameter and stricture rates following gastrointestinal anastomosis: systematic review and meta-analysis. World J Surg. 2018;42:3097–105.
42. Obermannová R, Alsina M, Cervantes A, Leong T, Lordick F, Nilsson M, van Grieken NCT, Vogel A, Smyth EC, ESMO Guidelines Committee. Oesophageal cancer: ESMO Clinical Practice Guideline for diagnosis, treatment and follow-up. Ann Oncol. 2022;33(10):992–1004.
43. Akiyama H, Miyazono H, Tsurumaru M, et al. Use of the stomach as an esophageal substitute. Ann Surg. 1978;188:606–10.
44. Grimminger PP, van der Sluis PC, Stein H, Lang H, van Hillegersberg R, Egberts JH. Feasibility of transcervical robotic-assisted esophagectomy (TC-RAMIE) in a cadaver study—a future outlook for an extrapleural approach. Appl Sci (Basel). 2019;9:3572.
45. van der Sluis P, Egberts JH, Stein H, Sallum R, van Hillegersberg R, Grimminger PP. Transcervical (SP) and transhiatal DaVinci robotic esophagectomy: a cadaveric study. Thorac Cardiovasc Surg. 2021;69(3):198–203.
46. Nakauchi M, Uyama I, Suda K, et al. Robot-assisted mediastinoscopic esophagectomy for esophageal cancer: the first clinical series. Esophagus. 2019;16(01):85–92.
47. He LR, Qiao W, Liao ZX, Komaki R, Ho L, Hofstetter WL, et al. Impact of comorbidities and use of common medications on cancer and non-cancer specific survival in esophageal carcinoma. BMC Cancer. 2015;15:1095.
48. Arends J, Bachmann P, Baracos V, Barthelemy N, Bertz H, Bozzetti F, et al. ESPEN guidelines on nutrition in cancer patients. Clin Nutr. 2017;36(1):11–48.
49. Hua R, Jiang H, Sun Y, Guo X, Yang Y, Li B, Ye B, Gu H, Mao T, Li Z. Postoperative complications and management of minimally invasive esophagectomy. Shanghai Chest. 2018;2:57.
50. Nishimura K, Tanaka T, Tsubuku T, Matono S, Nagano T, Murata K, Aoyama Y, Yanagawa T, Shirouzu K, Fujita H. Reflux esophagitis after esophagectomy: impact of duodenogastro-esophageal reflux. Dis Esophagus. 2012;25(5):381–5.
51. Markar S, Gronnier C, Duhamel A, Bigourdan JM, Badic B, du Rieu MC, et al. Pattern of postoperative mortality after esophageal cancer resection according to center volume: results from a large European multicenter study. Ann Surg Oncol. 2015;22(8):2615–23.
52. Ozawa S, Koyanagi K, Ninomiya Y, Yatabe K, Higuchi T. Postoperative complications of minimally invasive esophagectomy for esophageal cancer. Ann Gastroenterol Surg. 2020;4(2):126–34.
53. Miao L, Zhang Y, Hu H, Ma L, Shun Y, Xiang J, Chen H. Incidence and management of chylothorax after esophagectomy. Thorac Cancer. 2015;6(3):354–8.
54. Yang Y, Li B, Yi J, Hua R, Chen H, Tan L, Li H, He Y, Guo X, Sun Y, Yu B, Li Z. Robot-assisted versus conventional minimally invasive esophagectomy for resectable esophageal squamous cell carcinoma: early results of a multicenter randomized controlled trial: the RAMIE trial. Ann Surg. 2022;275(4):646–53.
55. Lambertz R, Hölscher AH, Bludau M, Leers JM, Gutschow C, Schröder W. Management of tracheo- or bronchoesophageal fistula after Ivor-Lewis esophagectomy. World J Surg. 2016;40(7):1680–7.
56. Abbas AE, Sarkaria IS. Specific complications and limitations of robotic esophagectomy. Dis Esophagus. 2020;33(Suppl_2):doaa109.
57. Alemzadeh H, Raman J, Leveson N, Kalbarczyk Z, Iyer RK. Adverse events in robotic surgery: a retrospective study of 14 years of FDA data. PLoS One. 2016;11(4):e0151470.

# Thoracoscopic Surgery of Esophagus Cancer

# 23

Kenan Can Ceylan and Arkın Acar

## 23.1 Introduction

Esophagectomy combined with lymphadenectomy is the most effective treatment approach in the multimodal treatment of operable esophageal cancer [1, 2]. However, high mortality and morbidity rates may occur after esophagectomy [3]. A study performed in the United States reported that the mortality rate due to esophagectomy is 8–23%, depending on the surgical volume of the center [4]. In addition, the high morbidity rates in transthoracic approaches stand out as a compelling factor in patients' preference for surgical treatment [5]. Therefore, minimally invasive approaches have begun to be adopted for this currently high-risk surgical method [6, 7].

Today, the thoracoscopic approach is routinely used in many intrathoracic surgical procedures. The minimally invasive approach to esophagectomy was first defined by Dallemagne et al. in the left lateral debit position in 1991 and in the prone position by Cuschieri et al. in 1992 with a series of five cases, as they performed laparoscopy and thoracoscopy on the patients [8]. In 1996, Akaishi et al. reported the first case of thoracoscopic total esophagectomy and mediastinal lymphadenectomy [9]. Kawahara described esophagectomy and extended lymphadenectomy using video-assisted thoracoscopic surgery (VATS) in 1999 [10]. Since this date, an increasing number of minimally invasive esophagectomies have been performed, and approximately half of the patients with esophageal cancer are operated on laparoscopically and thoracoscopically today [11]. Minimally invasive esophagectomy is possible in almost all esophageal cancer operations except high-grade

K. C. Ceylan (✉)
Department of Thoracic Surgery, University of Health Sciences, Dr. Suat Seren Chest Diseases and Surgery Medical Practice and Research Center, Izmir, Turkey

A. Acar
Department of Thoracic Surgery, Manisa Celal Bayar University, Manisa, Turkey


O. Engin (ed.), *Risk Factors and Therapy of Esophagus Cancer*,
https://doi.org/10.1007/978-3-031-47024-0_23

dysplasia, Barrett's esophagus, T4 tumor stage, and one-lung ventilation failure [12, 13].

Thoracoscopy is used as a minimally invasive approach in three-field esophagectomy (McKeown) and the Ivor Lewis method. This chapter reviews the role of thoracoscopy in esophagectomy methods, its technical features, and comparison with the open method.

## 23.2 Surgical Characteristics of the Thoracoscopic Approach

### 23.2.1 Anesthesia and Positioning of the Patient

Esophagectomy is performed with the right hemithorax approach. In doing so, one-lung ventilation is almost always used, with some exceptions, with double-lumen endotracheal tubes as well as endobronchial blockers. The patient is usually placed in the left lateral position. However, there are centers that operate in the prone position [14]. The patient can be tilted 30°–45° ventrally to visualize the posterior mediastinum better and retract the lung anteriorly using gravity. The order of laparoscopy and thoracoscopy should be determined in advance due to the position to be given to the patient. In the McKeown procedure, the patient is usually first started in the left lateral decubitus position. Initially, the thoracic phase is completed, and then the patient is placed in the supine position for the abdominal and cervical phases. On the other hand, the Ivor Lewis method generally starts with the abdominal phase when the patient is in the supine position. Afterward, the patient is taken to the lateral decubitus position, the thoracic phase starts, and the procedure is completed after the esophageal anastomosis [11]. However, if esophageal tumor invasion into intrathoracic structures or pulmonary metastasis is suspected, Ivor Lewis operations can also be started with the thoracic phase first [15].

### 23.2.2 Port Entry Locations

Different surgeons have different approaches to port entries when performing esophagectomy with VATS. The number and locations of ports vary according to patient characteristics and surgeon preferences. While a multiport approach is often used, uniportal VATS applications have also become more common [16, 17]. First, a utility port approximately 4 cm long is opened, usually at the intersection of the fifth intercostal space (ICS) with the posterior axillary line. Some centers can also prefer the sixth ICS for the utility incision. In addition, a port on the eighth ICS on the mid-axillary line for the camera and a third assistant port under the scapular tip or under the scapula on the eighth to ninth ICS can be used (Fig. 23.1). In some centers, four or even five port entries are adopted. The aim is to perform the operation within oncological principles so that the surgeon is most comfortable without placing a rib retractor.

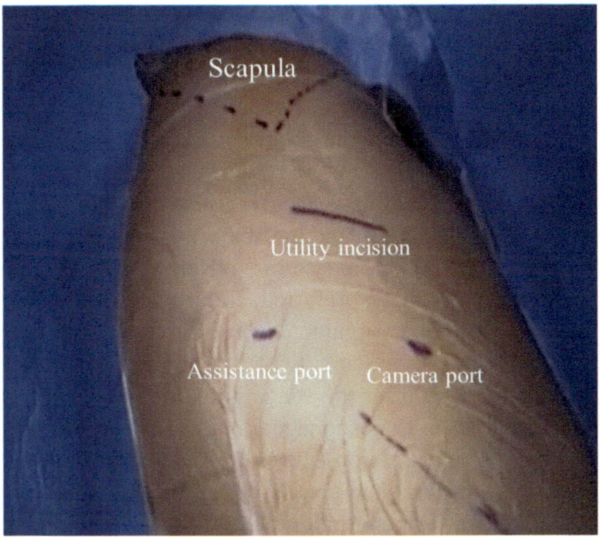


**Fig. 23.1** Port locations for VATS esophagectomy

### 23.2.3 Surgical Equipment

Although the author does not prefer it, some surgeons state that the lung and diaphragm are retracted more comfortably by using $CO_2$ insufflation in VATS operations [18]. However, in VATS operations performed without the use of $CO_2$ insufflation, all conventional surgical instruments used in the open method can also be used, which increases the comfort of the surgeon. In addition, endoscopic graspers, endoscopic scissors, long ovarian clamps, long snake dissectors, endoscopic knot pushers, and coated forceps may facilitate the operations. In addition, the wound retractor to be placed in the utility port both provides comfort and is beneficial when performing the anastomosis.

30° optics with a thickness of 5 or 10 mm are usually used for vision. 0°–120° adjustable optics on the market can also be beneficial in terms of surgeon comfort. High-resolution images can be obtained thanks to the full HD or 4K technology provided on the screens.

Long-tip or hook electrocautery is used as the standard for hemostasis. Furthermore, energy devices operating with ultrasonic or bipolar current principles provide comfort during both hemostasis and dissection (esophagus and lymph nodes) and shorten operation durations. Endoclips and hem-O-lock clips are useful when dissecting and cutting small vascular structures.

Finally, endoscopic staplers are indispensable for thoracoscopic operations. In the esophagectomy operation, the azygos vein is usually divided with a 45-mm endoscopic vascular stapler using a 2.5-mm (white) vascular cartridge. In addition, a 60-mm endoscopic stapler with a green (4.1-mm) cartridge is used when cutting the esophagus or during anastomosis. The use of circular staplers can be preferred while performing the anastomosis.

### 23.2.4 Thoracoscopic Approach in McKeown Esophagectomy

The three-field McKeown procedure, explicitly used for proximal or middle esophagus tumors, has cervical, thoracic, and abdominal phases. After the esophagus is dissected and freed in the abdomen and right hemithorax, the gastric tube is anastomosed in the cervical region [19]. First, the patient is placed in the left lateral decubitus position, and the thoracic phase is completed. Afterward, the patient is placed in the supine position, and the abdominal and cervical phases are performed.

When the thoracic phase of McKeown esophagectomy is achieved with VATS, the utility port and, if preferred, additional camera and assistance ports are opened. First, the pulmonary ligament is freed up to the inferior pulmonary vein. The azygos vein is then dissected and divided using an endoscopic vascular stapler. The procedure to be done after this stage is to free the esophagus by dissecting it from the thoracic inlet to the esophageal hiatus and performing the mediastinal lymphadenectomy. The dissection is usually initiated from the inferior and progressed to the superior. Subcarinal and paraesophageal lymph nodes are dissected and included in the specimen. Depending on the tumor localization, paratracheal lymph nodes can also be added, and lymph nodes on the pulmonary ligament and hilar lymph nodes, if any, are also collected. In the inferior posterior mediastinum, the mediastinal pleura is separated from the anterior and posterior esophagus using an energy device, and then the esophagus is encircled with the help of a dissector (Fig. 23.2). The esophagus is slung with the help of a nylon tape or Penrose drain. It is then completely dissected inferiorly to the diaphragmatic surface and superiorly to the thoracic inlet. During the dissection, it is vital to carefully cauterize the vascular and lymphatic vessels connected to the esophagus with an energy device for possible complications. Care should be taken against the risk of bleeding and chylothorax. Besides, dissections should be performed gently in the subcarinal area and above the tracheobronchial structures regarding possible airway injuries. Excessive traction should be avoided to not damage the recurrent laryngeal nerve at the azygos vein level; dissection should be performed as close to the esophagus as possible. After the esophagus is freed, the procedure is completed following the chest tube placement.

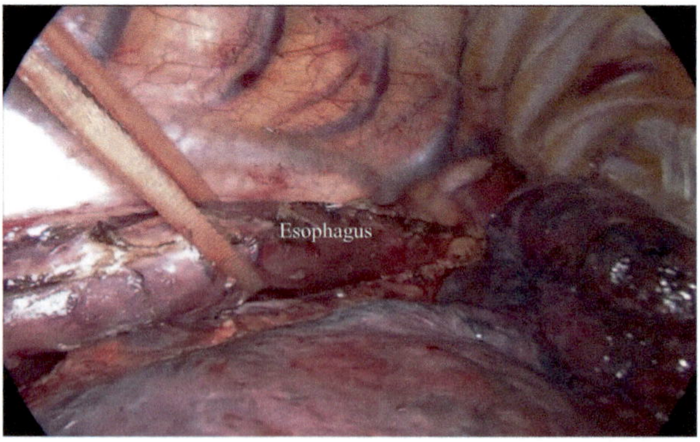


**Fig. 23.2** Encircling esophagus with the help of a nylon tape

### 23.2.5 Thoracoscopic Approach in Ivor Lewis Esophagectomy

The two-phase (abdominal and thoracic) esophagectomy was first described by Ivor Lewis in 1946. Accordingly, in the first operation, the gastric mobilization and creation of the gastric conduit were performed through an abdominal approach, and 15 days later, the thorax was entered with a second operation, the esophagectomy was completed, and the anastomosis was achieved [20]. As it continued to be applied, these two phases were first implemented in the same operative session, and then these phases were performed using minimally invasive methods.

After the abdominal phase is completed, the patient is placed in the left lateral decubitus position. According to the surgeon's preference, port entries are opened, and the thoracoscopic phase begins. The aim is primarily to dissect the esophagus from the thoracic inlet to the esophageal hiatus level and collect the mediastinal lymph nodes, as in the McKeown method. Afterward, an intrathoracic esophagogastric anastomosis is performed. The subcarinal, paraesophageal, and, if any, paratracheal, hilar, and lymph nodes on the pulmonary ligament are collected. The azygos vein is dissected and divided with an endoscopic vascular stapler. The mediastinal pleura is cut, and the tissues anterior and posterior to the esophagus are dissected using an energy device. The esophagus is encircled and slung with nylon tape or a Penrose drain. Then, with the help of the energy device, the esophagus is freed from the inferior to the superior. While dissecting, it is vital to care for the branches from the aorta to the esophagus, the lymphatic vessels, and the membranous wall in the tracheobronchial region. Anastomosis is usually performed at the level of the azygos vein. The proximal esophagus is transected with a 60-mm green endoscopic stapler, leaving a distance of at least 5 cm from the tumor. The gastric conduit prepared in the abdominal phase is gently pulled from the hiatus into the thorax. According to the prepared gastric tube, the distal esophagus-stomach is also cut with a 60-mm green endoscopic stapler, and the specimen is removed from the thorax. The order may vary depending on the anastomosis technique to be used. There are different approaches to esophagogastric anastomosis. VATS end-to-end transthoracic, VATS end-to-end transoral anvil, VATS side-to-side linear-stapled, and VATS hand-sewn anastomosis techniques have been described for the thoracoscopic approach in the literature [21].

The 25, 28, or 33 mm circular staplers are used in end-to-end anastomosis techniques. An anvil must be placed into the proximal esophagus in the transthoracic method. This procedure is usually achieved without cutting the proximal esophagus at full thickness with a stapler. A purse string is applied to the esophagus at the level of the azygos vein using 2–0 polyester or polypropylene sutures. Afterward, a vertical or partial esophagotomy is usually performed 5–10 mm below the purse suture, and the anvil is placed [21, 22]. The anvil is fixed by tying the purse suture, and the esophagotomy is completed (Fig. 23.3). The proximal esophagus is transected with a 60-mm green endoscopic stapler in the transoral anvil technique. Then, a small incision is made on the stapler midline, and the anvil, which is advanced transorally,

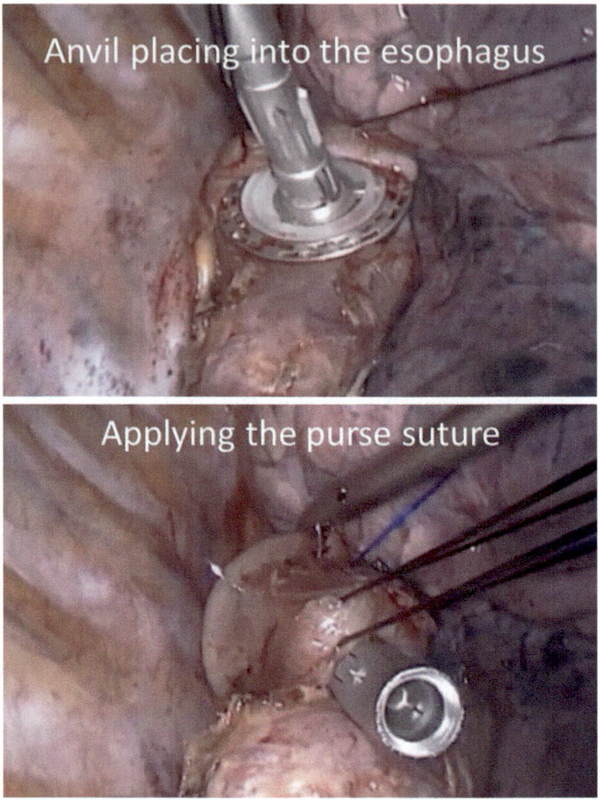


**Fig. 23.3** Preparing the proximal esophagus for the transthoracic anvil technique

is pushed out from the incision and placed (Fig. 23.4). There is currently a transoral anvil attached to a nasogastric tube (Orvil™ Device, Covidien, Dublin, Ireland) on the market. The nasogastric tube sutures to which Orvil™ is attached, which are pushed out of the proximal esophagotomy, are cut and ready for anastomosis [23]. The only disadvantage of the transoral anvil is that it is available in one size (25 mm) and unsuitable for the dilated esophagus. After the anvil is placed either in the transthoracic or transoral techniques, a gastrotomy is made over the gastric conduit, and a circular stapler is placed. After the anvil connection is established, the stapler is fired, and the anastomosis is created. The ring-shaped tissue in the stapler should be sent to the pathology unit to study the surgical margin.

Another commonly used esophagogastric anastomosis technique is side-to-side anastomosis using linear staplers. In this method, the specimen is first taken out of the thorax. An incision is then made on the staple line of the proximal esophagus, and a nasogastric tube is pushed out of the esophagus. The gastric conduit is then taken out through the utility incision, and a gastrotomy is performed at the distal end. Stay sutures are placed on both the esophagus and the gastric conduit in order to maneuver and place the stapler comfortably. A 60-mm endoscopic thick tissue stapler is prepared, and one leg is inserted into the gastric conduit. With the help of

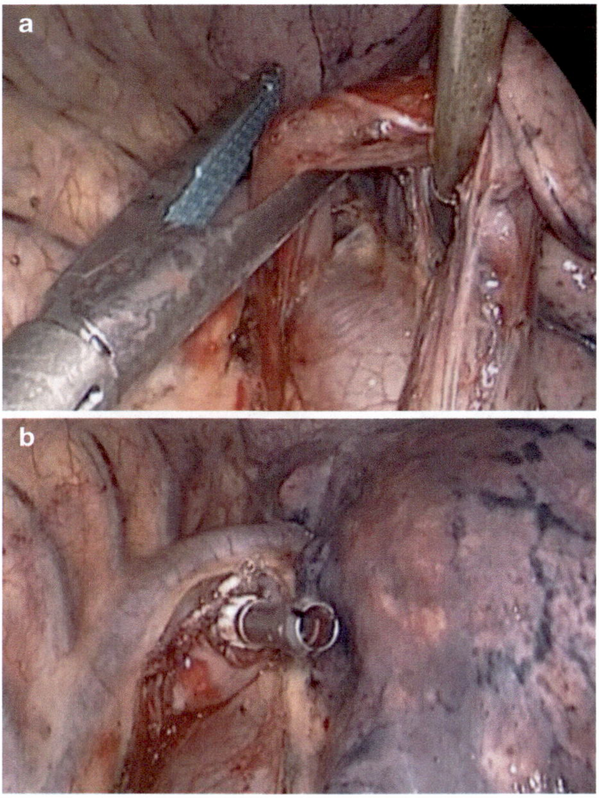


**Fig. 23.4** (**a**) Transecting the proximal esophagus with a stapler. (**b**) Pushing the transoral anvil through the esophagotomy under the stapler line

a stay suture, the gastric conduit is placed back into the thorax together with the stapler, and the other leg of the stapler is placed in the esophagus. With the help of stay sutures, both legs of the stapler are advanced at an equal distance, and then the stapler is fired (Fig. 23.5). Thus, the posterior of the anastomosis is completed. The anterior gastrotomy and esophagotomy lines are closed using another 60-mm endoscopic green stapler, and the anastomosis is completed [16].

Lastly, the anastomosis can be sutured end-to-side thoracoscopically in the hand-sewn technique. Here, high-level endoscopic-thoracoscopic suturing experience is required. A gastrotomy is performed over the gastric conduit to the greater curvature, and the posterior wall of the esophagus is sutured superiorly to the gastrotomy incision using interrupted sutures. Afterward, the anterior of the esophagus and the inferior of the gastrotomy are combined with continuous suturing, and the anastomosis is completed [21].

There are many factors when choosing the anastomosis technique, such as the surgeon's experience, the health status of the esophagus (such as neoadjuvant therapy), and the length of the gastric conduit. A meta-analysis published in 2022 reported that strictures developed less in linear-stapled anastomosis than in circular-stapled anastomosis [24]. However, it should not be forgotten that a longer gastric

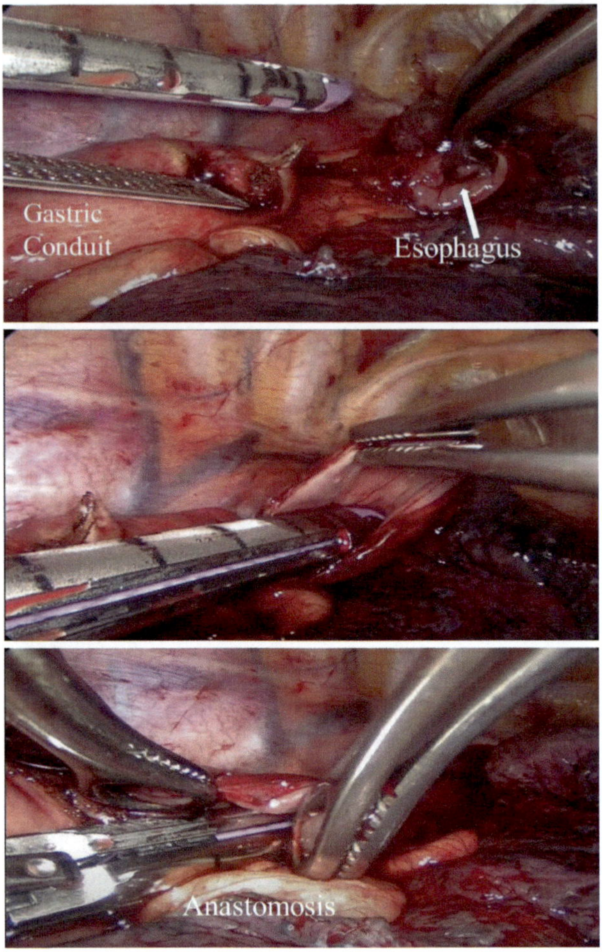


**Fig. 23.5** Performing the anastomosis in the side-to-side technique using an endoscopic stapler

conduit is needed to perform side-to-side with the linear stapler. In the short residual proximal esophagus and also in the presence of a short gastric conduit, a more comfortable anastomosis can be performed with a circular stapler. In a recently published meta-analysis, hand-sewn, linear-stapled, and circular-stapled anastomoses were compared, and it was reported that lower rates of anastomotic leakage were detected in circular-stapled anastomosis compared to the other two methods [25]. Whichever method is used, ensuring proper anastomosis tension and good blood supply to the tissues to be anastomized are considered the most crucial factors.

When the anastomosis is completed, supporting the anastomosis line with a healthy tissue flap is often recommended. After checking for anastomotic leakage by injecting air into a nasogastric tube in the esophagus, an omental flap to be pulled from the abdomen or an intrathoracic thymopericardial fatty tissue flap can be used to support the anastomosis line. Finally, chest tubes are placed, and VATS is terminated by closing the opened port entrances.

### 23.2.6 Advantages of Thoracoscopic Esophagectomy

Thoracotomy itself, together with the physiological changes it causes, may result in deterioration in respiratory functions in the patient even if no additional procedure is performed [26]. Therefore, choosing thoracoscopy instead of thoracotomy will inevitably lead to decreased respiratory complications such as atelectasis and pneumonia. Since its application became widespread, minimally invasive esophagectomies have been compared with the open method many times.

In 2013, Wu et al. compared VATS and the open method in esophagectomy and reported less intraoperative blood loss and faster recovery in the VATS group [27]. Moreover, in another study, higher quality of life scores were obtained in the first 6 months after esophagectomy with VATS compared to the open method [28]. Tan et al. on the other hand, stated that after esophagectomy with VATS, patients returned to their former immune system status more quickly compared to thoracotomy [29]. In the McKeown procedure, which is technically relatively easy, uniportal VATS and the open method were compared. Accordingly, similar oncological and survival outcomes were obtained in VATS group patients compared to the open method, and faster and uneventful recovery was reported. In addition, although it was uniportal, it was stated that there was a fast learning curve within the nature of the procedure [30].

Similar results have been obtained in the meta-analyses. A meta-analysis by Lv et al. demonstrated that a minimally invasive approach resulted in less blood loss, fewer respiratory complications, and better overall survival [31]. Guo et al. reported that thoracoscopic-laparoscopic esophagectomy groups had a lower rate of total complications, wound infections, and pulmonary complications. It was also emphasized that there was no compromise in the 5-year survival compared to the open method [32]. Finally, the TIME trial revealed no significant differences in disease-free and 3-year overall survival between the open and minimally invasive esophagectomy groups. Considering the short-term advantages, it was stated that minimally invasive methods should be preferred [33].

## 23.3 Conclusion

Esophagectomy operations may already cause high mortality and morbidity rates due to the physiological changes they cause, multi-phase and multi-site operation techniques, and often the presence of neoadjuvant therapy. Considering the burden that the thoracotomy method would create on the patient, thoracoscopy is an option that should be considered due to the advantages it provides. Thoracoscopy should be preferred for esophagectomy in experienced centers. However, as with any thoracoscopic operation, conversion to the open method is a possibility that should always be considered because of possible complications. The surgical team should prepare accordingly. Another point is that although the thoracoscopic method provides many advantages, oncological principles should always be followed. This way, patients may complete this challenging treatment with a more comfortable postoperative period, more satisfactory outcomes, and a faster recovery.

**Acknowledgments** The authors would like to thank Prof. Dr. Atila Eroglu for his valuable suggestions and contributions to the article.

## References

1. Ando N, Ozawa S, Kitagawa Y, Shinozawa Y, Kitajima M. Improvement in the results of surgical treatment of advanced squamous esophageal carcinoma during 15 consecutive years. Ann Surg. 2000;232(2):225–32. https://doi.org/10.1097/00000658-200008000-00013.
2. Altorki NK, Zhou XK, Stiles B, Port JL, Paul S, Lee PC, et al. Total number of resected lymph nodes predicts survival in esophageal cancer. Ann Surg. 2008;248(2):221–6. https://doi.org/10.1097/SLA.0b013e31817bbe59.
3. Markar S, Gronnier C, Duhamel A, Bigourdan JM, Badic B, du Rieu MC, et al. Pattern of postoperative mortality after esophageal cancer resection according to center volume: results from a large European multicenter study. Ann Surg Oncol. 2015;22(8):2615–23. https://doi.org/10.1245/s10434-014-4310-5.
4. Birkmeyer JD, Siewers AE, Finlayson EV, Stukel TA, Lucas FL, Batista I, et al. Hospital volume and surgical mortality in the United States. N Engl J Med. 2002;346(15):1128–37. https://doi.org/10.1056/NEJMsa012337.
5. Worrell SG, Gupta S, Alvarado CE, Sarode A, Luo X, Towe CW, et al. Morbidity after esophagectomy is higher for benign than malignant disease. Ann Thorac Surg. 2023;115(2):363–9. https://doi.org/10.1016/j.athoracsur.2022.08.043.
6. Luketich JD, Pennathur A, Awais O, Levy RM, Keeley S, Shende M, et al. Outcomes after minimally invasive esophagectomy: review of over 1000 patients. Ann Surg. 2012;256(1):95–103. https://doi.org/10.1097/SLA.0b013e3182590603.
7. Palanivelu C, Prakash A, Senthilkumar R, Senthilnathan P, Parthasarathi R, Rajan PS, et al. Minimally invasive esophagectomy: thoracoscopic mobilization of the esophagus and mediastinal lymphadenectomy in prone position—experience of 130 patients. J Am Coll Surg. 2006;203(1):7–16. https://doi.org/10.1016/j.jamcollsurg.2006.03.016.
8. Cuschieri A, Shimi S, Banting S. Endoscopic oesophagectomy through a right thoracoscopic approach. J R Coll Surg Edinb. 1992;37(1):7–11.
9. Akaishi T, Kaneda I, Higuchi N, Kuriya Y, Kuramoto J, Toyoda T, et al. Thoracoscopic en bloc total esophagectomy with radical mediastinal lymphadenectomy. J Thorac Cardiovasc Surg. 1996;112(6):1533–40.; discussion 40–1. https://doi.org/10.1016/s0022-5223(96)70012-0.
10. Kawahara K, Maekawa T, Okabayashi K, Hideshima T, Shiraishi T, Yoshinaga Y, et al. Video-assisted thoracoscopic esophagectomy for esophageal cancer. Surg Endosc. 1999;13(3):218–23. https://doi.org/10.1007/s004649900948.
11. Peng JS, Kukar M, Mann GN, Hochwald SN. Minimally invasive esophageal cancer surgery. Surg Oncol Clin N Am. 2019;28(2):177–200. https://doi.org/10.1016/j.soc.2018.11.009.
12. Eroglu A, Ulas AB, Aydin Y. Özofagus kanserleri. In: Gursoy S, editor. Göğüs Cerrahisinde Videotorakoskopi Uygulamaları. Ankara: Türkiye Klinikleri; 2021. p. 81–4.
13. Shichinohe T, Hirano S, Kondo S. Video-assisted esophagectomy for esophageal cancer. Surg Today. 2008;38(3):206–13. https://doi.org/10.1007/s00595-007-3606-5.
14. Booka E, Takeuchi H, Kikuchi H, Hiramatsu Y, Kamiya K, Kawakubo H, et al. Recent advances in thoracoscopic esophagectomy for esophageal cancer. Asian J Endosc Surg. 2019;12(1):19–29. https://doi.org/10.1111/ases.12681.
15. Eroglu A, Aydin Y. VATS esophageal surgery. Güncel Göğüs Hastalıkları Serisi. 2020;8(1):53–62.
16. Batirel H. Uniportal VATS approach in esophageal cancer—how to do it update. Front Surg. 2022;9:844796. https://doi.org/10.3389/fsurg.2022.844796.
17. Nachira D, Meacci E, Mastromarino MG, Pogliani L, Zanfrini E, Iaffaldano A, et al. Initial experience with uniportal video-assisted thoracic surgery esophagectomy. J Thorac Dis. 2018;10(Suppl 31):S3686–s95. https://doi.org/10.21037/jtd.2018.04.17.

18. Ninomiya I, Okamoto K, Fushida S, Oyama K, Kinoshita J, Takamura H, et al. Efficacy of $CO_2$ insufflation during thoracoscopic esophagectomy in the left lateral position. Gen Thorac Cardiovasc Surg. 2017;65(10):587–93. https://doi.org/10.1007/s11748-017-0816-7.
19. McKeown KC. Total three-stage oesophagectomy for cancer of the oesophagus. Br J Surg. 1976;63(4):259–62. https://doi.org/10.1002/bjs.1800630403.
20. Lewis I. The surgical treatment of carcinoma of the oesophagus; with special reference to a new operation for growths of the middle third. Br J Surg. 1946;34:18–31. https://doi.org/10.1002/bjs.18003413304.
21. Caso R, Wee JO. Esophagogastric anastomotic techniques for minimally invasive and robotic Ivor Lewis operations. Oper Tech Thorac Cardiovasc Surg. 2020;25(2):105–23.
22. Seong YW. Video-assisted thoracic surgery intrathoracic anastomosis technique. J Chest Surg. 2021;54(4):286–93. https://doi.org/10.5090/jcs.21.083.
23. Eroğlu A, Daharlı C, Bilal Ulaş A, Keskin H, Aydın Y. Minimally invasive Ivor-Lewis esophagectomy for esophageal cancer. Turk gogus kalp damar cerrahisi dergisi. 2022;30(3):421–30. https://doi.org/10.5606/tgkdc.dergisi.2022.22232.
24. Aiolfi A, Sozzi A, Bonitta G, Lombardo F, Cavalli M, Cirri S, et al. Linear- versus circular-stapled esophagogastric anastomosis during esophagectomy: systematic review and meta-analysis. Langenbecks Arch Surg. 2022;407(8):3297–309. https://doi.org/10.1007/s00423-022-02706-2.
25. Schlottmann F, Angeramo CA, Bras Harriott C, Casas MA, Herbella FAM, Patti MG. Transthoracic esophagectomy: hand-sewn versus side-to-side linear-stapled versus circular-stapled anastomosis: a systematic review and meta-analysis. Surg Laparosc Endosc Percutan Tech. 2022;32(3):380–92. https://doi.org/10.1097/sle.0000000000001050.
26. Sabanathan S, Eng J, Mearns AJ. Alterations in respiratory mechanics following thoracotomy. J R Coll Surg Edinb. 1990;35(3):144–50.
27. Wu X, He J, Jiang H, Song X, Tang X, Shen J, et al. Fully thoracoscopic versus conventional open resection for esophageal carcinoma: a perioperative comparison. Thoracic Cancer. 2013;4(4):369–72. https://doi.org/10.1111/1759-7714.12028.
28. Wang H, Feng M, Tan L, Wang Q. Comparison of the short-term quality of life in patients with esophageal cancer after subtotal esophagectomy via video-assisted thoracoscopic or open surgery. Dis Esophagus. 2010;23(5):408–14. https://doi.org/10.1111/j.1442-2050.2009.01025.x.
29. Tan JT, Zhong JH, Yang Y, Mao NQ, Liu DS, Huang DM, et al. Comparison of postoperative immune function in patients with thoracic esophageal cancer after video-assisted thoracoscopic surgery or conventional open esophagectomy. Int J Surg (London, England). 2016;30:155–60. https://doi.org/10.1016/j.ijsu.2016.04.052.
30. Nachira D, Congedo MT, Calabrese G, Tabacco D, Petracca Ciavarella L, Meacci E, et al. Uniportal-VATS vs. open McKeown esophagectomy: surgical and long-term oncological outcomes. Front Surg. 2023;10:1103101. https://doi.org/10.3389/fsurg.2023.1103101.
31. Lv L, Hu W, Ren Y, Wei X. Minimally invasive esophagectomy versus open esophagectomy for esophageal cancer: a meta-analysis. Onco Targets Ther. 2016;9:6751–62. https://doi.org/10.2147/ott.s112105.
32. Guo W, Ma X, Yang S, Zhu X, Qin W, Xiang J, et al. Combined thoracoscopic-laparoscopic esophagectomy versus open esophagectomy: a meta-analysis of outcomes. Surg Endosc. 2016;30(9):3873–81. https://doi.org/10.1007/s00464-015-4692-x.
33. Straatman J, van der Wielen N, Cuesta MA, Daams F, Roig Garcia J, Bonavina L, et al. Minimally invasive versus open esophageal resection: 3-year follow-up of the previously reported randomized controlled trial: the TIME trial. Ann Surg. 2017;266(2):232–6. https://doi.org/10.1097/sla.0000000000002171.

# 24 Management of Thoracic Esophagus Cancer

Omer Engin

The esophagus begins in the neck after the pharynx, runs in the thorax, enters the abdomen, and continues with the stomach. Esophageal cancer can occur in the cervical, thoracic, and abdominal regions, and treatment approaches for each region are different. While chemoradiotherapy is preferred instead of surgical treatment in cervical esophagus, surgical treatment is preferred in thoracic and abdominal region esophageal cancer [1].

In thoracic esophageal cancers, transhiatal esophagectomy (THE) can be performed by reaching the esophagus through the diaphragmatic hiatus, or a transthoracic esophagectomy (TTE) is performed under direct vision, including lymph node dissection, by reaching through the thoracic wall. Transhiatal and transthoracic esophagus surgery can be performed with the help of open surgery and minimally invasive surgery. As open surgery, laparotomy, left thoracotomy, right thoracotomy, bilateral thoracotomy, and transhiatal way without thoracotomy can be performed. As minimally invasive surgeries, laparoscopic or robotic abdominal surgery, thoracoscopic esophagectomy, robotic thoracic esophagectomy, and minimally invasive transhiatal esophagectomy are applied. These methods can also be combined, depending on the surgeon's preference. Since video-assisted thoracic surgery (VATS) and robotic esophagectomy are explained in detail in the relevant sections, they will not be mentioned in this section. In transhiatal esophagectomy, however, the esophagus is freed by blunt dissection and removed from the cervical region or the abdomen and anastomosis is made in the cervical region for gastrointestinal continuity. After the thoracic esophagus is removed, stomach, proximal jejunum, and colon can be used for gastrointestinal continuity and the anastomosis can be made in the thorax or in the cervical region [2–4].

O. Engin (✉)
Surgery Department, VM Medical Park Pendik Hospital, Istanbul, Türkiye



O. Engin (ed.), *Risk Factors and Therapy of Esophagus Cancer*, https://doi.org/10.1007/978-3-031-47024-0_24

## 24.1 Transhiatal Esophagectomies

Transhiatal esophagectomies can be performed as transhiatal esophagectomy with open surgery. The other method is a combined form of transhiatal esophagectomy with minimally invasive methods. Minimally invasive methods can be in the form of laparoscopic or robotic abdominal surgery. This method may be preferred for early-stage esophageal cancers or lesions that have shrunk after neoadjuvant therapy. In this method, intrathoracic lymph node dissection is not performed. Lower thoracic lymph node dissection can be performed because it is close to the abdomen. A similar incidence of anastomotic leak was detected in the comparison between the patients who underwent THE and TTE [5].

In a retrospective review by Chang et al. 868 patients underwent esophagectomy. Transhiatal esophagectomy was performed in 225 patients and transthoracic esophagectomy in 643 patients. A lower operative mortality rate was observed after a transhiatal operation than transthoracic esophagectomy. 5-year survival was higher in patients undergoing transhiatal rather than transthoracic esophagectomy. After adjusting for differences in esophageal cancer stage, provider factors, and patient, this survival advantage was no longer statistically significant [6].

In transhiatal esophagectomy with open surgery, the abdomen is entered with a midline laparotomy. The vagus nerve is cut, and the esophagus is freed. Entering the diaphragmatic hiatus, the esophagus is freed from the surrounding tissues with the fingers, and the upper cervical region is reached. It starts from the posterior wall of the esophagus first. When the posterior wall dissection is completed, the right and left esophageal walls are similarly dissected. After dissecting the posterior right and left walls of the esophagus, the anterior wall is finally dissected. Here, the posterior wall of the trachea and the anterior wall of the esophagus are adjacent. Care must be taken when separating the anterior wall of the esophagus from the posterior wall of the trachea, because the posterior wall of the trachea has a thin layer of tissue rather than cartilage, and this thin tracheal wall can be easily torn. Cervical region dissection is also similar. First, the posterior wall of the esophagus is dissected. Then the left lateral and then the right lateral are dissected. Then, the last anterior esophageal wall is separated from the trachea by blunt dissection. After the dissection is completed, the esophagus is removed from the cervical region, the gastric conduit is brought to the mediastinal region, and esophagogastrostomy is performed [7–9] (Fig. 24.1).

This blunt dissection requires experience. I would like to emphasize that in order to learn these dissection movements, it is necessary to perform transhiatal esophagectomy with an experienced surgeon who performs this dissection.

Esophagogastrostomy can be done end-to-end or end-to-side. This anastomosis can be performed with a surgical stapler or with a hand-sewn anastomosis. I prefer to do end-to-side anastomosis. In end-to-side anastomosis, the anterior surface of the gastric fundus is brought to the lower end of the esophagus. An incision is made for anastomosis to the anterior surface of the fundus, a few cm below the apex in the uppermost region of the fundus. The posterior margin of the lower end of the esophagus and the posterior margin of the fundus incision are sutured. Sutures are then

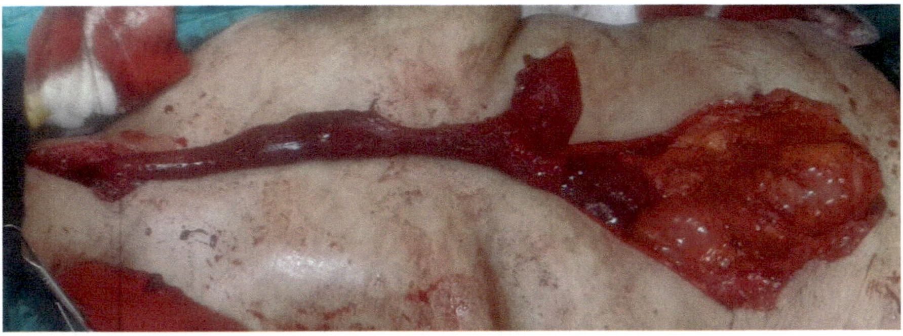

**Fig. 24.1** Patient who underwent transhiatal esophagectomy. Laparotomy was performed; after transection involving the cardia and part of the lesser curvature, the esophagus was removed from the cervical incision when the transhiatal esophageal dissection was completed with finger dissection. The esophagus was removed from the cervical incision and placed on the sternum. The incision line to be made from the cervical region is shown with silk sutures on the right and left of the esophagus

placed between the lateral and anterior margins of the lower end of the esophagus and the lateral and anterior margins of the fundus incision. In this way, since the fundus will cover the back of the esophagus by a few centimeters, suture safety in this area is increased. Suturing the gastric fundus to the prevertebral fascia with several sutures may prevent the stomach from descending by gravity, which may be effective in reducing anastomotic tension [10, 11].

There are different variations in minimally invasive transhiatel esophagectomy. The stomach is prepared as a gastric conduit by the laparoscopic method. A cervical incision is made, and the vein stripping "inversion" technique may be preferred for esophageal removal from the cervical region. Sometimes, for the stripping process, the entrance is made from the cervical region and the esophagus is removed through the abdominal way. Esophagogastrostomy is performed in the cervical region. Laparoscopic intra-abdominal preparation can also be performed with robotic surgery [12–14].

## 24.2 Transthoracic Esophagectomies

Transthoracic esophagectomies can be performed by open surgery or minimally invasive surgery (VATS and robotic surgery).

### 24.2.1 Transthoracic Operations with Open Surgeries

#### 24.2.1.1 Laparotomy Stage

A laparotomy can be performed with a midline incision. The lower part of the esophagus is released by the abdominal route. A gastric conduit is created, and pyloroplasty is performed. The abdominal phase can also be combined with a minimally invasive method [15].

### 24.2.2 Thoracic Open Surgery Stages

#### 24.2.2.1 Left Thoracotomy

Left thoracotomy and left thoracoabdominal intervention are methods of choice in lower esophageal tumors. However, the majority of people prefer laparotomy and right thoracotomy to obtain a tumor-free surgical margin in the esophageal wall. If gastric invasion is also present in lower esophageal tumors, the surgical method may be changed [16–20].

#### 24.2.2.2 Right Thoracotomy

Right thoracotomy is the most preferred method in open surgery of the esophagus. Right thoracotomy is used in two field (Ivor Lewis esophagectomy) and three field (McKeown esophagectomy) operations [21].

In the Ivor Lewis operation, the abdomen is entered with the midline, the peritoneum is opened around the esophagus, and the vagus is cut. After the esophagus is released, it is passed into the thoracic cavity. The thoracic cavity is entered with a right thoracotomy. The lung is pulled medially with the help of retractors, the pleura on the esophagus is opened, and the esophagus is dissected. In dissection, intra-abdominal and intrathoracic lymph nodes around the esophagus are also included. Resection is performed approximately 10 cm proximal to the tumor tissue. It is appropriate to see that the surgical margins are tumor-free with a frozen section after resection. After the esophagus is removed, the gastric conduit, colon, or proximal jejunum is brought to the intrathoracic space and a stapled or hand-sewn anastomosis is made. At the end of the surgery, the thoracic tube is placed into the thoracic cavity [22–24].

In the McKeown operation, after the completion of the abdominal and thoracic cavity stages, the anastomosis is performed in the cervical region. The proximal jejunum cannot reach the cervical region. Gastric conduit or colon is used for cervical anastomosis. In cervical esophageal resections, it may be more appropriate to use free jejunum graft [25].

#### 24.2.2.3 Bilateral Thoracotomy

Although not in routine practice, esophagectomies performed with bilateral thoracotomy are also reported in case reports for special cases [26, 27].

### 24.2.3 Transthoracic Operations With Minimally Invasive Surgeries

Transthoracic minimally invasive methods include VATS and robotic intrathoracic esophageal resection. Minimally invasive esophagectomy can be performed in two or three fields. The abdominal section can be done laparoscopically or robotically. The thoracic phase can be in the form of video-assisted thoracoscopic surgery (VATS) or robotic surgery. If the anastomosis is made in the thorax, it can be defined as two fields; if the anastomosis is made in the cervical region, it can be defined as three fields. These two methods will be examined in detail in other parts of the book [28, 29].

### 24.2.4 Salvage Esophagectomy

After patients are treated with chemotherapy and radiotherapy instead of surgery, if local regional relapse without distant metastasis, or if the primary tumor persists, esophagectomy is called salvage esophagectomy [30, 31].

Salvage esophagectomy has high postoperative morbidity. The risk of fistula development is higher in anastomoses. Salvage esophagectomies have poor survival outcomes [32, 33].

## References

1. Menezes MA, Sato RO, Schlottmann F, et al. Esophageal anatomy. In: Esophageal cancer: diagnosis and treatment. Springer; 2018. p. 1–13.
2. van der Sluis PC, Schizas D, Liakakos T, et al. Minimally invasive esophagectomy. Dig Surg. 2020;37(2):93–100.
3. Bao T, Wang YJ, Li KK, Zhao XL, Liu B, He XD, et al. Safety and feasibility of three-dimensional McKeown minimally invasive esophagectomy. In: Surgical endoscopy. Springer; 2023. p. 1–7.
4. Lin CH, Chuang CY, Ko JL, et al. Experiences in reverse sequence esophagectomy: a promising alternative for esophageal cancer surgery. Surg Endosc. 2023;37:1–12.
5. Schlottmann F, Strassle PD, Patti MG. Transhiatal vs. transthoracic esophagectomy: a NSQIP analysis of postoperative outcomes and risk factors for morbidity. J Gastrointest Surg. 2017;21:1757–63.
6. Chang AC, Ji H, Birkmeyer NJ, Orringer MB, et al. Outcomes after transhiatal and transthoracic esophagectomy for cancer. Ann Thorac Surg. 2008;85(2):424–9.
7. Orringer MB. Transhiatal esophagectomy: how I teach it. Ann Thorac Surg. 2016;102(5):1432–7.
8. Dubecz A, Kun L, Stadlhuber RJ, Peters JH, et al. The origins of an operation: a brief history of transhiatal esophagectomy. Ann Surg. 2009;249(3):535–40.
9. Melis M, Bizekis CS, Gouge TH. Minimally invasive esophagectomy. In: Chassins operative strategy in general surgery: an expositive atlas. Springer; 2014. p. 171–80.
10. Orringer MB, Marshall B, Iannettoni MD. Eliminating the cervical esophagogastric anastomotic leak with a side-to-side stapled anastomosis. J Thorac Cardiovasc Surg. 2000;119(2):277–88.
11. Bardini R, Bonavina L, Asolati M, Ruol A, Castoro C, et al. Single-layered cervical esophageal anastomoses: a prospective study of two suturing techniques. Ann Thorac Surg. 1994;58(4):1087–9.
12. Avital S, Zundel N, Szomstein S, et al. Laparoscopic transhiatal esophagectomy for esophageal cancer. Am J Surg. 2005;190(1):69–74.
13. Horgan S, Berger RA, Elli EF, et al. Robotic-assisted minimally invasive transhiatal esophagectomy. Am Surg. 2003;69(7):624–6.

14. Sanders G, Borie F, Husson E, Blanc PM, Mauro GD, Claus C, et al. Minimally invasive transhiatal esophagectomy: lessons learned. Surg Endosc. 2007;21:1190–3.
15. Sgourakis G, Gockel I, Radtke A, Musholt TJ, Timm S, Rink A, et al. Minimally invasive versus open esophagectomy: meta-analysis of outcomes. Dig Dis Sci. 2010;55:3031–40.
16. Ozkan M, Okten I. Özofagus kanserinde transtorasik özofagus rezeksiyonu. J Exp Clin Med. 2012;29(4S):233–6.
17. Yang Y, Xin X, Chen P, Shi X, Yang C, Fan J, et al. Left compared with right thoracic approach thoracotomy in esophageal cancer: a retrospective cohort study. J Cancer Res Clin Oncol. 2023;149:1–8.
18. Barreto JC, Posner MC. Transhiatal versus transthoracic esophagectomy for esophageal cancer. World J Gastroenterol WJG. 2010;16(30):3804.
19. Zheng Y, Li Y, Liu X, Zhang R, Sun H, et al. Right compared with left thoracic approach esophagectomy for patients with middle esophageal squamous cell carcinoma. Front Oncol. 2020;10:536842.
20. Yang D, Mao YS, He J, Gao SG, Sun KL, Mu JW, et al. Long-term survival of the middle and lower thoracic esophageal cancer patients after surgical treatment through left or right thoracic approach. J Thorac Dis. 2018;10(5):2648.
21. Kono K. McKeown esophagectomy. In: Lomanto D, Chen WTL, Fuentes MB, editors. Mastering endo-laparoscopic and thoracoscopic surgery. Singapore: Springer; 2023. https://doi.org/10.1007/978-981-19-3755-2_37.
22. Li B, et al. Esophagectomy with three-field versus two-field lymphadenectomy for middle and lower thoracic esophageal cancer: long-term outcomes of a randomized clinical trial. J Thorac Oncol. 2021;16(2):310–7.
23. Zheng Y-Z, et al. Impact of examined lymph node count for esophageal squamous cell carcinoma in patients who underwent right transthoracic esophagectomy. Ann Surg Oncol. 2021;28:3025–33.
24. Qaraqe TM, Low DE. Ivor Lewis esophagectomy. In: Atlas of esophageal surgery. Cham: Springer International Publishing; 2022. p. 125–38.
25. Sabra MJ, Alwatari YA, Wolfe LG, Xu A, Kaplan BJ, Cassano AD, et al. Ivor Lewis vs Mckeown esophagectomy: analysis of operative outcomes from the ACS NSQIP database. Gen Thorac Cardiovasc Surg. 2020;68:370–9.
26. Shimada Y, Kawabe A, Nakajima S, Hata K, Takahashi Y, Kume M, et al. A bilateral thoracic approach for esophageal cancer in the prone position. Surg Today. 2015;45:91–5.
27. Fujiwara H, Sato T, Okada N, Fujita T, Kojima T, et al. Thoracoscopic esophagectomy with three-field lymphadenectomy for thoracic esophageal cancer in a patient with a double aortic arch: a report of a case. Surg Case Rep. 2019;5(1):1–7.
28. Hu ZH, Li RX, Wang JT, Wang GJ, Deng XM, Zhu TY, et al. Thoracolaparoscopic esophagectomy for esophageal cancer with a cervical incision to extract specimen. Asian J Surg. 2023;46(1):348–53.
29. Zhang Y, Han Y, Gan Q, Xiang J, Jin R, Chen K, et al. Early outcomes of robot-assisted versus thoracoscopic-assisted Ivor Lewis esophagectomy for esophageal cancer: a propensity score-matched study. Ann Surg Oncol. 2019;26:1284–91.
30. Swisher SG, Wynn P, Putnam JB, Mosheim MB, Correa AM, Komaki RR, et al. Salvage esophagectomy for recurrent tumors after definitive chemotherapy and radiotherapy. J Thorac Cardiovasc Surg. 2002;123(1):175–83.
31. Hofstetter WL. Salvage esophagectomy. J Thorac Dis. 2014;6(Suppl 3):S341.
32. Broderick RC, Lee AM, Blitzer RR, Zhao B, Lam J, Cheverie JN, et al. It's not always too late: a case for minimally invasive salvage esophagectomy. Surg Endosc. 2021;35:4700–11.
33. Choe G, Molena D. Surgery versus active surveillance in clinical complete response. Ann Esophagus. 2021;4:31.

# Colon and Jejunum Interposition After Esophagectomy

# 25

Okan Demiray and Mehmet Lari Gedik

Total or long segmental esophagectomies in esophageal malignant tumors depend on the localization in cases where the endoscopic surgical boundaries are crossed. Following these operations, anastomosis is the most common procedure that involves the stomach being pulled up into the thorax or neck as a substitute for the esophagus. In this chapter, the methods employed to ensure continuity after esophageal removal in cases such as prior gastric surgeries or the requirement for gastrectomy due to tumor dissemination across the stomach are discussed [1].

The optimal conduit is always the patient's own esophagus; therefore, every effort should be made to preserve and use the native esophagus whenever possible. No peristalsis is observed since, instead of engaging in intrinsic peristaltic activity, all conduits used for esophageal replacement function as passive tubes. Consequently, a short and straight conduit is the best option. Typically, the posterior mediastinum is the shortest and straightest pathway. If the posterior mediastinum cannot be dissected safely, the presternal route can be used as an alternative. Preventing content from flowing back into the replaced segment is critical. An interpositional procedure connecting the normal distal esophageal junction to the gastrointestinal tract may be useful to prevent reflux complications. Although anastomotic strictures that may develop in this setting can be dilated, they often need to be revised. Rather than using complex, poorly functioning interpositions, the straightest, lowest resistance conduit is important [1, 2].

Gastric tubes are preferred in young individuals, while gastric transposition is preferred in the elderly. Usually, this preference can be explained by the simplicity of the technique and the resistance to acid. After removal of the esophagus, the stomach should be the first choice for the replacement tube. If the stomach cannot be used for a variety of reasons, the colon is used [3].

O. Demiray (✉) · M. L. Gedik
Department of General Surgery, Health Sciences University Taksim Training and Research Hospital, Istanbul, Turkey



O. Engin (ed.), *Risk Factors and Therapy of Esophagus Cancer*,
https://doi.org/10.1007/978-3-031-47024-0_25

The esophageal replacement procedure carries a number of predictable complications. Vascular insufficiency with graft necrosis is the most critical. This complication is most common when the jejunum or colon is used and is observed as a blue and pulseless graft after interposition. The most important cause of impaired blood flow is stretching or kinking of the vascular pedicle. Adjusting the graft to reduce this can help improve blood flow. Intraoperative hypotension may cause the graft to take on the appearance of vascular insufficiency. If the graft's form and the patient's blood pressure are satisfactory, the graft should be left in place since its vascularity might get better after the surgery [4].

## 25.1 Colon Interposition

When the stomach cannot be used or when the stomach must be resected for oncologic reasons, such as an adenocarcinoma involving most of the lesser curvature and the distal esophagus, colon interposition is employed as an alternate option [1, 5, 6].

The main advantage of using the colon is its versatility. It is freely available for replacement of the entire esophagus up to the pharyngeal region. The left colic artery has a substantial blood supply, and the presence of the artery of Drummond, a marginal artery near the colon, allows for a linear interposition procedure without mechanical kinking or redundancy. If anastomosis to the stomach is possible, this offers the potential to facilitate gastric emptying and reduce reflux. However, it is a complex procedure requiring at least three anastomoses. Therefore, longer surgery times and higher rates of necrosis, morbidity, and mortality have been reported [7, 8].

Colon use is contraindicated in the presence of an aortic aneurysm or extensive atherosclerosis involving the superior mesenteric artery, prior colon surgery, severe colonic inflammatory bowel disease, or tumors. Scattered diverticulosis is a relative contraindication. Prior colonoscopy is also recommended in patients in whom colon use is being considered [1, 5–11].

The advantages of the method [5–11]:

- It is technically relatively simple.
- It provides reliable blood flow (thanks to dual perfusion from the left colic and marginal arteries.).
- It allows you to adjust the length.

Disadvantages [5–11]:

- Requirement of three anastomoses.
- Bending, widening or the length of the graft may cause stasis over time.

Complications [5–11]:

- The mortality rate is between 1 and 5%.
- Fistula occurs at rates ranging from 7 to 29%.

- Anastomotic stricture affects 11–28% of patients. The most important causes of fistula and anastomotic stricture are ischemia and anastomotic tension.
- Redundancy/stagnation is reported in 10–16% of cases. The segment being longer than desired, that is, redundancy, contributes to this complication.
- Reflux is observed with a frequency of 12–38%.

Blood supply to the colon comes from both the superior and inferior mesenteric arteries. Typically, the middle, right, and ileocolic arteries originate from the superior mesenteric artery, while the inferior mesenteric artery supplies the left colic artery. The marginal arcades (Drummond artery) connect the colonic arteries. However, there are some variations that may compromise the use of the large intestine. The right colic artery may originate from the middle colic artery. Approximately 5–10% of cases have multiple right colic arteries with different origins from the middle, ileocolic, and superior mesenteric arteries. The marginal arcades are interrupted or interconnected by numerous small ramifications in about 10% of cases and are sometimes completely missing. A variation of the marginal artery of Drummond is the arc of Riolan, also known as the tortuous mesenteric artery or central anastomotic mesenteric artery. This is an arterioarterial anastomosis between the superior and inferior mesenteric arteries, proximal to the roots of the superior mesenteric artery, whereas the marginal of Drummond is found well distal to the roots of the mesenteric artery. The presence of an arc of Riolan often precludes the use of long-segment colon interposition [10].

There are two main graft types traditionally used for esophageal reconstruction among the many technical choices in colon interposition. In the right colon graft technique, the middle colic vessels are used as pedicles. This usually involves cutting and ligating the right colic and ileocolic vessels. A segment from the terminal ileum to the ascending colon is interposed isoperistaltically. The ascending branch of the left colic artery and the inferior mesenteric vein are used as pedicles to produce a left colon graft. The middle colic vessels should be split, preserving the connection between the right and left branches of these vessels. A segment from the transverse colon to the splenic flexure is used for interposition in an isoperistaltic way. In a long-segment interposition, the hepatic flexure is also included. This procedure may require cutting and ligating the right colic artery [11].

Technically, a transverse or left colon connected to the left colic artery is generally preferred. The right colon may also be used. The colon, which is prepared and mobilized by preserving the vessel, is pulled toward the neck, and a longitudinal esophageal colonic anastomosis is performed. Gastrocolic anastomosis is then performed. An anti-reflux procedure is subsequently added to prevent the development of reflux. As the vagus will be severed during esophageal dissection and resection, pyloroplasty is performed to ensure gastric emptying [12].

The colon is generally a well-blooded organ and makes an excellent esophageal replacement.

After ligation and transection of the left colic vessels, an antiperistaltic loop can be established by swinging the mobilized left colon upward so that it is supplied by the middle colic vessels. However, since this method does not always work well, it should be a last resort. The superior end of the anastomosed colon may show poor arterial circulation or bad venous return. In this case, arterial or venous anastomosis of the ligated colonic vessels to a suitable cervical vessel, performed by a team experienced in vascular surgery, can save the colon by improving organ perfusion. Sometimes both arterial and venous vascular anastomoses may be required [12, 13].

## 25.2 Preoperative Preparation

Preoperative angiography of the colic vessels is usually of no value, as the availability of the colon as reconstruction material can only be determined intraoperatively. Prior abdominal surgery with potential involvement of colonic vessels or prior surgery on major abdominal vessels may contradict the use of colon. Colonoscopy should be performed in elderly patients or those with a history of polyps or diverticula. The patient should be on a liquid, grain-free diet for 1–2 days preoperatively, and, in general, all patients should undergo mechanical bowel cleansing using polyethylene glycol or other substances. Enema is rarely required. Recently, the need for preoperative bowel preparation has been questioned. A study demonstrated that the frequency of cervical leaks was significantly reduced in the non-preparation arm versus the traditional preparation arm. Adding oral antibiotics may help lower the chance of infection even further, but this is debatable. Intravenous broad-spectrum antibiotics covering anaerobic organisms are administered immediately before surgery and for the next 48 h [14].

### 25.2.1 Advantages of the Right Colon for Esophageal Replacement [15]

Ileocecal valve prevents regurgitation.
Reservoir-like capacity of the cecum.
Close match in the diameters of the esophagus and ileum.

### 25.2.2 Disadvantages [15]

High rate of variation in blood vessels.
Large cecal volume and diameter.
Presence of more frequent regurgitation.

### 25.2.3 Advantages of the Left Colon for Esophageal Replacement [15]

Having a good blood supply.
Having sufficient length for reconstruction.
Smaller colon diameter.

### 25.2.4 Disadvantages [15]

The risk of atherosclerosis of the arteria mesenterica inferior may be considered a disadvantage.

### 25.2.5 Left Colon Interposition

This technique offers an isoperistaltic colon segment of sufficient length to anastomose with excellent vascular supply in the thorax or neck if no compromising anatomical variations are present [16, 17] (Figs. 25.1 and 25.2).

The left colon is almost completely mobilized from its peritoneal attachments by incising the Toldt's fascia down to where the inferior mesenteric artery is identified. The transverse colon is detached from the omentum, and the relevant colon segment is mobilized, including the splenic flexure. If a long-segment interposition is planned, the peritoneal fold on the right side is cut, and the hepatic flexure, right colon, and cecum are mobilized. Once the colon is totally mobilized, arterial vascularization is checked. Vessels can be easily seen in the colonic mesentery of lean patients. This procedure is more challenging for obese patients because the mesentery thickens. This can be resolved by using the transillumination technique with a light source. A thorough inspection of the vessels is performed, taking variations into account. It is necessary to locate the ascending branch of the left colic artery. In left colic transposition, this will be the artery on which the vascularization will be based. Vertical incisions are performed in the mesenterium alongside the middle and right colic arteries, which are also visualized. The required segment length is

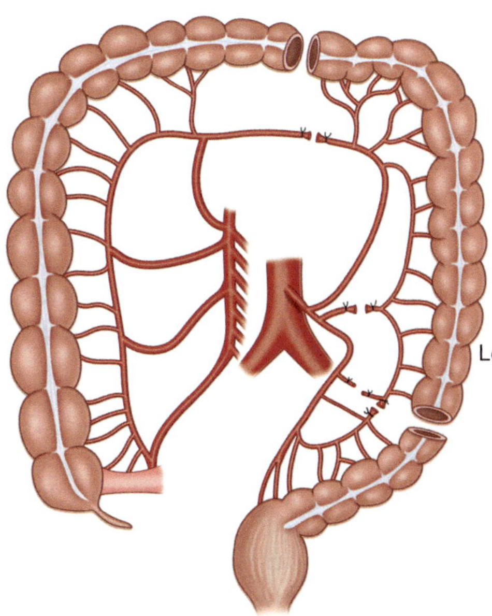


**Fig. 25.1** Left colon preparation and vascular pedicle isolation (Figure: left colon interposition 1–2)

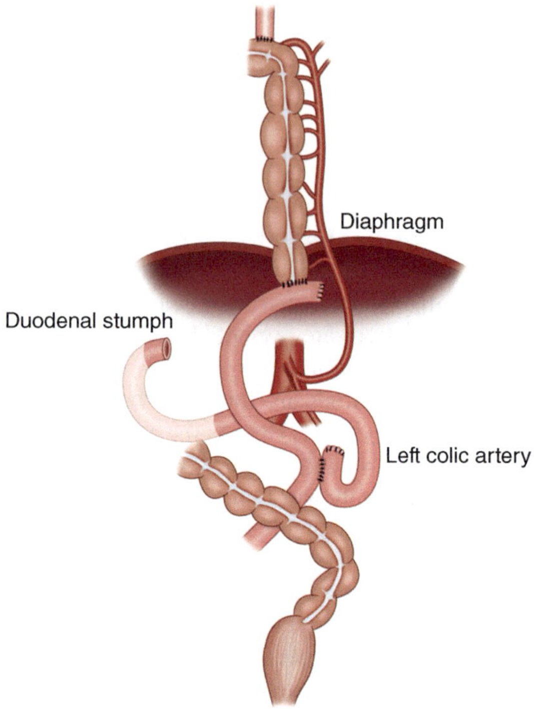


**Fig. 25.2** Left colon interposition

measured with white tape. The distance from the neck to the origin of the ascending branch of the left colic artery is measured with this tape. The length of the required segment is measured over the artery and marginal arteries, not by measuring the colon [16, 17].

Atraumatic vascular clamps such as bulldogs are placed at the base of the middle colic artery, or if greater length is required, they are also placed at the base of the right colic artery. The blood supply to the segment to be pulled up in place of the esophagus will now only come from the ascending branch of the left colic artery. Colon motions and blood flow should be checked both visually and by palpation. Doppler flow measurement may be used in cases of doubt. If there is no impairment in blood flow and supply after clamping, the roots of the middle colic artery and vein may be dissected, ligated, and severed. The marginal artery at the proximal transection point of the colon is clamped on the side that remains in place. Thus, flow to the non-clamped side can be immediately assessed after severing the marginal artery [17, 18].

The proximal part of the colon is transected, and the entire mobilized segment is moved upwards. Transection is performed using a linear cutting stapler. The colon is passed behind the stomach through an avascular opening in the lesser gastrohepatic omentum up to the level of the hiatus. It is attached to the distal esophagus before excision of the esophagus through a cervical incision. Care should be exercised to avoid rotating and twisting the colon's axis as it is being pulled upward [19].

The colon is gently stretched out into the chest cavity to determine the length required for anastomosis of the colon with the stomach. This ensures that the colon lies flat on the chest and that there is no redundancy. The risk of tension, which can be dangerous for the vascularization at the superior end, is also controlled. After the controls, the colon is transected with a linear cutting stapler [20].

The cologastric anastomosis is planned to be placed close to the greater curvature, 1/3 of the length down from the fundus to the pylorus on the posterior side of the stomach. Approximately 10 cm of the graft is retained underneath the diaphragm, forming an anti-reflux procedure [17, 18].

After the anastomosis is performed, the fundus wraps as a flap valve over the intra-abdominal part of the colon and acts as an effective secondary anti-reflux barrier against reflux colitis. This is an essential characteristic of the procedure. 3–0 absorbable material is used for the inner sutures of the anastomosis, and 3–0 non-absorbable material for the outer sutures [17, 20].

In cervical anastomosis, hand-sewn anastomosis is preferred due to the difference in diameter between the cervical esophagus and the colon. During the cervical anastomosis, a nasogastric tube is pushed down through the anastomosis into the colon and through the cologastric anastomosis to relieve the pressure in the stomach. A temporary placement of a gastrostomy for nutrition may also be useful [18].

Colocolic anastomosis is established between the right and left colons. As the colon is substantially mobilized, colocolic anastomosis can be performed with ease and without tension. The opening in the intestinal mesenterium should be sealed to prevent herniation and possible strangulation of the small intestine [21].

### 25.2.6 Right Colon

The principles of dissection and measurement of the required length are the same as for the left colon interposition [16]. The right colic artery is identified, and the mesenterium is dissected incisively along this artery. The marginal artery clamping technique may be used to assess vascularization at the anastomosis site of the cervical esophagus and colon, as in the left colon. If a long segment is required, the cecum and the last ileal loop may be used. In cases where the cecum and ileal loop are also used, the right ileocolic artery may be severed as well. The remainder of the surgery is similar to the transposition of the left colon [16] (Figs. 25.3 and 25.4).

An isoperistaltic anastomosis is generally preferred for colonic interposition. Antiperistaltic placement is believed to increase the risk of aspiration [15]. Antiperistaltic interposition may be the only option due to variations in vascular anatomy.

In cases of suspected impaired venous drainage, "super drainage" may be performed to prevent congestion of the transplant due to venous drainage insufficiency. The marginal vein is anastomosed to the anterior or exterior jugular vein or the internal thoracic vein using microsurgical techniques [16, 17].

"Supercharged colon interposition" is used for the technique of anastomosing arteries with microsurgical technique in suspicious cases to prevent ischemic

**Fig. 25.3** Right colon preparation and vascular pedicle isolation (Figure: right colon interposition 3–4)

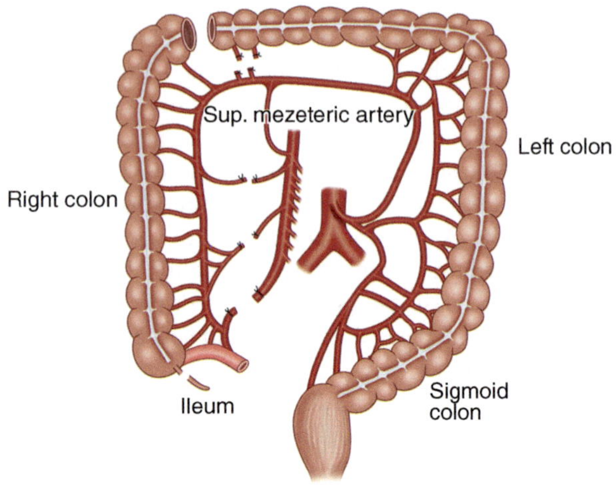


**Fig. 25.4** Right colon interposition

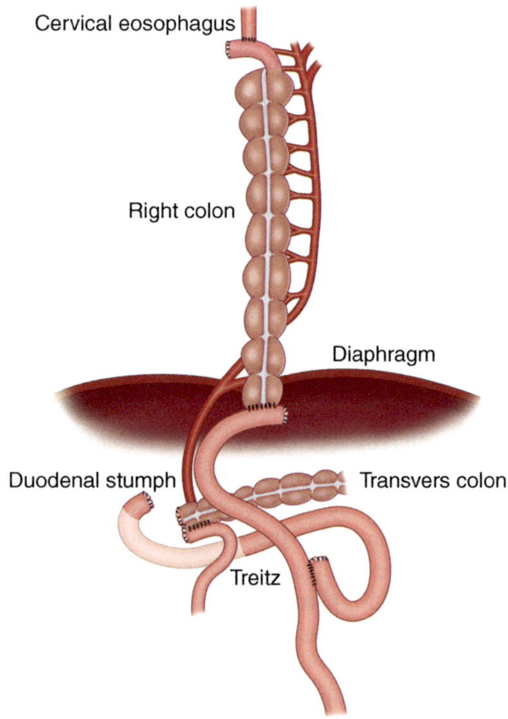

necrosis of the graft. Circulatory support is usually provided by an arterial anastomosis between the right or middle colic artery and the superior thyroid artery or internal mammary artery [19].

Colon interposition is a very complicated procedure, and after esophagectomy for cancer, postoperative mortality has been estimated to be 10–20%. This rate is higher than postoperative mortality after gastric pull-up. Graft necrosis, which occurs in approximately 5% of cases as per the literature, is one of the specific causes of mortality or severe morbidity. Common reasons include rupture of the vessels, rotation of the vascular pedicle at various time points during the surgery (in particular when bringing up the colon into the neck), and damaging the vessels by clamps or ligatures, which can result in thrombosis and subsequent necrosis. Too much narrowing of the hiatus during the same procedure may strangle the vascular pedicle, resulting in necrosis. When graft necrosis is diagnosed, the colon should be removed. Esophageal fistula from the neck and gastroscopy for feeding are used to control the condition. Then, when the patient has completely recovered, staged reconstruction must be performed [21, 22].

While anastomotic leak is rare in procedures for intrathoracic anastomosis using a short-segment colon, anastomotic leak after long-segment interposition with anastomosis in the cervical neck occurs in approximately 10% of cases. They can usually be managed conservatively and rarely require revisional surgery.

Another complication of long-segment anastomosis is the bulging of the supraclavicular region. The thin-walled colon bulges out due to air swallowed while talking or eating. This bulging in the neck creates aesthetic problems for the patient's appearance and may induce dysphagia in the long term. This complication will require revisional surgery by excising the protruded part [23, 24].

A colon segment that is longer than necessary is one of the complications that could arise, particularly in long-segment anastomoses. This complication is more common when using right-sided access for the esophagectomy after retrosternal interposition and, to a lesser extent, after left-sided or transhiatal esophagectomy. Follow-ups will reveal that the redundancy's size grows with time, eventually leading to mechanical kinking. Symptoms include dysphagia and aspiration due to stasis and regurgitation. These patients usually need revision surgery [23, 24].

Another example of late complications is the occurrence of fibrosis at the superior end of the graft. Fibrosis is believed to be caused by congestion of venous drainage. Dilation of such strictures is very difficult. Stricturoplasty may be planned for treatment [25].

Reflux-associated colitis may occur. The best way to prevent colitis is to adopt an appropriate surgical approach that reduces the risk of reflux, as previously mentioned. Reflux-associated colitis usually responds well to treatment with proton pump inhibitors. The development of reflux ulcers is rare. A cologastric stenosis requiring surgical revision may occur after an ulcer [24, 25].

Regurgitation and aspiration may develop due to reflux or stasis. If it fails to respond to conservative treatment, revisional surgery may be required to treat it [25].

The intervening complications, such as irritable bowel disease or colon cancer, in the colon segment in long-term follow-up have been described, albeit rarely [5–11]. The following complications rates have been reported in the literature [5–11]:

- Mortality rate 1–5%.
- Fistula 7–29%.
- Anastomotic stenosis 11–28%.
- Redundancy/stagnation 10–16%.
- Reflux 12–38%.

## 25.3 Jejunal Interposition

Jejunal interposition is the third most commonly used method for esophageal reconstruction. This is because preparing a long segment in the jejunum is more challenging vascularly than in the stomach and colon. The risk of ischemia and necrosis is higher. Jejunum can be used as an interposition, a Roux-en-Y loop, or a free vascular graft. It is used in esophageal cancer surgery in patients who have had prior gastrectomy or in patients who require total gastrectomy for oncologic reasons such as gastroesophageal junction tumors extending into the stomach [26].

A short-segment Roux-en-Y will be sufficient to provide an intrathoracic anastomosis at the level of the inferior pulmonary vein or slightly above the level of the aortic arch. The longer the length of the jejunum segment to be used, the greater the number of vascular structures to be ligated and severed [26, 27].

The jejunum receives blood supply from the superior mesenteric artery. Vascular anatomical variations causing technical challenges may be observed during jejunal loop preparation [26, 27].

The ligament of Treitz is identified, and vascularization is examined. In a thin patient, this will be quite easy, but in more obese patients with a fatty mesenterium, transillumination is required. The jejunal artery, which is necessary for the vascularization of the first 15-cm segment emerging from the ligament of Treitz, is exposed and preserved. In the next step, the length of the segment needed for anastomoses is identified and the proximal two to three segmental arteries of this segment are visualized. The arteries are gently dissected out of the mesenterium. The level of vascularization is assessed with atraumatic vascular clamps (bulldog, etc.). The vascular structures are individually ligated and severed. A segment long enough to raise the jejunum to the level of the inferior pulmonary vein or even the level of the aortic arch is obtained with two or three arteries divided. If a longer segment is needed, an additional artery can be ligated and severed, but the more arteries severed, the higher the risk of ischemia at the superior end of the canal [26, 28].

Some additional maneuvers may be performed to increase the length. When one or two of the primary arcades near the jejunum are ligated and severed, the secondary arcades close to the jejunum maintain vascular flow. After preparation of the jejunal loop, the jejunum is transected approximately 15 cm from the ligament of Treitz with a linear cutting stapler, and the jejunal loop is brought up into the thoracic cavity through the mesentery of the transverse colon transmesocolically. This is easy for a short segment, but if the loop needs to be longer, the surgery may be more challenging as the jejunum tends to retain its curved structure [28, 29].

Complications associated with the use of a long-segment jejunum include:

Regurgitation

Aspiration

Dysphagia

Stasis leading to distension.

A supercharged arterial anastomosis with the internal mammary artery or inferior thyroid artery may save the day in the absence of adequate blood flow at the superior end of the jejunum [30–32].

The esophago-jejunal anastomosis may be performed manually using two layers of either continuous or interrupted sutures or with a 25- or 28-mm circular stapler, depending on the patient's esophagus. The integrity of the anastomosis should be thoroughly examined. In anastomoses not performed end-to-end, the jejunal stump is sealed by using a linear cutting stapler very close to the circular anastomosis to prevent diverticulum development in the long term. Anastomosis may be performed using the VATS approach in the same way [33].

An alternative open surgical technique is to perform a semi-mechanical anastomosis. Two fixation sutures are placed between the superior end of the jejunum and the esophagus, approximately 4–5 cm above the incised end. A tiny incision is made on the antimesenteric side of the jejunum, and the two halves of a linear cutting stapler device are introduced into the esophagus and jejunum, respectively, and fired. Thus, the posterior wall of the anastomosis is now complete. The remaining open part of the esophageal circumference and the jejunal incision (i.e., the anterior wall) are sealed with double layers of sutures [33]. Such an anastomosis requires at least 4 cm of esophagus available proximal to the incised end of the esophagus. It also requires another 5 cm of esophagus proximal to the superior end of the tumor. Reconstruction is completed with jejuno-jejunal end-to-side anastomosis.

### 25.3.1 Merendino Procedure

It may be preferred when the colon cannot be used and preservation of gastric reservoir function is preferred. This method, also known as the Merendino operation, is seen as an alternative to Roux-en-Y surgery [30]. A jejunal ring is interposed in the operation. While it was preferred in early T1aN0M0 cases with high-grade dysplasia, this surgery is now rarely used in cancer surgery because of the increased experience and favorable outcomes with endoscopic resections [34].

Jejunal Roux-en-Y and interposition results are generally satisfactory. Postoperative mortality ranges from 3 to 5%, with a leakage rate of 5 to 10% [26]. Possible complications include dysphagia, regurgitation, diarrhea, and reflux. However, some patients with Roux-en-Y reconstruction may have persistent debilitating biliary reflux, even they adhere to a 70-cm distance from the proximal anastomosis to the distal anastomosis. Treatment of this complication may require revisional surgery that repositions the anastomosis more distally to the jejunum [35].

Given the technical challenges, long-segment jejunoplasty is rarely performed, but based on the available data in the literature, the outcomes seem to be comparable to those achieved after short-segment jejunoplasty [36, 37].

## References


1. Reinberg O. Esophageal replacements in children. Ann N Y Acad Sci. 2016;1381:104–412.
2. Napier KJ, Scheerer M, Misra S. Esophageal cancer: a review of epidemiology, pathogenesis, staging workup and treatment modalities. World J Gastrointest Oncol. 2014;6(5):112–20.
3. Mao WM, Zheng WH, Ling ZQ. Epidemiologic risk factors for esophageal cancer development. Asian Pac J Cancer Prev. 2011;12(10):2461–6.
4. Cross AJ, Freedman ND, Ren J, Ward MH, Hollenbeck AR, Schatzkin A, et al. Meat consumption and risk of esophageal and gastric cancer in a large prospective study. Am J Gastroenterol. 2011;106(3):432–42.
5. Lima M, Destro F, Contone N, et al. Long-term follow-up after esophageal replacement in children: 45-year single-center experience. J Pediatr Surg. 2015;50:1457–61.
6. Elfiky MM, El Tagy G, Mohamed W, et al. Gastric tube esophagoplasty for pediatric esophageal replacement. J Pediatr Surg. 2017;52:657–62.
7. Spitz L. Gastric transposition in children. Semin Pediatr Surg. 2009;18:30–3.
8. Cowles RA, Coran AG. Gastric transposition in infants and children. Pediatr Surg Int. 2010;26:1129–34.
9. Gupta L, Bhatnagar V, Gupta AK, et al. Long-term follow-up of patients with esophageal replacement by reversed gastric tube. Eur J Pediatr Surg. 2011;21:88–93.
10. Cauchi JA, Buick RG, Gornall P, et al. Oesophageal substitution with free and pedicled jejunum: short- and long-term outcomes. Pediatr Surg Int. 2007;23:11–9.
11. Bax KM. Jejunum for bridging long-gap esophageal atresia. Semin Pediatr Surg. 2009;18:34–9.
12. Larsson SC, Giovannucci E, Wolk A. Folate intake, MTHFR polymorphisms, and risk of esophageal, gastric, and pancreatic cancer: a meta-analysis. Gastroenterology. 2006;131:1271.
13. Orringer MB, Marshall B, Iannettoni MD. Transhiatal esophagectomy: clinical experience and refinements. Ann Surg. 1999;230(3):392–400. discussion 400–3.
14. Leal AJ, Tannuri AC, Tannuri U. Mechanical bowel preparation for esophagocoloplasty in children: is it really necessary? Dis Esophagus. 2013;26:475–8.
15. Thomas PA, Gilardoni A, Trousse D, et al. Colon interposition for oesophageal replacement. Multimed Man Cardiothorac Surg. 2009;2009:mmcts-2007.
16. Hamai Y, Hihara J, Emi M, et al. Esophageal reconstruction using the terminal ileum and right colon in esophageal cancer surgery. Surg Today. 2012;42:342–50.
17. Saeki H, Morita M, Harada N, et al. Esophageal replacement by colon interposition with microvascular surgery for patients with thoracic esophageal cancer: the utility of superdrainage. Dis Esophagus. 2013;26:50–6.
18. Chu KM, Law SY, Fok M, et al. A prospective randomized comparison of transhiatal and transthoracic resection for lower-third esophageal carcinoma. Am J Surg. 1997;174(3):320–4.
19. Shirakawa Y, Naomoto Y, Noma K, et al. Colonic interposition and supercharge for esophageal reconstruction. Langenbecks Arch Surg. 2006;391:19–23.
20. Rice TW, Rusch VW, Ishwaran H, Blackstone EH. Cancer of the esophagus and esophagogastric junction: data-driven staging for the seventh edition of the American Joint Committee on Cancer/International Union Against Cancer Staging Manuals. Cancer. 2010;116(16):3763–73.
21. Pompeo E, Nofroni I, Van Raemdonck D, et al. Esophagocoloplasty for congenital, benign and malignant diseases. Surgical and long-term functional results. Eur J Cardiothorac Surg. 1996;10:561–7.

22. Gust L, Ouattara M, Coosemans W, et al. European perspective in thoracic surgery-eso-coloplasty: when and how? J Thorac Dis. 2016;8:S387–98.
23. de Delva PE, Morse CR, Austen WG, et al. Surgical management of failed colon interposition. Eur J Cardiothorac Surg. 2008;34:432–7.
24. Gaur P, Blackmon SH. Jejunal graft conduits after esophagectomy. J Thorac Dis. 2014;6:S333–40.
25. Watanabe W, Mine S, Nishida K, et al. Reconstruction after esophagectomy for esophageal cancer patients with a history of gastrectomy. Gen Thorac Cardiovasc Surg. 2016;64:457–63.
26. Ascioti AJ, Hofstetter WL, Miller MJ, et al. Long-segment, supercharged, pedicled jejunal flap for total esophageal reconstruction. J Thorac Cardiovasc Surg. 2005;130:1391–8.
27. Nagasao T, Shimizu Y, Kasai S, Hatano A, Ding W, Jiang H, et al. Extension of the jejunum in the reconstruction of cervical oesophagus with free jejunum transfer using the thoracoacromial vessels as recipients. J Plast Reconstr Aesthet Surg. 2012;65(2):156–62.
28. Muller J, Erasmi H, Stelzner M, et al. Surgical therapy of oesophageal carcinoma. Br J Surg. 1990;77:845–57.
29. Putnam JB Jr, Suell DM, McMurtrey MJ, et al. Comparison of three techniques of esophagectomy within a residency training program. Ann Thorac Surg. 1994;57:319–25.
30. Blackmon SH, Correa AM, Skoracki R, et al. Supercharged pedicled jejunal interposition for esophageal replacement: a 10-year experience. Ann Thorac Surg. 2012;94:1104–11. [discussion 1111–1113].
31. Peracchia A, Rosati R. Chapter 57: Total gastrectomy and Roux-en-Y reconstruction. In: Patterson AG, Cooper JD, Deslauriers J, Lerut A, Luketich JD, Rice T, editors. Pearson's thoracic and esophageal surgery. Philadelphia: Churchill Livingstone; 2008. p. 613–9.
32. Merendino KA, Dillard DH. The concept of sphincter substitution by an interposed jejunal segment for anatomic and physiologic abnormalities at the esophagogastric junction; with special reference to reflux esophagitis, cardiospasm and esophageal varices. Ann Surg. 1955;142:486–506.
33. Stein H, Feith M, Siewert JR. Distal esophageal resection and jejunum interposition for early Barrett carcinoma. Zentralbl Chir. 2001;126:9–13.
34. Maier H, Pinter H, Tomaselli F, et al. Retrosternal pedicled jejunum interposition: an alternative for reconstruction after total esophago-gastrectomy. Eur J Cardiothorac Surg. 2002;22:661–5.
35. Ring WS, Varco RL, L'Heureux PR, et al. Esophageal replacement with jejunum in children: an 18–33 year follow-up. J Thorac Cardiovasc Surg. 1982;83:918.
36. Jurkiewicz MJ, Paletta CEL. Free jejunal graft. Current therapy in cardiothoracic surgery. Philadelphia: B.C. Decker; 1989. p. 206.
37. Jurkiewicz MJ. Vascularized intestinal graft for reconstruction of the cervical esophagus and pharynx. Plast Reconstr Surg. 1965;36:509–17.

# Use of Gastric Tube in Esophageal Replacement

# 26

Mehmet Yildirim

Although the prognosis of patients with esophageal cancer improves with multimodal therapies, esophageal cancer surgery continues to be one of the most extensive resection procedures in general surgery and thoracic surgery. While the 5-year life expectancy stood at 19% until the 1990s, it stood at 30–42% in the 2000s. The absence of serosa in the esophagus, involvement of lymph nodes located far from the tumor, and resection-related difficulties continue to be hallmarks of esophageal cancer surgery. Surgical approaches for esophageal resections differ for one-third upper and two-third lower esophageal cancers. Standard surgery is to perform esophageal anastomosis in the cervical area for cancers of the upper esophagus and intrathoracic anastomosis for two-third of cancers of the lower esophagus. After resection of the cancerous esophagus, the proximal esophagus is anastomosed with the stomach, jejunum, or colon segment. When the jejunum is used following esophageal resection, failure of the vascular pedicle and the formation of a jejunal ulcer occur. If the colon is used in interposition, ulcers develop due to the inability of the colon mucosa to tolerate fresh food. For these reasons, the stomach is used with a frequency of 80–90% due to the developed intramuscular vascular network in reconstruction after esophagectomy. For reconstruction, the whole stomach pulled up into the thoracic cavity or gastric tubes prepared from the stomach are used. The use of the whole stomach was first described by Levasseur and Couinaud. In 1955, Gavriliu prepared an isoperistaltic tube from the greater curvature of the stomach, followed by Hemlich and Gavriliu's reconstruction with an anisoperistaltic tube. In 1970, Yamagishi anastomosed the pedunculated gastric tube between the esophagus and the long limb of the Roux-en-Y, and in 1972, Akiyama described the

M. Yildirim (✉)
Department of General Surgery, University of Health Sciences, Izmir Bozyaka Training and Research Hospital, Izmir, Turkey


O. Engin (ed.), *Risk Factors and Therapy of Esophagus Cancer*,
https://doi.org/10.1007/978-3-031-47024-0_26

narrow gastric tube [1, 2]. In surgical practice, gastric tube procedures have been modified according to the proximity of the cancer to the stomach. Payne performed a right thoracotomy with Iwor-Lewis esophagectomy for cancers at all levels of the esophagus, Clagett-Sweet performed a left thoracotomy with distal cancers; and Orringer and Sloan performed gastric tube reconstruction after transhiatal esophagectomy. In cancers involving the upper esophagus and pharynx, complicated reconstructions are required with tubes prepared from the skin in addition to the gastric tube [3].

## 26.1 Rational of a Gastric Tube

The blood supply of the stomach is provided by the right and left gastric artery (LGA) at the lesser curvature, the right and left gastroepiploic artery at the greater curvature, and there is a rich intramural vascular network between these vessels. Even if all three of these arteries are ligated, one vessel is sufficient to supply the stomach. For replacement after esophagectomy, the whole stomach or the gastric tube formed from the greater curvature can be pulled into the chest. It is sufficient to protect the right gastroepiploic artery (RGEA) to ensure adequate blood flow to the gastric tube. The right gastroepiploic artery is approximately 14.5 cm long and represents 55% of the greater curvature. The left gastroepiploic artery is 3.4 cm in average and provides 12.7% of the length of the greater curvature [4]. The frequency of extramural anastomosis between two vessels was found to be between 23 and 100%. The rich blood flow of the gastric tube and its greater curvature are ideal features in the preparation of the gastric tube. The gastric tube should have an average length of 25–30 cm and a width of 4 cm. The gastric tubes are made isoperistically or anisoperistaltically. Gastric tubes can be used for intrathoracic and cervical anastomosis. Gastric tubes are passed subcutaneously in benign esophageal diseases, retrosternally in esophageal cancers, and nowadays through the posterior mediastinum. However, in Japanese studies, the subcutaneous route is preferred in patients with one-third upper esophageal cancers or lymph node metastases in the upper mediastinum [5].

## 26.2 Technique

The general anesthesia is applied in the supine position. The operation position for the patient should be supine with the patient's head at an extension. A left shoulder roll or gel ped should be placed at the level of the acromion process of the scapula to help expose the neck. The patient's skin, abdomen, thorax, and neck should be cleaned with antiseptics before surgery.

## 26.3 Preparation of the Cervical Region

The cervical part of the esophagus is approximately 5 cm long and descends between the trachea and the vertebral column. It lies in the midline but deviates to the left in the lower portion of the neck, where the lateral wall of the esophagus can be easily palpated. Therefore, it is easier to reach and dissect the esophagus with the left cervical incision in the right-facing position. First, an oblique incision is made on the neck skin along the medial edge of the left sternocleoid muscle. Then the thyroid tissue is pulled toward the midline as the anterior cervical muscles are retracted laterally. The cervical esophagus should be gently dissected from the posterior lining of the trachea and suspended with a tape band (Picture 26.1). At this exploration, care must be taken not to avoid damage to the recurrent nerve.

The strap muscles of the neck may be cut to prevent the gastric tube from being compressed in the cervical area. The esophagus should be cut with a scalpel or cautery. It is useful to suture the esophageal mucosa to the muscular layer in four quadrants so that the mucosa does not retract as the hand suture or anvil is placed (Picture 26.2).

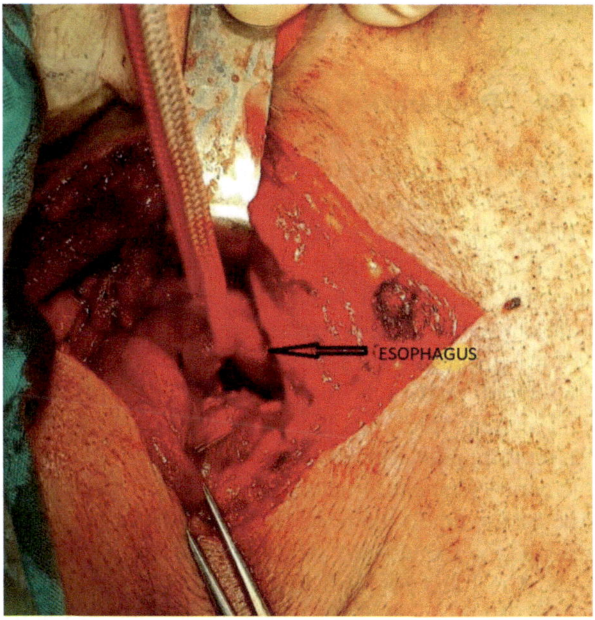


**Picture 26.1** Suspension of the esophagus in the cervical region (arrow, esophagus)

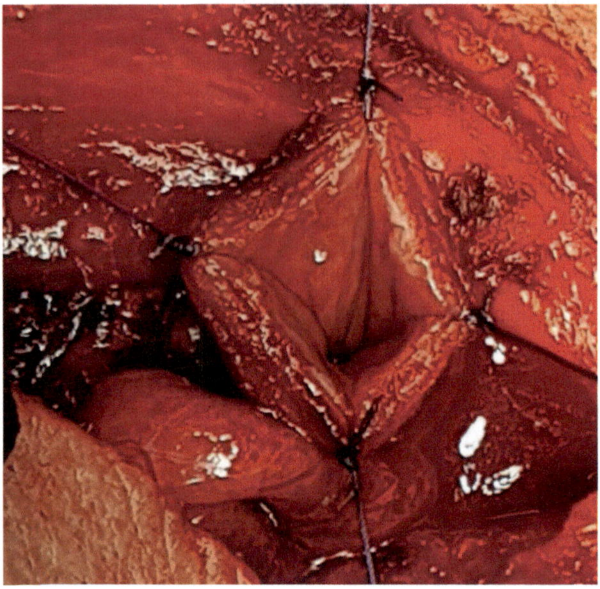

**Picture 26.2** Preparation of the cervical esophagus for anastomosis

## 26.4 Preparation of a Gastric Tube

Laparotomy is performed with a Chevron incision on the abdominal wall. A full exploration of the stomach and intraabdominal organs is performed. It is planned whether the whole stomach or gastric tube will be used for replacement [2]. Kocherization of the duodenum should be performed to ensure optimum length in the prepared stomach. A tunnel prepared in the retrosternal or posterior mediastinum is used to provide access from the gastric tube to the cervical region. Today, following transhiatal esophagectomy, the posterior mediastinum is the appropriate way to pull up the tube to the cervical region [6].

The creation of the tunnel in the posterior mediastinum should be performed in the surgical plan without blood loss by blunt dissection with the finger and cutting the periesophageal formations using vessel-sealing instruments in the visible area. The gastric tube's top point is knotted with tape or strong sutures. A long clamp is inserted via the thoracic inlet from the cervical region into the posterior mediastinum. The free ends of the tape or sutures attached to the tube are held with the clamp. While the clamp or tube is pulled upwards in the cervical region, the tube is pushed upwards from the abdomen to ensure that the gastric tube is passed from the mediastinum to the neck without tearing. At this time, care should be taken that the tube does not rotate around itself. Keeping the stapler line (SL) of the gastric tube posteriorly is helpful in preventing leaks. In patients who are planned for intrathoracic anastomosis, after thoracotomy, the lungs are pulled medially, while the parietal pleura is opened and the esophagus is suspended at the appropriate distance from the proximal side of the tumor. Then, the tumor segment is freed by blunt and sharp dissection. To obtain a tumor-free surgical margin, it is accepted that the proximal surgical margin is 12 cm [7]. However, this limit is up to 6 cm in Iwor-Levis esophagectomy [8]. An intraoperative frozen section of the incision line should be performed to show that the surgical margin is tumor-free. The resected esophagus is pulled via the diaphragmatic hiatus into the abdomen.

Esophagogastric anastomosis with the whole stomach or gastric tube can be done manually or with a stapler. Hand-sewn sutured anastomosis can be performed with single or two rows of sutures, and it is important to approximate the edge of mucosa to the edge of mucosa. In single-layer anastomosis, vertical mattress of the posterior side and Gambee sutures of the anterior sides are performed. A double anastomosis consists of an inner layer of continuous or interrupted absorbable suture and an outer layer of interrupted nonabsorbable suture. Hand-sewn cervical esophagogastric anastomosis should be performed in an end-to-side type. It can be done side-to-side using a linear cutter or end-to-side when using a circular stapler. If the esophagogastric anastomosis is to be performed with a stapler, an automatic purse string device can be used without cutting the esophagus since an anvil will be placed in the esophagus. In intrathoracic anastomoses, end-to-side, end-to-side double staplers, or side-to-side types are performed. The anastomosis site in the stomach tube should be placed at a distance of 4–5 cm from the stapler line to the area with good blood circulation [9, 10].

There should be no tension in the anastomosis line. For this, the uppermost point of the stomach should be determined. The end point of the upper stomach pinching between fingers should be pulled upward, and the section to be resected in the proximal stomach should be planned by checking whether it is of sufficient length (Fig. 26.1). Measures should be taken to prevent tension if the vascular arc of the gastric tube is not complete or if there is a history of prior gastric surgery. For this, it is required to clear the fibrotic bands that hinder the stomach tube from pulling, cut the hepatoduodenal ligament, execute a wide Kocher's maneuver and, if necessary, make relaxing incisions in the gastric serosa. The distal end of the gastric tube should be anastomosed to the jejunum limb using a shorter gastric tube if the supply of the gastric tube is impaired or uncertain. The additional procedures to prevent anastomotic leakage are to support the gastric tube with the omentum in the cervical anastomosis and with a pleural patch in the intrathoracic anastomosis. A Penrose drain should be placed in the cervical region. Pyloroplasty should be performed routinely in patients [11].

The blood supply of the gastric tube is important for the prevention of anastomotic leaks and strictures. Typical findings of a gastric tube with adequate blood flow are the pink-red color of the stomach that has been pulled up and active bleeding from the staple line. It should be examined whether the top avascular area of the gastric tube is ischemic. It should be remembered that because the anastomosis is done here in the gastric tube, cutting the vascular structures during the anastomosis incision will disrupt the gastric tube's distal end from feeding properly [9]. A small number of patients have undergone studies and found success with preoperative left

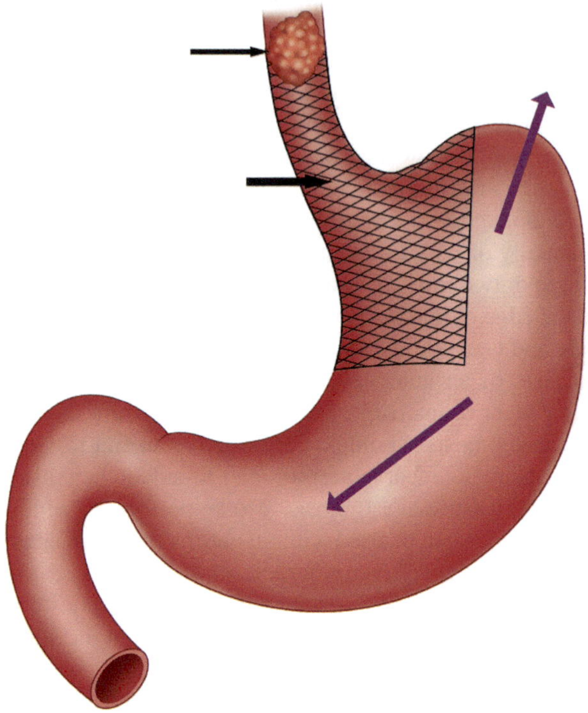

**Fig. 26.1** Forming the gastric tube with the least tension by pulling the stomach proximal and distally before resection. *Small arrow* tumor, *large arrow* area to be resected

gastric artery embolization or laparoscopic ligation to preserve the blood flow of the tissue in the stomach [12, 13]. There were different methods of measuring blood flow to detect ischemia in the gastric tube. The most widely utilized techniques are the laser Doppler flowmeter, near-infrared spectroscope, and fluorescent flowmeter [14]. The blood flow from the serosa to a depth of 1–6 mm can be measured using a laser Doppler. When determining the blood flow in the mucosa, the measurement from the serosa consistently yields reliable results [15]. Intraoperative safety measures should be implemented if it is found by these measurements that the gastric tube is passed subcutaneously and retrosternally, decreasing blood flow in the tube, or because less than 10 mL/min flow rate per 100 g graft may induce leakage after anastomosis. In cases where blood flow decreases, administration of prostaglandin E1 and dopamine has a corrective effect on blood flow in the gastric tube [16]. After surgery, inserting a nasogastric tube helps avoid complications caused by decreased blood flow in the undecompressed stomach, such as regurgitation and aspiration. No correlation was found between the frequency of anastomotic leaks and either early or late nasogastric withdrawal. However, it is possible to decompress the gastric tube percutaneously via transcervical or retrograde jejunostomy to prevent lung complications caused by prolonged holding of the nasogastric tube. Intraoperative pleural opening should be controlled in transhiatal intervention, and tube thoracostomy should be applied. Right tube thoracostomy should be performed in patients who underwent Iwor-Lewis esophagectomy, and left tube thoracostomy should be performed in left thoracotomy cases. Tube thoracostomy should be performed in all intrathoracic procedures [10, 17].

## 26.5 Using the Whole Stomach in Reconstruction

If the whole stomach is to be retracted into the thoracic cavity, the right gastric and right gastroepiploic arteries must be preserved, and the proximal part of the stomach must be resected, including the cardia and lesser curvature lymph nodes. In the resection procedure, the left gastric artery is ligated and cut from the root. The first and second branches of the artery and the lymph nodes around the left gastric artery should remain in the resected part. A sufficient arterial arc of lesser curvature helps the blood supply to the stomach. The right gastroepiploic artery is cut where it makes anastomoses (Demel's point) with the left gastroepiploic artery. After the gastrica brevis is cut, the dissection is continued up to the left edge of the esophagus. In order to prevent disruption of the blood supply, a 4–5 cm piece of omentum containing the artery and vein should be left at the greater curvature of the stomach (Fig. 26.2). In addition to the intramuscular vascular network, lateral branches

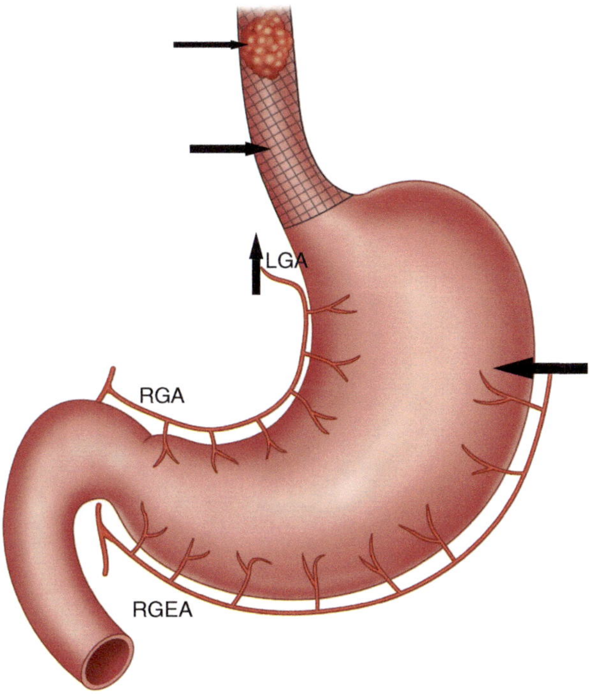


**Fig. 26.2** Using the whole stomach in reconstruction. *RGA* right gastric artery, *LGA* left gastric artery, *RGEA* right gastroepiploic artery, *small arrow* tumor, *large arrow* area to be resected

originating from the omental artery have an effect on the blood supply of the tube. Leaving a wider omentum may cause tension in the anastomosis and compression of the replaced stomach in the mediastinum by putting weight on the stomach [18].

## 26.6 Formation of the Gastric Tube (Gavriliu)

In one-third of upper cancers of the esophagus, approximately 25 cm of long gastric tube is required for anastomosis to the cervical region in the replacement procedure. The basic principle of surgery is the resection of the lesser curvature to make a gastric tube from the greater curvature approximately 4 cm wide, preserving the right gastroepiploic artery (Fig. 26.3). The ends of cut vessels should be fixed to the gastric serosa so that they do not cause bleeding by tearing while the gastric tube is pulled up into the mediastinal tunnel. In cases where the lesser curvature is short, the cardia and lesser curvature should be resected, which minimizes the area supplied by the gastroepiploic artery. Separation of the tube from the stomach is done by cutting the tissue between the clamps or with the help of a stapler (Pictures 26.3 and 26.4). Esophagogastric anastomosis is performed with end-to-side or side-to-side sutures [2].

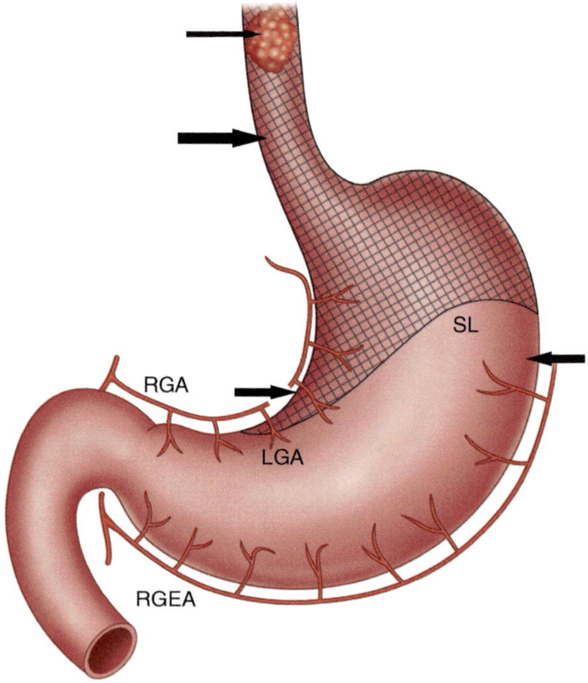


**Fig. 26.3** Preparation of a gastric tube. *RGA* right gastric artery, *LGA* left gastric artery, *RGEA* right gastroepiploic artery, *SL* stapler line, *small arrow* tumor, *large arrow* area to be resected

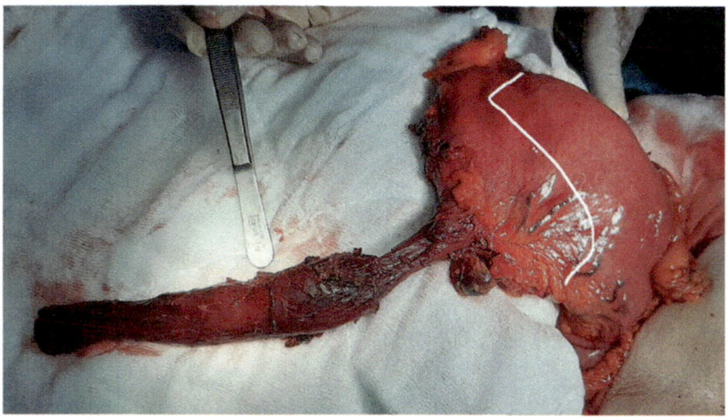

**Picture 26.3** Determination of the part to be prepared as a gastric tube (white line, stapled line)

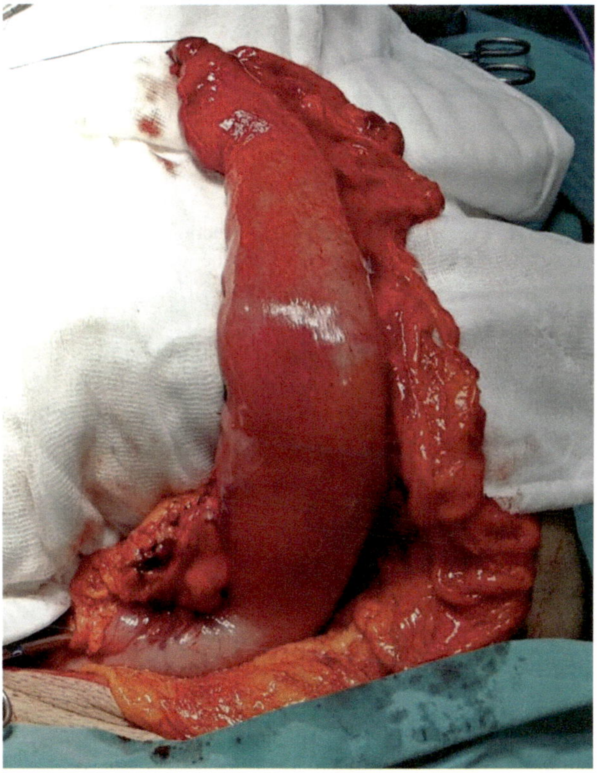

**Picture 26.4** Isoperistaltic gastric tube created after gastric resection

## 26.7 Pedunculated Isoperistaltic Tube

The gastric tube is prepared on the greater curvature side at a distance of 5 cm upwards from the pylorus by cutting with a stapler. The blood flow of the pedicled gastric tube provided by right gastroepiploic vessels. Since the gastric tube is prepared in a length of 40–50 cm, it can be easily pulled into the cervical region

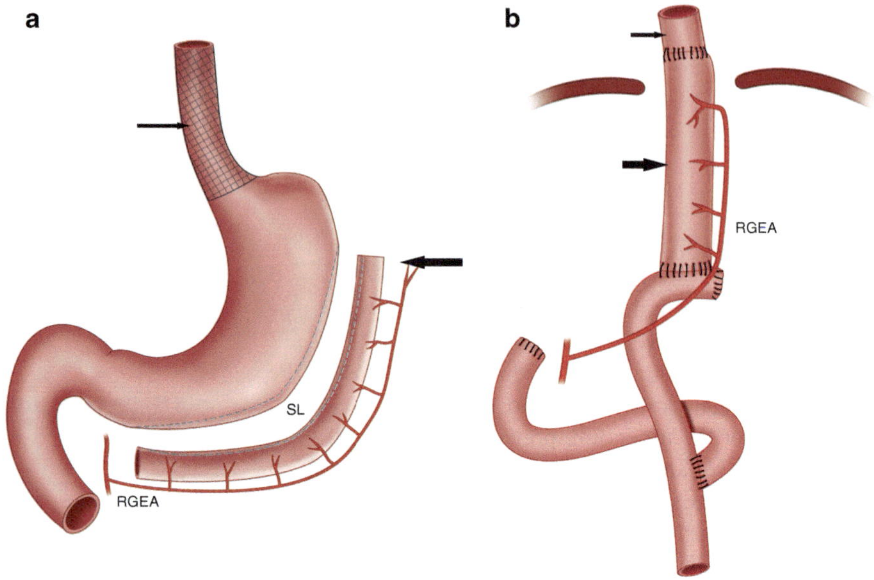


**Fig. 26.4** Free isoperstaltic tube construction with peduncle. *RGEA* right gastroepiploic artery. (**a**) Arrow, resection area. (**b**) Gastric tube interposition in the patient with total stomach. *Short arrow* esophagus, *long arrow* stomach tube

without tension (Fig. 26.4a). The proximal end of the gastric tube is anastomosed to the esophagus, and the distal end to the fundus of the stomach [19]. Care should be taken to place the gastroepiploic vessels in their anatomical position. Great care should be taken not to impair venous drainage. The continuity of the venous drainage of the tube should be especially checked. In patients who underwent total gastrectomy, the proximal end of the isoperistaltic tube is anastomosed to the cervical esophagus, and the distal end is anastomosed to the long limb of the prepared Roux-en-Y reconstruction (Fig. 26.4b) [20].

## 26.8 Anisoperistaltic (Reverse) Gastric Tube

The anisoperistaltic gastric tube (Heimlich–Gavriliu) is prepared by dividing between the clamps or linear staplers on the side of the greater curvature of the stomach. The double stapler method is also used while preparing the tube. The tube is prepared by cutting 5 cm from the pylorus parallel to the greater curvature, preserving the gastroepiploic vessels. The blood supply for the tube is provided by the gastroepiploic arc and the left gastric artery (Fig. 26.5). To ensure the freedom of the tube, the tail of the pancreas should be released and the vascular structures between the tube and spleen should be cut. While the base of the gastric tube is situated at the gastric fundus, the distal end of the tube is suitable for anastomosis to the esophagus in the neck. Thereafter, the gastric tube is passed through the

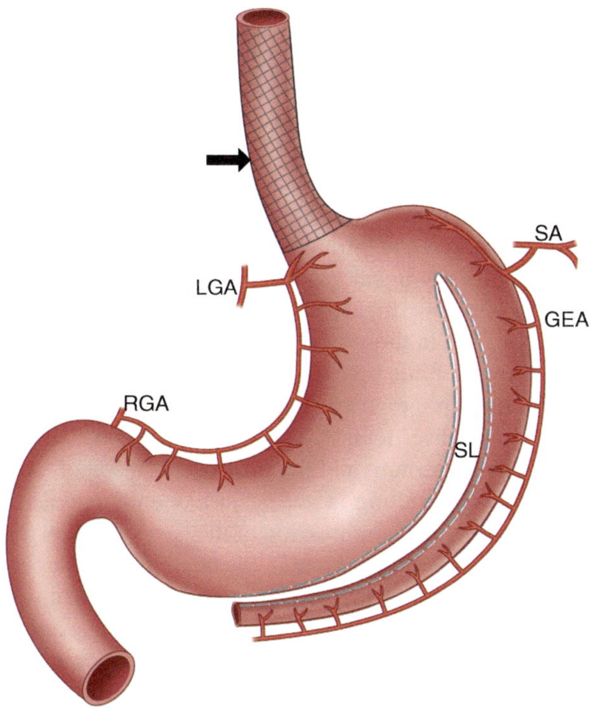


**Fig. 26.5** Preparation of an anisoperistaltic gastric tube from the greater curvature of the stomach. *RGA* right gastric artery, *LGA* left gastric artery, *GEA* gastroepiploic artery arch, *SL* stapler line

posterior mediastinum and pulled up to the cervical esophagus. If the thoracic inlet is closed, the subcutaneous route can be used. An end-to-side anastomosis is performed in the neck [21].

## 26.9 Advantages and Disadvantages of Gastric Tubes

In cases where the entire stomach is pulled into mediastinum, the stomach and omentum fill the posterior mediastinum. In cases where the stomach is filled with food and air, it causes compression in the heart and lungs. The symptoms seen in the patients are chest pain, tachycardia, and dyspnea, and changes are seen in the ECG. The complaints of the patients show improvement with hunger or vomiting. When the whole stomach is pulled into the thorax, reflux is common due to the absence of a sphincter mechanism, and peptic esophagitis occurs with the irritating effects of gastric juice in the esophagus. Negative intrathoracic and positive intraabdominal pressure play a role in the development of reflux in the first year. In procedures where the whole stomach is pulled up to the chest, vagotomy causes a decrease in gastric motility, but the presence of a large number of myenteric plexuses on the stomach causes an increase in contraction amplitudes and may cause nausea and vomiting due to the return of gastric motor function in the second year after surgery [10].

Isoperistaltic tubes can be prepared in sufficient length for cervical anastomosis, and anastomosis can be performed without tension in the neck. Ischemic complications occur less frequently in anastomoses. In cases of ischemia, the main reason is the insufficiency of the intramuscular vascular network that develops due to technical inadequacies during the gastric tubulization of greater curvature. Since the diameter of the narrow tube is similar to the diameter of the esophagus, the amount of gastric content retained is lower. The low gastric retention in the tube also helps to reduce reflux and intrathoracic stomach syndrome. Acid secretion was suppressed because of the truncal vagotomy. While the quality of life is better in the sixth and 12th months in patients who underwent gastric tube procedures, there is a similar quality of life in those who have had whole gastric pullup after 24 months [22, 23].

Anisoperistaltic tubes, on the other hand, are long enough to prolong the replaced gastric tube in the pharynx. The main complications are anastomotic leakage, dysphagia, and diverticula [24]. In the late period, between 1 and 3 years, adhesions between the sternum and the tube occur in 5% of cases, causing angulations in the gastric tube, resulting in achalasia-like enlargement of the tube. In addition, it has been thought that compression of the gastric tube in the hiatus causes tube dilatation [25]. Myotomy is beneficial in the treatment of dysphagia. Diverticulum formations due to weakness in the suture line or minor leaks may also be detected. Since the end of the anioperistaltic tube is formed from the antrum, the esophagitis is not seen because there is no acid secretion. However, since the proximal stomach remains in place in reverse tubes, it is not suitable for one-third lower esophageal tumors and benign pathologies that require proximal resection [26].

There was no difference in operation time, intraoperative blood loss, length of stay in the intensive care unit, or length of stay of the thoracic tube between the whole gastric pullup and the gastric tube procedure. Postoperative administration of proton pump inhibitors is beneficial [10, 27].

## 26.10 Early and Late Complications

The incidence of postoperative complications was 48% after reconstruction using the whole stomach, while it was 27% in the gastric tube. The main postoperative complications are pulmonary and anastomotic complications. Co-morbid conditions in oncological patients cause disruption of microperfusion [28]. For this reason, obesity, heart failure, chronic obstructive pulmonary disease, hypertension, and adverse effects related to steroid use should be eliminated before surgery. Preoperative nutritional disorders should be treated [14].

The most important life-threatening complication in cervical and intrathoracic anastomoses of the gastric tube is anastomotic leakage. Although cervical anastomotic leaks are more common than salivary fistulas, they cause less morbidity and mortality [29, 30]. The causes of leakage in cervical anastomoses are short tubes, tension or insufficient venous drainage in the anastomosis, and malnutrition. Preoperative neoadjuvant chemoradiotherapy has been shown to cause more frequent anastomotic leakage in patients with cardiorespiratory disease. No difference was found in patients who received only neoadjuvant chemotherapy [31]. There was no difference in the frequency of anastomotic leakage between the end-to-side construction of cervical anastomoses with a circular stapler and the side-to-side construction with a linear cutter [32]. However, while the leakage rate is 25% in manual end-to-side anastomosis, it is 11% in side-to-side linear anastomosis. In the intrathoracic anastomosis, the lowest leakage was found in the anastomoses made with the end-to-side purse string device [33]. In intrathoracic anastomosis, the most important cause of leakage is the longitudinal stress of the gastric tube. In addition to vascular diseases in the patient, calcifications of the vessels feeding the anastomosis, such as the aorta and celiac artery, also cause anastomotic leakage [34]. Opening the suture or stapler line on the long side of the gastric tube also causes life-threatening mediastinitis and requires immediate treatment (Picture 26.5). Endoluminal vacuum therapy is used for intraoperative or therapeutic purposes to prevent anastomotic leaks in the gastric tube with a high recovery rate [35]. The diagnosis of anastomotic leaks can be made by oral administration of methylene blue and color change in the drain fluid or by imaging tests with a contrast material dissolved in water [36]. The main anastomotic ischemia findings on endoscopy are black colorization of the mucosa, green or silvery mucus adhering to the mucosa, and a demarcation line on the mucosa. While one-third of patients with ischemic tubes recover completely, only one-third have anastomosis leakage and half of the remaining one-third have post-leak stricture. Conditions predisposing to ischemia are concomitant diseases such as diabetes mellitus, arrhythmias, and chronic obstructive pulmonary diseases that decrease tissue perfusion [14].

Dysphagia is less common in narrow gastric tubes and is a condition that occurs due to benign structure and ischemia or tumor recurrence in the late period. It is seen frequently in the sixth month after the operation, and the reason is benign strictures due to ischemia. Half of ischemic leaks heal with stricture. In obese patients, the tube becomes compressed due to adipose tissue and causes an increase in ischemia. Benign stenosis is a case where the 9-mm endoscope cannot pass. Although endoscopic dilatation is sufficient for benign strictures, the application of a stent in strictures that cannot benefit from dilatation provides benefits to the patient's quality of life [37, 38]. Although a single dilatation is usually sufficient in stenosis, a second dilatation is required in 16% of patients. When gastric tube and colon

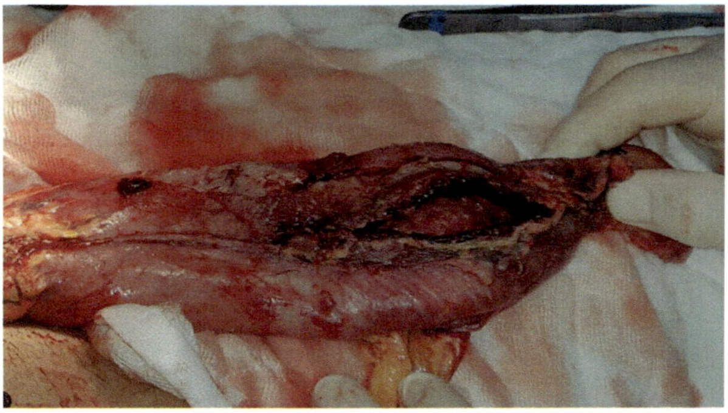

**Picture 26.5** Opening of stapler line in gastric tube

interposition are compared, anastomotic leakage is twice as common and stricture is four times more common in cases with gastric tubes [36]. The late complication is dysphagia of malignant origin, which occurs in the fifth year after surgery [37].

Metachronous cancer formation is observed in the gastric tube in patients with long-term surveillance. Gastric tube cancers are seen in the distal 1/3 of the tube and are of the adenocancer type. Annual gastric tube endoscopy is helpful in the early diagnosis of cancer. Endoscopic submucosal dissection is performed in gastric tube cancers detected at an early stage, and open or video-assisted tube resection of the gastric tube is performed in locally advanced lesions. In cases where distal tube resection is planned, since the right gastroepiploic artery will be cut, an arterial closure test can be performed beforehand. This method is to evaluate the feeding of the proximal tube by angiography, by occlusion of the artery with a ballooned catheter sent from the celiac trunk [39]. In cases where arterial supply is insufficient after resection of the distal tube, the right gastroepiploic artery should be anastomosed with an intact artery to prevent ischemia in the proximal tube. However, in cases where the blood flow of the proximal tube is not impaired, it is thought that there is bidirectional blood flow from the gastroepiploic artery or by capillary flow extending from the esophagogastric anastomosis to the gastric tube [40].

## 26.11 Gastric Tubes and Their Effect on Life Expectancy

While early death was reported with a frequency of 5% and a life expectancy of up to 24 months in the periods when gastric tubes were first defined, today the surveillance has been prolonged with multimodal treatments. Since the lymph nodes are excised during the preparation of the gastric tube, a suitable oncological surgery is performed. The prognosis is poor in patients who survived 5 years after whole stomach reconstruction since it is unknown whether there is a positive or micrometastasized lymph node in the region that cannot be resected [37]. Cancer recurrence occurs in 50% of patients 3 years after surgery. The main areas of recurrence are the mediastinum, liver, lung, and bones. Wide lymph node dissection during the preparation of narrow gastric tubes ensures that tumor recurrence and metastases are less common in the late period [41].

## References

1. Yamagishi M, Ikeda N, Yonemoto T. An isoperistaltic gastric tube. Arch Surg. 1970;100(6):689–92. https://doi.org/10.1001/archsurg.1970.01340240057012.
2. Akiyama H, Miyazono H, Tsurumaru M, Hashimato C, Kawamura T. Use of the stomach as an esophageal substitute. Ann Surg. 1978;188(5):606–10. https://doi.org/10.1097/00000658-197811000-00004. PMID: 718285; PMCID: PMC1396768.
3. Evans KFK, Mardini S, Salgado CJ, Chen HC. Esophagus and hypopharyngeal reconstruction. Semin Plast Surg. 2010;24(2):219–26. https://doi.org/10.1055/s-0030-1255339. PMID: 22550442; PMCID: PMC3324251.

4. Buunen M, Rooijens PPGM, Smaal HJ, Kleinrensink GJ, van der Harst E, Tilanius HW, et al. Vascular anatomy of the stomach related to gastric tube construction. Dis Esophagus. 2008;21(3):272–4. https://doi.org/10.1111/j.1442-2050.2007.00771.x.
5. Ikeda Y, Niimi M, Kan S, Shatari T, Takami H, Koairi S. Clinical significance of tissue blood flow during esophagectomy by laser Doppler flowmetry. J Thorac Cardiovasc Surg. 2001;122(6):1101–6. https://doi.org/10.1067/mtc.2001.117835.
6. Heitmiller RF. Impact of gastric tube diameter on upper mediastinal anatomy after transhiatal esophagectomy. Dis Esophagus. 2000;13(4):288–92. https://doi.org/10.1046/j.1442-2050.2000.00134.x.
7. Casson AG, Darnton SJ, Subramanian S, Hiller L. What is the optimal distal resection margin for esophageal carcinoma? Ann Thorac Surg. 2000;69(1):205–9. https://doi.org/10.1016/s0003-4975(99)01262-x.
8. Qureshi YA, Sarker SJ, Walker RC, Hughes SF. Proximal resection margin in Ivor-Lewis oesophagectomy for cancer. Ann Surg Oncol. 2017;24(2):569–77. https://doi.org/10.1245/s10434-016-5510-y.
9. Lai Y, Ye X, Wang X, Hu Y. The influence of anastomosis induced gastric wall defects on the blood supply to the gastric tube. J Thorac Cardiovasc Surg. 2020;159(4):e281–4. https://doi.org/10.1016/j.jtcvs.2019.10.157.
10. Zheng M, Wu QC, Li Q, Jiang YJ, Zhang C, Chen D. Comparison of the health-related quality of life in patients with narrow gastric tube and whole stomach reconstruction after oncologic esophagectomy: a prospective randomized study. Scand J Surg. 2013;102(2):77–82. https://doi.org/10.1177/1457496913482234.
11. Yuan Y, Zeng X, Hu Y, Xic T, Zhao Y. Omentoplasty for oesophagogastrostomy after oesophagostomy. Cochrane Database Syst Rev. 2014;10:CD008446. https://doi.org/10.1002/14651858.CD008446.pub3.
12. Akiyama S, Ito S, Sekiguchi H, Fujiwara M, Sakamoto J, Kondo K, et al. Preoperative embolization of gastric arteries for esophageal cancer. Surgery. 1996;120(3):542–6. https://doi.org/10.1016/s0039-6060(96)80075-4.
13. Berrisford RG, Veeramootoo D, Parameswaran R, Krishnadas R, Wajed SA. Laparoscopic ischaemic conditioning of the stomach may reduce gastric-conduit morbidity following total minimally invasive oesophagectomy. Eur J Cardiothorac Surg. 2009;36(5):888–93. discussion 893. https://doi.org/10.1016/j.ejcts.2009.01.055.
14. Vetter D, Gutschow CA. Strategies to prevent anastomotic leakage after esophagectomy and gastric conduit reconstruction. Langenbecks Arch Surg. 2020;405(8):1069–77. https://doi.org/10.1007/s00423-020-01926-8.
15. Hanashi T. An experimental study on circulation in stomach roll by laser-Doppler flowmetry. Teiko Med J. 1997;20:135–47.
16. Duda G, Huesken JE, Harmon JW. Effect of prostaglandins on esophageal blood flow. J Surg Res. 1998;44(4):371–81. https://doi.org/10.1016/0022-4804(88)90179-5.
17. Schuchert MJ, Pettiford BL, Landreneau JP, Waxman J, Kilic A, Santos RS, et al. Transcervical gastric tube drainage facilitates patient mobility and reduces the risk of pulmonary complications after esophagectomy. J Gastrointest Surg. 2008;12(9):1479–84. https://doi.org/10.1007/s11605-008-0541-8.
18. Settembre N, Labrousse M, Magnan PE, Branchereau A, Champsaur P, Bussani R, et al. Surgical anatomy of the right gastro-omental artery: a study on 100 cadaver dissections. Surg Radiol Anat. 2018;40(4):415–22. https://doi.org/10.1007/s00276-017-1951-7.
19. Acosta Suárez S, Mogollón Cruz G, Holguín Sanabria A, Luengas Pérez P. Isoperistaltic gastric tube: a surgical alternative in a pharyngoesophageal burn—a clinical case. Cir Pediatr. 2021;34(1):39–42.
20. Matsuki A, Kanda T, Kosugi SI, Suzuki T, Hatakeyama K. Gastric tube interposition for corrosive esophagitis associated with pyloric stenosis. Surg Today. 2009;39(3):261–4. https://doi.org/10.1007/s00595-008-3834-3.

21. Heimlich HJ. Esophagoplasty with reversed gastric tube. Review of 53 cases. Am J Surg. 1972;123(1):80–92. https://doi.org/10.1016/0002-9610(72)90315-7.
22. Zhang W, Yu D, Peng J, Xu J, Wei Y. Gastric-tube versus whole-stomach esophagectomy for esophageal cancer: a systematic review and meta-analysis. PLoS One. 2017;12(3):e0173416. https://doi.org/10.1371/journal.pone.0173416.
23. Poghosyan T, Gaujoux S, Chirica M, Munoz-Bongrand N, Sarfati E, Cattan P. Functional disorders and quality of life after esophagectomy and gastric tube reconstruction for cancers. J Visc Surg. 2011;148(5):e327–35. https://doi.org/10.1016/j.jviscsurg.2011.09.001.
24. Sitges AC, Sanchez-Ortega JM, Sitges AS. Late complications of reversed gastric tube oesophagoplasty. Thorax. 1986;41:61–5. https://doi.org/10.1136/thx.41.1.61.
25. Gavriliu D. Operation for functional obstruction of the cardia (cardiospasm-achalasia). Curr Probl Surg. 1975;12(10):29–36.
26. Schwartz B, Hall WW. Replacement of entire esophasus by reversed gastric tube procedure (Heimlich–Gavriliu operation). Am J Surg. 1961;102:79–82. https://doi.org/10.1016/0002-9610(61)90689-4.
27. Zhang M, Zhang C, Wu QC. Health-related quality of life and survival among 10-year survivors of esophageal cancer surgery: gastric tube reconstruction versus whole stomach reconstruction. J Thorac Dis. 2019;11(8):3284–91. https://doi.org/10.21037/jtd.2019.08.56.
28. Klevebro F, Elliot JA, Slaman A, Vermeulen BD, Kamiya S, Rosman C, et al. Cardiorespiratory comorbidity and postoperative complications following esophagectomy: a European multicenter cohort study. Ann Surg Oncol. 2019;26(9):2864–73. https://doi.org/10.1245/s10434-019-07478-6.
29. Biere SS, Maas KW, Cuesta MA, van der Peet DL. Cervical or thoracic anastomosis after esophagectomy for cancer: a systematic review and meta-analysis. Dig Surg. 2011;28(1):29–35. https://doi.org/10.1159/000322014.
30. Booka E, Takeuchi H, Suda K, Fukuda K, Nakamura R, Wada N, et al. Meta-analysis of the impact of postoperative complications on survival after oesophagectomy for cancer. BJS Open. 2018;2(5):276–84. https://doi.org/10.1002/bjs5.64.
31. Klevebro F, Friesland S, Hedman M, Tsai JA, Lindblad M, Rouvelas I, et al. Neoadjuvant chemoradiotherapy may increase the risk of severe anastomotic complications after esophagectomy with cervical anastomosis. Langenbecks Arch Surg. 2016;401(3):323–31. https://doi.org/10.1007/s00423-016-1409-0.
32. Zhou D, Liu QX, Deng XF, Min JX, Dai JG. Comparison of two different mechanical esophagogastric anastomosis in esophageal cancer patients: a meta-analysis. J Cardiothorac Surg. 2015;10:67. https://doi.org/10.1186/s13019-015-0271-4.
33. Schröder W, Raptis DA, Schmidt HM, Gisbertz SS, Moons J, Asti E, et al. Anastomotic techniques and associated morbidity in total minimally invasive transthoracic esophagectomy: results from the EsoBenchmark database. Ann Surg. 2019;270(5):820–6. https://doi.org/10.1097/SLA.0000000000003538.
34. Van Rossum PSN, Haverkamp L, Verkooijen HM, Van Leeuwen MS, van Hillegersberg R, Ruurda JP. Calcifications of arteries supplying the gastric tube: a new risk factor for anastomotic leakage after esophageal surgery. Radiology. 2015;274(1):124–32. https://doi.org/10.1148/radiol.14140410.
35. Gubler C, Vetter D, Schmidt HM, Müller PC, Morell B, Raptis D, et al. Preemptive endoluminal vacuum therapy to reduce anastomotic leakage after esophagectomy: a game-changing approach? Dis Esophagus. 2019;32(7):doy126. https://doi.org/10.1093/dote/doy126.
36. Briel JW, Tamhankar AP, Hagen JA, DeMeester SR, Johansson J, Choustoulakis E, et al. Prevalence and risk factors for ischemia, leak, and stricture of esophageal anastomosis: gastric pull-up versus colon interposition. J Am Coll Surg. 2004;198(4):536–41. https://doi.org/10.1016/j.jamcollsurg.2003.11.026.
37. Zheng M, Li Q, Tie HT, Jiang YJ, Wu QC. Methods of reconstruction after esophagectomy on long-term health-related quality of life: a prospective, randomized study of 5-year follow-up. Med Oncol. 2015;32(4):122. https://doi.org/10.1007/s12032-015-0568-0.

38. van Heijl M, Gooszen JA, Fockens P, Busch OR, van Lanschot JJ, van Berge Henegouwen MI. Risk factors for development of benign cervical strictures after esophagectomy. Ann Surg. 2010;251(6):1064–9. https://doi.org/10.1097/SLA.0b013e3181deb4b7.
39. Hayashi E, Yuasa N, Sasaki E, Kamiya J, Nagino M, Nimura Y, et al. Right gastroepiploic artery occlusion test for resection of recurrent lesion after esophageal reconstruction using a gastric tube. Am J Surg. 2004;187(3):446–9. https://doi.org/10.1016/j.amjsurg.2003.12.009.
40. Sakaki A, Kanamari J, Sato A, Okada N, Ishiyama K, Oguma J. Case report gastric tube cancer after esophagectomy retrograde perfusion after proximal resection of right gastroepiploic artery. Int J Surg Case Rep. 2019;59:97–100. https://doi.org/10.1016/j.ijscr.2019.03.020.
41. Chen G, Wang Z, Liu XY, Liu FY. Recurrence pattern of squamous cell carcinoma in the middle thoracic esophagus after modified Ivor-Lewis esophagectomy. World J Surg. 2007;31(5):1107–14. https://doi.org/10.1007/s00268-006-0551-1.

# Management of Esophagogastric Junction Cancer

# 27

Ahmet Akmercan, Tevfik Kivilcim Uprak, and Cumhur Yegen

## 27.1 Introduction

With 1.6 million cases annually, esophagogastric cancer (ESC) is the third most prevalent type of cancer worldwide. Adenocarcinomas, which are primarily found in the gastroesophageal junction and distal esophagus, have become more common [1, 2]. Esophageal cancer treatment is best reviewed within a multidisciplinary tumor board (MDT). A complete preoperative evaluation is essential for esophageal cancer management, including accurate tumor staging, evaluation of the patient's comorbidities and medical history (with particular attention to previous surgical history), and a patient-specific physiological evaluation. This should include a nutritional assessment, best performed using the European Society for Clinical Nutrition and Metabolism (ESPEN) criteria [3]. Pulmonary function testing should be routinely performed in preparation for one-lung ventilation. Selected objective cardiac testing is recommended in patients with documented coronary artery disease, congestive heart failure, or atrial or ventricular dysrhythmia.

## 27.2 Staging and Classification

Multimodality treatment strategies for esophagogastric junction (EGJ) cancer require accurate staging. The tumor (T), node (N), and metastasis (M) staging system used by the American Joint Committee on Cancer (AJCC) is the internationally accepted standard for EGJ cancer staging. The Eighth Edition of the AJCC Cancer Staging Manual includes staging of esophageal and esophagogastric epithelial cancers with clinical staging (cTNM), pathologic staging (pTNM), and post-neoadjuvant pathologic staging (ypTNM) stage groups [4] (Fig. 27.1). The tumor grade (G) is

A. Akmercan · T. K. Uprak (✉) · C. Yegen
Department of General Surgery, Marmara University School of Medicine, Istanbul, Turkey


O. Engin (ed.), *Risk Factors and Therapy of Esophagus Cancer*,
https://doi.org/10.1007/978-3-031-47024-0_27

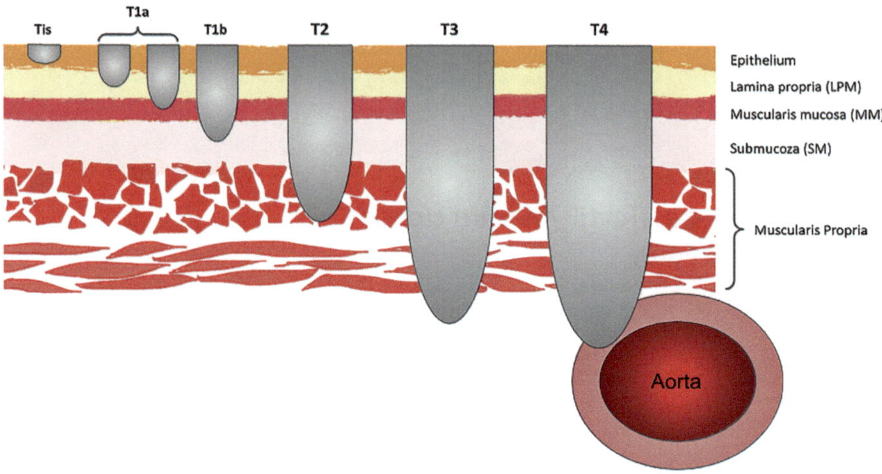


**Fig. 27.1** The Eighth Edition of the AJCC Cancer Manual TNM categories. *Tis* high-grade dysplasia, *T1a* tumor invades the lamina propria or muscularis mucosae, *T1b* tumor invades the submucosa, *T2* tumor invades the muscularis propria, *T3* tumor invades the adventitia, *T4a* tumor invades adjacent structures such as the pleura, pericardium, azygos vein, diaphragm, or peritoneum, *T4b* tumor invades the major adjacent structures, such as the aorta, vertebral body, or trachea

important for early-stage cancer staging (pTNM) in patients undergoing resection without neoadjuvant treatment. In addition, tumor location is necessary to subgroup pT3N0M0 squamous cell carcinoma [5].

In Japan Esophageal Society guidelines, mucosal invasion (T1a) depth is evaluated in three layers; M1 indicates the involvement of the epithelium, M2 is the invasion of the lamina propria, and M3 is the invasion of muscularis mucosa. Submucosal invasion depth (T1b) is also evaluated in three layers; SM1 describes the involvement of the upper third of the submucosa, SM2 is the involvement of the middle third of the submucosa, and SM3 is the involvement of the lower third of the submucosa [6] (Fig. 27.2).

EGJ adenocarcinomas were classified into three types by Siewert et al. based on the anatomic location of the tumor epicenter [7]. Siewert type I tumors are defined by the tumor epicenter located within 1–5 cm above the anatomic EGJ. Siewert type II tumors are defined by the tumor epicenter located within 1 cm above and 2 cm below the EGJ. Siewert type III tumors are defined with the tumor epicenter located between 2 and 5 cm below the EGJ, which infiltrates the EGJ and the distal esophagus from below (Fig. 27.3). The eighth edition of the AJCC Cancer Staging Manual also classified EGJ adenocarcinoma according to anatomic location. Based on this system, tumors involving the EGJ with an epicenter ≤2 cm into the proximal stomach are staged as esophageal carcinomas. Tumors with an epicenter located >2 cm into the proximal stomach are staged as gastric carcinomas, even if the EGJ is involved [4].

Initial clinical staging should include a complete physical examination, upper gastrointestinal (GI) tract endoscopy, endoscopic ultrasonography (EUS),

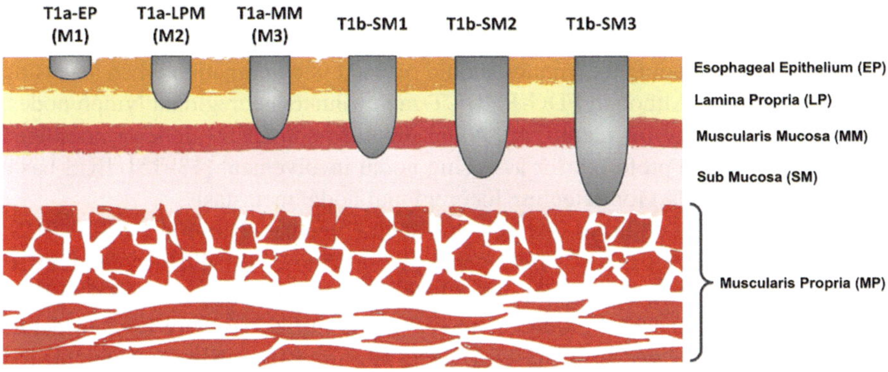


**Fig. 27.2** Japanese Classification of Esophageal Cancer 11th Edition Subclassification for Superficial Cancer. *T1a-EP(M1)* carcinoma in situ (Tis), *T1a-LPM(M2)* tumor invades the lamina propria mucosa, *T1a-MM(M3)* tumor invades the muscularis mucosa, *T1b-SM1* tumor invades the upper third of the submucosa, *T1b-SM2* tumor invades the middle third of the submucosa, *T1b-SM3* tumor invades the lower third of the submucosa

**Fig. 27.3** Siewert classification of esophagogastric cancer

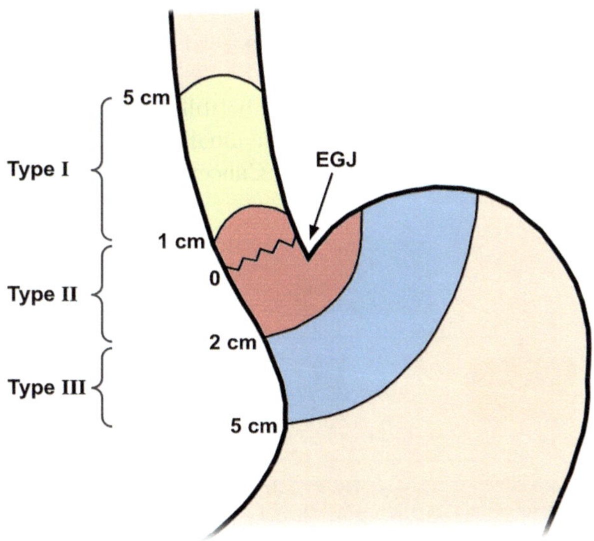


computed tomography (CT), or positron emission tomography (PET) with [$F^{18}$]2-fluoro-2-deoxy-D-glucose (FDG) [8]. EUS is considered the most reliable method for T staging; in a meta-analysis of 49 studies, EUS had excellent sensitivity (81–90%) and specificity (99%) for accurately determining the depth of the invasion in esophageal cancer [9]. A contrast-enhanced chest/abdominal CT scan or FDG-PET/CT can determine the location of the primary tumor and its invasion of adjacent structures. It plays an important role in the differentiation of T3 and T4 tumors [10]. FDG-PET/CT has higher sensitivity for detecting esophageal cancer than CT alone [11]. Nevertheless, CT and FDG-PET/CT have limited abilities in the diagnosis of early-stage tumors (Tis and T1) and in the differentiation of T1, T2, and T3 tumors [12]. Imaging techniques should be used in combination when assessing the clinic N stage. Although FDG-PET/CT can evaluate locoregional lymph nodes, it has low sensitivity for identifying nodal involvement. EUS (alone or combined with CT) should be preferred for assessing nodal involvement [13–15]. EUS has a high sensitivity (85%) for detecting locoregional nodal metastasis.

Furthermore, the addition of EUS-guided fine needle aspiration biopsy (EUS-FNA) increases the sensitivity of cN staging from 85 to 97% [9]. However, for distant lymph nodes, PET-CT has similar or better sensitivity and specificity than EUS [15]. Contrast-enhanced chest/abdomen CT is the initial modality used to detect distant metastasis. However, FDG-PET/CT is more sensitive than CT alone for cM staging and it may help identify distant metastases that are undetected by CT [10, 11, 14]. FDG-PET/CT should be done in esophageal cancer staging; thereby, it helps with proper patient selection for surgical resection [8, 16].

## 27.3 Treatment

### 27.3.1 Early-Stage Disease

The treatment scheme that can be followed in esophagogastric junction tumors is specified (Fig. 27.4). For individuals with clinical T1N0 (cT1N0) tumors, the National Comprehensive Cancer Network's (NCCN's) most recent

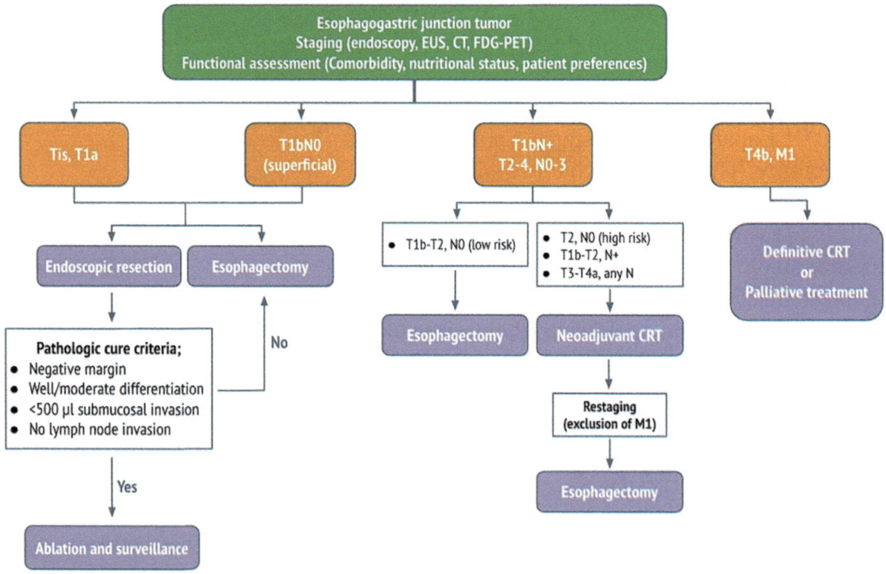


**Fig. 27.4** Treatment schema for esophagogastric junction tumors

recommendations suggest surgery initially. For individuals who have T2 lesions (less than 2 cm in size and well-differentiated), surgery alone may be an option. Early disease (cT1 N0 M0). For lesions with intraepithelial high-grade dysplasia and the majority of T1 tumors, endoscopic en bloc resection utilizing endoscopic mucosal resection (EMR) or endoscopic submucosal dissection (ESD) is the preferred method of care. The known risk factors for lymph node invasion include depth of invasion, lymphovascular invasion, low degree of differentiation, ulceration, and large tumor size [17, 18]. It can be used as a curative treatment for T1a malignancies and T1b tumors with superficial submucosal involvement (sm1, depth of invasion 500 μm, ulceration). EMR should typically be favored for small lesions, whereas ESD should be taken into consideration for lesions >15 mm, poorly confined tumors, and tumors at risk of submucosal invasion. Nevertheless, there is no evidence to suggest EMR or ESD for AC. While other risk factors are present, even deep intramucosal T1a tumors (m3) need extra therapy since the chance of lymph node metastasis in esophageal SCC is often high. 47 According to studies conducted in Asia, compared to EMR, ESD has a greater percentage of full resection and a lower risk of local recurrence [19–21].

Preoperative chemoradiation did not increase the rate of complete resection (R0) (93% in the surgery arm alone), disease-free survival (DFS), or overall survival in French research. However, the chemoradiation group had a considerably higher in-hospital postoperative mortality rate [22].

### 27.3.2 Local Advanced Disease

According to recent studies, individuals with locally advanced esophageal cancer who undergo surgery alone have 5-year OS rates between 23 and 33%. Multimodal treatment has become commonplace. Many studies have demonstrated that adding preoperative and postoperative techniques like chemotherapy or chemoradiation to surgery might enhance outcomes [23].

For both histological subtypes of locally advanced resectable esophageal cancer (cT2–T4a or cN1–3), surgery is the primary curative therapy. The recommended surgery is a radical transthoracic esophagectomy with lymphadenectomy. Reconstruction is done with a gastric tube conduit and an esophagogastric anastomosis in the upper mediastinum using abdominal and right chest access (Ivor Lewis procedure). Transhiatal esophagectomy without transthoracic access can be performed in elderly patients with distal tumors with lesser morbidity at the risk of a less thorough lymphadenectomy [24].

All patients with locally advanced resectable esophageal cancer should be considered for preoperative and perioperative treatment with chemotherapy or chemoradiotherapy, as it has been shown to increase tumor-free (R0) resection rates and survival rates in esophageal cancer. However, there are studies suggesting that it has adverse effects on postoperative mortality in stage 1–2 patients but does not improve R0 resection rates in patients receiving preoperative CT or CRT. There is insufficient data on the use of preoperative CT and CRT in clinical T2 n0 patients. Cases should be evaluated on an interdisciplinary and patient-specific basis [23, 25–28].

The standard of therapy for locally advanced esophageal cancer (AC) with OGJ is preoperative CRT [28]. In locally advanced AC of the OGJ, it has been found that preoperative and perioperative CT is another standard of care [25, 26, 29]. Phase III MAGIC research, which used a regimen of three preoperative and three postoperative epirubicin cisplatin5-FU (ECF) cycles, was the first to show the efficacy of perioperative KT. The R0 resection rate was achieved with improved survival [23]. In comparison with perioperative ECF (FLOT), the Phase II/III FLOT4 research found that FLOT had a better OS. Thus, for patients who can tolerate treatment, FLOT is the preferred perioperative regimen [30]. There haven't been many direct comparisons of KT with CRT; however, in 2021, the results of the phase III NeoAEGIS experiment, which evaluated two common regimens (MAGIC study ECF regimen or FLOT), were summarized. According to preliminary findings, the CRT arm had greater rates of tumor regression and pathological full responses. There was no difference in OS between the two therapies, but most patients in the CRT group received the old ECF regimen as opposed to the perioperative FLOT regimen, which is projected to have higher efficacy. We are waiting to collect results from the phase III ESOPEC research comparing the CROSS CRT regimen to FLOT [31, 32].

### 27.3.3 Surgical Margin

Providing a negative resection margin (longitudinal and circumferential) is mandatory in esophageal cancer surgery. It is known that a positive proximal resection margin is associated with poor prognosis [33]. Because of post-fixation shrinkage and intramural metastases, the determination of longitudinal margins is complicated. Gao et al. reported that 56% of the R+ patients had infiltration of the submucosa without infiltration of the mucosa, although a 5-cm proximal clear in vivo margin was achieved in a cohort of Siewert II and III patients without neoadjuvant treatment [34]. Khoshnevis et al. reported that the main shrinkage that occurs after 24 h is around 27% in formalin fixation [35]. Hence, some authors tried to describe optimal margins for safety and compatibility with clinical practice. A gross proximal esophageal margin greater than 5 cm is necessary for curative surgery of adenocarcinoma of the esophagogastric junction in clinical practice [36–38]. On the other hand, recent meta-analyses showed that a positive circumferential resection margin (CRM) is associated with a worse prognosis regardless of classification system, T category, tumor type, or neoadjuvant therapy [39, 40].

In summary, an initial proximal surgical margin of at least 5 cm and radical en bloc circumferential resection should be targeted.

### 27.3.4 Lymphadenectomy

Lymph node (LN) status is an important parameter in predicting survival for esophageal carcinoma. LN metastasis patterns depend on tumor characteristics such as location, invasion depth, histologic subtype, grade, and neoadjuvant chemotherapy. The effect of lymphadenectomy extent and the number of resected lymph nodes on prognosis has been studied widely. However, published studies on these subjects consist of heterogeneous groups. Evaluation of SCC and adenocarcinoma together, the use of different classification systems for LN stations, differences in lymphadenectomy types, study populations, and adjuvant or neoadjuvant treatment modalities can be considered among the reasons for this situation. Nevertheless, research has demonstrated that the degree of lymphadenectomy, the number of LN retrieved, and the number of involved LN are essential for an accurate staging system and survival prediction [41].

#### 27.3.4.1 Lymph Nodes Classification Systems

The AJCC eighth edition esophageal cancer staging and the JES 11th edition esophageal cancer staging (Fig. 27.5) are different categorization systems that are utilized in various nations to categorize LN stations surrounding the esophagus [4, 6].

### 27.3.5 Nodal Spread by Tumor Characteristic

LN involvement depends on the invasion depth of the primary tumor and progressively increases as the invasion depth rises. The incidence of nodal involvement in T1a tumors varies between 0 and 6% in published reports. The incidence of nodal metastases in T1b tumors is around 20% but peaks up to 45% in some studies. There have been reports of LN involvement in 50–60% of T2 tumors and up to 90% of T3/T4 tumors [42–48].

In Siewert type 1 tumors, lymphatic flow is mainly toward the abdomen. Abdominal lymph nodes are almost always involved in node-positive disease. Although they usually develop concomitant abdominal involvement, mediastinal nodes are frequently affected (17–77%). Nevertheless, mediastinal node involvement alone is rarely seen. Paracardial (stations 1 and 2), lesser curvature (station 3), and left gastric artery nodes (station 7) were the most frequently involved abdominal stations, while mid- and lower mediastinal paraoesophageal (stations 108 and 110) were the main mediastinal stations. Celiac trunk, splenic artery nodes (stations 9 and 11) can also be involved; thus, they should be dissected during lymphadenectomy. Supradiaphragmatic (station 111), posterior mediastinal (station 112), subcarinal (station 107), and main bronchus (station 109) lymph nodes are other stations that can be involved in the mediastinal region [43, 49–52]. Some studies of patients with Siewert-1 tumors treated with three-field lymphadenectomy described a relevant rate of cervical nodal involvement. Lerut et al. reported the presence of cervical metastatic nodes in 26% of Siewert type I cancers, while Altorki et al. reported 37% involvement of cervicothoracic nodes [53, 54]. In a recent study with middle and

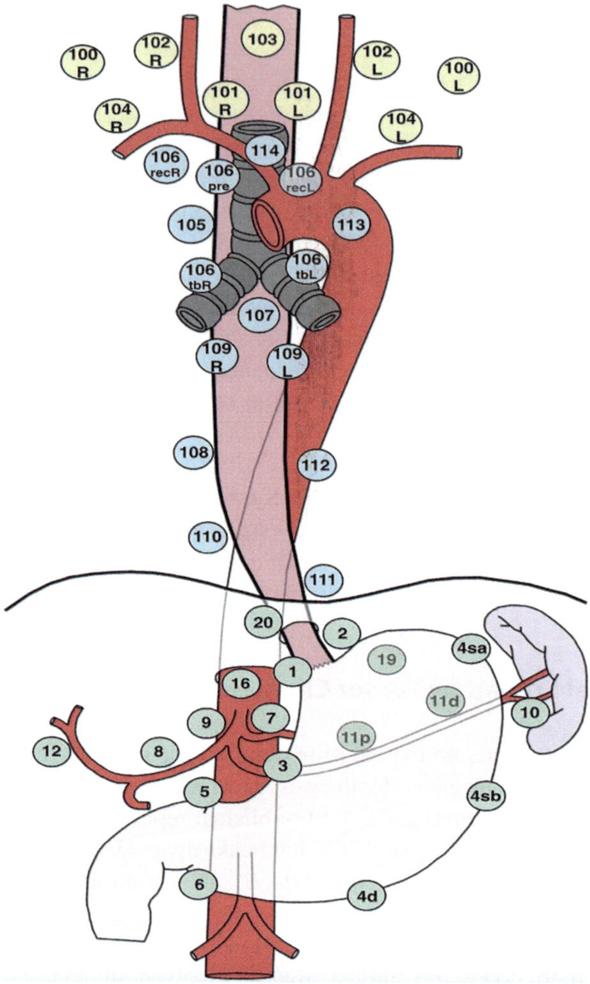


**Fig. 27.5** Japanese Classification of Esophageal Cancer 11th Edition, station number of regional lymph nodes. Cervical lymph nodes are classified as: 100, superficial lymph nodes of neck; 101, cervical paraesophageal lymph nodes; 102, deep cervical lymph nodes; 103, peripharyngeal lymph nodes; 104, supraclavicular lymph nodes. Thoracic lymph nodes are classified as 105, upper thoracic paraesophageal lymph nodes; 106, thoracic paratracheal lymph nodes; 107, subcarinal lymph nodes; 108, middle thoracic paraesophageal lymph nodes; 109, main bronchus lymph nodes; 110, lower thoracic paraesophageal lymph nodes; 111, supradiaphragmatic lymph nodes; 112, posterior mediastinal lymph nodes; 113, ligamentum arteriosum lymph nodes; 114, anterior mediastinal lymph nodes. Abdominal lymph nodes are classified as: 1, right paracardiac lymph nodes; 2, left paracardiac lymph nodes; 3, lesser curvature lymph nodes; 4, greater curvature lymph nodes; 5, suprapyloric lymph nodes; 6, infrapyloric lymph nodes; 7, left gastric artery lymph nodes; 8, common hepatic artery lymph nodes; 9, celiac trunk lymph nodes; 10, splenic hilum lymph nodes; 11, splenic artery lymph nodes; 12, hepatoduodenal ligament lymph nodes; 16, paraaortic lymph nodes; 19, infradiaphragmatic lymph nodes; 20, esophageal hiatus of the diaphragma lymph nodes

lower esophageal tumors, cervical node involvement was found at a rate of 21% [55]. However, relevance to cervical lymph nodes of Siewert 1 tumor is not common or at least not commonly studied.

In Siewert type 2 tumors, lymphatic flow is mainly toward the abdomen. Abdominal stations are the only metastatic sites in 64–95% of the patients, while concomitant mediastinal and abdominal involvement occurs in 5–30% of patients. Mediastinal node involvement alone has not been described. The mainly affected nodal stations are paracardial (stations 1 and 2), lesser curvature (station 3), and left gastric artery nodes (station 7) in the abdomen and mid- and lower mediastinal nodes in the mediastinum. Celiac trunk, common hepatic artery, and splenic artery nodes (stations 8, 9, and 11) are also frequently involved [43, 49–51, 56]. Also, para-aortic nodes are frequently affected. Mine et al. and Yoshikawa et al. reported 17% and 14% respectively involvement of para-aortic nodes around the left renal vein (station 16A2lat) [56, 57]. Lerut et al. and Kakeji et al. performing three-field lymphadenectomies for patients with type 2 tumors reported 18% and 2%, respectively, cervical node involvement [51, 53]. The recent prospective nationwide Japan study described 5% cervicothoracic node (106recR) involvement in type 2 tumors [52]. However, studies about three-field lymphadenectomy in type 2 tumors are limited and prevent making any conclusions. In patients with greater esophageal invasion, the involvement of mediastinal nodes increases. It has been reported that when esophageal invasion exceeds 2 cm, mediastinal node metastases increase significantly [58, 59]. Kurokawa et al. reported that inferior mediastinal nodes were markedly more affected when the esophageal invasion exceeded 2 cm, and upper and middle mediastinal nodes were markedly more affected when the esophageal invasion exceeded 4 cm [52].

### 27.3.6 Extend of Lymphadenectomy

The terminologies and types of lymphadenectomies for esophageal and esophagogastric junction cancer (EGJ) were defined at the 1995 Consensus Conference of the International Society for Diseases of the Esophagus (ISDE). Lymph node regions were divided into three fields: abdomen (field 1), thorax (field 2), and neck (field 3). Two-field lymphadenectomy includes abdominal and thoracic dissection, while in three-field lymphadenectomy, neck nodes are also dissected. Furthermore, thorax was also subdivided into three classes: standard, extended, and complete. Furthermore, thorax was also subdivided into three classes: standard, extended, and complete. Standard lymphadenectomy includes mid- and lower mediastinal nodes (stations 107, 108, 109, 110, and 111); extended lymphadenectomy also includes also upper mediastinum nodes (stations 101R, 105, 106tbR, 106pre, and 106recR) on the right site. Complete lymphadenectomy requires dissection of bilateral upper mediastinal lymph nodes [60].

Mid- and lower mediastinal nodes are commonly involved in both Siewert type 1 and type 2 tumors; therefore, a standard mediastinal lymphadenectomy is indicated [61, 62]. Furthermore, it has been reported that patients benefit from extended two-field lymphadenectomy over limited two-field lymphadenectomy. However, compared with two-field lymphadenectomy, three-field lymphadenectomy did not improve survival [55, 63].

Abdominal lymphadenectomy is usually performed according to Japanese guidelines for EGJ cancers. D1+ lymphadenectomy, in which the paracardial (stations 1 and 2), lesser curvature (station 3), left gastric artery (station 7), and celiac (station 9) lymph nodes are removed, and D2 lymphadenectomy, in which additional splenic (station 11) and common hepatic (station 8) lymph nodes are removed, have been described. In Siewert type 1 tumor, paracardial, lesser curvature, left gastric artery, and celiac nodes are commonly involved; therefore, D1+ lymphadenectomy should be performed. The risk of nodal metastasis is similar in Siewert type 2 tumors; in addition to splenic artery and common hepatic artery nodes, this is common. Hence, D2 lymphadenectomy is recommended for Siewert type 2 tumors. Splenectomy is not recommended for D2 dissection, given studies from both eastern and western centers [61, 64]. In Siewert type 2 tumors, mainly those with predominant gastric involvement, the incidence of para-aortic nodes (especially around the left renal vein) metastases is not negligible. Nevertheless, para-aortic dissection is not routinely recommended and can only be considered in selected patients [52, 56, 65].

### 27.3.7 Number of Resected Lymph Nodes

The number of resected LNs is indicative of sufficient lymphadenectomy. Accurate staging is made possible by retrieving more nodes. Reducing stage migration allows for the determination of efficient management strategies and the accurate prediction of survival. At the same time, increases in the retrieved nodes have been shown to be associated with better survival. It has been hypothesized that a reduction in stage migration and the elimination of micrometastases are responsible for the improvement in survival [66]. Several cut-off values have been reported for the minimal number of lymph nodes that should be harvested for maximizing survival and accurate staging [67–72].

Analysis of patients from the Memorial Sloan-Kettering Cancer Centre suggested retrieving at least 18 LNs for reliable staging [67]. An analysis of the Surveillance Epidemiology and End Results (SEER) database suggested retrieving at least 30 LNs to obtain optimal survival and staging [73]. Another recent SEER analysis suggested the same number of resected nodes for optimizing survival while suggesting 15 LNs for accurate staging [70]. Altorki et al. claimed that 16 nodes are sufficient for staging and to provide a survival benefit for N+ patients, while more than 40 nodes are required to provide a survival benefit for N0 patients [68]. Peyre et al. reported that survival was maximized with 23–29 nodes resected [69]. Analysis of Worldwide Esophageal Cancer Collaboration (WECC) data recommended that we retrieve at least 10, 20, and 30 nodes, respectively, for T1, T2, and T3. Moreover, according to this study, it is advised to retrieve at least 30 LN if the T stage and grade cannot be identified [66]. The number of lymph nodes that need to be removed is still controversial for patients without preoperative CRT. However, we believe that at least 15 LN should be retrieved for accurate staging and at least 30 LN should be retrieved to maximize survival.

The optimum number of nodes to be removed and examined after preoperative chemoradiation (CRT) is debated. Analysis of WECC data demonstrated a survival advantage with increased lymph node retrieval in patients who received preoperative CRT [72]. Guo et al. demonstrated that resection of 13–29 LN was associated with better survival in patients with locally advanced esophageal SCC receiving preoperative CRT [74]. Analysis of the USA National Cancer Database showed that resection of 25 or more LN was associated with longer median survival [75]. A recently published meta-analysis showed a survival benefit for increased lymph node retrieval from esophagectomy, regardless of whether or not patients had received preoperative CRT [76]. On the other hand, in the CROSS study population, there was no association between the number of LNs resected and survival for patients who had preoperative CRT [77]. In our opinion, preoperative CRT should not be a substitute for a proper lymphadenectomy, and a minimum of 15 LN should be resected for preoperative CRT received patients.

## 27.4 Surgical Approaches

With the variety of different surgical approaches currently available for esophagectomy, the choice of surgical approach should consider the individual patient and tumor characteristics. No single approach for esophageal resection is appropriate for all patients.

### 27.4.1 Ivor Lewis Transthoracic Esophagectomy

Ivor Lewis esophagectomy has advantages in middle and distal esophageal cancers. It offers optimal visualization during the dissection of the esophagogastric junction and thoracic esophagus and allows for a complete two-site thoracoabdominal lymphadenectomy. This approach uses two standard incisions, so trainees are relatively easy to teach, and unlike the transhiatal approach, all dissections are done under direct vision. It allows extensive abdominal and thoracic lymphadenectomy. Furthermore, it is easily adaptable to minimally invasive or robotic techniques [78].

The abdominal phase is started with a laparotomy or laparoscopy to exclude the presence of distant metastases. The stomach is dissected over the right gastroepiploic and right gastric arches, preserving the gastroepiploic arch. Complete freeing is achieved by dividing all posterior attachments of the stomach and duodenocolic ligament. The previously mentioned lymph node stations are dissected. During hiatal dissection, it is important to provide adequate space for the passage of the gastric conduit. The stomach is then stapled to form a conduit at the level of the right gastric artery from a lesser curvature using surgical staplers. The remaining stomach can be sutured to the esophagus, or it can be left to be pulled into the cervical area without a complete stapled incision. A gastric tube is created by resecting the specimen after the esophagus is separated along its length and the stomach and esophagus are transported to the abdomen on a band. A laparoscopic camera bag is typically used to extend the gastric tube into the neck through the rear of a Foley catheter for anastomosis. A feeding jejunostomy is routinely placed for postoperative feeding. The omentum close to the transverse colon may be sutured to the abdominal wall to prevent postoperative diaphragmatic herniation [79].

After the completion of the abdominal phase, the patient is placed in the left lateral decubitus position. The operating table is flexed to widen the intercostal space. It is performed through the fourth or fifth intercostal space via a right posterolateral thoracotomy. The operation can also be performed using minimally invasive surgery. The operation is started by dividing the arch of the azygos vein. The descending aorta and the adventitia fascia of the esophagus are separated by pleural incision. The thoracic duct is identified at the level of the azygos vein and can be dissected from the aorta. Paraaortic lymph nodes and thoracic ducts are mobilized, and the aortic branches are disconnected from the esophagus. The anterior plane of the dissection is along the pericardium, allowing suspension of the esophagus. The dissection continues caudally to the right pulmonary hilum, and the right bronchial, subcarinal, and left bronchial nodes are dissected. Care is taken in this area to avoid membranous injury to the tracheobronchial tree. The mediastinal pleura is dissected along the right vagus nerve toward the brachiocephalic and subclavian arteries. The right recurrent laryngeal nerve is preserved, and the adjacent lymph node chain is dissected. The pleura is incised along the border of the superior vena cava, and the right paratracheal lymph nodes between the trachea and vena cava are dissected. After the resection is completed, the esophagus is cut by observing the surgical margin. The proximal resection margin should be examined for Barrett's disease and cancer. The gastric conduit is positioned above the ligated azygos vein at the top of the chest, near the proximal esophagus. The conduit should not be under tension while it is in this position. Between the conduit and the esophagus, a suture is inserted. With a linear stapler, the proximal esophagus is incised. A 30 mm linear stapler is used to make anastomosis, with one arm in the esophagus and the other at the conduit. The anastomosis in the common walls of the esophagus and gastric tube is created by firing the stapler. A two layer of absorbable inner and nonabsorbable sutures in the outer layer are used to close the opening to finish the esophagogastric anastomosis [80–82].

### 27.4.2 Anastomosis and Choice of Conduit

A gastric tube is usually used after esophagectomy. It is generally preferred because it requires a single anastomosis and is easy to prepare. It is recommended to prepare an initial conduit of approximately 5 cm by preserving the right gastroepiploic arcade. Preservation of the right gastric artery is important in terms of preserving the intramural vascular arcade and preparing a well-blooded conduit. Pyloroplasty and pyloromyotomy can provide gastric drainage. Kocher maneuver is especially necessary in the presence of a long conduit [83, 84].

Colon interposition is preferred, especially in cases where the esophagus and stomach are to be resected or when the stomach cannot be used due to previous surgeries. It is generally less preferred because more anastomosis is needed and its long-term durability is less than that of gastric conduit. Isoperistaltic anastomoses are preferred. The vascular structure must be well determined. Generally, the transverse colon, in which the ascending branch of the left colic is protected, or the right colon, in which the middle colic artery is based, is used. After preoperative bowel cleansing, the whole colon should be mobilized, and variations should be paid attention to. After the colon to be used is selected, its proximal should be cut, and it should be extended toward the chest and neck, and it should be seen that it comes without tension [85].

## References


1. Bray F, et al. Global cancer statistics 2018: GLOBOCAN estimates of incidence and mortality worldwide for 36 cancers in 185 countries. CA Cancer J Clin. 2018;68(6):394–424.
2. Buas MF, Vaughan TL. Epidemiology and risk factors for gastroesophageal junction tumors: understanding the rising incidence of this disease. In: Seminars in radiation oncology. Elsevier; 2013.
3. Cederholm T, et al. ESPEN guidelines on definitions and terminology of clinical nutrition. Clin Nutr. 2017;36(1):49–64.
4. AJCC. AJCC Cancer Staging Manual. 8th ed. New York: Springer; 2017.
5. Rice TW, et al. Recommendations for pathologic staging (pTNM) of cancer of the esophagus and esophagogastric junction for the eighth edition AJCC/UICC staging manuals. Dis Esophagus. 2016;29(8):897–905.
6. Japan Esophageal Society. Japanese classification of esophageal cancer: part I. Esophagus. 2009;6(1):1–25.
7. Siewert J, Stein H. Carcinoma of the gastroesophageal junction-classification, pathology and extent of resection. Dis Esophagus. 1996;9(3):173–82.
8. National Comprehensive Cancer Network. Esophageal and Esophagogastric Junction Cancers NCCN Guidelines. Version 5.2022.
9. Puli SR, et al. Staging accuracy of esophageal cancer by endoscopic ultrasound: a meta-analysis and systematic review. World J Gastroenterol. 2008;14(10):1479–90.
10. Tirumani H, et al. Esophageal carcinoma: current concepts in the role of imaging in staging and management. Can Assoc Radiol J. 2015;66(2):130–9.
11. Kato H, et al. Comparison between positron emission tomography and computed tomography in the use of the assessment of esophageal carcinoma. Cancer. 2002;94(4):921–8.
12. Cuellar SL, et al. Clinical staging of patients with early esophageal adenocarcinoma: does FDG-PET/CT have a role? J Thorac Oncol. 2014;9(8):1202–6.
13. Kim TJ, et al. Multimodality assessment of esophageal cancer: preoperative staging and monitoring of response to therapy. Radiographics. 2009;29(2):403–21.
14. Pfau PR, et al. The role and clinical value of EUS in a multimodality esophageal carcinoma staging program with CT and positron emission tomography. Gastrointest Endosc. 2007;65(3):377–84.
15. Chowdhury F, Bradley K, Gleeson F. The role of 18F-FDG PET/CT in the evaluation of oesophageal carcinoma. Clin Radiol. 2008;63(12):1297–309.

16. Obermannová R, et al. Oesophageal cancer: ESMO Clinical Practice Guideline for diagnosis, treatment and follow-up*. Ann Oncol. 2022;33(10):992–1004.
17. Cao Y, et al. Meta-analysis of endoscopic submucosal dissection versus endoscopic mucosal resection for tumors of the gastrointestinal tract. Endoscopy. 2009;41(9):751–7.
18. Kato K, et al. Parallel-group controlled trial of surgery versus chemoradiotherapy in patients with stage I esophageal squamous cell carcinoma. Gastroenterology. 2021;161(6):1878–1886 e2.
19. Pimentel-Nunes P, et al. Endoscopic submucosal dissection for superficial gastrointestinal lesions: European Society of Gastrointestinal Endoscopy (ESGE) Guideline—Update 2022. Endoscopy. 2022;54(6):591–622.
20. Probst A, et al. Endoscopic submucosal dissection for early gastric cancer: are expanded resection criteria safe for Western patients? Endoscopy. 2017;49(9):855–65.
21. Yamashina T, et al. Long-term outcome and metastatic risk after endoscopic resection of superficial esophageal squamous cell carcinoma. Am J Gastroenterol. 2013;108(4):544–51.
22. Mariette C, et al. Surgery alone versus chemoradiotherapy followed by surgery for stage I and II esophageal cancer: final analysis of randomized controlled phase III trial FFCD 9901. J Clin Oncol. 2014;32(23):2416–22.
23. Cunningham D, et al. Perioperative chemotherapy versus surgery alone for resectable gastroesophageal cancer. N Engl J Med. 2006;355(1):11–20.
24. Hulscher JB, et al. Extended transthoracic resection compared with limited transhiatal resection for adenocarcinoma of the esophagus. N Engl J Med. 2002;347(21):1662–9.
25. Sjoquist KM, et al. Survival after neoadjuvant chemotherapy or chemoradiotherapy for resectable oesophageal carcinoma: an updated meta-analysis. Lancet Oncol. 2011;12(7):681–92.
26. Ronellenfitsch U, et al. Preoperative chemo(radio)therapy versus primary surgery for gastroesophageal adenocarcinoma: systematic review with meta-analysis combining individual patient and aggregate data. Eur J Cancer. 2013;49(15):3149–58.
27. Allum WH, et al. Long-term results of a randomized trial of surgery with or without preoperative chemotherapy in esophageal cancer. J Clin Oncol. 2009;27(30):5062–7.
28. van Hagen P, et al. Preoperative chemoradiotherapy for esophageal or junctional cancer. N Engl J Med. 2012;366(22):2074–84.
29. Ychou M, et al. Perioperative chemotherapy compared with surgery alone for resectable gastroesophageal adenocarcinoma: an FNCLCC and FFCD multicenter phase III trial. J Clin Oncol. 2011;29(13):1715–21.
30. Al-Batran SE, et al. Perioperative chemotherapy with fluorouracil plus leucovorin, oxaliplatin, and docetaxel versus fluorouracil or capecitabine plus cisplatin and epirubicin for locally advanced, resectable gastric or gastro-oesophageal junction adenocarcinoma (FLOT4): a randomised, phase 2/3 trial. Lancet. 2019;393(10184):1948–57.
31. Reynolds JV, et al. Neo-AEGIS (Neoadjuvant trial in Adenocarcinoma of the Esophagus and Esophago-Gastric Junction International Study): Preliminary results of phase III RCT of CROSS versus perioperative chemotherapy (Modified MAGIC or FLOT protocol). (NCT01726452). Wolters Kluwer Health; 2021.
32. Hoeppner J, et al. ESOPEC: prospective randomized controlled multicenter phase III trial comparing perioperative chemotherapy (FLOT protocol) to neoadjuvant chemoradiation (CROSS protocol) in patients with adenocarcinoma of the esophagus (NCT02509286). BMC Cancer. 2016;16:503.
33. Raziee HR, et al. Systematic review of the predictors of positive margins in gastric cancer surgery and the effect on survival. Gastric Cancer. 2012;15:116–24.
34. Gao F, et al. Incidence of microscopically positive proximal margins in adenocarcinoma of the gastroesophageal junction. PLoS One. 2014;9(2):e88010.
35. Khoshnevis J, et al. A study of contractility of proximal surgical margin in esophageal cancer. Iran J Cancer Prev. 2013;6(1):25.
36. Barbour AP, et al. Adenocarcinoma of the gastroesophageal junction: influence of esophageal resection margin and operative approach on outcome. Ann Surg. 2007;246(1):1–8.
37. DiMusto PD, Orringer MB. Transhiatal esophagectomy for distal and cardia cancers: implications of a positive gastric margin. Ann Thorac Surg. 2007;83(6):1993–9.

38. Ito H, et al. Adenocarcinoma of the gastric cardia: what is the optimal surgical approach? J Am Coll Surg. 2004;199(6):880–6.
39. Evans R, et al. Meta-analysis of the influence of a positive circumferential resection margin in oesophageal cancer. BJS Open. 2019;3(5):595–605.
40. Chan DS, et al. Systematic review and meta-analysis of the influence of circumferential resection margin involvement on survival in patients with operable oesophageal cancer. Br J Surg. 2013;100(4):456–64.
41. Herrera LJ. Extent of lymphadenectomy in esophageal cancer: how many lymph nodes is enough? Ann Surg Oncol. 2010;17:676–8.
42. Bollschweiler E, et al. High rate of lymph-node metastasis in submucosal esophageal squamous-cell carcinomas and adenocarcinomas. Endoscopy. 2006;38(02):149–56.
43. Pedrazzani C, et al. Lymph node involvement in advanced gastroesophageal junction adenocarcinoma. J Thorac Cardiovasc Surg. 2007;134(2):378–85.
44. Leers JM, et al. Clinical characteristics, biologic behavior, and survival after esophagectomy are similar for adenocarcinoma of the gastroesophageal junction and the distal esophagus. J Thorac Cardiovasc Surg. 2009;138(3):594–602.
45. Altorki NK, et al. Multifocal neoplasia and nodal metastases in T1 esophageal carcinoma: implications for endoscopic treatment. Ann Surg. 2008;247(3):434.
46. Barbour AP, et al. Risk stratification for early esophageal adenocarcinoma: analysis of lymphatic spread and prognostic factors. Ann Surg Oncol. 2010;17:2494–502.
47. Gertler R, et al. Prevalence and topography of lymph node metastases in early esophageal and gastric cancer. Ann Surg. 2014;259(1):96–101.
48. Akutsu Y, et al. The prevalence of overall and initial lymph node metastases in clinical T1N0 thoracic esophageal cancer: from the results of JCOG0502, a prospective multicenter study. Ann Surg. 2016;264(6):1009–15.
49. Meier I, et al. Adenocarcinoma of the esophagogastric junction: the pattern of metastatic lymph node dissemination as a rationale for elective lymphatic target volume definition. Int J Radiat Oncol Biol Phys. 2008;70(5):1408–17.
50. Dresner S, et al. The pattern of metastatic lymph node dissemination from adenocarcinoma of the esophagogastric junction. Surgery. 2001;129(1):103–9.
51. Kakeji Y, et al. Lymph node metastasis from cancer of the esophagogastric junction, and determination of the appropriate nodal dissection. Surg Today. 2012;42:351–8.
52. Kurokawa Y, et al. Mapping of lymph node metastasis from esophagogastric junction tumors: a prospective nationwide multicenter study. Ann Surg. 2021;274(1):120–7.
53. Lerut T, et al. Three-field lymphadenectomy for carcinoma of the esophagus and gastroesophageal junction in 174 R0 resections: impact on staging, disease-free survival, and outcome: a plea for adaptation of TNM classification in upper-half esophageal carcinoma. Ann Surg. 2004;240(6):962.
54. Altorki N, et al. Three-field lymph node dissection for squamous cell and adenocarcinoma of the esophagus. Ann Surg. 2002;236(2):177.
55. Li B, et al. Esophagectomy with three-field versus two-field lymphadenectomy for middle and lower thoracic esophageal cancer: long-term outcomes of a randomized clinical trial. J Thorac Oncol. 2021;16(2):310–7.
56. Mine S, et al. Lymphadenectomy around the left renal vein in Siewert type II adenocarcinoma of the oesophagogastric junction. J Br Surg. 2013;100(2):261–6.
57. Yoshikawa T, et al. Theoretical therapeutic impact of lymph node dissection on adenocarcinoma and squamous cell carcinoma of the esophagogastric junction. Gastric Cancer. 2016;19(1):143–9.
58. Nunobe S, et al. Benefit of mediastinal and para-aortic lymph-node dissection for advanced gastric cancer with esophageal invasion. J Surg Oncol. 2008;97(5):392–5.
59. Hosokawa Y, et al. Clinicopathological features and prognostic factors of adenocarcinoma of the esophagogastric junction according to Siewert classification: experiences at a single institution in Japan. Ann Surg Oncol. 2012;19:677–83.

60. Fumagalli U. Resective surgery for cancer of the thoracic esophagus. Results of a Consensus Conference held at the VIth World Congress of the International Society for Diseases of the Esophagus. Dis Esophagus. 1996;9:30–8.
61. Mariette C, et al. Oesophagogastric junction adenocarcinoma: which therapeutic approach? Lancet Oncol. 2011;12(3):296–305.
62. Lutz MP, et al. Highlights of the EORTC St. Gallen International Expert Consensus on the primary therapy of gastric, gastroesophageal and oesophageal cancer-differential treatment strategies for subtypes of early gastroesophageal cancer. Eur J Cancer. 2012;48(16):2941–53.
63. D'Journo XB, et al. Transthoracic esophagectomy for adenocarcinoma of the oesophagus: standard versus extended two-field mediastinal lymphadenectomy?*. Eur J Cardio-Thorac Surg. 2005;27(4):697–704.
64. Goto H, et al. Value of splenectomy in patients with Siewert type II adenocarcinoma of the esophagogastric junction. Gastric Cancer. 2013;16:590–5.
65. Sasako M, et al. Left thoracoabdominal approach versus abdominal-transhiatal approach for gastric cancer of the cardia or subcardia: a randomised controlled trial. Lancet Oncol. 2006;7(8):644–51.
66. Rizk NP, et al. Optimum lymphadenectomy for esophageal cancer. Ann Surg. 2010;251(1):46–50.
67. Rizk N, et al. The prognostic importance of the number of involved lymph nodes in esophageal cancer: implications for revisions of the American Joint Committee on Cancer staging system. J Thorac Cardiovasc Surg. 2006;132(6):1374–81.
68. Altorki NK, et al. Total number of resected lymph nodes predicts survival in esophageal cancer. Ann Surg. 2008;248(2):221–6.
69. Peyre CG, et al. The number of lymph nodes removed predicts survival in esophageal cancer: an international study on the impact of extent of surgical resection. Ann Surg. 2008;248(4):549–56.
70. Mariette C, et al. The number of metastatic lymph nodes and the ratio between metastatic and examined lymph nodes are independent prognostic factors in esophageal cancer regardless of neoadjuvant chemoradiation or lymphadenectomy extent. Ann Surg. 2008;247(2):365–71.
71. Groth SS, et al. Determination of the minimum number of lymph nodes to examine to maximize survival in patients with esophageal carcinoma: data from the Surveillance Epidemiology and End Results database. J Thorac Cardiovasc Surg. 2010;139(3):612–20.
72. Stiles BM, et al. Worldwide Oesophageal Cancer Collaboration guidelines for lymphadenectomy predict survival following neoadjuvant therapy†. Eur J Cardio-Thorac Surg. 2012;42(4):659–64.
73. Schwarz RE, Smith DD. Clinical impact of lymphadenectomy extent in resectable esophageal cancer. J Gastrointest Surg. 2007;11(11):1384–94.
74. Guo J-C, et al. Number of resected lymph nodes and survival of patients with locally advanced esophageal squamous cell carcinoma receiving preoperative chemoradiotherapy. Anticancer Res. 2018;38(3):1569–77.
75. de Geus SWL, et al. Lymphadenectomy and survival after neoadjuvant chemoradiation for esophageal adenocarcinoma: is more better? J Gastrointest Surg. 2020;24(11):2447–55.
76. Visser E, et al. Prognostic value of lymph node yield on overall survival in esophageal cancer patients: a systematic review and meta-analysis. Ann Surg. 2019;269(2):261–8.
77. Koen Talsma A, et al. Lymph node retrieval during esophagectomy with and without neoadjuvant chemoradiotherapy: prognostic and therapeutic impact on survival. Ann Surg. 2014;260(5):786–93.
78. Caso R, Wee JO. Esophagogastric anastomotic techniques for minimally invasive and robotic Ivor Lewis operations. Oper Tech Thorac Cardiovasc Surg. 2020;25(2):105–23.
79. Slaman AE, et al. Improved anastomotic leakage rates after the "flap and wrap" reconstruction in Ivor Lewis esophagectomy for cancer. Dis Esophagus. 2023;36(1):doac036.
80. Egberts J-H, et al. Impact of the site of anastomosis after oncologic esophagectomy on quality of life—a prospective, longitudinal outcome study. Ann Surg Oncol. 2008;15:566–75.

81. Orringer MB, Marshall B, Iannettoni MD. Eliminating the cervical esophagogastric anastomotic leak with a side-to-side stapled anastomosis. J Thorac Cardiovasc Surg. 2000;119(2):277–88.
82. Lerut T, et al. Anastomotic complications after esophagectomy. Dig Surg. 2002;19(2):92–8.
83. Akiyama H, et al. Use of the stomach as an esophageal substitute. Ann Surg. 1978;188(5):606.
84. Arya S, et al. The impact of pyloric drainage on clinical outcome following esophagectomy: a systematic review. Dis Esophagus. 2015;28(4):326–35.
85. DeMeester TR, et al. Indications, surgical technique, and long-term functional results of colon interposition or bypass. Ann Surg. 1988;208(4):460–74.

# 28 The Management of Esophageal Cancer with Pericardial Involvement and the Vascular Reconstruction of Jejunal Interposition Grafts After Cervical Esophagectomy

Lutfi Cagatay Onar, Ufuk Ciloglu, and Ugur Filizcan

## 28.1 Historical Aspect

Very early in the history of man, it must have been quite obvious that things left standing would deteriorate. Thousands of years ago, human beings weren't in need of biological elimination for foods. Rats, cockroaches, termites, fungi, bacteria, and countless other species are natural contributors to our biological food cycle. In those years, fresh food was rarely kept for more than a day, whereas fermentation, curdling, fumigation, and salifying provided a longer shelf life for it. After many milestones in human population were reached, the rules of healthy food production changed dramatically, and of course, not in a proper way. At that stage of human history, surely the most strident voice of the industrial world obliged an increasing human population to consume processed or ultraprocessed food with a very extended shelf life. Besides the frequent use of tobacco and alcohol, processed food is another high-risk lifestyle based factor. These factors increase the number of esophageal cancer patients, which also increases the surgical experience related to the large volume of patients [1]. Nowadays, surgical resection of the esophagus is complemented with more than three alternative surgical steps, including the interposition of an autograft [1, 2]. After the first successful resection of esophagus was carried out by Torek in 1913 [3], so many things changed. Unfortunately, frequent use of drugs for gastrointestinal symptoms (heartburn, epigastric, or back pain) may hide symptoms of esophageal cancer, which leads to a late diagnosis and an advanced stage of the disease with metastasis at the time of diagnosis. In this expensive era of

L. C. Onar (✉)
Department of Cardiovascular Surgery, Tekirdag Dr. Ismail Fehmi CUMALIOĞLU City Hospital, Tekirdag, Türkiye
e-mail: lutficagatay.onar@saglik.gov.tr

U. Ciloglu · U. Filizcan
Department of Cardiovascular Surgery, Medical Park Pendik Hospital, Istanbul, Türkiye


O. Engin (ed.), *Risk Factors and Therapy of Esophagus Cancer*,
https://doi.org/10.1007/978-3-031-47024-0_28

pandemics, climate change, water, and food scarcity, the number of esophageal cancer patients is increasing, but not in a slow way, whereas the current availability of improved surgical techniques and driver mutation targeting therapies increases survival rates [4].

As defined well before, the mediastinum is responsible for hosting vital cardiac chambers, big vessels, and the surrounding pericardium, which may be directly affected by the primary tumor of the esophagus; therefore, the first or second symptom of the cancer may be related to the circulation system [5].

In recent years, due to the fact that scientific interest has been more focused on genomic alterations and the molecular biology of tumors, surgical approaches have been assumed to be developing treatment options in only selected cases. But in current practice, game-changing immunotherapies provide a better survival outcome, treat advanced disease, and/or limit the disease; therefore, the number of patients requiring complementary R0 surgery increases day by day [6].

## 28.2 Definition and Morphology

Despite the relatively rare involvement of pericardium and the circulatory system in esophageal carcinoma, it is especially important in driver mutation-based, slow progressing invasive tumors of the esophagus after definitive chemoradiotherapy and immunotherapy and locally advanced and/or advanced cases [4–6].

Esophagus enters the thoracic cavity right after its' proximal one-third formed by laryngeal pharynx. Thoracal segment starts in the superior mediastinum, whereas the aortic arch pushes it to the midline of the mediastinal cavity between the superior and posterior mediastinum borders. In the posterior mediastinum, except some anatomical variations, the esophagus and the left atrium are in close proximity and separated by the pericardium. Besides the left atrium and the pericardium, the esophagus is anatomically related to many structures, such as trachea, left laryngeal recurrent nerve, left main bronchus, the thoracic duct, azygos veins, the origins of right posterior intercostal arteries, mediastinal pleura, the thoracic aorta, and the terminal branch of the azygos vein [7].

The arterial supply of one third of the proximal part of the esophagus originates from inferior thyroidal artery, the mid one third originates from the thoracic aorta, and the distal one third originates from the left gastric artery. The venous drainage occurs in the inferior thyroidal vein for the proximal one third, the azygos veins for the mid one third, and the lower one third, the left gastric vein, and the portal vein, respectively. These anatomical conditions are crucially important regarding the vascular reconstructions during the jejunal interposition after esophagectomy [7] (Fig. 28.1a, b).

Pericardial involvement or invasion is thought to be a sign of advanced disease in esophageal carcinoma. Once a careful history has been taken from an esophageal cancer patient, it is easy to diagnose pericardial, cardiac, or great vascular involvement because of their early-appearing symptoms. Extremity edema with jugular venous congestion and dyspnea on exertion may be the first symptoms of the

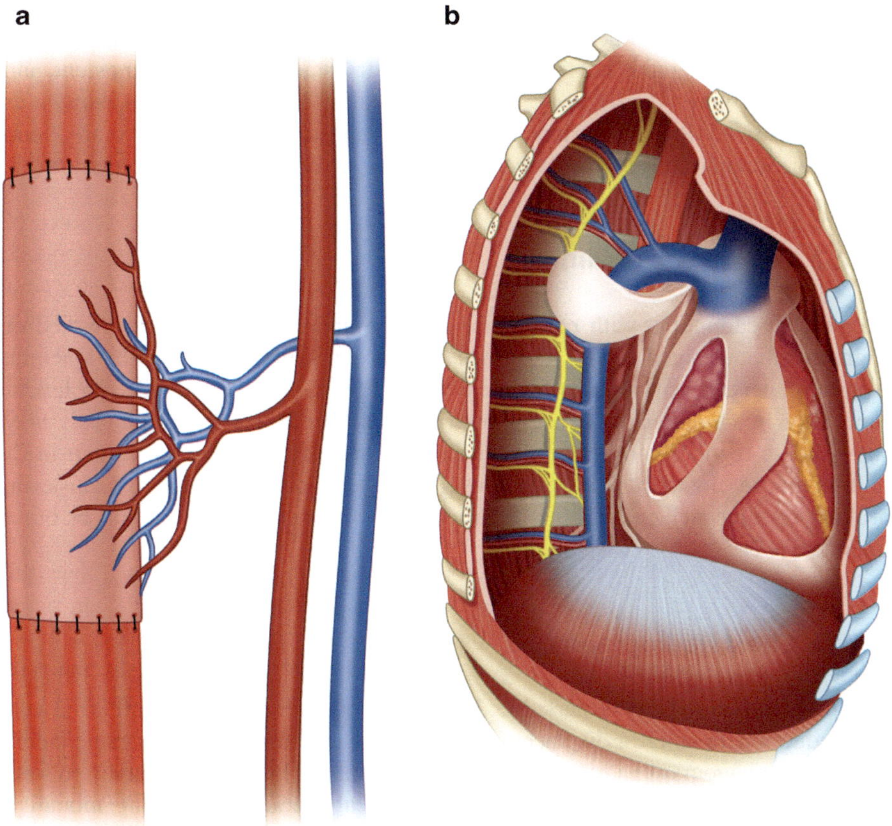


**Fig. 28.1** (**a**) Illustration of the jejunal interposition graft as an autograft in esophageal position. (**b**) Illustration of the thoracic cavity with posterior pericardial flap, which is the most involved pericardial part in esophageal cancers

clinical condition. In severe cases, cardiac tamponade may occur [5, 8], which is going to be discussed later on.

### 28.2.1 Clinical Findings

As it is discussed above, classically, symptoms of pericardial effusion due to tumor cell invasion may be observed in the late stages of the disease. Chemoradiotherapy receiving patients are more likely to develop pericardial effusions compared to immunotherapy-receiving patients. In both therapy modalities, pericardial effusion-related pseudo-progression of the disease has been reported in a few cases [9]. Besides the pseudo-progression, it is also important to distinguish between the involvement of common parapericardial lymph nodes and the direct invasion of the pericardium by the tumor. Multimodal imaging of the mediastinum may be beneficial for this distinction. In cases of direct pericardial invasion. When the pericardial effusion or constriction is not severe, clinical findings are modest but persistent, and hepatomegaly may occur slowly. Ascites, pleural effusion, and pulsus paradoxus may be observed. Rapid ventricular filling in the diastole with a usually early, loud third heart sound referred to as "pericardial knock" may be heard in auscultation [8].

### 28.2.2 Laboratory Findings

Esophageal carcinoma with pericardial invasion and effusion leads to marked or slight anemia, elevated hepatic enzymes, hypoproteinemia, and hypoalbuminemia. Approximately 1/3 of patients have elevated CEA, CA19–9, and CA-125 levels, especially in squamous cell carcinoma. Besides, this Western blot analysis may show the up-regulation of total procathepsin D and high-mannose procathepsin D, high-mannose clusterin. The serum levels of glycosylated fractions of clusterin, proline–arginine-rich end leucine-rich repeat protein, and haptoglobin may be other findings [1, 2, 5, 8].

### 28.2.3 Chest Radiography

Chest-ray film may be unremarkable. However, pericardial effusion, left atrial volume reduction, or anterior displacement may cause increased cardio-thoracic index. Barium esophagogram and single or double multiphase lateral radiography following barium swallowing may be a less invasive and practical imaging modality. Barium entrapping or difficulty with contrast cleaning may be an objective finding of an extensive esophageal tumor [1, 2, 5].

### 28.2.4 Electrocardiography

The electrocardiography (ECG) of esophageal carcinoma patients with pericardial involvement is usually abnormal. Low voltage QRS complexes and non-specific ST-segment or T-wave changes are predominant in half of the patients [1, 2, 8].

### 28.2.5 Definitive Imaging Studies

Two- or three-dimensional echocardiography may show posterior pericardial thickening, restriction, or underpressure mass effect of left atrium and cardiac tamponade findings. Corrupted Systolic Myocardial Velocity (Sa), diminished Mitral Annulus Systolic Excursion (MAPSE), and Tricuspid Annular Plane Systolic Excursion (TAPSE) may be other supportive echocardiographic parameters for cardiopericardial effects of the esophageal tumor [10].

Contrast-enhanced computed tomography, magnetic resonance imaging (MRI), and positron emission computed tomography (PET-CT) are other definitive high-resolution imaging modalities showing great sensitivity for pericardial invasion. Regarding the patients who undergo serial imaging after the diagnosis in follow-up period, deep learning artificial intelligence may predict pericardial invasion before it occurs [11]. Determining the accurate site of the esophageal wall thickening may bring out a good aspect in order to carry out other treatment options like surgery or SBRT (Stereotactic Body Radiation Therapy) to prevent pericardial invasion [12].

## 28.3 Surgical Techniques for Esophageal Carcinoma with Pericardial Invasion

Cardiac invasion or metastasis of tumors originating from the esophagus are rare and atypical if the histopathological type is squamous cell carcinoma. That presentation is generally associated with poor prognosis and most treatment options are still palliative [13]. For this reason, according to the aim of the surgery, we are going to discuss the surgical methods in two main captions (Table 28.1).

1. Definitive surgery for esophageal carcinoma with pericardial invasion
2. Obligatory and palliative surgical options

**Table 28.1** The indications for the definitive and palliative surgical approaches for neoplastic and non-neoplastic conditions are summarized below

| Definitive surgery | | Palliative surgery |
|---|---|---|
| Neoplastic | Non-neoplastic | Neoplastic |
| *Esophageal cancer<br>*Proximal gastric cancer<br>Laryngeal cancer<br>Thyroid cancer<br>Malignant carcinoid | Stricture<br>Caustic<br>*Radiation<br>Congenital atresia<br>Motility disorder | Esophageal cancer with massive pericardial effusion |
| *Potentially coexist with pericardial involvement | | |
| Surgical technique | | Surgical technique |
| Esophagectomy/esophagoplasty | | Pericardiosynthesis/pericardiostomy |
| Esophagocoloplasty w/wo pericardiectomy | | Esophagocoloplasty with pericardiectomy |
| Esophagojejunoplasty w/wo pericardiectomy | | Esophagojejunoplasty with pericardiotomy/pericardiectomy |
| **Free jejunal transfer, short segment colon interposition** | | **Free jejunal transfer, short segment colon interposition, with pericardiotomy/pericardiectomy** |

## 28.4 Operative Techniques in Pericardial and Paracardial Involvement

Restriction of pericardial compliance may deteriorate the patient's overall status quickly and critically. Most of the patients in the literature underwent surgical pericardiostomy or pericardiectomy in unstable clinical conditions. Arterial line and central venous line must be inserted before the operation. Once the right ventricular wall is freed, a rapid fluid shift occurs and may cause altered right ventricular filling pressure, pulmonary edema, and cardiac arrhythmia. The surgical approach may be via median sternotomy or left anterolateral thoracotomy (Fig. 28.2). If the median sternotomy preferred on pump beating heart may provide better cardiac decompression and the patient won't be affected by any arrhythmia that may be a result of using electrocautery or injury of sinus node. The pericardial flaps are dissected through the medial–lateral axis and the superior–inferior axis. If posterior pericardial invasion strikes over the left atrium, a posterior pericardiotomy may be necessary. Posterior pericardiectomy usually requires slow and careful dissection, in which cardiopulmonary bypass (CPB) is essential. The most convenient routes to initiate the CPB are the femoral artery and the femoral vein. Pericardial flaps are excised about 1.5–2 cm anterior to the bilateral phrenic nerves. During the posterior pericardiectomy, opening a posterior pericardial window in the undamaged area may provide good cleavage. For opening this window, holding the pericardium with a long Pean Rochester Curved Clamp and placing a superficial single silk suture may be useful for guiding the dissection plan. During this procedure, in order to

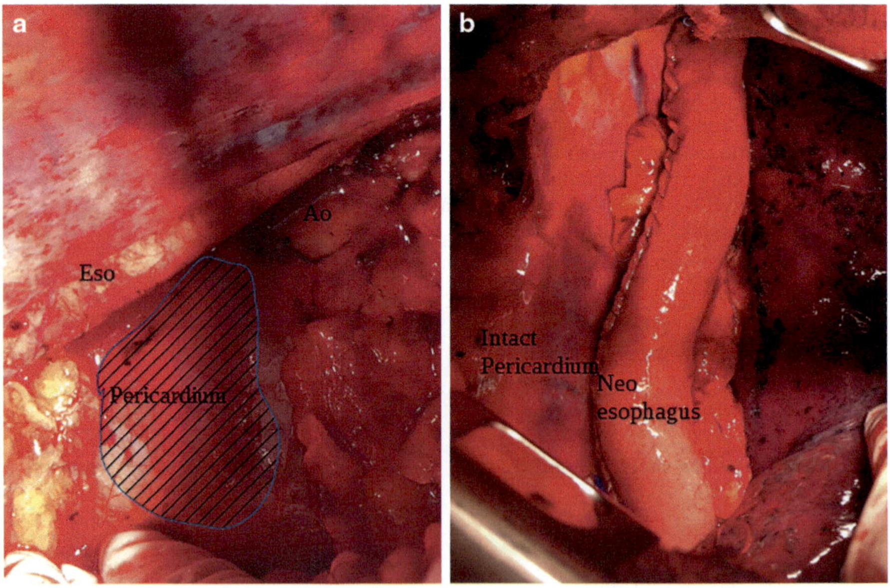


**Fig. 28.2** The anatomic positioning of the esophagus, aorta, and pericardium via left anterolateral thoracotomy, and the new esophagus formed by transposition and tube shaped stomach

protect the organs lying behind the pericardium, the position of the descending aorta must be kept in mind. This guiding suture eases getting and maintaining the proper dissection cleavage plane by providing manipulation of the dissected pericardial flap [13, 14].

The left anterolateral thoracotomy approach may provide a better exposure for posterior pericardiectomy, and the dissection may be easier. But using CPB and managing arrythmias may be difficult. Therefore, self-adhesive defibrillation pads must be placed before the surgery [15, 16].

In both incision methods, usually a pericardial fluid-filled space is found to open the pericardial cavity without damaging the epicardium, the great vessels, or the heart. When the infiltration causes constrictive pericarditis, there may be no space to open the pericardium in a proper way. The pericardium may be thick; dense scarring and calcification islands may be observed. It is important not to open the pericardium close to the coronary vessels. Once the pericardium is opened and a pericardial flap is procured, abrupt maneuvers may cause coronary injuries. Therefore, some calcification islands may be left in their place. The anterior and posterior pericardial flaps must be left long until the dissection is completed, so they may be used temporarily to tamponade any bleeding from the epicardium and the myocardium. Placing a Jackson Pratt drain into the pericardial space may be useful after the procedure, considering the drainage capability and lower volumetric features compared to conventional chest tubes. One or two left pleural tubes are usually necessary, one is to be placed posterior and inferiorly and the other anterior and superiorly [15, 16].

## 28.5 Operative Techniques After Esophageal Resection and Vascular Reconstruction

In most patients undergoing esophageal resection for esophageal cancer, reconstruction involves lengthening and transposition of the stomach (gastric conduit) through the diaphragm into the thoracic cavity. This method requires no additional vascular anastomosis. Also, gastric arteries are known to be resistant to atherosclerotic disease. The major handicap in this method is the complete lack of peristaltic activity of the gastric tube, which may lead to persistent reflux of the gastric contents to the cervical esophagus. Anastomose acid secreting from the stomach directly to the cervical esophagus is quite a predisposing factor for Barret esophagus. When the patient is unfit for orthotopic gastric transposition, esophagocoloplasty and esophagojejunoplasty operations are lifesaving methods due to their isoperistaltic nature. Performing these two methods requires careful vascular reconstruction to provide adequate blood flow to the interposition grafts. Jejunum is usually the third surgical option for esophageal replacement because the jejunal interposition graft cannot replace the entire esophagus. It is often used for proximal tumors. Esophagojejunoplasty may be performed using three alternative techniques, the first is free jejunal graft, the second is pedicled graft, and the third is Roux and Y replacement. So that the jejunal Roux and Y replacement is usually done for the distal esophageal tumors, we are going to discuss the methodology of free jejunal interposition grafts and their blood supply in this section of the book [1, 2, 13, 17].

Pedicled Jejunal graft (Fig. 28.3) is an interposition graft retaining its vascular supply with the branches originating from the superior mesenteric artery and vein.

During the graft harvesting, a left thoracoabdominal incision extending to the costal border of the rectus muscle is a convenient way. Transillumination of the jejunum provides an accurate estimation of the graft length. The first jejunal artery must be identified and preserved to provide the vascular integrity of the 10–12 cm of jejunum adjacent to the Treitz Ligament (Fig. 28.3). During the harvesting, local injections of heparinized saline may provide better patency. Following the injection of heparinized saline, the other 3–4 jejunal arteries must be exposed and sequentially occluded with atraumatic bulldog clamps to test the reliability of the first jejunal artery and whether it may supply adequate arterial blood circulation or not. The proximal jejunum is transected via a stapler, and the mesentery is divided down each side toward the feeding artery and the collecting vein. The preservation of the highest jejunal artery is essential for graft viability. If there is no adequate blood flow in the feeding artery, especially in cervical esophagojejunoplasty, there is always a good alternative vascular enhancement method. The left internal mammary artery or superior thyroid artery may provide good arterial blood flow to the

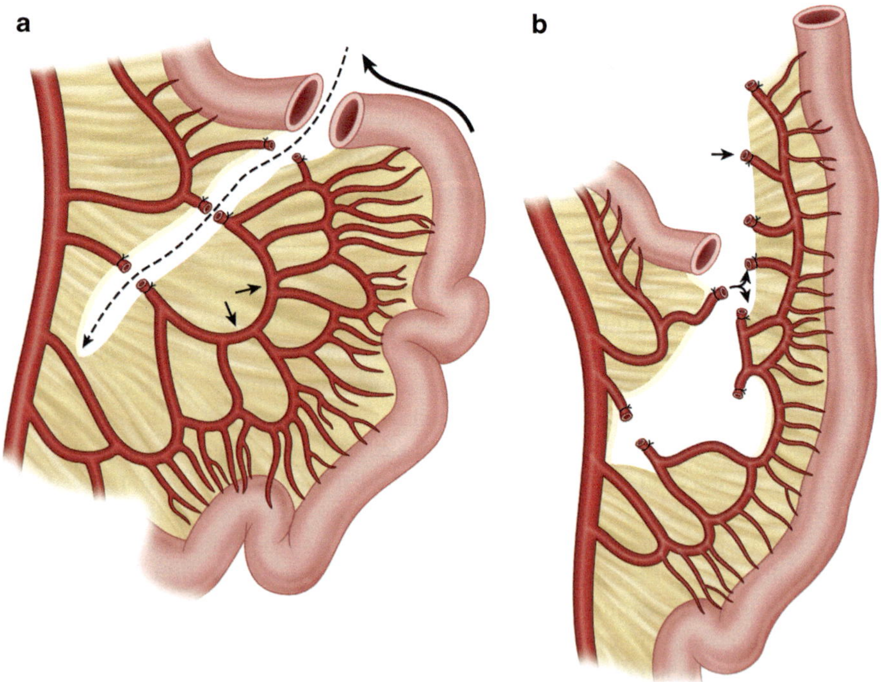


**Fig. 28.3** (**a**, **b**) The preparation of pedicled jejunal graft with preserving feeding artery and collecting vein

graft. The main and subsequent (if needed) microvascular anastomoses may be carried out with 8/0 or 9/0 non-absorbable monofilament polypropylene suture material [1, 2, 13, 17, 18].

Free jejunal transfer is needed when the pedicle is not sufficient in length. The procurement of the jejunal autograft must be done by a well-experienced "harvesting team." It is important to decide on the suitable segment of the jejunum, preferably at least 40 cm distal to the ligament of Treitz (Fig. 28.4). This segment is the cardinal part of the jejunum regarding the appropriate length of the jejunal artery and the vein for vascular reconstructions following jejunal interposition. Kinking of the feeding artery, short and tight arterial grafts and superposition of the surrounding tissues over the vein anastomosis may cause graft ischemia and necrosis. Therefore, the length of the vessels is another important point. After the graft harvesting, a left cervical incision is made to isolate the carotid artery, jugular vein, and esophagus. The most dominant artery as it is in the pedicled jejunal grafts, must be identified and divided (Fig. 28.4). After the division and harvesting of the jejunal graft are done (Fig. 28.5), the artery and the vein are flushed with heparinized saline,

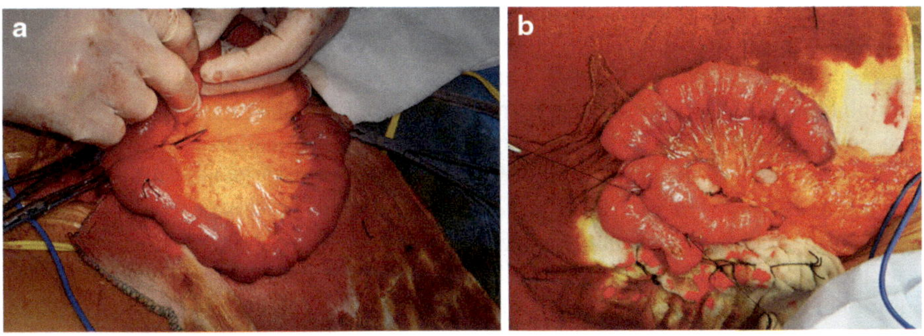


**Fig. 28.4** (**a**, **b**) The operation view of jejunal graft of two different patients during the harvesting procedure

**Fig. 28.5** Jejunal graft with its pedicle, including feeding artery and the collecting vein

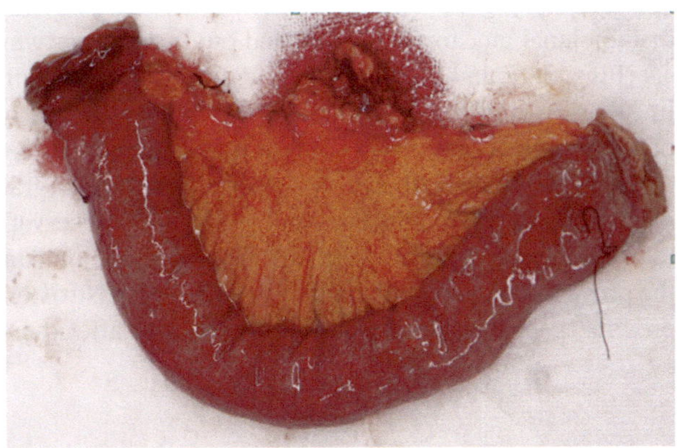

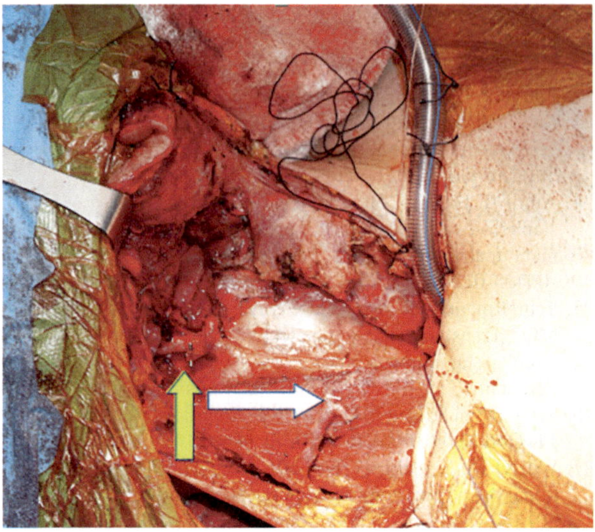

**Fig. 28.6** The Cervical bed of esophagus after it is resected. The transverse cervical artery (yellow arrow) and the branch of jugular vein (white arrow) are prepared, and local heparinized flush injected into the vascular stumps

and they must be clamped with atraumatic bulldog clamps. The interposition graft is placed in the esophageal bed. The proximal jejunal anastomosis is performed first on the cervical esophagus or hypopharynx with two layers of 4/0 silk to provide enough fixation and to avoid torsion or tension. After the placement of the interposition graft, an appropriate neck artery must be chosen, considering the diameter of the feeding artery of the graft (Fig. 28.6). Proper selection of the neck artery depends on various factors. The inferior thyroid artery and the transverse cervical artery are resistant to atherosclerosis but may be affected from previous history of radiotherapy. Indeed, if there is a requirement for adjuvant radiotherapy or a providence of additional therapy, the common carotid artery itself may be chosen to provide better perfusion pressure considering the disruptive effect of radiation on vascular responsiveness. The arterial anastomosis is performed with 9/0 or 10/0 polypropylene or nylon monofilament sutures under the microscope. Following arterial reconstruction, venous anastomosis is accomplished using the middle thyroid vein, facial vein, or one of the jugular veins with identical 9/0 or 10/0 monofilament sutures. After the distal jejunal anastomosis is carried out in a similar way as the proximal anastomosis (Figs. 28.7 and 28.8), the cervical incision is usually closed without a drainage line. Graft viability is another key point in the early postoperative period. For observing graft viability, different methods may be used. The least invasive technique is to place a thermistor probe around the graft. Alternative methods are meshed skin graft or silastic window for direct observation. It is not found to be safe to place a nasogastric tube through the cervical jejunal interposition graft. Therefore, the procedure is accomplished with a feeding gastrostomy or jejunostomy. This also provides gastric drainage and decompression after the operation [17–19].

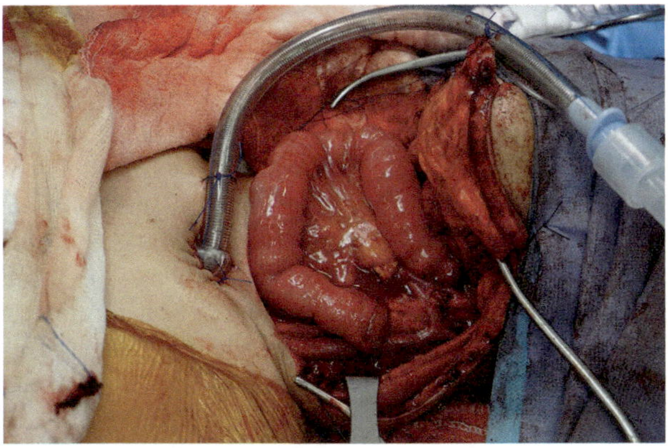

**Fig. 28.7** The jejunal graft before the vascular reconstruction and the distal anastomosis is done

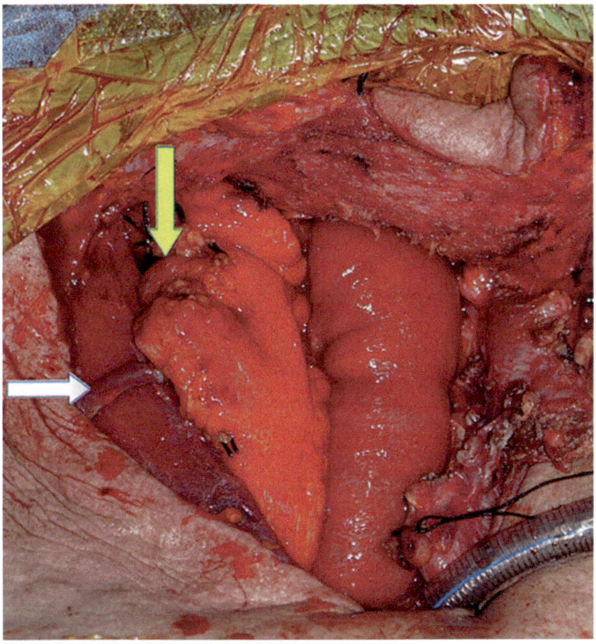

**Fig. 28.8** The new position of jejunal graft with two luminal and two vascular anastomosis. The yellow arrow shows the feeding artery (transverse cervical artery), and the white arrow shows the collecting vein (inferior thyroidal vein)

## 28.6 Complications

The pericardiectomy requires particular postoperative care. Even in well-experienced medical centers, the mortality rates vary from 1% up to 28%. As described before, resection of the esophagus with the pericardium is usually for an advanced disease. If this surgical method is required, the impaired preoperative functional status is a powerful risk factor for death in the early period after the operation. Related to this ascites, the severity of the peripheral edema is usually associated with poor functional class and is also strongly correlated with late mortality. If impaired left and right ventricular function is observed before the operation, they are related to a very high right ventricular end-diastolic pressure and a serious risk factor for mortality. Previous history of pulmonary hypertension, history of radiation, peripheral vascular disease, diabetes, and malnutrition are other independent risk factors. Congestive heart failure and acute pulmonary edema may occur instantly, right after the operation. Therefore, the fluid replacement and diuretic treatment strategies must be closely followed up. Postoperative bleeding, atrial fibrillation, pulmonary or peripheral embolism, and death are other reported complications of the surgery [17–19].

The complications of the jejunal interposition after esophageal resection with or without pericardiectomy depend on the factors related to the patient. The most frequent complications are graft thrombosis, anastomotic leak, anastomotic stricture, respiratory complications, and bleeding. Bleeding following esophagectomy occurs about 5%, regardless of the vascular anastomotic technique. Vascular thrombosis of the graft may be observed via a retaining silastic window or a skin mesh graft adjunct to the skin incision (Figs. 28.8 and 28.9). The use of antiplatelets should be stopped before the surgery. Perioperative administration of low-molecular-weight heparin does not increase bleeding-related complications. The bleeding of the azygos vein and its branches, besides the innominate vein, is difficult to stop. Another common bleeding site is the intercostal vessels inferior to the incision. Therefore, a good inspection should be carried out after the retractor is removed [20].

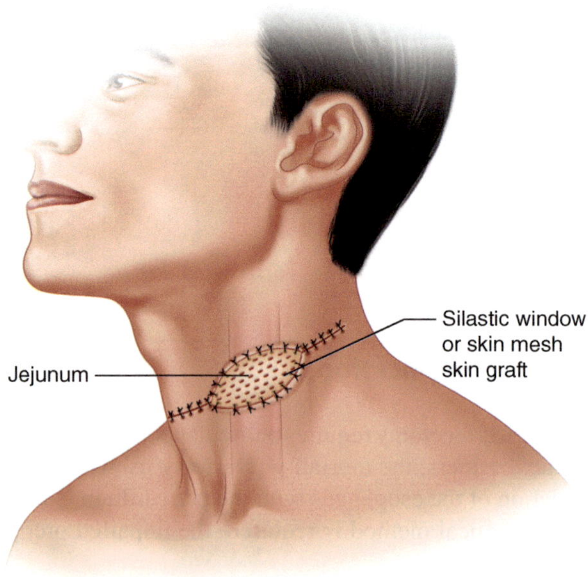


**Fig. 28.9** After the procedure, a silastic skin mesh window is retained to observe the jejunal graft. Early thrombosis of the artery or the vein causes rapid pallor of the graft

## References


1. Dimick JB, Wainess RM, Upchurch GR Jr, Iannettoni MD, Orringer MB. National trends in outcomes for esophageal resection. Ann Thorac Surg. 2005;79(1):212–6.; discussion 217–8. https://doi.org/10.1016/j.athoracsur.2004.06.044.
2. Napier KJ, Scheerer M, Misra S. Esophageal cancer: a review of epidemiology, pathogenesis, staging workup and treatment modalities. World J Gastrointest Oncol. 2014;6(5):112–20. https://doi.org/10.4251/wjgo.v6.i5.112. PMID: 24834141; PMCID: PMC4021327.
3. Torek F. The first successful case of resection of the thoracic portion of the oesophagus for carcinoma. Surg Gynecol Obstet. 1913;16:614–7.
4. Yar Saglam AS, Alp E, Elmazoglu Z, Menevse S. Treatment with cucurbitacin B alone and in combination with gefitinib induces cell cycle inhibition and apoptosis via EGFR and JAK/STAT pathway in human colorectal cancer cell lines. Hum Exp Toxicol. 2016;35:526–43.
5. Zhang J, Zhang Q, Chen X, Zhang N. Management of neoplastic pericardial disease. Herz. 2020;45(Suppl 1)):46–51. https://doi.org/10.1007/s00059-019-4833-4. Epub 2019 Jul 11.
6. Karimata H, Shimoji H, Nishimaki T. Clinicopathological factors predicting R0 resection and long-term survival after esophagectomy in patients with T4 esophageal cancer undergoing induction chemotherapy or chemoradiotherapy. Surg Today. 2015;45(4):479–86. https://doi.org/10.1007/s00595-014-0980-7. Epub 2014 Jul 25.
7. Patti MG, Gantert W, Way LW. Surgery of the esophagus. Anatomy and physiology. Surg Clin N Am. 1997;77(5):959–70. https://doi.org/10.1016/s0039-6109(05)70600-9.
8. Marnejon T, Kassis H, Gemmel D. The constricted heart. Postgrad Med. 2008;120(1):8–10. https://doi.org/10.3810/pgm.2008.04.1754.
9. Ma Y, Wang Q, Dong Q, Zhan L, Zhang J. How to differentiate pseudoprogression from true progression in cancer patients treated with immunotherapy. Am J Cancer Res. 2019;9(8):1546–53. PMID: 31497342; PMCID: PMC6726978.
10. Chalikias G, Samaras A, Ziakas A, Kikas P, Thomaidis A, Drosos I, Giannakoulas G, Karvounis H, Konstantinides S, Tziakas D. Novel echocardiographic prognostic markers for cardiac tamponade in patients with large malignant pericardial effusions: a paradigm shift from flow to tissue imaging. Echocardiography. 2017;34(9):1315–23. https://doi.org/10.1111/echo.13620. Epub 2017 Jul 7.
11. Horie Y, Yoshio T, Aoyama K, Yoshimizu S, Horiuchi Y, Ishiyama A, et al. Diagnostic outcomes of esophageal cancer by artificial intelligence using convolutional neural networks. Gastrointest Endosc. 2019;89(1):25–32. https://doi.org/10.1016/j.gie.2018.07.037.
12. Seyedin SN, Gannon MK, Plichta KA, Abushahin L, Berg DJ, Arshava EV, Parekh KR, Keech JC, Caster JM, Welsh JW, Allen BG. Safety and efficacy of stereotactic body radiation therapy for locoregional recurrences after prior chemoradiation for advanced esophageal carcinoma. Front Oncol. 2020;10:1311. https://doi.org/10.3389/fonc.2020.01311. PMID: 32850412; PMCID: PMC7412633.
13. Allum WH, Bonavina L, Cassivi SD, Cuesta MA, Dong ZM, Felix VN, Figueredo E, Gatenby PA, Haverkamp L, Ibraev MA, Krasna MJ, Lambert R, Langer R, Lewis MP, Nason KS, Parry K, Preston SR, Ruurda JP, Schaheen LW, Tatum RP, Turkin IN, van der Horst S, van der Peet DL, van der Sluis PC, van Hillegersberg R, Wormald JC, Wu PC, Zonderhuis BM. Surgical treatments for esophageal cancers. Ann N Y Acad Sci. 2014;1325:242–68. https://doi.org/10.1111/nyas.12533. PMID: 25266029; PMCID: PMC4384171.
14. Kishino T, Kumamoto K, Matsukawa H, Kondo A, Ando Y, Uemura J, Suto H, Asano E, Oshima M, Chiba Y, Ueno M, Nakagawa S, Kitamoto S, Yamashita Y, Horii T, Okano K. Constrictive pericarditis caused by pericardial metastasis from esophageal squamous cell carcinoma: a case report. Int Cancer Conf J. 2022;11(3):172–7. https://doi.org/10.1007/s13691-022-00543-0. PMID: 35669905; PMCID: PMC9163270.
15. Vistarini N, Chen C, Mazine A, Bouchard D, Hebert Y, Carrier M, Cartier R, Demers P, Pellerin M, Perrault LP. Pericardiectomy for constrictive pericarditis: 20 years of experience at

the Montreal Heart Institute. Ann Thorac Surg. 2015;100(1):107–13. https://doi.org/10.1016/j.athoracsur.2015.02.054. Epub 2015 May 13.
16. Gaudino M, Sanna T, Ballman KV, Robinson NB, Hameed I, Audisio K, Rahouma M, Di Franco A, Soletti GJ, Lau C, Rong LQ, Massetti M, Gillinov M, Ad N, Voisine P, DiMaio JM, Chikwe J, Fremes SE, Crea F, Puskas JD, Girardi L, PALACS Investigators. Posterior left pericardiotomy for the prevention of atrial fibrillation after cardiac surgery: an adaptive, single-centre, single-blind, randomised, controlled trial. Lancet. 2021;398(10316):2075–83. https://doi.org/10.1016/S0140-6736(21)02490-9. Epub 2021 Nov 14.
17. Pandolfo N, Spigno L, Guiddo G, Tronfi G, Villavecchia G, Mattioli FP. Valutazione funzionale dell'impianto gastrico e digiunale dopo esofagectomia [Functional evaluation of gastric and jejunal transplant after esophagectomy]. Minerva Chir. 1991;46(7 Suppl):253–62.
18. Mohan AT, Mardini S, Blackmon SH. Supercharged jejunal interposition. Thorac Surg Clin. 2022;32(4):529–40. https://doi.org/10.1016/j.thorsurg.2022.07.007.
19. Ascioti AJ, Hofstetter WL, Miller MJ, Rice DC, Swisher SG, Vaporciyan AA, Roth JA, Putnam JB, Smythe WR, Feig BW, Mansfield PF, Pisters PW, Torres MT, Walsh GL. Long-segment, supercharged, pedicled jejunal flap for total esophageal reconstruction. J Thorac Cardiovasc Surg. 2005;130(5):1391–8. https://doi.org/10.1016/j.jtcvs.2005.06.032. Epub 2005 Oct 13.
20. Veenstra MMK, Smithers BM, Visser E, Edholm D, Brosda S, Thomas JM, Gotley DC, Thomson IG, Wijnhoven BPL, Barbour AP. Complications and survival after hybrid and fully minimally invasive oesophagectomy. BJS Open. 2021;5(1):zraa033. https://doi.org/10.1093/bjsopen/zraa033. PMID: 33609389; PMCID: PMC7893474.

# 29 Endoscopic Management of Esophagogastric Anastomotic Leak

Ahmet Akmercan, Mumin Coskun, Sakir Karpuz, and Cumhur Yegen

## 29.1 Endoscopic Management

In recent years, endoscopic interventions have evolved into a successful alternative to surgery for esophageal anastomotic leaks. Endoscopic procedures, such as endoscopic suturing, clip placement, over-the-scope clips, and fibrin glue application, have been utilized for small-sized lesions with maintained tissue perfusion and in the absence of systemic inflammation [1, 2]. Afterward, the use of self-expanding fully or partially covered metal or plastic stents (SEMS or SEPS) has been established as the first-line treatment for more significant leakages or perforations in clinically stable patients [3–5].

## 29.2 Esophageal Stents

The first published clinical studies were conducted in the 1960s, when clinicians began researching esophageal stents for the treatment of malignant dysphagia in small cohorts [6]. Currently, esophageal stent placement is used for a wide range of indications. The features of stents vary with regard to the following: mechanic characteristics, such as the material (metal, plastic, or biodegradable); radial and axial forces acting on the lumen; and the kind of coating. Covered, self-expendable metal and plastic stents (SEMS and SEPS) are widely employed in esophageal diseases. Covered esophageal stents have emerged as the treatment of choice in the palliative treatment of patients with advanced esophageal cancer and benign esophageal strictures. Those have also been utilized to treat esophageal perforation or malignant esophago-pleural fistulas with good outcomes and short-term quality of life [7, 8]. Afterward, Bruckner et al. reported the effective treatment of esophageal

A. Akmercan · M. Coskun (✉) · S. Karpuz · C. Yegen
Department of General Surgery, Marmara University School of Medicine, Istanbul, Turkey


O. Engin (ed.), *Risk Factors and Therapy of Esophagus Cancer*,
https://doi.org/10.1007/978-3-031-47024-0_29

anastomotic leakage with a transnasally fixed Celestin tube in a small cohort [9]. In 2001, SEMS was used to successfully treat 14 patients with esophageal anastomotic leakage [10]. Subsequently, several reports have reported using SEMS and SEPS to treat esophageal leakages [11–17].

Esophageal stents are used as the initial option in the management of esophageal leakages in many centers [2]. The reported success rates of esophageal stents vary (59–92%) in anastomotic leakages. Moreover, many studies are based on small cohorts in which the focus has been on the technical success and healing rates without further analysis of benign esophageal perforation or anastomotic leakages [10–17]. A recent review reported that the technical and clinical success rates are 91.4% and 81.1%, respectively. Subgroup analysis in the same study revealed no significant differences in the technical and clinical success rates [4]. It should be kept in mind that endoscopic reinterventions and more than one stent placement may be required to increase the success rate of treatment. The treatment protocol should also include pleural and mediastinal drainage procedures for effective sepsis control [2]. The most important benefit of esophageal stenting is that it allows early oral feeding in addition to limiting leakage. Nevertheless, in some cases, additional procedures such as surgical jejunostomy or parenteral nutrition may be necessary for nutritional support [4]. The determination of the optimal time for esophageal stent removal is still debated. Published studies show significant variability regarding the time to stent removal. While some centers removed the stents after a mean of 4 weeks, some centers could leave the stents in place for a longer period of time [11, 14–17]. Freeman et al. reported an increase in stent-related complication rates when stents were removed in place for more than 4 weeks in the treatment of acute perforations or more than 2 weeks in the treatment of anastomotic leaks [18]. A recent review recommended that small esophageal defects should be treated for 10–14 days, while larger esophageal wall lesions should be treated for up to 8 weeks [19].

The reasons for stent failure have been investigated in many studies. Freeman et al. described four reasons that markedly reduce the success rate of stent therapy in overall esophageal leakages: (1) a defect larger than 6 cm in length; (2) a defect that traversed the esophagogastric junction; (3) cervical esophageal leakages; and (4) leakage in the gastric conduit in esophagectomy patients [20]. Perrson et al. associated stent failures with persistent leakage after initial stent placement, poor physical performance, severe comorbidities, and esophago-respiratory fistulas [19]. Additionally, the anatomical condition around an esophagogastric anastomosis frequently makes it unsuitable for esophageal stents to be effective. Specially manufactured stents could be used in order to address these challenging scenarios. Nevertheless, there is no data about the superiority of these specialized stents [21].

Due to utilizing a combination of different surgical repairs and interventions in available studies, ascertaining the accurate mortality rates after stent placement is difficult in patients with esophageal anastomotic leakage. Nevertheless, Dasari et al. reported that the overall mortality was 13% [4]. This study did not evaluate in-hospital, 30-day, 90-day, or even long-term mortality rates. On the other hand, Perrson et al. reported an in-hospital mortality rate of 17% [21].

The complication rates of esophageal stent placement vary substantially between published series. The complication rate related to the procedure varies between 26 and 52% in the literature. Moreover, the mortality rate related to procedures is 2–3% [22]. Complications related to stent placement include stent migration, bleeding, reflux, perforation, prolonged esophageal intubation, chest pain or foreign body sensation, and recurrent dysphagia. Stent migration is accepted as the main complication associated with stent placement.

## 29.3 The Over-the-Scope Clip System

The over-the-scope clip (OTSC) system is a novel mechanical clipping instrument that is applied as a nonsurgical choice to endoscopically treat insistent gastrointestinal bleeding, perforations/luminal defects, and fistulas [23]. When compared to standard hemostatic clips, its primary advantage is its strong and continuous tissue-grasping force. Moreover, using specialized forceps, even large luminal defects and perforation areas can also be stitched up. On the other hand, it is challenging to remove or replace the clip once it has been positioned on the target lesion. Therefore, the endoscopist should be trained and familiar with the device prior to application [24].

Although increasing failure rates for defects >13 mm have been reported, the use of OTSC is indicated in the case of acute anastomose leakages characterized by minimal inflammation and for minor defects up to 15 mm. A successful OTSC insertion requires viable, non-inflammatory mucosal edges, which could technically be reached with the OTSC placed at the tip of the scope and easily grasped with the forceps or twin grasper [25, 26].

The OTSC system includes a hand wheel, a thread retriever, and an applicator cap with an attached clip (Fig. 29.1). The clip is made of a shape-memory nitinol material that, when removed from the applicator, returns to its original shape. Rotating the wheel connected to the working channel of the scope, the thread connected to the end cap is pulled, and this releases the clip to the target (Fig. 29.2). The deployed clip permits complete hemostasis and close perforations through a mechanism that involves the four prongs of the clip to fix the lesion from the left side to the other side, which provides continuous compression of the tissue. Through a mechanism that uses the clip's four prongs to secure the lesion from the left to the other side and continuously pressure the tissue, the deployed clip enables full hemostasis and the closure of perforations. In addition to the inter-prong space of the clip,

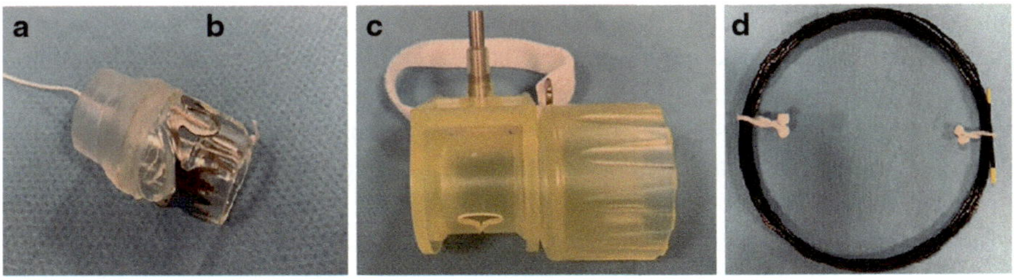


**Fig. 29.1** The OTSC system consists of an applicator cap (**a**), a mounted clip (**b**), a hand wheel (**c**), and a thread retriever (**d**)

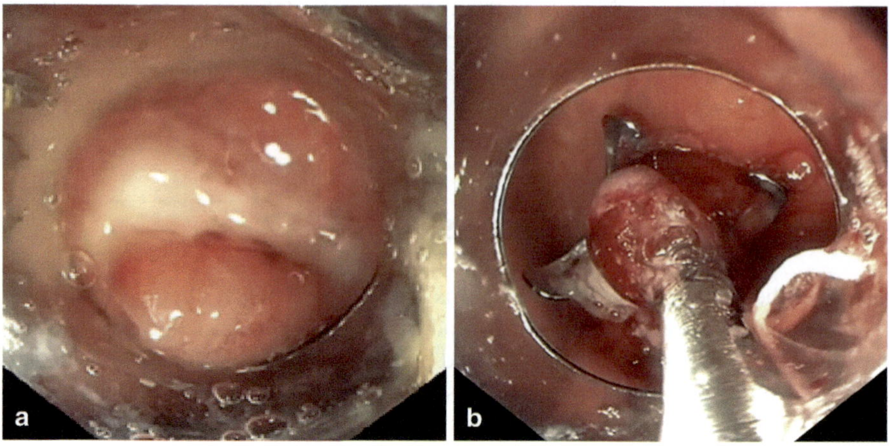


**Fig. 29.2** Endoscopic view of esophagogastric anastomosis leakage before (**a**) and after (**b**) OTSC

which maintains the normal flow of blood, the OTSC is able to prevent tissue necrosis and accelerate wound healing. Although the effectiveness and safety of this approach have been confirmed in some studies, there have been no large studies that examined the effectiveness of OTSC clips until now. The success rate is higher for acute compared to chronic lesions. The main reason for the low clinical success rate in the treatment of chronic lesions is possibly due to the lesions' fibrotic edges. OTSC system is considered as a safe device. Because device-related complications are rare, they include OTSC deviation, jejunal stenosis or obstruction, esophageal laceration or perforation, and fistulas. In order to avoid these complications, using a maximum of two clips in the narrow lumen, and releasing the clip by aspiration of the entire defect into the cap are recommended [27].

## 29.4 Endoscopic Vacuum Therapy

Endoscopic vacuum therapy (EVT) has been recently introduced as an effective treatment for anastomotic leakages following esophageal resections. For the first time in 2008, Wedemeyer et al. described the endoscopic insertion of a polyurethane sponge to the defect side and the application of an external vacuum in upper gastro-intestinal tract anastomotic leakages [28]. Negative pressure therapy prevents bacterial contamination of the wound, clears the secretions, decreases local edema, and promotes the perfusion and finally granulation of the anostomotic defect [29].

According to defect size, the open-pore sponge can be either applied by placing it into the cavity (intracavitary) or placed into the lumen of the esophagus (intraluminal) to cover the defect in cases with small defects without a cavity (Fig. 29.3). Moreover, sponge placement can be modified from its original intracavitary position to an intraluminal position with shrinking defect size. Under conscious sedation, a nasogastric tube is inserted nasally and exteriorized orally. A sponge, trimmed

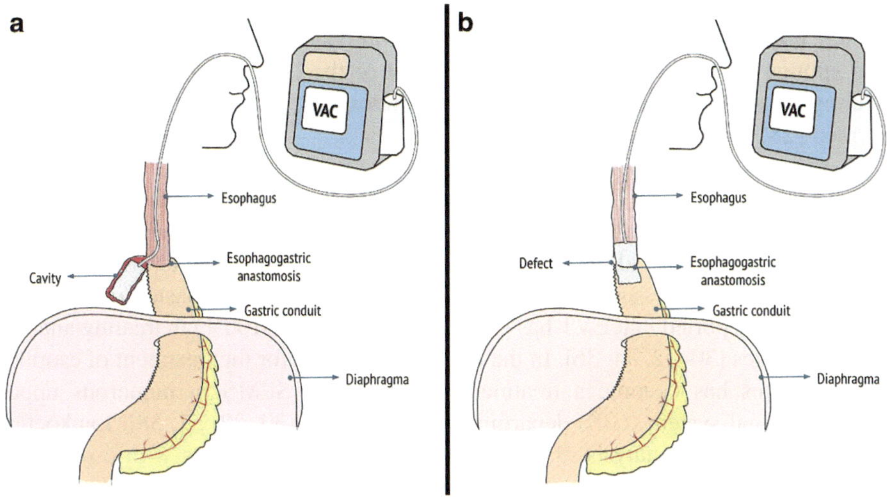


**Fig. 29.3** EVT can be either performed intracavitary (**a**) or intraluminally (**b**), depending on the characteristics of the defect

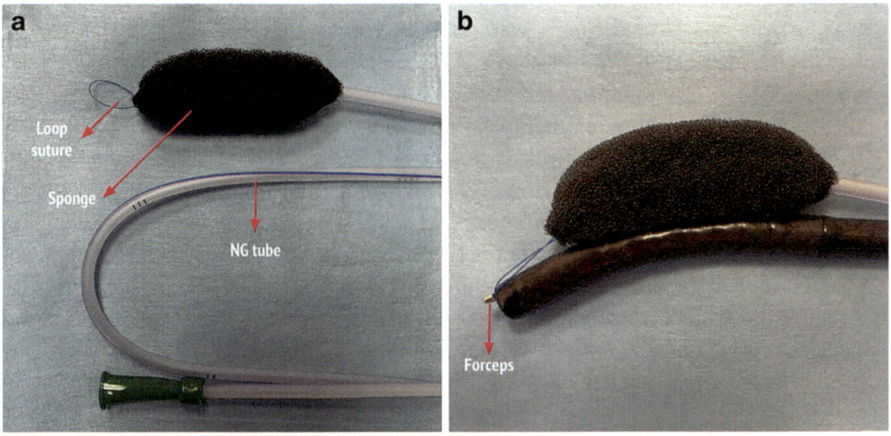


**Fig. 29.4** The sponge is placed at the end of the nasogastric tube and fixed with a non-absorbable suture. An additional suture loop is placed at the end of the sponge (**a**). This loop is grasped with endoscopic forceps, pulled close to the endoscope, and the sponge drainage system is guided in parallel to the endoscope ("backpack-method") and placed (**b**)

to the size of the defect, is placed at the end of the nasogastric tube and fixed with a non-absorbable suture. A second suture loop is placed at the top of the sponge. The suture loop is grasped with forceps, pulled close to the endoscope, and the sponge drainage system is guided in parallel to the endoscope ("backpack method") and placed in the leakage cavity or intraluminally under the endoscopic view (Fig. 29.4). Another method is to adjust the position of the sponge system endoscopically after insertion using an overtube and pusher. The controlled negative pressure generated by an electronic vacuum pump system is applied via the nasogastric tube. Generally, sponge change is repeated twice a week to minimize the risk of severe hemorrhage and sponge attachment to the esophagus wall or the leakage cavity. Thus, defect healing or worsening can be checked, and endoscopic re-application can be performed [28, 30–32] (Fig. 29.5).

For many years, the placement of SEMS has been accepted as the initial treatment for esophageal leakages [2]. In recent years, there has been increasing data on the efficiency and feasibility of EVT as first-line treatment for esophageal leakages. Furthermore, Müller et al. introduced preemptive endoluminal EVT (pEVT) in Ivor Lewis esophagectomy, and they reported that pEVT improved anastomotic healing [33]. Studies reported that EVT has good success rates (66–100%) in treating anastomotic leakages [30–32, 34–36]. In the last decades, EVT for the treatment of esophageal leakages has become a treatment alternative to SEMS in numerous upper gastrointestinal system (GIS) departments in Germany [30, 32, 37, 38]. Laukoetter et al. published the analysis of prospective data from 52 patients with esophageal leaks; after the EVT, the defects were closed in 94% of cases without further surgery [30]. Analysis of University Hospital of Heidelberg patients showed an 89% successful healing rate with EVT in esophageal leaks [32]. Hwang et al. performed the first retrospective analysis in Asia on seven patients with esophageal leakage; all cases were healed successfully with EVT [39]. The first small cohort on EVT for upper GI leakages from the United States was published in 2015. According to this report, defects were successfully closed with EVT in all the patients [35]. Additionally, it has been shown that inflammatory parameters returned to normal during the EVT and markedly decreased following therapy when compared to before treatment [30, 32].

In the first years, one of the disadvantages of EVT was the requirement for multiple endoscopic interventions. However, this problem seems to disappear with the development of endoscopic techniques. Early oral feeding is considered to be a significant benefit of stent insertion, but it is also very simple to utilize a second nasogastric or jejunal feeding tube in combination with EVT for enteral nutrition [40]. EVT should not be performed in patients with suspected bronchial or pleural fistulas and cases of proximity to major vascular structures of the cavity. Overall procedure-related complication rates are low (0–14.8%) in EVT [30–32, 37, 41]. Bleeding in

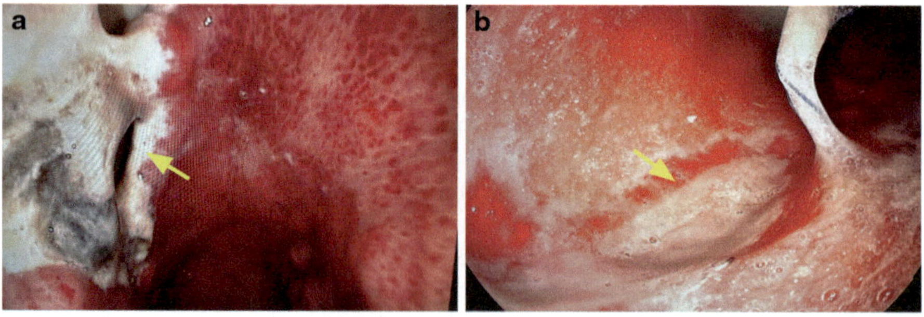


**Fig. 29.5** Endoscopic view of esophagogastric anastomosis leakage before (**a**) and after (**b**) EVT. The yellow arrow shows the defect area

the short term and anastomotic stenosis in the long term are the most important procedure-related complications, despite their low incidence rates. Until recently, death due to procedure-related major bleeding had been reported in only three patients [30]. One of these patients had severe hemorrhage due to an aorto-esophageal fistula that happened during dilatation therapy 6 weeks after the end of EVT [42]. In the review by Kuehn et al. the overall stenosis rate was reported as 7.6% (3–14%). The in-hospital mortality rate during EVT varies between 5.7 and 9.6%.

Several studies have shown that EVT has a greater success rate than stent placement in treating esophageal anastomotic leakages. Brangewitz et al. evaluated patients with intrathoracic leakages and compared 39 stent-treated patients and 32 EVT-treated patients. EVT had a markedly higher success rate compared to stent placement (84.4% vs 53.8%) in this study. They also detected markedly higher stricture rates in the stent group (28.2% vs. 9.4%). However, there was no difference observed in in-hospital mortality [40]. Mennigen et al. reported that EVT has a noticeably better success rate in esophageal leakages compared to SEMS placement (84.4% vs. 53.8%, respectively). On the other hand, there was no difference detected in the in-hospital mortality rate (stent vs. EVT: 26.7% vs. 6.7%) [43]. Recent meta-analyses reported that EVT has a significantly better healing rate, fewer major complications, and a lower hospital mortality rate compared to esophageal stents for esophageal leakages [44, 45]. These results showed that EVT could potentially replace stent therapy as the gold standard for treating esophageal anastomotic leaks. However, data regarding EVT for esophageal anastomosis leakages are still rare and lacking. Studies are mostly retrospective and have a small number of patients. Keep in mind that, randomized controlled studies comparing stents and EVT are necessary [46].

## 29.5 Sealant

The two main groups of sealants consist of cyanoacrylates and fibrin glues. The endoscopic application of these tissue sealants seems to be a favorable option to avoid surgery. However, the use of sealants for treating postoperative anastomotic leakage was only slightly discussed in the literature. This approach generally seems to be more appropriate for small defects (<15 mm) and persisting small fistulas after the use of stents or EVT. Moreover, the benefits of combined treatments using sealants were reported in some studies. So, these sealants are currently seen as more suitable for combined treatments in addition to treatments such as clips, stents, or EVT [25, 47].

## References

1. Licht E, et al. Endoscopic management of esophageal anastomotic leaks after surgery for malignant disease. Ann Thorac Surg. 2016;101(1):301–4.
2. Ong GK, Freeman RK. Endoscopic management of esophageal leaks. J Thorac Dis. 2017;9(Suppl 2):S135.

3. Tuebergen D, et al. Treatment of thoracic esophageal anastomotic leaks and esophageal perforations with endoluminal stents: efficacy and current limitations. J Gastrointest Surg. 2008;12:1168–76.
4. Dasari BV, et al. The role of esophageal stents in the management of esophageal anastomotic leaks and benign esophageal perforations. Ann Surg. 2014;259(5):852–60.
5. Aryaie AH, et al. Efficacy of endoscopic management of leak after foregut surgery with endoscopic covered self-expanding metal stents (SEMS). Surg Endosc. 2017;31:612–7.
6. Celestin L. Permanent intubation in inoperable cancer of the oesophagus and cardia: a new tube. Ann R Coll Surg Engl. 1959;25(2):165.
7. Morgan RA, et al. Malignant esophageal fistulas and perforations: management with plastic-covered metallic endoprostheses. Radiology. 1997;204(2):527–32.
8. Sarper A, et al. The efficacy of self-expanding metal stents for palliation of malignant esophageal strictures and fistulas. Eur J Cardiothorac Surg. 2003;23(5):794–8.
9. Brückner M, et al. Experience with a transnasally fixed endoprosthesis for treating esophageal anastomotic leakage. Surg Endosc. 1991;5:185–8.
10. Roy-Choudhury SH, et al. Symptomatic malignant gastroesophageal anastomotic leak: management with covered metallic esophageal stents. Am J Roentgenol. 2001;176(1):161–5.
11. Hünerbein M, et al. Treatment of thoracic anastomotic leaks after esophagectomy with self-expanding plastic stents. Ann Surg. 2004;240(5):801–7.
12. Langer FB, et al. Management of postoperative esophageal leaks with the Polyflex self-expanding covered plastic stent. Ann Thorac Surg. 2005;79(2):398–403.
13. D'Cunha J, et al. Esophageal stents for anastomotic leaks and perforations. J Thorac Cardiovasc Surg. 2011;142(1):39–46.e1.
14. Al-Issa MA, et al. The role of esophageal stent placement in the management of postesophagectomy anastomotic leak. Saudi J Gastroenterol. 2014;20(1):39.
15. Hoeppner J, et al. Covered self-expanding stent treatment for anastomotic leakage: outcomes in esophagogastric and esophagojejunal anastomoses. Surg Endosc. 2014;28:1703–11.
16. Doniec J, et al. Therapy of anastomotic leaks by means of covered self-expanding metallic stents after esophagogastrectomy. Endoscopy. 2003;35(08):652–8.
17. Freeman RK, Ascioti AJ, Wozniak TC. Postoperative esophageal leak management with the Polyflex esophageal stent. J Thorac Cardiovasc Surg. 2007;133(2):333–8.
18. Freeman RK, et al. An assessment of the optimal time for removal of esophageal stents used in the treatment of an esophageal anastomotic leak or perforation. Ann Thorac Surg. 2015;100(2):422–8.
19. Persson S, et al. Treatment of esophageal anastomotic leakage with self-expanding metal stents: analysis of risk factors for treatment failure. Endosc Int Open. 2016;4(04):E420–6.
20. Freeman RK, et al. Analysis of unsuccessful esophageal stent placements for esophageal perforation, fistula, or anastomotic leak. Ann Thorac Surg. 2012;94(3):959–65.
21. Persson S, et al. Outcomes following the main treatment options in patients with a leaking esophagus: a systematic literature review. Dis Esophagus. 2017;30(12):1–10.
22. McLoughlin MT, Byrne MF. Endoscopic stenting: where are we now and where can we go? World J Gastroenterol. 2008;14(24):3798–803.
23. Bartell N, et al. Clinical efficacy of the over-the-scope clip device: a systematic review. World J Gastroenterol. 2020;26(24):3495–516.
24. Kobara H, et al. Over-the-scope clip system: a review of 1517 cases over 9 years. J Gastroenterol Hepatol. 2019;34(1):22–30.
25. Fabbi M, et al. Anastomotic leakage after esophagectomy for esophageal cancer: definitions, diagnostics, and treatment. Dis Esophagus. 2021;34(1):doaa039.
26. Hagel AF, et al. Over-the-scope clip application yields a high rate of closure in gastrointestinal perforations and may reduce emergency surgery. J Gastrointest Surg. 2012;16(11):2132–8.
27. Donatelli G, et al. Closure of gastrointestinal defects with Ovesco clip: long-term results and clinical implications. Ther Adv Gastroenterol. 2016;9(5):713–21.
28. Wedemeyer J, et al. Endoscopic vacuum-assisted closure of upper intestinal anastomotic leaks. Gastrointest Endosc. 2008;67(4):708–11.

29. Weidenhagen R, et al. Endoscopic vacuum-assisted closure of anastomotic leakage following anterior resection of the rectum: a new method. Surg Endosc. 2008;22:1818–25.
30. Laukoetter MG, et al. Successful closure of defects in the upper gastrointestinal tract by endoscopic vacuum therapy (EVT): a prospective cohort study. Surg Endosc. 2017;31(6):2687–96.
31. Jung CFM, et al. Impact of endoscopic vacuum therapy with low negative pressure for esophageal perforations and postoperative anastomotic esophageal leaks. Digestion. 2021;102(3):469–79.
32. Zhang CC, et al. Feasibility, effectiveness, and safety of endoscopic vacuum therapy for intrathoracic anastomotic leakage following transthoracic esophageal resection. BMC Gastroenterol. 2021;21(1):72.
33. Müller PC, et al. Preemptive endoluminal vacuum therapy to reduce morbidity after minimally invasive Ivor Lewis esophagectomy: including a novel grading system for postoperative endoscopic assessment of GI-anastomoses. Ann Surg. 2021;274(5):751–7.
34. Kuehn F, et al. Endoscopic vacuum therapy for various defects of the upper gastrointestinal tract. Surg Endosc. 2017;31(9):3449–58.
35. Smallwood NR, et al. The use of endoluminal vacuum (E-Vac) therapy in the management of upper gastrointestinal leaks and perforations. Surg Endosc. 2016;30:2473–80.
36. Min YW, et al. Endoscopic vacuum therapy for postoperative esophageal leak. BMC Surg. 2019;19(1):37.
37. Schorsch T, Müller C, Loske G. Endoscopic vacuum therapy of perforations and anastomotic insufficiency of the esophagus. Chirurg. 2014;85:1081–93.
38. Bludau M, et al. Results of endoscopic vacuum-assisted closure device for treatment of upper GI leaks. Surg Endosc. 2018;32(4):1906–14.
39. Hwang JJ, et al. Comparison of endoscopic vacuum therapy and endoscopic stent implantation with self-expandable metal stent in treating postsurgical gastroesophageal leakage. Medicine. 2016;95(16):e3416.
40. Brangewitz M, et al. Endoscopic closure of esophageal intrathoracic leaks: stent versus endoscopic vacuum-assisted closure, a retrospective analysis. Endoscopy. 2013;45(06):433–8.
41. Berlth F, et al. Self-expanding metal stents versus endoscopic vacuum therapy in anastomotic leak treatment after oncologic gastroesophageal surgery. J Gastrointest Surg. 2019;23:67–75.
42. Ahrens M, et al. Drainage of esophageal leakage using endoscopic vacuum therapy: a prospective pilot study. Endoscopy. 2010;42(09):693–8.
43. Mennigen R, et al. Comparison of endoscopic vacuum therapy versus stent for anastomotic leak after esophagectomy. J Gastrointest Surg. 2015;19:1229–35.
44. Rausa E, et al. Comparison of endoscopic vacuum therapy versus endoscopic stenting for esophageal leaks: systematic review and meta-analysis. Dis Esophagus. 2018;31(11):doy060.
45. Scognamiglio P, et al. Endoscopic vacuum therapy versus stenting for postoperative esophago-enteric anastomotic leakage: systematic review and meta-analysis. Endoscopy. 2020;52(08):632–42.
46. Tachezy M, et al. Endoscopic vacuum therapy versus stent treatment of esophageal anastomotic leaks (ESOLEAK): study protocol for a prospective randomized phase 2 trial. Trials. 2021;22(1):377.
47. Ojima T, et al. Successful treatment of esophageal fistulas with endoscopic injection of alpha-cyanoacrylate monomer. Endoscopy. 2014;46:E62–3.

# Surgical Management of Esophageal Cancer Complications

# 30

Yahya Ozel and Samet Yardimci

As diagnostic and therapeutic utilities for esophageal cancer improve, so does the number of complications, particularly those associated with invasive procedures. Having a thorough understanding of the anatomy and physiology of the esophagus and establishing experienced teams in this field become important to prevent complications. Although we take every measure to avoid complications, unfortunately, a complication-free medical life is simply inconceivable. Timely diagnosis and treatment of complications can be life-saving for patients.

Esophagectomy is the most effective treatment for esophageal cancer without local invasion or distant metastasis. There are 3 different esophagectomy methods most commonly used depending on tumor localization: transhiatal esophagectomy, Ivor Lewis esophagectomy (right thoracotomy and laparotomy), and McKeown esophagectomy (right thoracotomy, laparotomy, and neck incision, cervical anastomosis) [1, 2]. There are studies showing the survival benefit of Ivor Lewis and McKeown esophagectomy, which allows en bloc esophagectomy, over the transhiatal approach [3]. Esophagectomies may be performed using open or minimally invasive methods, and no difference has been found between the two methods in terms of oncologic outcomes. In addition, minimally invasive methods have benefits such as less blood loss, reduced postoperative hospitalization and pain, and fewer pulmonary complications [4, 5]. This section discusses some of the after-esophagectomy complications, prevention methods, and diagnosis and treatment management in the event of complications.

Y. Ozel
VM Medical Park Pendik Hospital, Istanbul, Turkey

S. Yardimci (✉)
Istinye University Medical Faculty, VM Medical Park Pendik Hospital, Istanbul, Turkey


O. Engin (ed.), *Risk Factors and Therapy of Esophagus Cancer*,
https://doi.org/10.1007/978-3-031-47024-0_30

## 30.1 Delayed Emptying of the Gastric Conduit (DGCE)

Delayed emptying of the gastric conduit after esophagectomy occurs between 10 and 20% [6–8]. Patients with lung disorders, patients with muscle diseases, patients undergoing operations in which the entire stomach is used as a gastric conduit, and patients with anastomotic leaks are more likely to experience it [9, 10]. It is less common in patients in whom a pyloric drainage method such as pyloromyotomy or pyloroplasty has been used [11].

Denervation of the stomach and pylorus as a result of transection of the vagus nerve during surgery and disruption of the celiac and mesenteric sympathetic axes at various levels during lymph node dissection leads to DGCE. Although there is no complete consensus, there are two types of early DGCE and late DGCE based on the time of onset of symptoms [12, 13]. Symptoms include nausea, vomiting, dysphagia after solid food, oral intolerance, early satiety, loss of appetite, regurgitation, weight loss due to malnutrition, pain, cough, and recurrent pneumonia [14].

Upper gastrointestinal radiographs with water-soluble contrast agent are useful in the diagnosis. These investigations, albeit insightful into the passage of liquids, fall short of capturing the passage of solids. Barium is a more viscous substance and therefore better at demonstrating the passage of solids. However, the use of barium is not recommended because aspiration of barium into the respiratory tract causes far more severe lung damage than water-soluble contrast agents [15, 16]. An endoscopic examination is necessary for differential diagnosis. Anastomotic stricture or other causes of upper GI obstruction should be excluded. The presence of food remnants despite adequate fasting time and a narrow pyloric orifice supports the diagnosis [17]. Gastric scintigraphy and paracetamol absorption tests can be used as problem solvers in cases with difficulties in diagnosis [18, 19].

Prokinetic agents, proton pump inhibitors, and macrolide-group antibiotics are used in medical treatment. Many surgeons perform pyloric drainage procedures such as pyloromyotomy or pyloroplasty on every patient receiving a vagotomy to prevent DGCE. Some studies show the opposite, despite meta-analyses that claim that such interventions decrease the incidence of DGCE without increasing the incidence of other complications [11, 20]. Problems such as bile reflux, esophagitis, and dumping syndrome seen in the late period after pyloric drainage procedures have recently prompted surgeons to embark on a quest. Perioperative intra-pyloric botulinum toxin injection was aimed to accomplish early pyloric muscular paralysis and comfortable pyloric passage and to prevent late biliary reflux and dumping syndrome due to the temporary effect. However, patients receiving intrapyloric botulinum toxin have been shown to require a higher rate of endoscopic pyloric dilatation and develop more reflux than patients undergoing other pyloric drainage procedures, so it has not been introduced into routine practice [21].

Pyloric drainage procedures have also started to be used less frequently with the increasing use of minimally invasive methods in esophageal surgery. Instead, preoperative or postoperative endoscopic balloon dilatations are used. Repeated dilatations with 12–22-mm-diameter balloons used as through the scope (TTS) are known to be effective [22]. Using 30-mm-diameter balloons, which are generally used for achalasia, is known to be more effective under fluoroscopic guidance. Re-dilatation needs are less compared to TTS balloons [7]. Although successful results with gastric per oral endoscopic myotomy (G-POEM) have been reported in persistent cases, further research is needed before it can be widely used [23, 24].

## 30.2 Anastomotic Leak or Fistula

One of the most serious complications, an anastomotic leak (AL), prolongs hospital stays and significantly increases mortality and morbidity. In the long term, AL is known to be associated with poorer quality of life and an increased risk of cancer recurrence, which has a negative impact on long-term survival. After esophageal cancer surgery, the incidence of AL is 11.4–21.2%, with an associated mortality rate of 7.2–35% [25–29].

Esophagectomy Complications Consensus Group (ECCG) defined anastomotic leak as a full-thickness defect involving the esophagus anastomosis line, staple line, or gastric conduit, irrespective of clinical presentation. Three levels have been defined according to the severity of the disease and treatment modalities. Type 1 leaks do not necessitate a modification in the patient's medical or dietary treatment; type 2 leaks necessitate interventional radiology drainage, stent, or bedside abscess drainage; and type 3 leaks necessitate surgical intervention [30].

### 30.2.1 Risk Factors

Risk factors affecting AL include the presence of comorbidities, neoadjuvant treatment, anastomotic location, surgical technique, and perioperative monitoring techniques and therapies. Malnutrition (albumin <3.0 g/dL), obesity (body mass index [BMI] >30 kg/m$^2$), or cachexia (BMI <18.5 kg/m$^2$) enhance the risk of AL, as do heart failure, hypertension, diabetes, renal failure, steroid use, and tobacco use [25]. The correlation between neoadjuvant chemoradiation and the risk of AL has not been clearly demonstrated. Although chemoradiation is known to impair microcirculation and suppress the immune system, the results of studies on how this affects the incidence of AL are controversial. It has been found that while 31 Gy increases the incidence of AL, 24.2 Gy radiation exposure has no effect on the risk of anastomotic leak in cervical anastomoses [31]. Another study reported that radiation up to 45 Gy did not raise the risk of AL [32].

Cervical anastomoses are known to be 5 times more at risk for AL compared to intrathoracic anastomoses. This is due to the need for a longer gastric conduit, a greater extension of the fundus, where blood supply is usually the worst, and tension and/or pressure on the anastomosis [33]. However, since cervical AL has a milder clinical course, the mortality rate is the same as that of intrathoracic anastomosis [26]. Performing the surgery with an open or minimally invasive method has no impact on the incidence of AL [34]. However, one should keep in mind that minimally invasive methods are technically more difficult and take more time to gain adequate competence. Omentoplasty is a factor that reduces the risk of an anastomotic leak [35]. Although comparative studies between hand-sewn or stapled anastomosis or a circular-stapled (25–29 mm) anastomosis have been conducted, no factor has been identified to increase or decrease the risk of AL [36–38].

Intraoperative or postoperative hemodynamic alterations that may impair tissue perfusion pose a risk for AL. This requires careful monitoring of adequate oxygen levels in the blood and blood pressure, as well as fluid therapy and the use of vasopressor therapies when necessary. Although fluid restriction has recently been widely suggested, particularly for preventing pulmonary complications and lowering the risk of AL, it is evident that excessive fluid restriction will lead to hypotension and perfusion problems due to dehydration. Goal-directed therapy should therefore be employed intraoperatively or in the early postoperative period to optimize fluid therapy. In this method, three major hemodynamic parameters [stroke volume, mean arterial pressure (MAP), and cardiac output (CO)] should be closely monitored. Stroke volume is the amount of blood pumped with each ventricular contraction. In other words, it is the difference between end-diastolic ventricular volume and end-systolic ventricular volume. Thus, it is directly proportional to pulse pressure. Cardiac output (CO) is the total volume of blood pumped by the left ventricle in a minute. MAP is the mean arterial pressure during one cardiac cycle (systole/diastole). It is influenced by CO and systemic vascular resistance [39].

Thoracic epidural analgesia (TEA) has also been shown to increase intestinal micro perfusion and decrease the likelihood of AL after esophagectomy. It should, however, be used with caution due to the possibility of sympathetic block and hypotension [40].

### 30.2.2 Clinical Presentation

The clinical presentation of an anastomotic leak may be asymptomatic or fulminant sepsis. The most common and early symptoms include fever, abscess discharge from the incision (particularly in cervical anastomosis), and tachycardia [41]. Chest pain, dyspnea, bronchopneumonia, mediastinitis, and respiratory failure may occur when there is an intrathoracic AL. Sepsis may progress to multiorgan failure. Elevated acute phase reactants [C-reactive protein (CRP), procalcitonin, and white blood cell counts] are remarkable. Drain amylase level is a useful indicator for early diagnosis. A high amylase level in the drain fluid indicates contamination with saliva [42].

### 30.2.3 Diagnostic Imaging

Oral contrast-enhanced esophagography, computed tomography (CT), and endoscopy are the diagnostic modalities. Esophagography is a cost-effective and safe modality that reveals the presence of AL with high specificity. Extravasation of oral contrast agents through the anastomosis is diagnostic [43]. However, false-negative results are considerable, with a sensitivity of 33–52% [44]. CT is a noninvasive, safe, and most widely used modality for the diagnosis of AL. This method is the most preferred modality due to its ability to visualize the neck, thorax, and abdomen concurrently, its applicability in patients with limited postoperative mobility or in critically ill patients, its ability to provide information about the amount and localization of possible fluid collections, and its ability to adequately diagnose concomitant pulmonary pathologies or other diagnoses in the differential diagnosis [45]. AL findings on the CT scan are the appearance of extraluminal air and fluid and/or the presence of oral contrast agent in the mediastinum, as well as direct imaging of the esophageal wall defect [46]. Upper gastrointestinal endoscopy is a safe and useful modality for both the diagnosis and treatment of AL. It was demonstrated that, contrary to fears, increased intraluminal pressure at endoscopy does not increase the risk of anastomotic separation [47]. Endoscopy has very high sensitivity and specificity, especially in intrathoracic anastomoses. Its advantages are the assessment of the viability of the gastric conduit, its bedside applicability in intubated and intensive care patients, and the lack of a requirement for oral contrast agents [48].

### 30.2.4 Leakage Management

The purpose of anastomotic leak management is to close or contain the leak line and drain the contaminated area [49]. The type of treatment depends on the size of the leak and the patient's clinical condition. A small leak may be resolved by drainage of the infected area, stopping oral intake, and medical supportive therapy, whereas larger leaks and patients who do not respond well to first-line treatment may require endoscopic and/or surgical intervention.

Some endoscopic interventions are intended to achieve primary closure of the defect. These are clips, endoscopic sutures, or fibrin glue injections. Stents and endoscopic vacuum therapy also target secondary closure. In the early period (first 72 h), endoscopic primary closure may be a good choice for leaks smaller than 3 cm. In other cases, secondary closure methods should be preferred. The patient's general condition must be stable for stent treatment or vacuum treatment. Therefore, these procedures should be postponed until after the drainage of infected collections [50].

More than 90% of esophageal anastomotic leaks can be repaired with endoscopic stenting. The major limitations are stent migration and pain. The mean duration of the stent staying in the esophagus is 6–8 weeks. Although stent migration occurs in one-fifth of patients, the likelihood of complications (bleeding and perforation) due to this migration is lower but should be kept in mind. Esophageal stents are the best option for leaks that do not have diffuse necrosis and have less than 30% circumferential dehiscence [51].

Endoscopic endoluminal vacuum therapy was first described by Loske [52] in 2007. Its use in esophageal anastomotic leaks was also reported in 2010. A sponge is placed by endoscopy into the defect in the anastomosis and attached to a pump that provides negative pressure during this procedure. The internal drainage of collections and secondary closure are provided by changing the sponge every 3–6 days [53].

Indications for surgical treatment of anastomotic leaks [54]:

- Presence of uncontrolled sepsis,
- Failure to recover adequately with conservative treatments.
- Early leaks within the first 72 h.
- Uncontrolled intrathoracic leaks.

If the defect in the anastomosis is very small and there is no widespread contamination around it, surgical primary repair may be the best option. Flaps made of chest wall muscle, omentum, pleural, or pericardial adipose tissue may be employed to strengthen this line. If the leak line is too wide or there is necrosis of the gastric conduit, complete resection of the anastomosis followed by an esophagostomy and gastrostomy is recommended. Reconstructive surgery may be planned after the patient's general condition improves. A feeding jejunostomy must be established in patients operated on for anastomotic leaks. Enabling enteral nutrition during the postoperative follow-up period is of vital importance in some patients. The mortality rate is between 12 and 15% in patients requiring reoperation for an esophageal anastomotic leak. Pre- or postoperative intensive care follow-up is often required until the patient's general condition stabilizes [54, 55].

## 30.3 Anastomotic Stenosis

After radical esophageal cancer surgery, 3–40% of patients develop anastomotic stenosis. Although it is not a life-threatening complication, it has a negative impact on quality of life. Anastomotic stenoses may be associated with the anastomotic technique. Scar contraction, multiple sutures in the anastomosis, tight sutures, and mucosal layers that are not completely end-to-end may cause stenosis. Late stenosis may occur when the anastomotic leak is closed by secondary healing. Factors that increase the risk of stenosis are anastomotic leak, multilayered anastomosis, circular stapler anastomosis with a narrow diameter, and long-term continuation of a liquid diet [56, 57].

Randomized controlled trials compared three different anastomosis techniques. Anastomotic stenosis was found to be the least with the linear stapler compared to hand-sewn anastomosis, circular stapled anastomosis, and "side-to-side" anastomosis with a linear stapler. No increase in leak and reflux rate was observed in anastomoses with linear staplers [58]. Repeated endoscopic balloon dilatations and/or esophageal stents are highly effective in treatment.

## 30.4 Chylothorax

Chylothorax after esophageal cancer surgery is an important cause of prolonged hospitalization and reoperation. It results from intraoperative injury to the ductus thoracicus and usually presents with chylous drainage from the catheter on postoperative days 2–10. The thoracic duct emerges from the cisterna chyli at the level of the second lumbar vertebra and travels upward lateral to the aorta, draining 75% of the body's lymphatics into the brachiocephalic vein. The incidence of chylothorax after esophagectomy is between 0.9 and 18.6% [59, 60]. Patients with a low body mass index, those who received excess fluid intraoperatively, and patients having neoadjuvant chemoradiotherapy are at higher risk for chylothorax [61, 62].

The ECCG group classified chylothorax by type of treatment and amount of daily drainage (Table 30.1). Those who respond to conservative therapy are referred to as type 1, those who require TPN as type 2, and those who require surgical or interventional intervention as type 3. If the daily drainage is less than 1 L, A is added, and if it is more than 1 L, B is added. For example, a chylothorax with daily drainage of over 1 L requiring TPN is classified as Type 2B [30].

Treatment of chylothorax is long term. Monitoring the respiratory functions and ensuring adequate drainage should be the primary goals. The amount of drainage should be closely monitored, a medium-chain fatty acid diet should be given, and fluid electrolyte balance should be maintained. Partial or total parenteral nutrition should be added if necessary. An octreotide subcutaneous injection may be given to reduce lymphatic drainage. Some of the patients recover with this conservative treatment [63]. If drainage does not fall below 1000 cc/day after 2 days of octreotide treatment, alternative treatment methods should be sought [64]. There are small series of successful pleurodesis using a high concentration of glucose solution in the chest tube [65].

The lymphoscintigraphy and coil embolization method described by Cope et al. in 1997 [66] involve percutaneous catheterization and embolization of the ductus thoracicus. It has been shown to treat 71–74% of chylothorax. However, one should keep in mind that complications such as foot lymphedema, wound infection, and pulmonary artery embolization may occur [67].

**Table 30.1** Chylothorax classification by ECCG group [30]

| |
|---|
| Chyle leak |
| Type I: treatment—enteric modifications |
| Type II: Treatment—total parenteral nutrition |
| Type III: Treatment—interventional or surgical therapy |
| Severity level |
| (A) <1 L output/day |
| (B) >1 L output/day |

If these treatments fail, open or minimally invasive thoracic exploration should be performed to locate and connect the leaking lymphatic duct [68]. Preoperative feeding of cream and butter or drinking methylene blue will help to visualize the ductus more easily. Maximum effort is required to locate the site of the lymphatic leak. If it cannot be located, fibrin glue should be applied to suspicious areas. Some sites recommend routine ligation of the ductus thoracicus during primary surgery to reduce the risk of postoperative chylothorax [68], but this method remains controversial.

## 30.5 Recurrent Laryngeal Nerve Palsy

The recurrent laryngeal nerve (RLN) originates from the nervus vagus and plays a major role in vocal cord coordination. It has a key role in talking, swallowing, and breathing. Although it can also be injured at the time of thoracic paratracheal lymph node dissection during esophagectomy, it is usually injured during cervical dissection or anastomosis. Anastomosis should be planned at the lowest possible level to reduce the risk of RLN injury [69]. The incidence of RLN injury during esophagectomy is between 0 and 29.3%.

RLN injury is less common in transthoracic esophagectomy compared to the other two methods. Laryngeal nerve monitoring is routinely performed at many sites. Although it allows identification of the laryngeal nerve by 87%, there is no conclusive evidence that it reduces the rate of RLN injury [70, 71].

Initial treatment of RLN injuries is conservative. Voice physiotherapy may be provided. Medialization of the paralyzed vocal cord may be achieved by injections into the paraglottic space. However, this method is of limited benefit, and its effect is temporary. The injected material is expected to be absorbed within 3–6 months. It does, however, improve the outcome of conservative treatment by keeping the paralyzed vocal cord more medially [72]. Temporary medialization provides an improvement in 65% of patients in 6–12 months without the need for further treatment [73].

If paralysis persists despite this treatment, transcervical permanent medialization is recommended. Under local anesthesia and sedation, a material (usually polytetrafluoroethylene, silastic, hydroxyapatite, titanium, or Gore-Tex) is implanted through a cartilage window at the level of the vocal fold on the paralytic side [74].

## 30.6 Trans-Hiatal Herniation with Obstruction

It is the herniation and incarceration of the gastric conduit or small intestine through the hiatus esophageal. Although rare, it is very important to keep in mind as it can have life-threatening consequences. It may appear right away following an esophagectomy or years later. It is more common in the male gender and in patients who underwent diaphragmatic crus resection during primary surgery. The patient may experience vomiting, dysphagia, tachyarrhythmia, shortness of breath, and chest pain. Thoracic and abdominal oral contrast-enhanced CT reveal gastric or intestinal obstruction at the level of the hiatus. Endoscopy may be used for differential diagnosis. The treatment is emergency surgery. After retrieval of the herniated organs into the abdomen by laparotomy or laparoscopy under general anesthesia, the defect must be repaired with primer or mesh [75].

## 30.7 Reflux Esophagitis

Reflux esophagitis is a common complication after esophageal cancer surgery. Reflux of acid, bile, or food, especially when lying down at night, causes discomfort in the patient. Post-sternal burning, pain, and dysphagia may be observed. Medical treatments and lifestyle changes should be recommended [76, 77].

## References


1. Wright CD. Esophageal cancer surgery in 2005. Minerva Chir. 2005;60(6):431–44.
2. Rentz J, et al. Transthoracic versus transhiatal esophagectomy: a prospective study of 945 patients. J Thorac Cardiovasc Surg. 2003;125(5):1114–20.
3. Hagen JA, Peters JH, DeMeester TR. Superiority of extended en bloc esophagogastrectomy for carcinoma of the lower esophagus and cardia. J Thorac Cardiovasc Surg. 1993;106(5):850–8. discussion 858–9.
4. Mariette C, Markar SR, Dabakuyo-Yonli TS, et al. Hybrid minimally invasive esophagectomy for esophageal cancer. N Engl J Med. 2019;380(2):152–62.
5. Straatman J, van der Wielen N, Cuesta MA, et al. Minimally invasive versus open esophageal resection: 3-year follow-up of the previously reported randomized controlled trial: the TIME trial. Ann Surg. 2017;266(2):232–6.
6. Lanuti M, de Delva PE, Wright CD, et al. Post-esophagectomy gastric outlet obstruction: role of pyloromyotomy and management with endoscopic pyloric dilatation. Eur J Cardiothorac Surg. 2007;31:149–53.
7. Maus MK, Leers J, Herbold T, et al. Gastric outlet obstruction after esophagectomy: retrospective analysis of the effectiveness and safety of postoperative endoscopic pyloric dilatation. World J Surg. 2016;40:2405–11.
8. Fritz S, Feilhauer K, Schaudt A, et al. Pylorus drainage procedures in thoracoabdominal esophagectomy—a single-center experience and review of the literature. BMC Surg. 2018;18:13.
9. Benedix F, Willems T, Kropf S, et al. Risk factors for delayed gastric emptying after esophagectomy. Langenbecks Arch Surg. 2017;402:547–54.
10. Zhang L, Hou SC, Miao JB, et al. Risk factors for delayed gastric emptying in patients undergoing esophagectomy without pyloric drainage. J Surg Res. 2017;213:46–50.
11. Young JE, et al. Pyloric drainage (pyloroplasty) or no drainage in gastric reconstruction after esophagectomy: a meta-analysis of randomized controlled trials. Dig Surg. 2002;19:160–4.
12. Deng B, Tan QY, Jiang YG, et al. Prevention of early delayed gastric emptying after high-level esophagogastrostomy by "pyloric digital fracture". World J Surg. 2010;34:2837–43.
13. Martin JT, Federico JA, McKelvey AA, et al. Prevention of delayed gastric emptying after esophagectomy: a single center's experience with botulinum toxin. Ann Thorac Surg. 2009;87:1708–13. discussion 1713–4.
14. Konradsson M, Nilsson M. Delayed emptying of the gastric conduit after esophagectomy. J Thorac Dis. 2019;11(Suppl 5):S835–44.
15. Fok M, Cheng SW, Wong J. Pyloroplasty versus no drainage in gastric replacement of the esophagus. Am J Surg. 1991;162:447–52.

16. Siddiqui MT, Litts JK, Cheney DM, et al. The effect of aspirated barium sulfate, iodixanol, and diatrizoic acid on survival and lung injury in a lagomorph model. Laryngoscope. 2017;127:E148–52.
17. Sutcliffe RP, Forshaw MJ, Tandon R, et al. Anastomotic strictures and delayed gastric emptying after esophagectomy: incidence, risk factors and management. Dis Esophagus. 2008;21:712–7.
18. Djerf P, Brundin M, Bajk M, et al. Validation of the paracetamol absorption test for measuring gastric tube emptying in esophagectomized patients versus gold standard scintigraphy. Scand J Gastroenterol. 2015;50:1339–47.
19. Kim JH, Lee HS, Kim MS, et al. Balloon dilatation of the pylorus for delayed gastric emptying after esophagectomy. Eur J Cardiothorac Surg. 2008;33:1105–11.
20. Palmes D, Weilinghoff M, Colombo-Benkmann M, et al. Effect of pyloric drainage procedures on gastric passage and bile reflux after esophagectomy with gastric conduit reconstruction. Langenbecks Arch Surg. 2007;392:135–41.
21. Eldaif SM, Lee R, Adams KN, et al. Intrapyloric botulinum injection increases postoperative esophagectomy complications. Ann Thorac Surg. 2014;97:1959–64. discussion 1964–5.
22. Lanuti M, DeDelva P, Morse CR, et al. Management of delayed gastric emptying after esophagectomy with endoscopic balloon dilatation of the pylorus. Ann Thorac Surg. 2011;91:1019–24.
23. Malik Z, Kataria R, Modayil R, et al. Gastric per oral endoscopic myotomy (G-POEM) for the treatment of refractory gastroparesis: early experience. Dig Dis Sci. 2018;63:2405–12.
24. Chung H, Dallemagne B, Perretta S, et al. Endoscopic pyloromyotomy for postesophagectomy gastric outlet obstruction. Endoscopy. 2014;46(Suppl 1):E345–6.
25. Kassis ES, Kosinski AS, Ross P, et al. Predictors of anastomotic leak after esophagectomy: an analysis of the Society of Thoracic Surgeons general thoracic database. Ann Thorac Surg. 2013;96:1919–26.
26. van Workum F, van der Maas J, van den Wildenberg FJH, et al. Improved functional results after minimally invasive esophagectomy: intrathoracic versus cervical anastomosis. Ann Thorac Surg. 2017;103(1):267–73.
27. Seesing MFJ, Gisbertz SS, Goense L, et al. A propensity score matched analysis of open versus minimally invasive transthoracic esophagectomy in The Netherlands. Ann Surg. 2017;266:839–46.
28. Schmidt HM, Gisbertz SS, Moons J, et al. Defining bench-marks for transthoracic esophagectomy: a multicenter analysis of total minimally invasive esophagectomy in low risk patients. Ann Surg. 2017;266(5):814–21.
29. Low DE, Kuppusamy MK, Alderson D, et al. Benchmarking complications associated with esophagectomy. Ann Surg. 2019;269:291–8.
30. Low DE, Alderson D, Cecconello I, et al. International consensus on standardization of data collection for complications associated with esophagectomy: Esophagectomy Complications Consensus Group (ECCG). Ann Surg. 2015;262:286–94.
31. Koeter M, Kathiravetpillai N, Gooszen JA, et al. Influence of the extent and dose of radiation on complications after neoadjuvant chemoradiation and subsequent esophagectomy with gastric tube reconstruction with a cervical anastomosis. Int J Radiat Oncol Biol Phys. 2017;97:813–21.
32. Gronnier C, Tréchot B, Duhamel A, et al. Impact of neoadjuvant chemoradiotherapy on postoperative outcomes after esophageal cancer resection results of a European Multicenter Study. Ann Surg. 2014;260:764–71.
33. Markar SR, Arya S, Karthikesalingam A, et al. Technical factors that affect anastomotic integrity following esophagectomy: systematic review and meta-analysis. Ann Surg Oncol. 2013;20(13):4274–81.
34. Biere SS, van Berge HMI, Maas KW, et al. Minimally invasive versus open oesophagectomy for patients with oesophageal cancer: a multicentre, open-label, randomised controlled trial. Lancet. 2012;379:1887–92.
35. Zhou D, Liu QX, Deng XF, et al. Anastomotic reinforcement with omentoplasty reduces anastomotic leakage for minimally invasive esophagectomy with cervical anastomosis. Cancer Manag Res. 2018;10:257–63.

36. Rostas JW, Graffree BD, Scoggins CR, et al. Long-term outcomes after hand-sewn versus circular-stapled (25 and 29 mm) anastomotic technique after esophagogastrectomy for esophageal cancer. J Surg Oncol. 2018;117(3):469–72.
37. Price TN, Nichols FC, Harmsen WS, et al. A comprehensive review of anastomotic technique in 432 esophagectomies. Ann Thorac Surg. 2013;95(4):1154–60.
38. Honda M, Kuriyama A, Noma H, et al. Hand-sewn versus mechanical esophagogastric anastomosis after esophagectomy: a systematic review and meta-analysis. Ann Surg. 2013;257(2):238–48.
39. Feldheiser A, Conroy P, Bonomo T, et al. Development and feasibility study of an algorithm for intraoperative goal directed haemodynamic management in noncardiac surgery. J Int Med Res. 2012;40(4):1227–41.
40. Feltracco P, Bortolato A, Barbieri S, et al. Perioperative benefit and outcome of thoracic epidural in esophageal surgery: a clinical review. Dis Esophagus. 2018;31(5):dox135.
41. Stippel DL, Taylan C, Schröder W, Beckurts KT, Hölscher AH. Supraventricular tachyarrhythmia as early indicator of a complicated course after esophagectomy. Dis Esophagus. 2005;18(4):267–73.
42. Miller DL, Helms GA, Mayfield WR. Evaluation of esophageal anastomotic integrity with serial pleural amylase levels. Ann Thorac Surg. 2018;105(1):200–6.
43. Lantos JE, Levine MS, Rubesin SE, et al. Comparison between esophagography and chest computed tomography for evaluation of leaks after esophagectomy and gastric pull-through. J Thorac Imaging. 2013;28:121–8.
44. Jones CM, Clarke B, Heah R, et al. Should routine assessment of anastomotic integrity be undertaken using radiological contrast swallow after oesophagectomy with intra-thoracic anastomosis? Best evidence topic (BET). Int J Surg. 2015;20:158–62.
45. Kim TH, Kim JH, Shin CI, et al. CT findings suggesting anastomotic leak and predicting the recovery period following gastric surgery. Eur Radiol. 2015;25(7):1958–66.
46. Goense L, Stassen PMC, Wessels FJ, et al. Diagnostic performance of a CT-based scoring system for diagnosis of anastomotic leakage after esophagectomy: comparison with subjective CT assessment. Eur Radiol. 2017;27(10):4426–34.
47. Page RD, Asmat A, McShane J, et al. Routine endoscopy to detect anastomotic leakage after esophagectomy. Ann Thorac Surg. 2013;95(1):292–8.
48. Hogan BA, Winter DC, Winter D, et al. Prospective trial comparing contrast swallow, computed tomography and endoscopy to identify anastomotic leak following oesophagogastric surgery. Surg Endosc. 2008;22:767–71.
49. Schaheen L, Blackmon SH, Nason KS. Optimal approach to the management of intrathoracic esophageal leak following esophagectomy: a systematic review. Am J Surg. 2014;208:536–43.
50. Chevallay M, Jung M, Chon SH, Takeda FR, Akiyama J, Mönig S. Esophageal cancer surgery: review of complications and their management. Ann N Y Acad Sci. 2020;1482(1):146–62.
51. Dasari B, Neely D, Kennedy A, et al. The role of esophageal stents in the management of esophageal anastomotic leaks and benign esophageal perforations. Ann Surg. 2014;259:852–60.
52. Loske G, Schorsch T, Müller C. Endoscopic vacuum sponge therapy for esophageal defects. Surg Endosc. 2010;24:2531–5.
53. Weidenhagen R, Hartl WH, Gruetzner KU, et al. Anastomotic leakage after esophageal resection: new treatment options by endoluminal vacuum therapy. Ann Thorac Surg. 2010;90:1674–81.
54. Martin LW, Swisher SG, Hofstetter W, et al. Intrathoracic leaks following esophagectomy are no longer associated with increased mortality. Ann Surg. 2005;242:392–402.
55. Page RD, Shackcloth MJ, Russell GN, Pennefather SH. Surgical treatment of anastomotic leaks after esophagectomy. Eur J Cardiothorac Surg. 2005;27:337–43.
56. Jun L, Jibiao H. Experiences in prevention and management of anastomotic stenosis during esophageal cancer surgery. J Pract Med. 2003;19(9):1062.
57. Petrin G, Ruol A, Battaglia G, Buin F, Merigliano S, Constantini M, Pavei P, Cagol M, Scappin S, Ancona E. Anastomotic stenoses occurring after circular stapling in esophageal cancer surgery. Surg Endosc. 2000;14(7):670–4.

58. Wang WP, Gao Q, Wang KN, Shi H, Chen LQ. A prospective randomized controlled trial of semi-mechanical versus hand-sewn or circular stapled esophagogastrostomy for prevention of anastomotic stricture. World J Surg. 2013;37(5):1043–50.
59. Dugue L, Sauvanet A, Farges O, et al. Output of chyle as an indicator of treatment for chylothorax complicating oesophagectomy. Br J Surg. 1998;85:1147–9.
60. Merigliano S, Molena D, Ruol A, et al. Chylothorax complicating esophagectomy for cancer: a plea for early thoracic duct ligation. J Thorac Cardiovasc Surg. 2000;119:453–7.
61. Ohkura Y, Ueno M, Shindoh J, et al. Risk factors for postoperative chylothorax after radical subtotal esophagectomy. Ann Surg Oncol. 2018;25:2739–46.
62. Zhang SS, Yang H, Luo KJ, et al. The impact of body mass index on complication and survival in resected oesophageal cancer: a clinical-based cohort and meta-analysis. Br J Cancer. 2013;109:2894–903.
63. de Gier HH, et al. Systematic approach to the treatment of chylous leakage after neck dissection. Head Neck. 1996;18(4):347–51.
64. Fujita T, Daiko H. Efficacy and predictor of octreotide treatment for postoperative chylothorax after thoracic esophagectomy. World J Surg. 2014;38:2039–45.
65. Fujino K, Motooka Y, Koga T, et al. Novel approach to pleurodesis with 50% glucose for air leakage after lung resection or pneumothorax. Surg Today. 2016;46:599–602.
66. Cope C, Timms I, Pavcnik D. Percutaneous transthoracic duct catheterization to the neck and esophagus: a feasibility study. J Vasc Interv Radiol. 1997;8:845–9.
67. Cope C, Kaiser LR. Management of unremitting chylothorax by percutaneous embolization and blockage of retroperitoneal lymphatic vessels in 42 patients. J Vasc Interv Radiol. 2002;13:1139–48.
68. Lagarde SM, et al. Incidence and management of chyle leakage after esophagectomy. Thorac Surg. 2005;80(2):449–54.
69. Wright C, Zeitels S. Recurrent laryngeal nerve injuries after esophagectomy. Thorac Surg Clin. 2006;16:23–33.
70. Hikage M, Kamei T, Nakano T, et al. Impact of routine recurrent laryngeal nerve monitoring in prone esophagectomy with mediastinal lymph node dissection. Surg Endosc. 2017;31:2986–96.
71. Gelpke H, Grieder F, Decurtins M, et al. Recurrent laryngeal nerve monitoring during esophagectomy and mediastinal lymph node dissection. World J Surg. 2010;34:2379–82.
72. Yung KC, Likhterov I, Courey MS. Effect of temporary vocal fold injection medialization on the rate of permanent medialization laryngoplasty in unilateral vocal fold paralysis patients. Laryngoscope. 2011;121:2191–4.
73. Friedman AD, Burns JA, Heaton JT, et al. Early versus late injection medialization for unilateral vocal fold paralysis. Laryngoscope. 2010;120:2042–6.
74. Isshiki N, Morita H, Okamura H, et al. Thyroplasty as a new phonosurgical technique. Acta Otolaryngol. 1974;78:451–7.
75. Oppelt PU, Askevold I, Hörbelt R, Roller FC, Padberg W, Hecker A, Reichert M. Trans-hiatal herniation following esophagectomy or gastrectomy: retrospective single-center experiences with a potential surgical emergency. Hernia. 2022;26(1):259–78.
76. Rostas JW 3rd., Mai TT, Richards WO. Gastric motility physiology and surgical intervention. Surg Clin N Am. 2011;91(5):983–99.
77. Sakai M, et al. Impact of the level of anastomosis on reflux esophagitis following esophagectomy with gastric tube reconstruction. World J Surg. 2017;41(3):804–9.

# Interventional Radiological Procedures for Esophageal Cancer

# 31

Yavuz Metin and Kivilcim Yavuz

The esophageal cancer is the seventh most commonly diagnosed cancer worldwide [1]. Despite significant progress in the treatment of this disease in recent years, due to the silent course of the disease, advanced-stage tumors are often encountered.

The application and importance of radiological interventional procedures in the treatment of esophageal cancer are increasing day by day. The most important reasons for this are that these procedures are performed by minimal invasive methods and the rates of minor and major complications associated with the procedures are quite low. Radiological procedures play a role in both the treatment of the primary tumor and the complications or systemic spread arising from the primary tumor [2].

This chapter of the book will discuss the interventional radiological procedures applied in the treatment of esophageal cancer, both in the primary treatment and in the treatment of secondary conditions related to this cancer.

## 31.1 Interventional Radiological Procedures Used in the Local Treatment of Esophageal Cancer

### 31.1.1 Esophageal Stenting

Esophageal cancer is a malignancy with a very poor prognosis, and patients typically receive a diagnosis at advanced stages. One of the most important findings and complications of esophageal cancer is dysphagia and advanced narrowing or obstruction secondary to the tumor or metastatic lymph nodes. The most important method applied for this purpose is esophageal stenting.

Y. Metin (✉) · K. Yavuz
Radiology Department, Medicine Faculty, Ankara University, Ankara, Turkey
e-mail: kyavuz@ankara.edu.tr


O. Engin (ed.), *Risk Factors and Therapy of Esophagus Cancer*,
https://doi.org/10.1007/978-3-031-47024-0_31

Stenting for esophageal cancer is primarily applied for palliation of advanced esophageal cancer, but sometimes it is also performed as a supportive preparation for chemoradiotherapy. Other indications for stenting include esophageal compression due to primary or secondary mediastinal tumors or lung cancer, tracheoesophageal fistulas, and esophageal perforations. Especially in the treatment of malignant strictures, esophageal stenting has been used for over a century [3, 4]. The structure and design of the stent to be used in the palliative treatment of esophageal cancer are primarily determined based on the localization of the tumor [5]. Esophageal stents can be classified into various categories based on the material used (plastic, silicone, stainless steel, etc.), expansion properties (self-expandable, memory stents), and coating status (bare, partially covered, and fully covered) [6]. Additionally, special types have been developed in recent years that have the potential to play a role in local medical treatment, such as radioactive and chemotherapy drug slow-release stents [7].

The stenting procedure can be performed under endoscopy guidance, but during this procedure, both the endoscope and stent need to be passed through the pharynx simultaneously, and the procedure is performed blindly in terms of the position of the guide wire and the delivery system distal to the stricture. This can result in malpositioning of the stent. Stenting performed under interventional radiology guidance is a less traumatic, accurate, and cost-effective method that provides the opportunity to avoid the contraindications or complications of endoscopic procedures [3–7].

### 31.1.2 Self-Expandable Metallic Stents (SEMS)

Self-expandable metallic stents (SEMS) are cylindrical metallic frames that apply forces on their own until they reach their maximum width. These stents, which are used in the palliative treatment of esophageal cancer, were first applied by Domschke et al. in 1990 [8] (Fig. 31.1).

There are two types of self-expanding metallic stents commonly used in routine treatment today. One is the traditional stainless steel stent, and the other is a nickel-titanium alloy stent. The Wallstent and Z-stent are examples of traditional stainless steel stents. The most significant disadvantage of these two types of stents is their weak histological compatibility, which can cause significant inflammation and fibrosis in esophageal tissues. Currently, the stents most commonly used in clinical practice are made of a nickel-titanium alloy and have a morphological memory effect. Compared to stainless steel stents, these stents have better tissue compatibility, excellent flexibility, moderate durability, and a special softness. With technological improvements and developments, these stents now come in three main types: covered, partially covered, and uncovered. SEMS stents are completely or partially covered with a membrane made of various materials (e.g., silicone and expanded polytetrafluoroethylene [ePTFE]) to prevent tumor growth into the stent (Fig. 31.2). The three types of metallic stents have common complications such as stent migration and tumor tissue growth into the stent. However, various publications have not

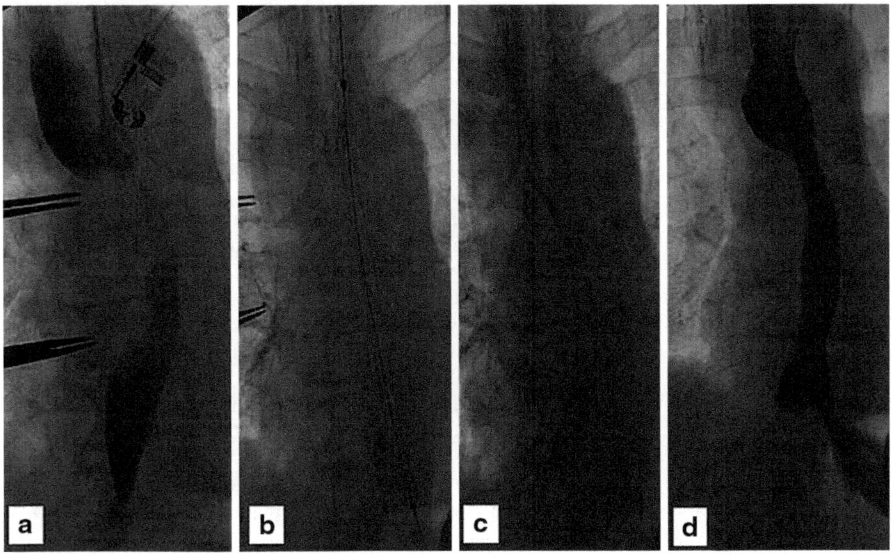


**Fig. 31.1** In the interventional radiology unit, the procedure of placing a self-expandable metallic esophageal stent for palliative purposes is being observed in a patient diagnosed with esophageal cancer (**a**–**c**). Following the placement of the stent, restoration of passage in the esophagus is achieved (**d**). (This image has been used with the permission of Prof. Dr. Türkmen Çiftçi from the Department of Radiology at Hacettepe University)

found statistically significant differences in stent migration rates between stent types [9].

Most SEMS have developed anti-migration features (e.g., flared ends and double-layer design) to reduce stent migration, which is a significant complication [6]. Some manufacturers have developed SEMS variants with reflux-preventing features such as sleeves and flaps to reduce gastroesophageal reflux [6].

### 31.1.3 Radioactive Self-Expandable Metallic Stents (SEMS)

Radioactive self-expandable metallic stents (SEMS) are one of the preferred methods for the treatment of advanced esophageal cancer. While stents provide relief from dysphagia and maintain patency of the passage, they can also carry I-125 radioactive particles that help in the treatment of esophageal tumors. Compared to conventional external radiotherapy, radioactive SEMS allows for increased radiation dose to the target area by preventing dose attenuation caused by distant radiation, thus increasing treatment effectiveness. Multicenter randomized controlled clinical trials have shown that I-125 radioactive SEMS is a safer and more effective method than conventional esophageal stents, significantly improving patient survival [10, 11].

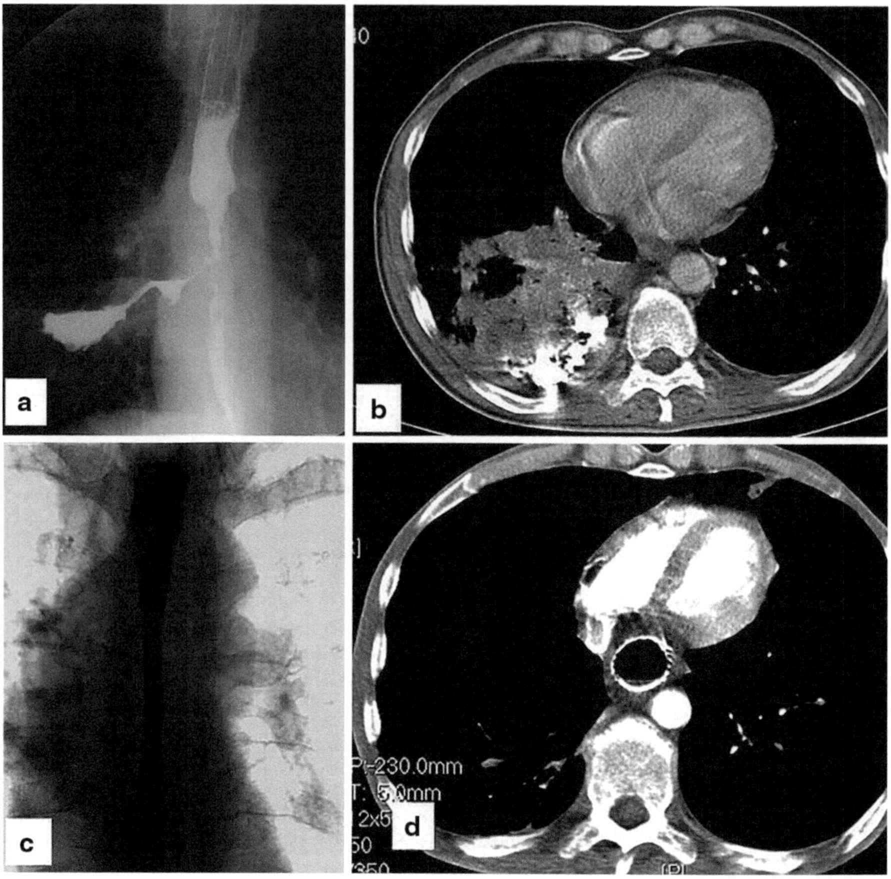


**Fig. 31.2** In the case of secondary perforation due to esophageal cancer, extravasation of contrast material is observed during endoscopic examination (**a**), and on CT imaging, consequent abscess formation is identified (**b**). Following the placement of a cover stent under fluoroscopic guidance in the interventional radiology unit (**c**), a follow-up CT scan reveals complete resolution of the abscess (**d**). (This image has been used with the permission of Prof. Dr. Türkmen Çiftçi from the Department of Radiology at Hacettepe University)

Although the use of radioactive SEMS has become more widespread, there is still no consensus on the size of the radioactive particles to be used, the total dose of particles, or how they should be distributed.

### 31.1.4 Drug-Eluting SEMS

Recently, drug-eluting self-expandable metal stents (DE-SEMS) have been tested for not only palliative treatment of esophageal obstruction but also for medical treatment of primary tumors. These stents, coated with a drug-loaded polymer membrane, provide mechanical support to expand the obstructed esophagus while also releasing various anticancer drugs to inhibit tumor growth [12].

Stents with different anticancer drug releases are currently under development, and various animal studies have shown significant potential in preventing tumor growth [13, 14].

## 31.2 Nonstent Applications

### 31.2.1 Arterial Infusion Chemotherapy

The insensitivity of esophageal tumor cells to radiotherapy and chemotherapy significantly limits the success of medical treatment. Most patients with advanced esophageal cancer die within a year of diagnosis, and the 5-year survival rate varies only between 10 and 25% [15].

Arterial infusion chemotherapy is a local chemotherapy method in which chemotherapeutic drugs are directly delivered to the tumor tissue by catheterizing the vessels that directly feed the tumor, following femoral artery puncture. Compared to traditional intravenous chemotherapy, arterial infusion chemotherapy can significantly increase the concentration of chemotherapeutic drugs in local tumor regions, reduce the toxicity and side effects of chemotherapeutic drugs, and allow damage to surrounding tissues to occur at the lowest possible levels [15, 16].

There are two significant limitations to arterial infusion chemotherapy. First, the specific catheterization and infusion of the tumor-feeding artery may not be achievable as esophageal cancer may not exhibit rich vascularity. Second, even if attempting to apply the optimal dose of the chemotherapeutic agent, it may not be possible to reach a sufficient treatment duration to sustain the effective dose of the drug [17].

Although serious complications are rare after arterial perfusion chemotherapy, the most common complications that may occur include esophageal perforation, spinal cord injury, and esophagitis. Transarterial chemoembolization (TACE) is applied as a palliative treatment method for unresectable or recurrent esophageal cancer and gastrointestinal bleeding associated with this tumor [18].

Conventional TACE enables the increased concentration of chemotherapy drugs through localized-selective transarterial infusion, but the main problems encountered are the slow release of the drug and the inability to maintain high concentration continuity for a long time. As a new drug delivery system, drug-eluting beads allow for the slow release of chemotherapy drugs in DEB-TACE, thereby improving the safety and efficacy of the treatment [19, 20]. There are studies in the literature regarding the effectiveness of transarterial infusion chemotherapy in patients with T3-stage squamous cell carcinoma of the esophagus after radical surgical treatment [21].

In order for transarterial embolization treatment to be effectively performed, knowledge of the main feeding vessels of the tumor and their catheterization is required. For tumors often located in the esophagogastric junction, the left gastric artery is frequently the major tumor-feeding vessel, while for upper and middle esophageal carcinomas, the bronchial artery is the major tumor-feeding vessel. Transarterial embolization can be applied via these main vascular structures in patients with esophageal cancer who develop secondary bleeding complications [22, 23]. DEB-TACE can embolize the artery feeding the tumor to block blood flow and enable controlled release of chemotherapy drugs, thereby allowing for improved clinical outcomes [20, 24]. A recent study has reported that DEB-TACE may be a safe and feasible option for the treatment of unresectable or recurrent esophageal cancer, which can be considered as an alternative option [25].

## 31.3 Interventional Radiological Procedures in Metastatic Esophageal Cancer

Almost 50% of patients with esophageal cancer present with advanced or metastatic disease at the time of diagnosis, primarily due to the aggressive biology of the tumor, and the 5-year survival rate for patients with advanced or metastatic esophageal cancer is only 3–5% [26]. The most common distant organ metastases of esophageal cancer are to the lungs, liver, and bone. It has been shown that patients with liver recurrence after esophagectomy have worse survival rates than those with distant metastases to other organs [27]. Therefore, there are important consequences of local control for liver metastases secondary to esophageal cancer. Since most patients with liver metastasis are not suitable for surgical treatment, systemic chemotherapy and radiotherapy are mainly used for palliative purposes. Considering the low surgical resection rates and unsatisfactory results of systemic chemotherapy, there is an urgent need for effective local-regional treatments to improve survival and provide local control in metastatic disease. Currently, ablative therapies are considered a promising treatment method for metastatic liver diseases due to their minimally invasive nature, high efficacy, and low complication rates [28].

### 31.3.1 Interventional Radiological Procedures in the Treatment of Liver Metastases Secondary to Esophageal Cancer

The liver is one of the most common sites of metastasis, with metastatic lesions detected in 35–40% of patients at the time of diagnosis. In addition, the liver is the organ where the first recurrence is observed in 6–25% of cases after esophagectomy [29, 30].

In general, ablative therapies continue to be a complementary treatment method for patients who cannot be surgically resected due to cancer-specific factors and accompanying comorbidities. These treatment methods are especially preferred for small liver lesions with a high surgical risk.

### 31.3.2 Microwave Ablation (MWA) Therapy for Liver Metastases

In recent years, microwave ablation (MWA) has been used as a promising method due to its minimally invasive nature, effectiveness, repeatability, and low complication rates. The effectiveness of MWA has been demonstrated in patients with primary and metastatic liver tumors. In a study conducted by Zhou et al., it was found that combined MWA therapy with systemic chemotherapy provided better survival outcomes than systemic chemotherapy alone in patients with unresectable esophageal cancer and metastatic lesions in the liver. The repeatability and low complication rates of MWA provide a longer survival chance, especially for esophageal cancer patients with recurrent liver metastases [31] (Fig. 31.3).

In the past, patients with esophageal cancer and liver metastases located in anatomically high-risk areas (e.g. major blood vessels, liver hilum, gallbladder, diaphragm, gastrointestinal tract) were considered "unresectable" and only received systemic chemotherapy as palliative treatment. However, nowadays, the reliability and effectiveness of MWA have been confirmed in patients with liver metastases located near these risk areas [32, 33] (Fig. 31.4).

### 31.3.3 Transarterial Radioembolization (TARE) for Esophageal Cancer Metastasis to Liver

Traditionally, the role of radiation in the treatment of liver malignancies has been limited due to the inability to deliver high doses of radiation to tumors. Yttrium-90 microsphere (TheraSphere, MDS Nordion) therapy allows for high doses of radiation to be delivered to tumors while relatively sparing normal liver tissue. In this treatment technique, transarterially delivered 90Y microspheres are primarily retained within the tumor bed [34].

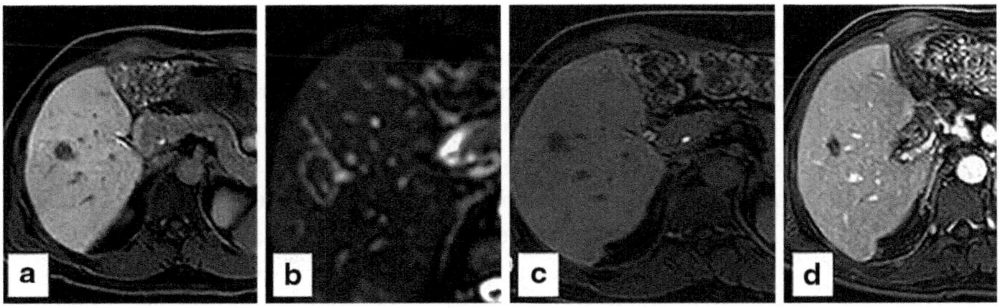


**Fig. 31.3** The patient, who developed liver metastasis due to esophageal cancer (**a**, **b**), underwent MWA therapy under US guidance in the interventional radiology unit. The patient's post-procedural MRI image is shown, followed by the 1-year (**c**) and 3-year follow-up MRI images (**d**). Reduction in lesion size was observed during the follow-up examinations. (This image has been used with the permission of Prof. Dr. Türkmen Çiftçi from the Department of Radiology at Hacettepe University)

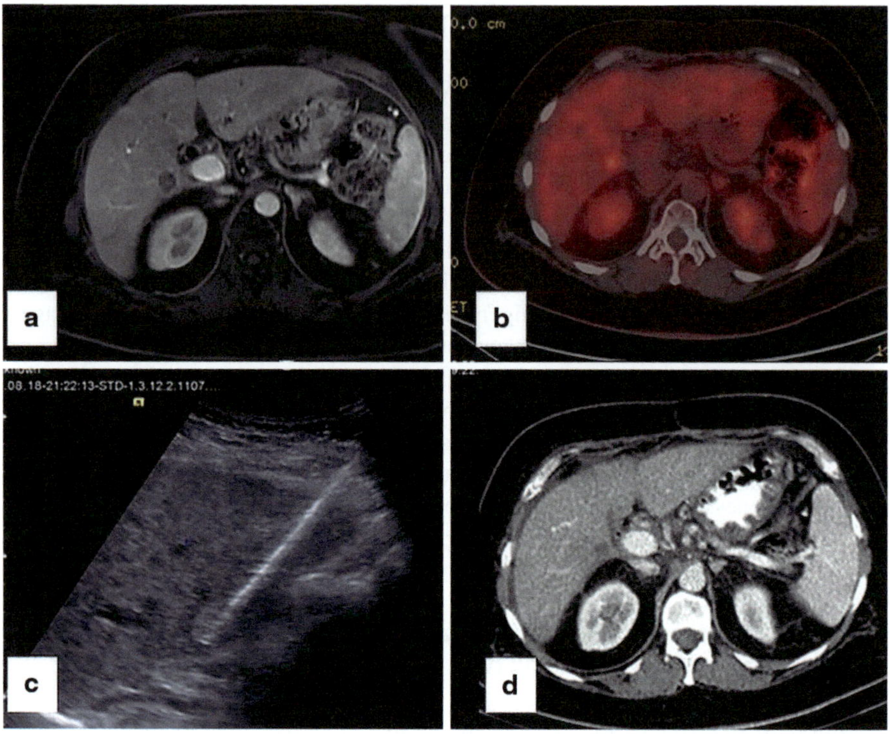


**Fig. 31.4** In a case of esophageal cancer with secondary liver metastasis, pre-treatment MRI (**a**) and PET-CT (**b**) images are being observed ultrasound-guided microwave ablation (**c**). Following ultrasound-guided microwave ablation (MWA) treatment, significant regression of the lesion is detected in the post-treatment image (**d**). (These images have been used with the permission of Prof. Dr. Fatih Boyvat from the Department of Radiology at Ankara Baskent University)

Radioembolization has been proven to have an effective role mainly in the treatment of liver metastases secondary to colon cancer, but recent studies have shown that TARE is also effective in some other primary liver tumors and in the treatment of metastatic diseases. Generally, radioembolization is applied only in cases where standard treatment has failed or where certain criteria required for standard treatment are not met. In patients with large or multiple lesions, radioembolization may be preferred over surgical resection to control disease progression. In patients who have failed systemic treatments or cannot tolerate further chemotherapy, radioembolization can be used as an alternative treatment option as a salvage therapy. Several researchers have reported their experiences with TARE in the treatment of liver metastases arising from primary tumors other than colon cancer (including esophageal cancer). The majority of these cases consisted of patients with unresectable tumors selected on a case-by-case basis. The experiences gained through these studies indicate that TARE can be applied to almost any liver tumor, whether primary or metastatic [35, 36] (Fig. 31.5).

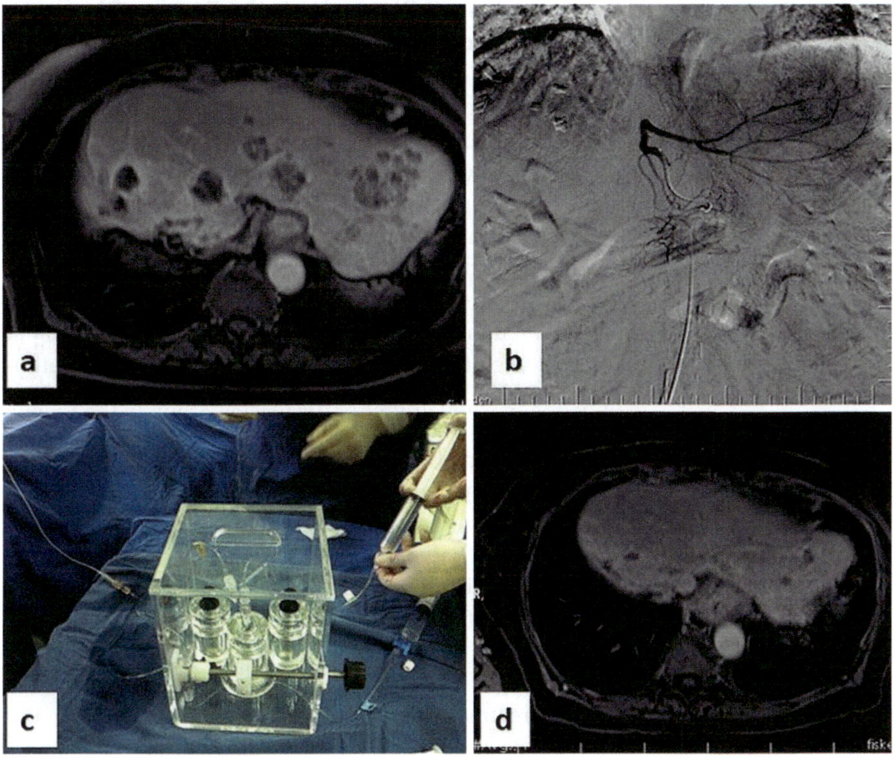

**Fig. 31.5** The patient with multiple metastases in the liver due to esophageal cancer (**a**) underwent transarterial radioembolization (TARE) (**c**) guided by digital subtraction angiography (**b**) by interventional radiologists. Subsequent follow-up imaging revealed a significant reduction and disappearance of the metastatic lesions (**d**). (These images have been used with the permission of Prof. Dr. Fatih Boyvat from the Department of Radiology at Ankara Başkent University)

Collecting data for each tumor type will take time, but as studies and applications increase, radioembolization will become a standard treatment option for unresectable liver diseases, including those with metastatic disease due to esophageal tumors. It should also be noted that TARE is a well-tolerated procedure with post-embolization syndrome symptoms reported in 67–100% of cases, but without any serious adverse effects. Although hepatic insufficiency induced by radioembolization is a valid side effect, it only occurs in 0–4% of cases, which is evidence of TARE's reliability as a treatment alternative [37, 38].

## 31.4 Radiological Interventional Procedures in Cases of Lung Metastases Secondary to Esophageal Cancer

Metachronous pulmonary metastasis constitutes 18–41% of hematogenous recurrence of esophageal squamous cell carcinomas and is one of the major recurrence patterns of this cancer. Systemic chemotherapy is always used as the initial treatment in these patients due to the multiple number of lung metastases and/or concomitant involvement of other extrapulmonary organs. Surgical excision of metastatic lesions is another treatment option in selected patients [39]. Image-guided percutaneous radiofrequency ablation (RFA) is a minimally invasive treatment method for solid tumors. Although this treatment is often used in the treatment of liver tumors, it has also started to be frequently used in the treatment of intrathoracic malignancies [40, 41].

In their study, Baba et al. found that percutaneous CT-guided RFA provides relatively high local control rates with acceptable complication rates in the treatment of pulmonary metastases secondary to esophageal cancer [42].

In conclusion; thanks to technological advancements, minimally invasive interventional radiological procedures have become an increasingly important alternative to surgical and medical treatments in cases where traditional approaches prove inadequate. These procedures offer effective treatment options for both primary tumors and metastatic tumors that have developed as a result of the primary tumor. While primarily considered palliative treatments, they are expected to become increasingly effective as primary treatment methods in the coming years.

## References


1. Parkin DM, Laara E, Muir CS. Estimates of the worldwide frequency of sixteen major cancers in 1980. Int J Cancer. 1988;41:184–97.
2. Bancewicz J. Palliation in oesophageal neoplasia. Ann R Coll Surg Engl. 1999;81:382–6.
3. Atkinson M, Ferguson R. Fibreoptic endoscopic palliative intubation of inoperable oesophagogastric neoplasms. Br Med J. 1977;1:266–7.
4. Frimberger E. Expanding spiral—a new type of prosthesis for the palliative treatment of malignant esophageal stenoses. Endoscopy. 1983;15(suppl 1):213–4.
5. Rana F, Dhar A. Oesophageal stenting for benign and malignant strictures: a systematic approach. Frontline Gastroenterol. 2015;6(2):94–100. https://doi.org/10.1136/flgastro-2015-100559. Epub 2015 Mar 6
6. Kim KY, Tsauo J, Song HY. Self-expandable metallic stent placement for the palliation of esophageal cancer. J Korean Med Sci. 2017;32:1062–71.
7. Mao A. Interventional therapy of esophageal cancer. Gastrointest Tumors. 2016;3(2):59–68. https://doi.org/10.1159/000447512. Epub 2016 Aug 27
8. Varadarajulu S, Banerjee S, Barth B, Desilets D, Kaul V, Kethu S, Pedrosa M, Pfau P, Tokar J, Wang A, et al. Enteral stents. Gastrointest Endosc 2011; 74: 455-64. 6. Domschke W, Foerster EC, Matek W, Rödl W. Self-expanding mesh stent for esophageal cancer stenosis. Endoscopy. 1990;22:134–6.
9. Jang S, Parsi M, Collins J, Vargo J. Predictors of esophageal self-expandable metal stent migration: an academic center study. Gastrointest Interv. 2016;5:72–9.

10. Wang ZM, Huang XB, Cao J. Intraluminal radioactive stent compared with covered stent alone for the treatment of malignant esophageal stricture. Cardiovasc Intervent Radiol. 2012;35:351–8.
11. Tian D, Wen H, Fu M. Comparative study of self-expanding metal stent and intraluminal radioactive stent for inoperable esophageal squamous cell carcinoma. World J Surg Oncol. 2016;14:18–25.
12. Suk KT, Kim JW, Kim HS. Human application of a metallic stent covered with a paclitaxel-incorporated membrane for malignant biliary obstruction: multicenter pilot study. Gastrointest Endosc. 2007;66(4):798–803. https://doi.org/10.1016/j.gie.2007.05.037.
13. Kim SY, Kim M, Kim MK, Lee H, Lee DK, Lee DH, Yang SG. Paclitaxel-eluting nanofiber-covered self-expanding nonvascular stent for palliative chemotherapy of gastrointestinal cancer and its related stenosis. Biomed Microdevices. 2014;16:897–904.
14. Lei L, Liu X, Guo S, Tang M, Cheng L, Tian L. 5-fluorouracil-loaded multilayered films for drug controlled releasing stent application: drug release, microstructure, and ex vivo permeation behaviors. J Control Release. 2010;146:45–53.
15. Mariette C, Piessen G, Triboulet JP. Therapeutic strategies in oesophageal carcinoma: role of surgery and other modalities. Lancet Oncol. 2007;8:545–53.
16. Yin MP, Xie PF, Zhao Y, He W, Ma YZ, Li CX, Li Z, Zeng YW, Wu G. Clinical evaluation of Transarterial infusion chemotherapy for advanced esophageal cancer. J Cancer. 2021;12(5):1493–8. https://doi.org/10.7150/jca.46877.
17. Tanohata S. The clinical investigation of esophageal arteriography in esophageal cancer—with special reference to proper esophageal arteriography—(author's transl). Newsl Int Coll Dent India Sect. 1977;37:103–24.
18. Gaur P, Kim MP, Dunkin BJ. Esophageal cancer: recent advances in screening, targeted therapy, and management. J Carcinog. 2014;13:11.
19. Park S, Shin JH, Gwon DI, Kim HJ, Sung KB, Yoon HK, Ko GY, Ko HK. Transcatheter arterial embolization for gastrointestinal bleeding associated with gastric carcinoma: prognostic factors predicting successful hemostasis and survival. J Vasc Interv Radiol. 2017;28(7):1012–21.
20. Melchiorre F, Patella F, Pescatori L, Pesapane F, Fumarola E, Biondetti P, Brambillasca P, Monaco C, Ierardi AM, Franceschelli G, et al. DEB-TACE: a standard review. Future Oncol. 2018;14(28):2969–84.
21. Wu B, Zhou J, Ling G, Zhu D, Long Q. CalliSpheres drug-eluting beads versus lipiodol transarterial chemoembolization in the treatment of hepatocellular carcinoma: a short-term efcacy and safety study. World J Surg Oncol. 2018;16(1):69.
22. Liu BD, Zhi XY, Xu QS. The value of postoperative arterial infusion chemotherapy in patients with T3 esophageal squamous carcinoma after radical surgery. Zhonghua Yi Xue Za Zhi. 2005;85(9):586–9.
23. Aoki M, Tokue H, Koyama Y, Tsushima Y, Oshima K. Transcatheter arterial embolization with N-butyl cyanoacrylate for arterial esophageal bleeding in esophageal cancer patients. World J Surg Oncol. 2016;14:54.
24. Nagase H, Kawasaki H, Wajima N, Nakai M, Kimura A, Nakayama Y, Hakamada K. Two cases of bleeding from locally advanced esophageal cancer successfully treated by transcatheter arterial embolization. Gan To Kagaku Ryoho. 2013;40:2167–9.
25. Kunisada K, Ishikawa H, Takafuji J, Komuta K. A case of a 91-year-old patient with advanced squamous cell lung cancer complicated with renal dysfunction successfully treated with transarterial chemo-embolization. Gan To Kagaku Ryoho. 2013;40(7):917–9.
26. Bi Y, Shi X, Ren J, Yi M, Han X, Song M. Clinical outcomes of doxorubicin-eluting CalliSpheres® beads-transarterial chemoembolization for unresectable or recurrent esophageal carcinoma. BMC Gastroenterol. 2021;21(1):231. https://doi.org/10.1186/s12876-021-01816-3.
27. Rustgi AK, El-Serag HB. Esophageal carcinoma. N Engl J Med. 2014;371:2499–509.
28. Ichida H, Imamura H, Yoshimoto J, Sugo H, Kajiyama Y, Tsurumaru M, et al. Pattern of post-operative recurrence and hepatic and/or pulmonary resection for liver and/or lung metastases from esophageal carcinoma. World J Surg. 2013;37:398–407.

29. Liang P, Wang Y, Yu X, Dong B. Malignant liver tumors: treatment with percutaneous microwave ablation—complications among cohort of 1136 patients. Radiology. 2009;251:933–40.
30. Quint LE, Hepburn LM, Francis IR, Whyte RI, Orringer MB. Incidence and distribution of distant metastases from newly diagnosed esophageal carcinoma. Cancer. 1995;76:1120–5.
31. Mariette C, Balon JM, Piessen G, Fabre S, Van Seuningen I, Triboulet JP. Pattern of recurrence following complete resection of esophageal carcinoma and factors predictive of recurrent disease. Cancer. 2003;97:1616–23.
32. Zhou F, Yu X, Liang P, Cheng Z, Han Z, Yu J, Liu F, Tan S, Dai G, Bai L. Combined microwave ablation and systemic chemotherapy for liver metastases from oesophageal cancer: preliminary results and literature review. Int J Hyperth. 2016;32(5):524–30. https://doi.org/10.3109/02656736.2016.1155758. Epub 2016 Apr 7
33. Li M, Yu X, Liang P, Dong B, Liu F. Ultrasound-guided percutaneous microwave ablation for hepatic malignancy adjacent to the gallbladder. Int J Hyperth. 2015;31:579–87.
34. Li M, Yu XL, Liang P, Liu F, Dong B, Zhou P. Percutaneous microwave ablation for liver cancer adjacent to the diaphragm. Int J Hyperth. 2012;28:218–26.
35. Campbell AM, Bailey I, Burton M. Analysis of the distribution of intra-arterial microspheres in human liver following hepatic yttrium-90 microsphere therapy. Phys Med Biol. 2000;45:1023–33.
36. Stuart JE, Tan B, Myerson RJ, Garcia-Ramirez J, Goddu SM, Pilgram TK, et al. Salvage radioembolization of liver-dominant metastases with a resin-based microsphere: initial outcomes. J Vasc Interv Radiol. 2008;19(10):1427–33. https://doi.org/10.1016/j.jvir.2008.07.009.
37. Sato KT, Lewandowski RJ, Mulcahy MF, Atassi B, Ryu RK, Gates VL, et al. Unresectable chemorefractory liver metastases: radioembolization with 90Y microspheres—safety, efficacy, and survival. Radiology. 2008;247(2):507–15. https://doi.org/10.1148/radiol.2472062029.
38. Zurkiya O, Ganguli S. Beyond hepatocellular carcinoma and colorectal metastasis: the expanding applications of radioembolization. Front Oncol. 2014;4:150.
39. Nakagawa S, Kanda T, Kosugi S, Ohashi M, Suzuki T, Hatakeyama K. Recurrence pattern of squamous cell carcinoma of the thoracic esophagus after extended radical esophagectomy with three-field lymphadenectomy. J Am Coll Surg. 2004;198(2):205–11.
40. Lanuti M, Sharma A, Willers H, Digumarthy SR, Mathisen DJ, Shepard JA. Radiofrequency ablation for stage I non-small cell lung cancer: management of locoregional recurrence. Ann Thorac Surg. 2012;93(3):921–7. discussion 7–88.
41. Lencioni R, Crocetti L, Cioni R, et al. Response to radiofrequency ablation of pulmonary tumours: a prospective, intention-to-treat, multicentre clinical trial (the RAPTURE study). Lancet Oncol. 2008;9(7):621–8.
42. Baba Y, Watanabe M, Kawanaka K, Iwagami S, Ishimoto T, Iwatsuki M, Yoshida N, Yamashita Y, Baba H. Radiofrequency ablation for pulmonary metastases from esophageal squamous cell carcinoma. Dis Esophagus. 2014;27(1):36–41. https://doi.org/10.1111/dote.12034. Epub 2013 Feb 5.

# 32 Surgical Treatment of Liver Metastases in Esophageal Cancer

Ozhan Cetindag and Omer Engin

## 32.1 Introduction

According to epidemiological data, the incidence of liver metastasis in esophageal cancer varies between 20 and 50%. Liver metastases are a significant factor worsening prognosis in patients with esophageal cancer. In patients with esophageal cancer, liver metastases are generally seen in advanced stages of the disease and the chances of surgical intervention are lower [1].

Esophageal cancer patients with liver metastases require a multidisciplinary approach when it comes to treatment options. The aim of the treatment is to halt the progression of the disease and to prolong life. For this purpose, surgical treatment, chemotherapy, radiotherapy, or combinations thereof may be used. However, surgical intervention for liver metastases in esophageal cancer patients is rarely applied. Surgical intervention can only be applied in a limited number of metastasis cases, and the selection of these cases is crucial.

The option of surgical treatment depends on the number, size, and location of the liver metastases. The surgical intervention should not only include the metastases in the liver but also the esophageal cancer itself [2].

O. Cetindag (✉)
Private Clinic, Izmir, Turkey

O. Engin
Surgery Department, VM Medical Park Pendik Hospital, Istanbul, Türkiye


O. Engin (ed.), *Risk Factors and Therapy of Esophagus Cancer*,
https://doi.org/10.1007/978-3-031-47024-0_32

## 32.2 Liver Metastases and Their Management

### 32.2.1 Diagnostic Methods

When a diagnosis of esophageal cancer is made, several diagnostic methods can be employed to determine whether there are metastases in the patient's liver. These methods may include:

### 32.2.2 Imaging Methods

Computed tomography (CT) scans are quite effective in detecting any abnormal growth in the liver. These scans use X-rays to create cross-sectional images, thereby allowing for a precise examination of tissues.

Magnetic resonance imaging (MRI) scans can provide more detailed images than CT scans. MRI scans create cross-sectional images using magnetic fields and radio waves.

A small amount of radioactive material is used in PET-CT, and this substance is stored more in cancer cells than in normal cells. In this way, cancer cells appear brighter. These scans can be used to detect metastases in the liver of patients diagnosed with esophageal cancer [3].

## 32.3 Biopsy

A biopsy can be performed to directly examine abnormal cells in the liver. This procedure is done by taking a sample of liver tissue using a thin needle. The biopsy sample is then examined under a microscope, and if cancer cells are detected, the diagnosis can be confirmed and the patient's treatment can be planned [3, 4].

## 32.4 Management

Esophageal cancer (EC) is one of the lethal types of cancer worldwide and can often metastasize to other organs. This spread can most often lead to the formation of liver metastases. Liver metastases are a significant prognostic factor affecting the treatment process and outcomes of patients with esophageal cancer [3].

In the past 20 years, the number of EC cases has rapidly increased, reaching about half a million new cases. EC still represents an aggressive disease associated with a poor prognosis. Currently, the preferred treatment method is a surgical approach combined with chemotherapy (ChT)/chemoradiotherapy. The 5-year survival rate for patients undergoing surgical resection reaches approximately 50%. Advanced metastatic patients are generally considered suitable only for palliative care, with a 5-year estimated survival time of less than 5%. The liver is one of the most common sites of metastasis in 35–40% of patients during EC diagnosis and is the first site of recurrence after esophagectomy [3–6].

The optimal management of liver oligometastatic EC patients is still a controversial issue. Surgical resection for liver metastases is not usually performed due to oncological reasons. Alternative therapeutic options generally include ChT and local regional treatments. More recent studies have reported that patients with a low liver tumor burden have a favorable prognosis with liver resection after ChT. In fact, the prognosis of nonsurgical liver oligometastatic EC patients is still largely unknown. Although primary EC is often sensitive to multimodal treatment, metastatic EC does not usually respond well to ChT; therefore, medical treatment alone does not offer a chance of treatment. A full response with the current ChT regimen is rare, the response time is short, typically 6–8 months. Therefore, in selected patients with liver oligometastatic EC resistant to standard medical treatments, a multimodal approach including liver resection and/or other local treatments can be considered [3, 4].

Oligometastatic disease, despite the lack of a precise and consistent definition, is generally considered a relatively favorable clinical condition with slower-progressing biology, a limited number of disease sites, and potential for long-term disease control. Oligometastatic gastric cancer, although the tumor burden is defined as fewer than five nodules [4], this is not the case for EC. Therefore, it seems mandatory to establish definition criteria to determine the correct treatment. Reviews of literature have shown that the definition is based only on personal opinions. However, the main factor to determine the correct definition is having a maximum of three lesions in the disease that can be radically treated with surgical and/or local treatments [4].

## 32.5 Surgical

Currently, there are no randomized trials comparing palliative and multimodal approaches (chemotherapy versus chemotherapy + surgical/ablative treatment) for liver metastases in primary esophageal cancer, and there are no comparative studies with propensity score matching and meta-analyses. The existing data mostly rely on a few case reports or anecdotal information from Eastern centers and are therefore not suitable for forming robust recommendations [5, 6].

Although a general consensus has not been reached, small studies report that patients with a low hepatic tumor burden (less than three lesions) have a favorable prognosis after liver resection, regardless of synchronous or metachronous disease. There are some studies related to synchronous disease [7–9].

In one study [7], the median follow-up period after surgery was 22 months, and the overall survival (50%) and disease-free survival (33%) of the patients were reported. One-third of the patients analyzed in the study underwent metastasectomy of one to two liver metastases during the same session as esophageal cancer surgery. These findings closely reflect a 60% 5-year survival after liver resection in a cohort of 48 patients. In another retrospective study [8], it was reported that 14 patients treated with a multimodal approach involving liver resection showed a more favorable prognosis compared to patients who did not undergo surgery. The most common surgeries are represented by peritoneal (29%), hepatic (24%), and distant lymph node (11%) resections [10]. In the liver metastasized EC patients, one or two lesions were resected in 82% of the patients, and 92% of the patients received chemotherapy before surgery. In this patient subgroup, the median overall survival was 17 months, while the 1-year and 3-year disease-free survival rates were 42% and 35%, respectively. Another study [11] reported that the mean survival was 12.5 months in patients treated with metastasectomy.

There are some studies indicating a positive effect of surgical treatment on the prognosis of liver metastatic disease. However, there are not yet large-scale randomized studies that are comparable, especially with palliative treatment. However, small-scale studies have reported that patients with one or two lesions have a favorable prognosis with liver resection, regardless of metachronous or synchronous disease [10, 11]. Similar results are also available in the literature for metachronous disease [5, 12].

Today, there is no guideline indicator regarding the treatment of metachronous distant metastases of esophageal cancer. Deciding to remove distant metastases is often recommended by tumor boards as a personalized treatment proposal for patients with good general conditions and long tumor-free survival. In a recent retrospective study, Hiyoshi and colleagues [12] assessed the clinical significance of surgery for recurrence after radical esophagectomy. Of 100 patients treated with different treatments for esophageal cancer, 14 patients with 22 lesions responded to surgical treatment—one of them underwent metastasectomy only for a single liver metastasis. The group that underwent surgical treatment showed a more favorable survival both after esophagectomy and after the first recurrence. The survival times between patients with and without liver metastasectomy were 35 and 23 months, respectively. Similarly, Liu et al. [13] showed the positive effect of surgery on survival compared to other locoregional treatments for a single liver metastasis.

The authors also demonstrated that a longer disease-free interval longer than 12 months after esophagectomy could be considered as a potential positive prognostic factor for patient selection for liver resection. Similarly, another study [5] concluded that a good response to chemotherapy and operability of liver disease were biologically positive predictors and therefore potential selection criteria for curative liver resection.

## 32.6 Ablative Therapy

Over the past decade, radiofrequency ablation (RFA) has secured a solid place for itself in the treatment algorithm for liver tumors that cannot be surgically removed [14].

In small lesions, RFA is considered a standard technique that can achieve a complete response rate of up to 97% and 5-year survival rates that can reach up to 51% [15–17].

Many studies comparing RFA with resection showed no difference in terms of overall and local tumor progression-free survival [18–21].

However, although these data are not definitive due to methodological limitations, the superiority of surgery in terms of local disease control has been proven even for lesions with a diameter of 2–3 cm, compared to RFA, in large retrospective series [15, 21–24].

There are many studies demonstrating the potential benefits of aggressively applying a multitreatment approach. Emphasis is placed on the role of surgical treatment (both staged and simultaneous esophageal-liver resection) especially in patients with a low tumor burden (less than three lesions). For these patients, the 5-year survival rate after liver resection has been reported to be 50%, compared to 8–12% in patients receiving only chemotherapy. These results show that surgery has a significant impact on the prognosis of patients with esophageal cancer [15, 20, 21, 25]. However, the increased use of modern systemic chemotherapy suggests that some of the survival increase after surgical treatment may be due to these chemotherapeutics. It has been reported that chemotherapy, when applied in addition to surgery, has positive effects that make the tumor suitable for surgery and reduce recurrence characteristics. Therefore, in the treatment of patients with a low tumor burden and suitable for surgical treatment, surgical and systemic therapy should be used together. However, the appropriate timing of systemic therapy in resectable disease is still controversial and requires further study. For small liver lesions, RFA may be preferred even if the surgical risk is high or surgery is not possible. However, there is no definitive evidence as to whether RFA is a preferable alternative to surgery in patients with resectable liver esophageal cancer. Therefore, further studies are needed. In summary, there is no difference in efficacy between surgical and ablation therapies in the treatment of patients with esophageal cancer, but surgery can be preferred considering the anatomical location or size of the tumor. Stereotactic body radiation therapy (SBRT) can be preferred in patients with unresectable disease. More studies need to be done in this field. Limitations of this review include a small patient sample and mostly based on retrospective studies. However, the results should be considered in the treatment of patients with liver esophageal cancer with surgical and local-regional treatments [23–25].

In conclusion, an aggressive, multidisciplinary approach has been seen to increase survival in patients with liver esophageal cancer. However, while the data are weak, there are examples of good results obtained from surgery. If not applicable, local treatments can be considered. However, there is a serious need for better patient selection and clarification of treatment protocols so that a chance for recovery can be given, or at least the prognosis can be optimized. Considering the risk of tumor recurrence, strict follow-up protocols and a recurring multidisciplinary approach are required [25].

## References


1. Sehdev A, Catenacci DVT. Gastroesophageal cancer: focus on epidemiology, classification, and staging. Discov Med. 2013;16(87):103–11.
2. Wu PC, Posner MC. The role of surgery in the management of oesophageal cancer. Lancet Oncol. 2003;4(8):481–8.
3. Sehdev A, Catenacci DV. Gastroesophageal cancer: focus on epidemiology, classification, and staging. In: El-Zein RA, editor. Esophageal cancer—recent scientific Progress and clinical application. Springer International Publishing; 2013. p. 1–20. https://doi.org/10.1007/978-3-319-69269-3_1.
4. Ichida H, Imamura H, Yoshimoto J, Sugo H, Kajiyama Y, Tsurumaru M, et al. Pattern of postoperative recurrence and hepatic and/or pulmonary resection for liver and/or lung metastases from esophageal carcinoma. World J Surg. 2013;37:398–407.
5. Huddy JR, Thomas RL, Worthington TR, et al. Liver metastases from esophageal carcinoma: is there a role for surgical resection? Dis Esophagus. 2015;28(5):483–7.
6. Mudan SS, Giakoustidis A, Giakoustidis D, et al. Synchronous oesophagectomy and hepatic resection for metastatic oesophageal cancer: report of a case. Hippokratia. 2010;14(4):291.
7. Van Daele E, Scuderi V, Pape E, Van de Putte D, Varin O, Van Nieuwenhove Y, Ceelen W, Troisi R, Pattyn P. Long-term survival after multimodality therapy including surgery for metastatic esophageal cancer. In: Mishra NN, editor. Oesophageal cancer. Springer Singapore; 2018. p. 65–78. https://doi.org/10.1007/978-981-13-1299-6_5.
8. Wang J, Suri JS, Allen PK, Liao Z, Komaki R, Ho L, et al. Factors predictive of improved outcomes with multimodality local therapy after palliative chemotherapy for stage IV esophageal cancer. Am J Clin Oncol. 2016;39(3):228–35.
9. Gandy RC, Bergamin PA, Haghighi KS. Hepatic resection of non-colorectal non-endocrine liver metastases. ANZ J Surg. 2017;87:810–4.
10. Carmona-Bayonas A, Jiménez-Fonseca P, Echavarria I, Sánchez Cánovas M, Aguado G, Gallego J, Custodio A, Hernández R, Viudez A, Cano JM, et al. Surgery for metastases for esophageal-gastric cancer in the real world: data from the AGAMENON national registry. Eur J Surg Oncol. 2018;44:1191–8.
11. Slotta JE, Schuld J, Distler S, Richter S, Schilling MK, Kollmar O. Hepatic resection of non-colorectal and non-neuroendocrine liver metastases—survival benefit for patients with non-gastrointestinal primary cancers—a case-controlled study. Int J Surg. 2014;12:163–8.
12. Hiyoshi Y, Morita M, Kawano H, Otsu H, Ando K, Ito S, Miyamoto Y, Sakamoto Y, Saeki H, Oki E, et al. Clinical significance of surgical resection for the recurrence of esophageal cancer after radical esophagectomy. Ann Surg Oncol. 2015;22:240–6.
13. Liu J, Wei Z, Wang Y, Xia Z, et al. Hepatic resection for post-operative solitary liver metastasis from oesophageal squamous cell carcinoma. ANZ J Surg. 2018;88(4):E252–6.
14. Machi J, Oishi AJ, Sumida K, Sakamoto K, Furumoto NL, Oishi RH, Kylstra JW. Long-term outcome of radiofrequency ablation for unresectable liver metastases from colorectal cancer: evaluation of prognostic factors and effectiveness in first- and second-line management. Cancer J. 2006;12:318–26.
15. Abdalla EK, Vauthey JN, Ellis LM, Ellis V, Pollock R, Broglio KR, Hess K, Curley SA. Recurrence and outcomes following hepatic resection, radiofrequency ablation, and combined resection/ablation for colorectal liver metastases. Ann Surg. 2004;239:818–25.
16. Agcaoglu O, Aliyev S, Karabulut K, El-Gazzaz G, Aucejo F, Pelley R, Siperstein AE, Berber E. Complementary use of resection and radiofrequency ablation for the treatment of colorectal liver metastases: an analysis of 395 patients. World J Surg. 2013;37:1333–9.
17. Solbiati L, Ahmed M, Cova L, Ierace T, Brioschi M, Goldberg SN. Small liver colorectal metastases treated with percutaneous radiofrequency ablation: local response rate and long-term survival with up to 10-year follow-up. Radiology. 2012;265:958–68.

18. Hammill CW, Billingsley KG, Cassera MA, Cassera MA, Wolf RF, Ujiki MB, Hansen PD. Outcome after laparoscopic radiofrequency ablation of technically resectable colorectal liver metastases. Ann Surg Oncol. 2011;18:1947–54.
19. Otto G, Duber C, Hoppe-Lotichius M, König J, Heise M, Pitton MB. Radiofrequency ablation as first-line treatment in patients with early colorectal liver metastases amenable to surgery. Ann Surg. 2010;251:796–803.
20. Elias D, Baton O, Sideris L, Matsuhisa T, Pocard M, Lasser P. Local recurrences after intraoperative radiofrequency ablation of liver metastases: a comparative study with anatomic and wedge resections. Ann Surg. 2004;11:500–5.
21. Evrard S, Becouarn Y, Fonck M, Brunet R, Mathoulin-Pelissier S, Picot V. Surgical treatment of liver metastases by radiofrequency ablation, resection, or in combination. Eur J Surg Oncol. 2004;30:399–406.
22. Lee H, Heo JS, Cho YB, Yun SH, Kim HC, Lee WY, Choi SH, Choi DW. Hepatectomy vs radiofrequency ablation for colorectal liver metastasis: a propensity score analysis. World J Gastroenterol. 2015;21:3300–7.
23. Weng M, Zhang Y, Zhou D, Yang Y, Tang Z, Zhao M, Quan Z, Gong W. Radiofrequency ablation versus resection for colorectal cancer liver metastases: a meta-analysis. PLoS One. 2012;7:e45493.
24. Bai H, Huangz X, Jing L, Zeng Q, Han L. The effect of RFA and hepatic resection on the long-term survival outcomes of colorectal cancer patients with liver metastases: a systematic review and meta-analysis. Cancer Manag Res. 2019;11:331–42.
25. Procopio F, Marano S, Gentile D, Da Roit A, Basato S, Riva P, et al. Management of liver oligometastatic esophageal cancer: overview and critical analysis of the different loco-regional treatments. Cancers. 2019;12(1):20.

# 33 Management of Esophageal Cancer with Head and Neck Cancer

Banu Atalay Erdogan

## 33.1 Pathophysiology

Esophageal squamous cell carcinoma (ESCC) commonly occurs alongside other cancers, including those of the head, neck, and stomach [1]. Heavy smoking and drinking are well-known risk factors for squamous cell carcinoma in the head and neck region. These same habits also increase the risk of developing squamous cell carcinoma in other areas of the upper respiratory-digestive tract, such as the esophagus [2–4]. Heavy smoking and drinking have a synergistic effect on the development of multiple cancers in the upper aerodigestive tract [5], leading to the frequent observation of multifocal squamous cell carcinoma in the head, neck, and esophagus. One explanation for this phenomenon is the concept of field cancerization, which suggests that genetically altered fields can lead to the development of multiple tumors in the same or different locations [6]. These cancers can occur either simultaneously (within 6 months of diagnosis) or sequentially [7, 8]. The most common locations for second primary malignancies in head and neck cancer patients are the esophagus, lung, and head and neck area [9]. Esophageal cancer is an aggressive malignancy, with higher incidence rates in Asia than in the United States [10]. The global incidence of synchronous esophageal cancer with head and neck squamous cell carcinoma (HNSCC) ranges from 2.7 to 12.5% [10–12]. In Thailand, the incidence of synchronized ESCC in HNSCC patients was 12.4% between 2009 and 2011 [13].

B. A. Erdogan (✉)
Department of Otorhinolaryngology Head and Neck Surgery, Istinye University, VM Medicalpark Pendik Hospital, Istanbul, Turkey
e-mail: banuatalay81@gmail.com


O. Engin (ed.), *Risk Factors and Therapy of Esophagus Cancer*,
https://doi.org/10.1007/978-3-031-47024-0_33

## 33.2 Diagnosis

Regular screening and vigilant monitoring of patients with esophageal or head and neck cancer are crucial for detecting both primary and secondary malignancies. Timely identification of a second cancer, whether synchronous or metachronous, is of utmost importance.

Early detection of a secondary cancer allows for less invasive treatment options, such as endoscopic resection and larynx preservation, which yield more favorable outcomes [14–16]. To detect second cancers in patients with head and neck cancer, triple endoscopy, which includes laryngoscopy, bronchoscopy, and esophagoscopy, is recommended for routine screening and close follow-up [17].

There is some controversy surrounding the use of routine triple endoscopic screening due to its high cost. For instance, a French study suggested that routine esophagoscopy may suffice for patients with hypopharyngeal cancer, while questioning the role of bronchoscopy and esophagoscopy in the presence of a normal thoracic computed tomography scan due to the low incidence of second cancers of the esophagus and lungs [18]. Similarly, a US study found no benefit from routine panendoscopy in never-smokers with oral cavity or oropharyngeal cancer [19]. Lugol-stained endoscopy is a potent tool not only for detecting small superficial carcinomas but also for evaluating the intraepithelial spread of esophageal squamous cell carcinoma [20, 21]. While Lugol's solution was initially used to diagnose cervical cancer through the Schiller test, it has also been applied for early detection of esophageal cancer [20]. In addition, endoscopy using Lugol's staining is an effective screening method for detecting esophageal cancer and secondary cancers of the esophagus associated with head and neck cancer, both synchronously and metachronously [22–27]. More recently, narrowband imaging combined with magnifying endoscopy has been touted as a promising tool for detecting secondary primary cancer [28–31]. Lugol's staining has some adverse side effects, including severe chest pain and discomfort [27] and a risk of aspiration, which is why narrow-band imaging is preferable. In conclusion, narrowband imaging combined with Lugol's stained endoscopy and magnifying endoscopy is a potent tool for early detection of esophageal cancer. Shiozaki et al. found nine esophageal cancers among 178 patients with head and neck cancer detected by endoscopic screening with the iodine dye method. For early detection of secondary cancer, it is advisable to conduct careful examinations at 6–12 month intervals [23, 32].

Patients with synchronous cancers of the thoracic esophagus and head and neck frequently necessitate highly complicated and invasive surgical procedures to remove both tumors. However, squamous cell carcinoma of the upper respiratory-digestive system is relatively responsive to anticancer drugs like 5-fluorouracil and cisplatin, as well as radiotherapy [33]. Esophagectomy and reconstruction in patients with a history of head and neck cancer are challenging due to prior neck surgery or irradiation.

Treatment options for patients with esophageal cancer associated with head and neck cancer include aggressive surgical resections using appropriate procedures like staged operations and microvascular surgery, with closure using muscle flaps [34]. However, these operations are highly invasive and carry significant morbidity and mortality risks.

Managing patients with double esophageal and head and neck cancers can be complicated, and various factors need to be considered while deciding on the treatment strategy. It is crucial to evaluate such patients multidisciplinary, particularly if surgical approaches are being considered [35, 36].

In determining the appropriateness of surgical treatment, it is essential to consider the curability of both cancers carefully. If both tumors can be treated, each should be addressed separately. In patients with metachronous dual cancers, previous treatment of the first primary carcinoma can impact the treatment of the second cancer. Therefore, a multidisciplinary approach for dual cancers and close collaboration among medical staff for complex surgeries are essential. Every case requires appropriate techniques, such as careful dissection, staged operations, muscle flaps, and microvascular anastomosis. When contemplating surgical resection for esophageal cancer associated with head and neck cancer, several factors must be considered, including the curability of both cancers, surgical invasiveness, and the patient's general condition [34]. Patients with synchronous cancers of the thoracic esophagus and head and neck often necessitate extremely complicated and invasive surgical procedures to remove both lesions.

If both tumors are treatable, each lesion should be planned for individually as if it were a single primary lesion. In patients with metachronous dual cancer, the previous treatment of the first primary carcinoma can interfere with the treatment of the second cancer, as previous surgery can result in the formation of adhesions in surrounding organs, complicating subsequent surgery. Planning treatment for patients with synchronous double cancers can present two challenges: total pharyngo-laryngo-esophagectomy may be considered for optimal treatment of both lesions, or treatment may be planned for each cancer separately. The surgical process involving resection and subsequent reconstruction of both cancers is highly invasive and complex in the former case. However, timing of treatments becomes a concern in the latter case. Therefore, a multidisciplinary approach is essential for synchronous double cancer surgery, with close collaboration between medical staff members, including the esophageal surgeon, head and neck surgeon, and plastic surgeon. Microvascular anastomosis and muscle flaps are often required [34–36]. Since both head and neck cancer and esophageal cancer respond relatively well to radiation and anticancer drugs like 5-fluorouracil and cisplatin [33], definitive chemoradiotherapy is often an option, but it can lead to residual lesions or recurrent tumors. Salvage surgery may be considered for such lesions. However, it is essential to keep in mind that the surgical risk remains high, particularly in cases of salvage esophagectomy and pharyngo-laryngectomy [35].

## 33.3 Total Pharyngo-Laryngo-Esophagectomy for Synchronous Double Cancer

Total pharyngo-laryngo-esophagectomy is a highly invasive procedure for synchronous double cancer of the head-neck and thoracic esophagus, and it often results in various issues such as loss of voice function and high surgical stress. To minimize the surgical stress in esophageal surgery, minimally invasive surgery can be used. Thoracoscopic approach with total pharyngo-laryngo-esophagectomy is an example of this approach, which allows mediastinal lymphadenectomy and esophageal mobilization [37, 38].

After total pharyngo-laryngo-esophagectomy, reconstruction of a long canal is required, but the blood flow to the distal end of the organ can be poor for both arterial blood supply and venous return. Various organs, such as gastric tube interposition, colonic interposition, and jejunal interposition, can be used for reconstruction. Techniques called "supercharge" and "superdrainage" in the neck have also been reported to be helpful for microvascular anastomosis to maintain blood flow [39] (Fig. 33.1). Another alternative method is the elongated stomach roll with microvascular anastomosis, in which the stomach is incised with a linear stapler, and the left gastric vessels are anastomosed to the cervical vessels.

A new surgical technique was introduced by Kawahara et al. [40] to restore both voice and swallowing functions after cervical esophagectomy combined with pharyngo-laryngectomy. In this technique, a free ileocolic flap was harvested and brought to the neck, and the cecum and ascending colon were used for reconstruction of the alimentary segment. To create a phonatory shunt, an end-to-end anastomosis was made between the terminal ileum and tracheal stump, directing airflow to the neo-pharynx. This procedure offers several advantages, including a strong air supply (trachea), a biological airway (terminal ileum), a vibrating mechanism, and a mechanism to prevent aspiration (ileocecal valve) [41, 42]. Chen et al. [43] made modifications to Kawahara's technique to facilitate voice rehabilitation after total pharyngo-laryngo-esophagectomy in patients with synchronous double cancer of the esophagus and head and neck. They utilized a pedicled ileocolic flap to perform the procedure.

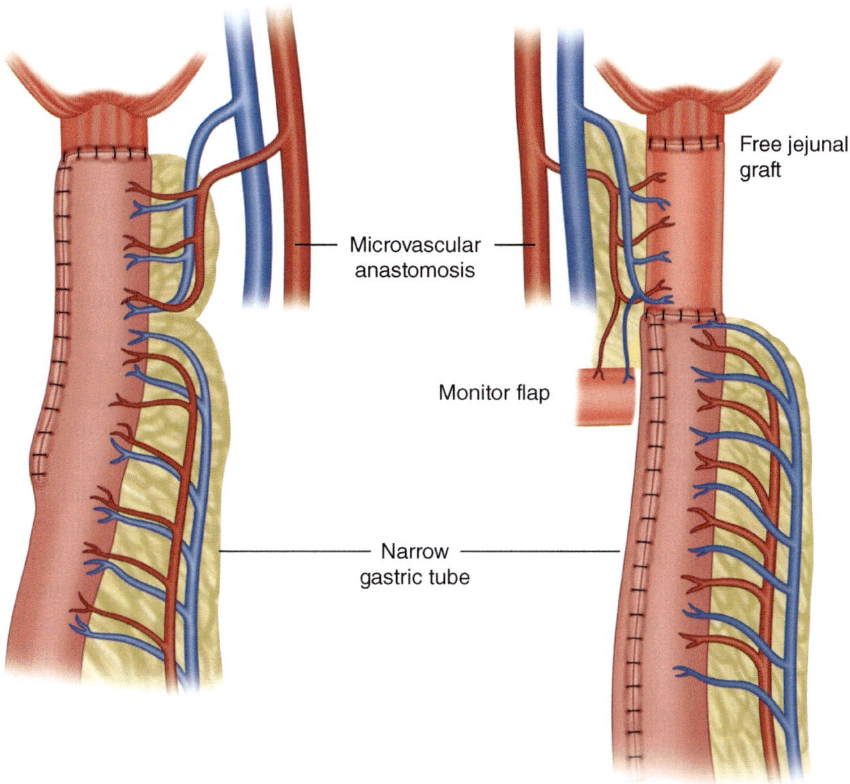


**Fig. 33.1** Reconstruction after total pharyngo-laryngo-esophagectomy. (**a**) Reconstruction with gastric tube. A reconstructed long canal is required. The distal end of the organ tends to have poor blood flow. A narrow gastric tube is pulled up through the posterior mediastinal route. It is attached to the neck by microvascular anastomosis. (**b**) Intervention of the free jejunal graft. When the length of the gastric tube is insufficient, a free jejunal graft can be placed between the pharynx and the gastric tube

## 33.4 Esophagectomy and Reconstruction for Metachronously Developed Cancer

For patients with a prior history of esophagectomy, the previous tumor and its treatment must be taken into account when planning treatment. Second hypopharyngeal or cervical esophageal cancers can be treated using free jejunal transfer and gastric pull-up, but anastomosis of the distal portion of the jejunal graft can be challenging due to tight adhesions and narrow spaces, especially with retrosternal gastric tube pull-up [37]. In cases where primary esophageal cancer develops after pharyngo-laryngectomy for head and neck cancer, reconstruction and dissection in the cervicothoracic region can pose challenges [1].

During surgery, special attention should be given to tracheal circulation, with care taken to protect the bronchial arteries and vascular networks around the tracheal stumps [2]. The dead space in the thoracocervical region should be filled, and the area between the tracheal stump and brachiocephalic artery should be separated with a muscle flap [44]. The use of an omental pedicle graft can provide reliable protection for the exposure of great vessels, although it may increase the procedure time slightly [45].

The cervicothoracic region is often characterized by tight adhesions, and the thoracic outlet is typically narrow. As such, it is important to enlarge this outlet under direct vision without injuring large vessels and tracheal blood supply. In cases where secondary cancer is located in the mid- or lower esophagus, distal esophagectomy may be a viable option to avoid adhesion around the cervicothoracic region [37]. Surgical intervention for double cancers of the head and neck and esophagus is a complex and invasive procedure that carries a high risk of complications. Some of the most common complications associated with the surgery include wound infections, tracheal tears, and necrosis, as well as stomal stenosis, empyema thoracis, cutaneous fistula, pulmonary edema, atelectasis, gastric necrosis and leakage, and gastric outlet obstruction. It is important to carefully monitor patients for these potential complications in the postoperative period, as they can significantly impact patient outcomes. Additionally, following total pharyngo-laryngo-esophagectomy, a long-reconstructed conduit is necessary, but the blood flow to the distal end of the organ is often poor due to limited arterial blood supply and venous return [46]. To minimize the risk of complications and optimize patient outcomes, it is essential to closely monitor patients during the postoperative period and take appropriate measures to address any potential issues that arise.

## References


1. Abemayor E, Moore DM, Hanson DG. Identification of synchronous esophageal tumors in patients with head and neck cancer. J Surg Oncol. 1988;38:94–6.
2. Morita M, Kuwano H, Ohno S, et al. Multiple occurrence of carcinoma in the upper aerodigestive tract associated with esophageal cancer: reference to smoking, drinking and family history. Int J Cancer. 1994;58:207–10.
3. Morita M, Kuwano H, Nakashima T, et al. Family aggregation of carcinoma of the hypopharynx and cervical esophagus: special reference to multiplicity of cancer in upper aerodigestive tract. Int J Cancer. 1998;76:468–71.
4. Morita M, Saeki H, Mori M, Kuwano H, Sugimachi K. Risk factors for esophageal cancer and the multiple occurrence of carcinoma in the upper aerodigestive tract. Surgery. 2002;131:S1–6.
5. Yoshinaga K, Saeki H, Emi Y, Kakeji Y, Sakaguchi Y, Toh Y, Maehara Y. Alcohol drinking, cigarette smoking, and the development of squamous cell carcinoma of the esophagus: epidemiology, clinical findings, and prevention. Int J Clin Oncol. 2010;15:126–34.
6. Slaughter DP, Southwick HW, Smejkal W. "Field cancerization" in oral stratified squamous epithelium. Cancer. 1953;6:963–8.
7. Morita M, Saeki H, Ito S, Kimura Y, Yamashita N, Ando K, Hiyoshi Y, Tokunaga E, Oki E, Ikeda T, Yoshida S, Nakashima T, Maehara Y. Surgical strategies for esophageal cancer associated with head and neck cancer. Surg Today. 2014;44:1603–10.

8. Braakhuis BJ, Tabor MP, Leemans CR, van der Waal I, Snow GB, Brakenhoff RH. Second primary tumors and field cancerization in oral and oropharyngeal cancer: molecular techniques provide new insights and definitions. Head Neck. 2002;24(2):198–206.
9. Vaamonde P, Martin C, Labella T. Second primary malignancies in patients with cancer of the head and neck. Otolaryngol Head Neck Surg. 2003;129(1):65–70.
10. Scherübl H, Von Lampe B, Faiss S, Däubler P, Bohlmann P, Plath T, et al. Screening for oesophageal neoplasia in patients with head and neck cancer. Br J Cancer. 2002;86(2):239–43.
11. Fukuzawa K, Noguchi Y, Yoshikawa T, Saito A, Doi C, Makino T, et al. High incidence of synchronous cancer of the oral cavity and the upper gastrointestinal tract. Cancer Lett. 1999;144(2):145–51.
12. Kim DH, Gong EJ, Jung H-Y, Lim H, Ahn JY, Choi K-S, et al. Clinical significance of intensive endoscopic screening for synchronous esophageal neoplasm in patients with head and neck squamous cell carcinoma. Scand J Gastroenterol. 2014;49(12):1486–92.
13. Laohawiriyakamol S, Sunpaweravong S, Leelamanit V, Pruegsanusak K, Sinkijcharoenchai W. Evaluating synchronous esophageal cancer in head and neck cancer patients using Lugol dye chromoendoscopy. J Med Assoc Thail. 2014;97(11):1164–70.
14. Matsubara T, Yamada K, Nakagawa A. Risk of second primary malignancy after esophagectomy for squamous cell carcinoma of the thoracic esophagus. J Clin Oncol. 2003;21:4336–41.
15. Natsugoe S, Uchino Y, Kijima F, Shimada M, Shirao K, Kusano C, et al. Synchronous and metachronous carcinomas of the esophagus and head and neck. Dis Esophagus. 1997;10:134–8.
16. Kohmura T, Hasegawa Y, Matsuura H, Terada A, Takahashi M, Nakashima T. Clinical analysis of multiple primary malignancies of the hypopharynx and esophagus. Am J Otolaryngol. 2001;22:107–10.
17. Weaver A, Fleming SM, Knechtges TC, Smith D. Triple endoscopy: a neglected essential in head and neck cancer. Surgery. 1979;86:493–6.
18. Guardiola E, Pivot X, Dassonville O, Poissonnet G, Marcy PY, Otto J, et al. Is routine triple endoscopy for head and neck carcinoma patients necessary in light of a negative chest computed tomography scan? Cancer. 2004;101:2028–33.
19. Rodriguez-Bruno K, Ali MJ, Wang SJ. Role of panendoscopy to identify synchronous second primary malignancies in patients with oral cavity and oropharyngeal squamous cell carcinoma. Head Neck. 2011;33:949–53.
20. Sugimachi K, Ohno S, Matsuda H, Mori M, Kuwano H. Lugol-combined endoscopic detection of minute malignant lesions of the thoracic esophagus. Ann Surg. 1988;208:179–83.
21. Sugimachi K, Tsutsui S, Kitamura K, Morita M, Mori M, Kuwano H. Lugol stain for intraoperative determination of the proximal surgical margin of the esophagus. J Surg Oncol. 1991;46:226–9.
22. Hashimoto CL, Iriya K, Baba ER, Navarro-Rodriguez T, Zerbini MC, Eisig JN, et al. Lugol's dye spray chromoendoscopy establishes early diagnosis of esophageal cancer in patients with primary head and neck cancer. Am J Gastroenterol. 2005;100:275–82.
23. Shiozaki H, Tahara H, Kobayashi K, Yano H, Tamura S, Imamoto H, et al. Endoscopic screening of early esophageal cancer with the Lugol dye method in patients with head and neck cancers. Cancer. 1990;66:2068–71.
24. Shimizu Y, Tukagoshi H, Fujita M, Hosokawa M, Kato M, Asaka M. Metachronous squamous cell carcinoma of the esophagus arising after endoscopic mucosal resection. Gastrointest Endosc. 2001;54:190–4.
25. Hori K, Okada H, Kawahara Y, Takenaka R, Shimizu S, Ohno Y, et al. Lugol-voiding lesions are an important risk factor for a second primary squamous cell carcinoma in patients with esosphageal cancer or head and neck cancer. Am J Gastroenterol. 2011;106:858–66.
26. Katada C, Muto M, Nakayama M, Tanabe S, Higuchi K, Sasaki T, et al. Risk of superficial squamous cell carcinoma developing in the head and neck region in patients with esophageal squamous cell carcinoma. Laryngoscope. 2012;122:1291–6.
27. Muto M, Hironaka S, Nakane M, Boku N, Ohtsu A, Yoshida S. Association of multiple Lugol-voiding lesions with synchronous and metachronous esophageal squamous cell carcinoma in patients with head and neck cancer. Gastrointest Endosc. 2002;56:517–21.

28. Takenaka R, Kawahara Y, Okada H, Hori K, Inoue M, Kawano S, et al. Narrow-band imaging provides reliable screening for esophageal malignancy in patients with head and neck cancers. Am J Gastroenterol. 2009;104:2942–8.
29. Nonaka S, Saito Y, Oda I, Kozu T, Saito D. Narrow-band imaging endoscopy with magnification is useful for detecting metachronous superficial pharyngeal cancer in patients with esophageal squamous cell carcinoma. J Gastroenterol Hepatol. 2010;25:264–9.
30. Muto M, Minashi K, Yano T, Saito Y, Oda I, Nonaka S, et al. Early detection of superficial squamous cell carcinoma in the head and neck region and esophagus by narrow band imaging: a multicenter randomized controlled trial. J Clin Oncol. 2010;28:1566–72.
31. Katada C, Tanabe S, Koizumi W, Higuchi K, Sasaki T, Azuma M, et al. Narrow band imaging for detecting superficial squamous cell carcinoma of the head and neck in patients with esophageal squamous cell carcinoma. Endoscopy. 2010;42:185–90.
32. Yoshino K, Endo M, Ishikawa N, Takahashi Y. Diagnosis and treatment of metachronous cancers in the esophagus and head and neck region. J Surg Oncol. 1995;58:246–51.
33. Cooper JS, Guo MD, Herskovic A, et al. Chemoradiotherapy of locally advanced esophageal cancer: long-term follow-up of a prospective randomized trial (RTOG 85-01). Radiation Therapy Oncology Group. JAMA. 1999;281:1623–7.
34. Morita M, Kawano H, Otsu H, Kimura Y, Saeki H, Ando K, et al. Surgical resection for esophageal cancer synchronously or metachronously associated with head and neck cancer. Ann Surg Oncol. 2013;20:2434–9.
35. Tachimori Y, Watanabe H, Kato H, Ebihara S, Ono I, Nakatsuka T, et al. Treatment for synchronous and metachronous carcinomas of the head and neck and esophagus. J Surg Oncol. 1990;45:43–5.
36. Wind P, Roullet MH, Quinaux D, Laccoureye O, Brasnu D, Cugnenc PH. Long-term results after esophagectomy for squamous cell carcinoma of the esophagus associated with head and neck cancer. Am J Surg. 1999;178:251–5.
37. Watanabe M, Baba Y, Nagai Y, Baba H. Minimally invasive esophagectomy for esophageal cancer: an updated review. Surg Today. 2013;43:237–44.
38. Cense HA, Law S, Wei W, Lam LK, Ng WM, Wong KH, et al. Pharyngo laryngo esophagectomy using the thoracoscopic approach. Surg Endosc. 2007;21:879–84.
39. Sekido M, Yamamoto Y, Minakawa H, Sasaki S, Furukawa H, Sugihara T, et al. Use of the "supercharge" technique in esophageal and pharyngeal reconstruction to augment microvascular blood flow. Surgery. 2003;134:420–4.
40. Kawahara H, Shiraishi T, Yasugawa H, Okamura K, Shirakusa T. A new surgical technique for voice restoration after laryngo pharyngo esophagectomy with a free ileocolic graft: preliminary report. Surgery. 1992;111:569–75.
41. Motoyama S, Saito R, Maruyama K, Okuyama M, Sasaki K, Wako M, et al. Sound spectrogram analysis in patients receiving Kawahara's surgical voice restoration for advanced carcinoma of the hypopharynx and cervical esophagus. Dis Esophagus. 2007;20:42–6.
42. Rampazzo A, Salgado CJ, Gharb BB, Mardini S, Spanio di Spilimbergo S, Chen HC. Donor-site morbidity after free ileocolon flap transfer for esophageal and voice reconstruction. Plast Reconstr Surg. 2008;122:186e–94e.
43. Chen HC, Gharb BB, Rampazzo A, Perrone F, Chen SH, Trignano E. Simultaneous restoration of voice function and digestive tract continuity in patients with synchronous primaries of hypopharynx and thoracic esophagus with pedicled ileocolon flap. Surgery. 2011;149:662–71.
44. Hosoya Y, Sarukawa S, Matsumoto S, Zuiki T, Hyodo M, Abe K, et al. Esophagectomy and gastric pull-up in patients with previous free jejunal transfer. Ann Thorac Surg. 2009;87:647–9.
45. Martins AS, Lage HT, Lopes LR, Brandalise NA. Use of omentum pedicled graft to protect great vessels in gastric transposition for pharyngoesophageal cancer. J Surg Oncol. 1999;70:181–4.
46. Puttawibul P, Pornpatanarak C, Sangthong B, Boonpipattanapong T, Peeravud S, Pruegsanusak K, Leelamanit V, Sinkijcharoenchai W. Results of gastric pull-up reconstruction for pharyngolaryngo-oesophagectomy in advanced head and neck cancer and cervical oesophageal squamous cell carcinoma. Asian J Surg. 2004;27(3):180–5. https://doi.org/10.1016/S1015-9584(09)60029-4.

# Esophageal Cancer and Infections 34

Sukran Kose and Muge Ozguler

## 34.1 Introduction

In the current literature, 572.034 new diagnoses and 508.585 related deaths are seen due to esophageal cancer (EC) worldwide [1]. Esophageal cancer is the sixth leading cause of cancer-related mortality globally because of its high malignant potential and poor prognosis [2]. The most observed histological types of esophageal cancer are esophageal adenocarcinoma (EAC) and esophageal squamous cell carcinoma (ESCC) [3]. In high-income countries, the majority of esophageal cancer patients have esophageal adenocarcinoma [4].

The relationship between infections and development of esophageal cancer is evaluated in many studies. The results show that bacterial derangement plays an important role in the emergence of cancers such as esophageal cancers [5]. In particular, while changes in the microbiome have been well described in esophageal adenocarcinoma, it is not yet clear for esophageal squamous cell carcinoma [6]. In this study, we aimed to determine the role of infections at development of esophageal cancer and post-diagnostic infections associated with esophageal cancer.

S. Kose (✉)
Department of Clinical Microbiology and Infectious Diseases, Faculty of Medicine, Dokuz Eylul University, İzmir, Turkey

M. Ozguler
Department of Clinical Microbiology and Infectious Diseases, University of Health Sciences, Hamidiye Medical Faculty, Elazig Fethi Sekin Health Training and Research Hospital, Elazig, Turkey



O. Engin (ed.), *Risk Factors and Therapy of Esophagus Cancer*,
https://doi.org/10.1007/978-3-031-47024-0_34

## 34.2 Pathogenesis

### 34.2.1 Microbiome

The definition of microbiome means to the community of microorganisms that live in the human body as commensal, symbiotic, and pathogenic [7]. Mouth, skin, vagina, and gastrointestinal tract are regions with microbiota. The esophagus was thought to be sterile based on conventional culture methods and contains only oral ingested bacteria [8].

With PCR-based metagenomic analysis; bacterial DNA extraction, sequencing, and analysis of 16S rRNA genes can be used to analyze the microbiota and identify microorganisms existing in the microbiome. In metagenomic analysis of normal esophageal biopsies, Firmicutes (phylum containing bacteria with gram-positive cell wall) has been detected in 69% and Bacteroidetes (phylum containing gram-negative anaerobic rods without spores) have been detected in 20.2%. *Streptococcus* was most common in Firmicutes and Prevotella was most common in Bacteroidetes [9].

As an oral bacterium, *S. anginosus* has often been found in the oral cavity, gastrointestinal tract, and genitourinary tract [10]. Alive *S. anginosus* can be isolated from esophageal cancer tissues [11]. Specifically, a higher presence of *S. anginosus* has been identified in esophageal squamous cell carcinoma (E-SCC) tissues. Presence of *S. anginosus* in tissues in head and neck squamous cell carcinomas, esophageal dysplasia, esophageal, and gastric cancer suggests that *S. anginosus* is involved in the carcinogenic process [12]. Streptolysin S was supposed to be responsible for the cytotoxicity of *S. anginosus* [13].

The microbial dysbiosis of esophageal squamous cell carcinoma tissues was characterized by decreased *Faecalibacterium*, *Bacteroides*, *Curvibacter*, and *Blautia* and increased Fusobacteria [14]. Yang et al. [15] have demonstrated significantly enriched Bacteroides in E-SCC. Bacteroides had a bidirectional role in the esophageal squamous cell carcinoma oncogenesis. An increase in *Fusobacterium* is another common anaerobic Gram-negative bacteria of the oral cavity, it has been also observed in esophageal squamous cell carcinoma tissues [6]. However, Li et al. [6] have found no significant difference between esophageal squamous cell carcinoma and healthy controls in terms of *Fusobacterium*. An increase in *Fusobacterium nucleatum* in esophageal cancer is considered as a poor prognostic marker. It has been shown that *F. nucleatum* can promote carcinogenesis by stimulating chemokines [16].

### 34.2.2 Physiopathogenesis

It has been suggested that the microbiome contributes to gastroesophageal reflux and esophageal adenocarcinoma by inducing chronic inflammation and gastroesophageal reflux [17]. It is stated that antibiotics/probiotics can play an important role in this process [18].

It has been emphasized that another factor is mucin production. In the case of malignancy, different mucin expressions are observed in terms of both type and amount [19]. Mucins act as a mucosal barrier. Mucins coat surfaces exposed to the external environment. The mucus layer allows the passage of nutrients and immune factors while blocking toxins and pathogens [20]. Mucins are produced by epithelial cells. They are big molecular glycoproteins. Two subtypes of mucins can be mentioned. These are the cell surface mucins, which are attached to the cell membrane and the secreted mucins, which impart viscous properties to the mucus gel [21]. Mucins may also play a direct role in tumor progression. Membrane-bound mucins can interact with epidermal growth factor receptor families [19]. Mucins are thought to have potential roles in the development of epithelial malignancies through their role in bacterial control and regulation of inflammation. However, they also have the potential to be involved in signal transduction in epithelial cells in cases of dysplasia and malignancy. Cell growth, proliferation, and differentiation are thought to be affected by mucins [22]. Normal squamous mucosa in the esophagus does not excrete mucin. In the case of dysplasia, mucin expression may vary [23].

Bacteria are general stimulators for both the production of inflammatory cytokines and mucin production. For example, butyrate produced by anaerobic bacteria has been shown to stimulate MUC2 production [24]. Both Gram-positive and Gram-negative bacteria can upregulate mucin production [25]. Mediators and cytokines for the inflammatory response, particularly IL-1, TNF-alpha, IL-4, and IL-6, can also be bound by mucins. In addition, mucin production is also affected by these cytokines [19]. It has been shown that there is a gradual increase in the expression of NF-B, IL-8, and IL-1 from normal to Barrett's epithelium toward adenocarcinoma [18].

### 34.2.3 Infections That Can Progress to Esophageal Cancer

#### 34.2.3.1 Esophagitis

While esophagitis is generally a benign disease, it is a risk factor for esophageal squamous cell carcinoma [26]. Infectious esophagitis is the third leading cause of esophagitis behind gastroesophageal reflux disease and eosinophilic esophagitis and It can be caused by bacterial, viral, fungal, and parasitic infections [27].

Infectious esophagitis most commonly occurs in immunosuppressed patients (HIV/AIDS, diabetes, and immunosuppressive drug users). However, it can sometimes affect immunocompetent individuals [28]. The most common cause of infectious esophagitis is *Candida.* The other etiological agents are herpes simplex virus (HSV) and cytomegalovirus (CMV). Less commonly observed agents are human immunodeficiency virus (HIV), tuberculosis, varicella zoster virus (VZV), human papillomavirus (HPV), and various bacterial and parasitic organisms [29].

#### 34.2.3.2 Esophageal Candidiasis

Esophageal candidiasis is the most common cause of infectious esophagitis, and *Candida albicans* is the most common organism among all candida species [29]. AIDS is the most frequently associated risk factor for esophageal candidiasis. AIDS patients with esophageal candidiasis were found to have lower CD4 counts compared to AIDS patients with fewer oropharyngeal lesions [30]. A recent large cohort study evaluated the prevalence of esophageal candidiasis in 80.219 patients between 2002 and 2014. The prevalence of esophageal candidiasis was found in total, HIV patients, and non-HIV patients 1.7%, 9.8%, and 1.6%, respectively [31]. A general decrease in the prevalence of esophageal candidiasis has been found in AIDS patients with highly active antiretroviral therapy (HAART) [32].

Common risk factors for the development of esophageal candidiasis in the non-HIV patient population; antibiotics, proton pump inhibitors (PPIs), H2 blockers, alcohol, malignancy, topical and systemic corticosteroids, and motility disorders [29]. Drugs alter the microenvironment of the esophageal mucosa and may predispose to candida colonization and infection. The most important drugs are antibiotics and corticosteroids [33, 34]. Hypochlorhydria after PPI and H2 blockers may cause *Candida* colonization and infection [35].

Esophageal candidiasis is diagnosed by detecting characteristic findings after endoscopic and histopathological examination. Endoscopically, the esophageal mucosa displays thick, white plaques. The diagnosis is made by the appearance of thick white plaques in the esophageal mucosa endoscopically and the budding yeast and pseudohyphae or hyphae invading the epithelium in the obtained histopathological material [29].

Treatment is not required in all patients with esophageal candidiasis [36]. There are studies showing that systemic antifungal therapy may not be necessary in asymptomatic, immune-competent esophageal candidiasis patients. One study evaluated the clinical course of patients with asymptomatic esophageal candidiasis Improvement was observed in repeated endoscopy in 81.0% of cases, and recurrent esophageal candidiasis was detected in repeated endoscopy in the remainder. Only 6.3% of cases in which esophageal candidiasis persisted developed esophageal symptoms or no worsening disease was detected endoscopically in the others, suggesting that asymptomatic esophageal candidiasis may be a self-limiting disease in the majority of cases [37].

It is recommended that esophageal candidiasis occurring in immunocompromised patients be treated with systemic antifungal drugs. Fluconazole is one of the essential drug in the first line of treatment. Empirical fluconazole is the most cost-effective treatment option for HIV patients with esophageal symptoms [38]. Identification of *Candida* species may be clinically important in terms of the possibility of azole resistance [39]. Prolonged use of antifungal therapy increases the rate of drug-resistant *C. albicans* species in the gastrointestinal tract [29]. In fluconazole-resistant esophageal candidiasis, other azoles such as echinocandins, amphotericin, and posaconazole can be considered as treatment options [40].

As a matter of fact, in a case–control study evaluating patients aged 65 years and over with esophageal candidiasis, the 6-month mortality rate of patients with esophageal candidiasis was found to be significantly higher than the control group [41].

#### 34.2.3.3 Herpes Simplex Virus Esophagitis

A large proportion of the adult population is HSV seropositive and latent. HSV-1 causes herpes simplex esophagitis (HSE) at a higher rate than HSV-2 in adults. Infection can occur with primary infection or reactivation of the latent virus [42]. Hematologic malignancy, solid tumors, extensive burns, autoimmune disease, and HIV infection are most known risk factors for herpes simplex esophagitis [29].

Endoscopy and histopathology are beneficial for the diagnosis of HSV esophagitis. Multiple small, perforated ulcers, and fibrin exudates are the characteristic endoscopic findings of HSV esophagitis. Multinucleated giant cells and nuclear chromatin with ground glass appearance or Cowdry A inclusion bodies may be seen in histological investigation [43].

Acyclovir, famciclovir, or valacyclovir are the treatment options available for HSE in the immunocompromised host. In immunocompetent patients, there is less evidence for antiviral therapy. Herpes simplex esophagitis is a self-limiting clinical picture, usually within 1–2 weeks in an immunocompetent host. However, even if the immune system is competent, acyclovir treatment is required in some cases [42].

#### 34.2.3.4 Cytomegalovirus Esophagitis

Immunosuppressed individuals such as AIDS, organ transplants, long-term dialysis patients, and those using chemotherapy, corticosteroids, or immunosuppressive drugs are in the risk group for CMV esophagitis. But, CMV esophagitis has been reported in patients without immunodeficiency [44].

Clinical history, endoscopic findings, and histologic findings are important for the diagnosis of CMV esophagitis. Odynophagia, fever, nausea, emesis, dysphagia, epigastric pain, substernal chest pain, and gastrointestinal bleeding are the complaints in CMV esophagitis [44]. The endoscopic findings of CMV esophagitis may vary. It usually presents with plural ulcers that may extend from the mid to the distal esophagus. Cytomegalovirus esophageal ulcers are typically either superficial or of intermediate profundity, some of the patients have deep ulcers. The ulcers tend to be linear and separate with normal mucosa. Diffusely erosive and mimicking of reflux esophagitis and HSV may be seen rarely in CMV esophagitis [29]. Necrosis and strictures may appear in the course of CMV esophagitis [45].

CMV and HSV co-infection may be observed in some individuals [46]. In CMV esophagitis, inflammation findings, nuclear and cytoplasmic inclusion bodies are detected in the histopathological examination. Sight of a basophilic intranuclear inclusion enclosed by an explicit halo "owl's eyes" and intracytoplasmic inclusion bodies is distinctive for cytomegalic cells [29].

Before antiviral therapy, CMV infection was considered mortal in patients diagnosed with AIDS. However, significant improvements in prognosis have been observed with highly active antiretroviral therapy [47]. Currently, CMV infection is observed in patients with AIDS who do not use highly active antiretroviral therapy, are not compatible with antiretroviral therapy, have intolerance or resistance to antiretroviral therapy, and do not receive CMV prophylaxis when clinically indicated. These patients have a poor prognosis for CMV [29].

Patients at high risk for CMV esophagitis should be treated in the presence of severe clinical symptoms, even if pathological results have not been reported. Agents with similar efficacy, such as ganciclovir or foscarnet, are used for 3–6 weeks of induction therapy. Ganciclovir is preferred to foscarnet due to cost and renal side effects of foscarnet. When ganciclovir is contraindicated (moderate-to-severe thrombocytopenia or ganciclovir resistance), foscarnet can be used for treatment. Oral valganciclovir may be taken into account in patients with moderate symptoms and no problem in oral intake [29].

#### 34.2.3.5 Human Papilloma Virus Esophagitis

Human papillomavirus infection is commonly responsible for genital verrucas and cervical cancer. Mucosal damage due to acid effects in the esophagus allows the virus to reach the basal layer in the mucosal transformation zone. HPV can reach basal cells, especially in the squamocolumnar transformation zone [48].

Esophageal manifestations of HPV infection are ulcers, hyperkeratosis, and papillomas. Diffuse esophageal papillomatosis may be observed asymptomatically or symptomatically [49]. Presence of koilocytosis, perinuclear sheen, and giant and multinucleated cells are known microscopic characteristics of HPV lesions [29].

The development of esophageal squamous papillomas has been emphasized to be associated with HPV. The presence of HPV infection in esophageal squamous papillomas varies among studies. In a study, HPV was detected in 87.5% of 19 cases of esophageal squamous papillomas [50]. But, in another study from France, HPV has not been observed in any of the cases of esophageal squamous papillomas [51].

Although the prevalence of HPV in esophageal squamous papillomas varies in the literature, there are studies and meta-analysis suggesting that HPV infections especially types 16 and 18 have an effect on the pathogenesis of squamous cell carcinoma [50–52].

The togetherness of HPV and esophageal carcinoma is a topic that has been studied for a long time. It has been suggested that there is a high prevalence of HPV in esophageal squamous cell carcinoma and its role in esophageal carcinogenesis. In a large meta-analysis including 5755 cases previously reported, it was emphasized that there is a significant relationship between HPV16 and esophageal squamous cell carcinoma, but its role in esophageal carcinogenesis is not clear, and the same relationship is not found with HPV 18 [52]. Similarly, an association between esophageal squamous cell carcinoma and HPV has been expressed in another meta-analysis. In this meta-analysis, studies that screened HPV DNA in tissue in esophageal squamous cell carcinoma have been evaluated and the risk of ESCC has been found three-times increased [53].

In a meta-analysis of 66 cases, a significant relationship has been found between HPV infection and squamous cell carcinoma [54]. An analysis evaluating a total of 16.484 patients recently examined the chance, frequency, and prognosis of HPV-16 and 18-related esophageal squamous cell carcinoma in adults. DNA-based, generally polymerase chain reaction methods have been applied for HPV search, and a remarkably increased risk of esophageal squamous cell carcinoma associated with HPV infection has been found in this analysis. However, when individuals diagnosed with esophageal squamous cell carcinoma were evaluated collectively, the prevalence of HPV 16/18 was found to be only 18.2% [55].

The effect of HPV in esophageal adenocarcinoma is not clear [56]. There are some studies in which active HPV infection is associated with Barrett's dysplasia and squamous cell carcinoma. The prevalence of viral infection in esophageal adenocarcinoma has been detected as low as 13–35% compared to other virus-induced cancers [57].

In a study, transcriptionally active high-risk HPV has been found strongly associated with esophageal adenocarcinoma, and a potential role in esophageal carcinogenesis has been emphasized. In this study, increased high-risk HPV viral load has been found significantly associated with Barrett's esophagus—Barrett's dysplasia—esophageal adenocarcinoma disease severity. The high risk HPV has been detected more commonly at the transformation zone [48].

#### 34.2.3.6 *Helicobacter Pylori* Infection

*Helicobacter pylori* is an important spiral formed microorganism in the etiology of cancer. It is considered to be responsible for thereabout 5% of the total cancers worldwide. In the course of *H. pylori* infection, patients with atrophic corpus gastritis face the minimal risk of gastroesophageal reflux disease. In contrast, patients with antrum-dominant gastritis and those with normal or high acidity face the top of the risk for gastroesophageal reflux disease [58].

It has been suggested that the opposite relationship between *H. pylori* and EAC is decreasing in gastric acidity secondary to atrophic gastritis [59]. It is thought that the presence of *Helicobacter* may have a protective effect on esophageal and gastric cardia adenocarcinomas [60]. However, there is still no clear evidence whether *H. pylori* has a positive or negative effect on cardia carcinoma. More inflammation and the ability to produce ulcers, atrophy, and carcinoma have been observed in some subtypes of *Helicobacter* infections [22].

Significant relationship has been emphasized between gastric cardia adenocarcinoma and *Helicobacter pylori* [61]. There are two types of gastroesophageal adenocarcinomas. One of them is linked to atrophic gastritis. It is more common in countries where the prevalence of *H. pylori* is high [22]. Gastric cardia adenocarcinoma has been relatively associated with gastric atrophy caused by *H. pylori* and not early *H. pylori* infection [62]. The other type is related to Barrett's esophageal cancer. It has been suggested that these differences between studies may be explained by the relative prevalence of *H. pylori* between regions [63].

Observation of *Helicobacter pylori* colonizing the area of gastric metaplasia in the esophagus suggested that it may play a potential role in the pathogenesis of esophageal AC. However, several studies demonstrated that *H. pylori* is not more common and does not have a different distribution in patients with Barrett's esophagus than in controls [64]. In contrast, *H. pylori* may be a significant factor for cardia inflammation and intestinal metaplasia. However, distinguishing cardia adenocarcinoma from cancers originating from the distal esophagus can be difficult as the disease progresses [65]. The absence of *H. pylori* is thought to be a risk factor for the development of esophageal adenocarcinoma [66]. A meta-analysis has noted a significant opposite link between esophageal adenocarcinoma and the prevalence of *H. pylori* infection. However, it has not been detected for squamous cell carcinoma. Similarly, a substantial inverse relationship has been also observed for patients with Barrett's esophagus [67].

#### 34.2.3.7 Other Infectious Esophagitis

**Other Fungal Esophagitis:** Candida species are the prevalent reason for fungal esophagitis. However, other fungi besides *Candida*, such as *Aspergillus* and *Histoplasma* species, can also cause infectious esophagitis. *Aspergillus* is frequently seen in immunocompromised patients with previous lung pathology [29]. The cytological scrub or biopsy is valuable in the diagnosis of *Aspergillus*-related esophagitis [68]. Voriconazole and amphotericin B in some cases are recommended for treatment [69].

Primary esophageal infection by *Histoplasma capsulatum* is rare. Esophageal ulceration may emerge in the course of the disseminated disease and may result in esophageal stricting due to mediastinal lymph node involvement and enlarged lymph node compression [70]. Itraconazole is recommended for mild to moderate esophageal infection with *Histoplasma capsulatum* and amphotericin B is recommended for severe disease [71].

**Bacterial Esophagitis:** Bacterial esophagitis may progress with gram-positive, gram-negative, and anaerobic organisms that create the normal oropharyngeal flora. The most common bacterial agent in the esophagus is *Streptococci* [72]. In patients with long-standing reflux, inflammation can cause an increase in gram-negative anaerobes and thus changes in the normal microbiome [73].

Although bacterial esophagitis mostly occurs in immunocompromised hosts such as malignancy and neutropenia, there are case reports indicating that it is rarely observed in individuals with normal immunity. Broad-spectrum antibiotics should be started after the diagnosis in patients with bacterial esophagitis, and de-escalation should be performed with appropriate antibiotherapy according to the culture results [29].

**Esophageal Tuberculosis:** Esophageal tuberculosis can be considered in patients with dysphagia and immunodeficiency, especially in developing countries [74]. Esophageal tuberculosis may present with tracheoesophageal fistula, local invasion, or ulceration. Standard antituberculous therapy is recommended in patients with esophageal tuberculosis [75]. *Mycobacterium avium* complex has rarely been defined as the causative agent of esophagitis [76].

**Other Viral Esophagitis:** HIV, VZV, and Epstein-Barr virus (EBV) are the other agents of viral esophagitis other than HPV [77]. *Primary HIV ulceration* is usually seen in untreated and newly diagnosed patients with HIV, but it is less common in patients treated with highly active antiretroviral therapy. In the acute HIV seroconversion syndrome or AIDS stage, HIV-associated esophagitis may develop. In an HIV-diagnosed patient with esophageal symptoms, HIV-associated idiopathic esophageal ulcers are considered when there is no response to antifungals or antivirals or a histopathological diagnosis cannot be established [29].

**Varicella Zoster Virus Esophagitis** is rare and should be considered in the diagnosis of patients with VZV dermatological findings [29]. Patients may present with esophagitis clinic due to dysphagia or esophagobronchial fistula secondary to multiple cranial nerve damage [78]. Observation of vesicles and ulcers with endoscopy and observation of multinucleated giant cells histopathologically are helpful in diagnosis. Acyclovir, valacyclovir, or famciclovir should be started within 72 h in patients with or at risk of complications from herpes zoster [79].

**Epstein-Barr Virus,** which is the causative agent of infectious mononucleosis, can also cause esophagitis. Most studies have shown that EBV-associated esophageal carcinoma demonstrates similar morphologic findings. Histopathological findings similar to nasopharyngeal lymphoepithelial carcinoma are observed [80].

There are limited studies in the literature on the relationship between EBV and esophageal cancer. These studies contain quite different results from each other. While there are studies showing that there is no relationship between EBV infection and esophageal carcinoma, there are studies showing that EBV association in esophageal carcinoma is 1.8–35.5% [81, 82]. In most cases, East Asia has been shown to have a higher rate of EBV-related esophageal carcinoma than in Western countries [80, 82]. Symptomatic EBV esophageal disease may require treatment with acyclovir [29].

### 34.2.4 Infections at Esophageal Cancer; Post Diagnostic-Post Surgical Infections

Esophagectomy is still an important treatment approach in esophageal cancers [83]. The most important infectious complications that can be observed after esophagectomy are pulmonary complications [84]. Apart from this, other hospital-acquired infections (HAI) can also be seen during the care of the patient, especially in the intensive care unit. Most observed HAI infections are central line-associated bloodstream infections, hospital-acquired pneumonia, ventilator-associated pneumonia, surgical site infections (SSI), and catheter-associated urinary tract infections [85].

In a study, the infection rates have been detected as pneumonia (21.8%), surgical site infections (21.8%), gastrointestinal infections (17.1%), urinary tract infections (12.9%), and primary bloodstream infections (9.9%), respectively [86].

In the diagnosis of infections that observed after esophageal surgery; elevated, elevated bands, thrombocytopenia, C-reactive protein (CRP), procalcitonin, hypoglycemia, hyperglycemia, lactic acidosis, higher liver transaminases and prothrombin time elevation in blood urea nitrogen (BUN), and serum creatinine should be evaluated in order to define the focus of infection and evaluate the infectious approach. In addition, blood gas analysis should be performed to evaluate tissue oxygenation and metabolic balance. It is important to collect sufficient samples for culture and two sets of blood cultures, one from a peripheral venous site and the other from the central venous catheter site before starting antibiotics to determine the causative pathogen and its antimicrobial susceptibility [87].

Especially in patients with systemic inflammatory response syndrome criteria, the selection and early initiation of antibiotics are vital. Antibiotics or antibiotic combinations with sufficient spectrum according to risk factors for MDR pathogens and clinical stability of the patient should be started empirically. In addition to antibiotic therapy in the presence of sepsis, additional treatments such as fluid resuscitation and close follow-up and treatment for organ dysfunction should be started as soon as possible. In patients with a central catheter with unexplained hypotension, hypoperfusion, or organ dysfunction, the catheter should be removed without delay and the catheter tip should be cultured [88].

#### 34.2.4.1 Postoperative Pulmonary Infections

Acquired pneumonia is defined as "pneumonia occurring ≥48 h or more after admission to hospital and in which the infectious agent is not in the incubation period at the time of admission." Ventilator-associated pneumonia is defined as "pneumonia that develops 48–72 h after endotracheal intubation" [87]. Globally, hospital/ventilator-associated pneumonia has been associated with adverse outcomes and significant morbidity and mortality rates [89].

Risk factors for hospital-acquired pneumonia include advanced age, intensive care unit stay, immunodeficiency, length of hospital stay, multiple comorbidities, mechanical ventilation, recent invasive procedures, and medical devices [90].

Patients in this risk group are also susceptible to resistant pathogens that cause nosocomial infections. Intravenous antibiotic administration in the last 90 days is one of the most important risk factors for the development of multiple antimicrobial drug resistance [91]. The presence of septic shock, acute renal replacement therapy prior to the onset of VAP, prolonged hospital stay, acute respiratory distress syndrome has been suggested as other risk factors for MDR VAP [87]. The most common pathogens in the etiology of HAP and VAP are *Staphylococci* and *Pseudomonas aeruginosa*, *E. coli*, *Klebsiella pneumonia*, and *Acinetobacter* spp. [92].

Postoperative pulmonary complications are particularly related to the patient's prognosis and pulmonary infections in the postoperative period are a major problem in patients with esophageal cancer. In recent years, the incidence and mortality of esophageal cancer have decreased due to medical advances and perioperative management [93]. It has been reported that the frequency of pulmonary infections is seen in 16–40% of patients with esophageal carcinoma. It has been emphasized that it is related to death [94, 95]. Therefore, it is important to distinguish patients with the highest risk of pulmonary infections and early intervention. In studies, it has been stated that factors such as age, smoking, preoperative comorbidity, low hemoglobin, high creatinine, and postoperative dysphagia are risk factors for pulmonary infections [96]. In one study, the frequency of pulmonary infections after esophageal cancer resection has been found to be 20.6% [97]. Length of hospital stay, albumin, intraoperative bleeding, and administration of perioperative blood transfusion were reported to be independent factors for pulmonary infections [97]. In one study, the relationship between length of hospital stay and healthcare-associated infection has been determined, and pulmonary infection was observed in 1.039 of 51.691 patients [98]. Studies have shown that the rate of respiratory tract infection increases significantly in patients with hypoalbuminemia after radical esophagectomy. Hypoalbuminemia causes a decrease in plasma osmotic pressure and pulmonary interstitial edema occurs [99].

Fever, chills, mental status change, productive cough, respiratory distress, tachycardia, abdominal pain, and back pain can be observed in these patients. Also, gas exchange is affected and abnormal ventilation makes patients with esophageal cancer susceptible to pulmonary infections. In addition, hypoalbuminemia impairs the immunity of patients and makes them susceptible to pulmonary infection [99]. CRP, procalcitonin, and blood gas analysis should be performed in addition to routine laboratory tests for diagnosis. Noninvasive tracheal aspirate samples should be obtained for culture in intubed patients [88].

In addition, systemic inflammatory response syndrome (SIRS) is frequently observed after esophagectomy, which is a highly invasive procedure. It has also been reported that SIRS is mostly associated with pulmonary complications after esophagectomy [100]. Hypothermia or hyperthermia, tachypnea, tachycardia, and hypotension, which are signs of systemic inflammatory response or sepsis, can be detected. In a study, the association of postoperative pneumonia with SIRS was found to be significantly higher [101].

#### 34.2.4.2 The Surgical Site Infections (SSIs)

The surgical site infections (SSIs) are the most common hospital-acquired infection (HAI) in the postoperative period. However, these cases have not been reported in the literature after esophageal cancer surgery [102]. The incidence of SSI after open esophageal cancer surgery is indefinite. In a study, the rate of SSI has been found to be 20.5% in 711 patients who applied esophagectomy and cervical anastomosis [103].

Factors such as age, malnutrition, obesity, diabetes, previous colonization, concomitant infections, antimicrobial prophylaxis, skin antisepsis, duration of the procedure, and surgical technique are factors that affect the development of SSI. *S. aureus*, coagulase-negative staphylococcus, *Enterococcus*, *E coli*, *Pseudomonas aeruginosa*, *Enterobacter*, *Klebsiella pneumoniae* are the most commonly detected pathogens for CAE [104]. In a study conducted in patients after surgery for esophageal or esophageal-gastric junction (EGJ) cancer, the most common organisms observed in culture-positive SSI were MSSA (32%), *Candida albicans* (29%), *Escherichia coli* (14%), *Enterococcus faecium* (11%) and *Klebsiella pneumoniae* (7%) [105].

#### 34.2.4.3 Hospital-Acquired Bloodstream Infections

Hospital-acquired bloodstream infections may be observed in patients associated with central venous catheters after esophagectomy. Bacteremia may occur secondary to catheter-related urinary tract infections, pneumonia, and surgical site infections. Since the risk of infection is higher in catheters applied to the femoral region, catheter applications to this region should be avoided [106]. *Staphylococcus aureus* and *Staphylococcus epidermidis* are common organisms associated with biofilm formation in catheters. Coagulase-negative staphylococci are the common cause of colonization in central lines, and these highlighted pathogens are major causes of central line-associated bloodstream infections [107].

#### 34.2.4.4 Hospital-Acquired Catheter-Related Urinary Tract Infections (CRUTI)

Urinary tract infections may occur in association with urinary catheters applied to patients. Common pathogens that are known to cause CRUTI are *Enterococcus*, *Staphylococcus aureus*, *Pseudomonas*, *Proteus*, *Klebsiell*a, and *Candida* [108]. Urine samples should be obtained prior to initiating empirical antibiotic therapy. Empirical antimicrobial therapy should be initiated based on the patient's condition, the presence of systemic symptoms, and the risk of MDR from CRUTI. Antibiotic selection should be narrowed according to the agent and antibiotic susceptibility [109].

#### 34.2.4.5 Prevention of Hospital-Acquired Infections After Esophagectomy

Standard infection control measures, such as proper hand washing or use of alcohol-based disinfectants before and after patient examination, reduce the incidence of postoperative infection. In order to prevent infections after esophagectomy, appropriate hand washing, antibiotic prophylaxis, skin decontamination, and infection prevention procedures should be applied during surgical site care. In some cases, it may be necessary to use prophylactic antibiotics effective against MRSA and carbapenemase-producing Enterobacteriaceae [104].

Patients undergoing minimally invasive esophagectomy have a lower risk of postoperative complications compared to patients undergoing open esophagectomy. Minimally invasive esophagectomy is a better approach in suitable patients [110].

## 34.3 Conclusion

Infectious agents may play a role in the development of cancer with the physiopathological changes and may adversely affect the prognosis of patients by causing various infectious complications after esophagectomy in the post-diagnosis period. We believe that multidisciplinary approaches are necessary in these patients.

## References

1. Bray F, Ferlay J, Soerjomataram I, Siegel RL, Torre LA, Jemal A. Global cancer statistics 2018: GLOBOCAN estimates of incidence and mortality worldwide for 36 cancers in 185 countries. CA Cancer J Clin. 2018;68(6):394–424.
2. Sung H, Ferlay J, Siegel RL, Laversanne M, Soerjomataram I, Jemal A, Bray F. Global cancer statistics 2020: GLOBOCAN estimates of incidence and mortality worldwide for 36 cancers in 185 countries. CA Cancer J Clin. 2021;71(3):209–49.
3. Arnold M, Soerjomataram I, Ferlay J, Forman D. Global incidence of oesophageal cancer by histological subtype in 2012. Gut. 2015;64(3):381–7.

4. Abnet CC, Arnold M, Wei WQ. Epidemiology of esophageal squamous cell carcinoma. Gastroenterology. 2018;154(2):360–73.
5. Garrett WS. Cancer and the microbiota. Science. 2015;348(6230):80–6.
6. Li M, Shao D, Zhou J, Gu J, Qin J, Chen W, et al. Signatures within esophageal microbiota with progression of esophageal squamous cell carcinoma. Chin J Cancer Res. 2020;32(6):755–67.
7. Lederberg J, McCray AT. 'Ome sweet 'Omics—a genealogical treasury of words. Scientist. 2001;15:8–8.
8. Wang ZK, Yang YS. Upper gastrointestinal microbiota and digestive diseases. World J Gastroenterol. 2013;19(10):1541–50.
9. Pei Z, Bini EJ, Yang L, Zhou M, Francois F, Blaser MJ. Bacterial biota in the human distal esophagus. Proc Natl Acad Sci USA. 2004;101(12):4250–5.
10. Morita E, Narikiyo M, Yano A, Nishimura E, Igaki H, Sasaki H, et al. Different frequencies of Streptococcus anginosus infection in oral cancer and esophageal cancer. Cancer Sci. 2003;94(6):492–6.
11. Narikiyo M, Tanabe C, Yamada Y, Igaki H, Tachimori Y, Kato H, et al. Frequent and preferential infection of Treponema denticola, Streptococcus mitis, and Streptococcus anginosus in esophageal cancers. Cancer Sci. 2004;95(7):569–74.
12. Tateda M, Shiga K, Saijo S, Sone M, Hori T, Yokoyama J, et al. Streptococcus anginosus in head and neck squamous cell carcinoma: implication in carcinogenesis. Int J Mol Med. 2000;6(6):699–703.
13. Asam D, Mauerer S, Spellerberg B. Streptolysin S of Streptococcus anginosus exhibits broad-range hemolytic activity. Med Microbiol Immunol. 2015;204(2):227–37.
14. Gilbert JA, Blaser MJ, Caporaso JG, Jansson JK, Lynch SV, Knight R. Current understanding of the human microbiome. Nat Med. 2018;24(4):392–400.
15. Yang W, Chen CH, Jia M, Xing X, Gao L, Tsai HT, et al. Tumor-associated microbiota in esophageal squamous cell carcinoma. Front Cell Dev Biol. 2021;9:641270.
16. Yamamura K, Baba Y, Nakagawa S, Mima K, Miyake K, Nakamura K, et al. Human microbiome fusobacterium nucleatum in esophageal cancer tissue is associated with prognosis. Clin Cancer Res. 2016;22(22):5574–81.
17. Yang L, Francois F, Pei Z. Molecular pathways: pathogenesis and clinical implications of microbiome alteration in esophagitis and Barrett esophagus. Clin Cancer Res. 2012;18(8):2138–44.
18. O'Riordan JM, Abdel-latif MM, Ravi N, McNamara D, Byrne PJ, McDonald GS, et al. Proinflammatory cytokine and nuclear factor kappa-B expression along the inflammation-metaplasia-dysplasia-adenocarcinoma sequence in the esophagus. Am J Gastroenterol. 2005;100(6):1257–64.
19. Hollingsworth MA, Swanson BJ. Mucins in cancer: protection and control of the cell surface. Nat Rev Cancer. 2004;4(1):45–60.
20. Thornton DJ, Sheehan JK. From mucins to mucus: toward a more coherent understanding of this essential barrier. Proc Am Thorac Soc. 2004;1(1):54–61.
21. Thornton DJ, Rousseau K, McGuckin MA. Structure and function of the polymeric mucins in airways mucus. Annu Rev Physiol. 2008;70:459–86.
22. Al-Haddad S, El-Zimaity H, Hafezi-Bakhtiari S, Rajendra S, Streutker CJ, Vajpeyi R, et al. Infection and esophageal cancer. Ann N Y Acad Sci. 2014;1325:187–96.
23. Glickman JN, Blount PL, Sanchez CA, Cowan DS, Wongsurawat VJ, Reid BJ, et al. Mucin core polypeptide expression in the progression of neoplasia in Barrett's esophagus. Hum Pathol. 2006;37(10):1304–15.
24. Hatayama H, Iwashita J, Kuwajima A, Abe T. The short chain fatty acid, butyrate, stimulates MUC2 mucin production in the human colon cancer cell line, LS174T. Biochem Biophys Res Commun. 2007;356(3):599–603.
25. Dohrman A, Miyata S, Gallup M, Li JD, Chapelin C, Coste A, et al. Mucin gene (MUC 2 and MUC 5AC) upregulation by gram-positive and gram-negative bacteria. Biochim Biophys Acta. 1998;1406(3):251–9.

26. Hamilton SR, Aaltonen LA. World Health Organization classification of tumors. Pathologyand genetics of tumors of the digestive system. Lyon: IARC Press; 2000. p. 203–19.
27. Wilcox CM. Overview of infectious esophagitis. Gastroenterol Hepatol (N Y). 2013;9(8):517–9.
28. Hoversten P, Otaki F, Katzka DA. Course of esophageal candidiasis and outcomes of patients at a single center. Clin Gastroenterol Hepatol. 2019;17(1):200–2.
29. Hoversten P, Kamboj AK, Katzka DA. Infections of the esophagus: an update on risk factors, diagnosis, and management. Dis Esophagus. 2018;31(12).
30. López-Dupla M, Mora Sanz P, Pintado García V, Valencia Ortega E, Uriol PL, Khamashta MA, et al. Clinical, endoscopic, immunologic, and therapeutic aspects of oropharyngeal and esophageal candidiasis in HIV-infected patients: a survey of 114 cases. Am J Gastroenterol. 1992;87(12):1771–6.
31. Takahashi Y, Nagata N, Shimbo T, Nishijima T, Watanabe K, Aoki T, et al. Long-term trends in esophageal candidiasis prevalence and associated risk factors with or without HIV infection: lessons from an endoscopic study of 80,219 patients. PLoS One. 2015;10(7):e0133589.
32. Raufman JP. Declining gastrointestinal opportunistic infections in HIV-infected persons: a triumph of science and a challenge for our HAARTs and minds. Am J Gastroenterol. 2005;100(7):1455–8.
33. Chocarro Martínez A, Galindo Tobal F, Ruiz-Irastorza G, González López A, Alvarez Navia F, Ochoa Sangrador C, et al. Risk factors for esophageal candidiasis. Eur J Clin Microbiol Infect Dis. 2000;19(2):96–100.
34. Yakoob J, Jafri W, Abid S, Jafri N, Islam M, Hamid S, et al. Candida esophagitis: risk factors in non-HIV population in Pakistan. World J Gastroenterol. 2003;9(10):2328–31.
35. Choi JH, Lee CG, Lim YJ, Kang HW, Lim CY, Choi JS. Prevalence and risk factors of esophageal candidiasis in healthy individuals: a single center experience in Korea. Yonsei Med J. 2013;54(1):160–5.
36. Min YW, Kim E, Son HJ, Kim JJ, Rhee PL. Antifungal treatment is not required for immunocompetent individuals with asymptomatic esophageal candidiasis. Medicine (Baltimore). 2015;94(45):e1969.
37. Lee SP, Sung IK, Kim JH, Lee SY, Park HS, Shim CS. The clinical course of asymptomatic esophageal candidiasis incidentally diagnosed in general health inspection. Scand J Gastroenterol. 2015;50(12):1444–50.
38. Pappas PG, Kauffman CA, Andes DR, Clancy CJ, Marr KA, Ostrosky-Zeichner L, et al. Clinical practice guideline for the management of candidiasis: 2016 update by the Infectious Diseases Society of America. Clin Infect Dis. 2016;62(4):e1–50.
39. Wilson A, Delport J, Ponich T. Candida glabrata esophagitis: are we seeing the emergence of a new azole-resistant pathogen? Int J Microbiol. 2014;2014:371631.
40. Skiest DJ, Vazquez JA, Anstead GM, Graybill JR, Reynes J, Ward D, et al. Posaconazole for the treatment of azole-refractory oropharyngeal and esophageal candidiasis in subjects with HIV infection. Clin Infect Dis. 2007;44(4):607–14.
41. Weerasuriya N, Snape J. A study of candida esophagitis in elderly patients attending a district general hospital in the UK. Dis Esophagus. 2006;19(3):189–92.
42. Kadayakkara DK, Candelaria A, Kwak YE, Loeser C. Herpes simplex virus-2 esophagitis in a Young immunocompetent adult. Case Rep Gastrointest Med. 2016;2016:7603484.
43. Wong RC, Abdul-Karim FW. Atypical herpes simplex esophagitis. Gastrointest Endosc. 2005;61(2):291–2.
44. Wang HW, Kuo CJ, Lin WR, Hsu CM, Ho YP, Lin CJ, et al. The clinical characteristics and manifestations of cytomegalovirus esophagitis. Dis Esophagus. 2016;29(4):392–9.
45. Olmos M, Sanchez Basso A, Battaglia M, Concetti H, Magnanini F. Esophageal strictures complicating cytomegalovirus ulcers in patients with AIDS. Endoscopy. 2001;33(9):822.
46. Albuquerque A, Cardoso H, Ribeiro A, Rios E, Silva R, Magalhães J, Macedo G. Herpes and cytomegalovirus esophagitis. Endoscopy. 2012;44 Suppl 2 UCTN:E242–3.

47. Salzberger B, Hartmann P, Hanses F, Uyanik B, Cornely OA, Wöhrmann A, et al. Incidence and prognosis of CMV disease in HIV-infected patients before and after introduction of combination antiretroviral therapy. Infection. 2005;33(5–6):345–9.
48. Rajendra S, Wang B, Snow ET, Sharma P, Pavey D, Merrett N, et al. Transcriptionally active human papillomavirus is strongly associated with Barrett's dysplasia and esophageal adenocarcinoma. Am J Gastroenterol. 2013;108(7):1082–93.
49. Gençdal G, Degirmencioglu S, Akyıldız M. Diffuse esophageal squamous papillomatosis covering the entire esophagus. Clin Gastroenterol Hepatol. 2018;16(6):A28.
50. Bohn OL, Navarro L, Saldivar J, Sanchez-Sosa S. Identification of human papillomavirus in esophageal squamous papillomas. World J Gastroenterol. 2008;14(46):7107–11.
51. d'Huart MC, Chevaux JB, Bressenot AM, Froment N, Vuitton L, Degano SV, et al. Prevalence of esophageal squamous papilloma (ESP) and associated cancer in northeastern France. Endosc Int Open. 2015;3(2):E101–6.
52. Yong F, Xudong N, Lijie T. Human papillomavirus types 16 and 18 in esophagus squamous cell carcinoma: a meta-analysis. Ann Epidemiol. 2013;23(11):726–34.
53. Liyanage SS, Rahman B, Ridda I, Newall AT, Tabrizi SN, Garland SM, et al. The aetiological role of human papillomavirus in oesophageal squamous cell carcinoma: a meta-analysis. PLoS One. 2013;8(7):e69238.
54. Li X, Gao C, Yang Y, Zhou F, Li M, Jin Q, Gao L. Systematic review with meta-analysis: the association between human papillomavirus infection and oesophageal cancer. Aliment Pharmacol Ther. 2014;39(3):270–81.
55. Petrick JL, Wyss AB, Butler AM, Cummings C, Sun X, Poole C, et al. Prevalence of human papillomavirus among oesophageal squamous cell carcinoma cases: systematic review and meta-analysis. Br J Cancer. 2014;110(9):2369–77.
56. Iyer A, Rajendran V, Adamson CS, Peng Z, Cooper K, Evans MF. Human papillomavirus is detectable in Barrett's esophagus and esophageal carcinoma but is unlikely to be of any etiologic significance. J Clin Virol. 2011;50(3):205–8.
57. Kunzmann AT, Graham S, McShane CM, Doyle J, Tommasino M, Johnston B, et al. The prevalence of viral agents in esophageal adenocarcinoma and Barrett's esophagus: a systematic review. Eur J Gastroenterol Hepatol. 2017;29(7):817–25.
58. Plummer M, de Martel C, Vignat J, Ferlay J, Bray F, Franceschi S. Global burden of cancers attributable to infections in 2012: a synthetic analysis. Lancet Glob Health. 2016;4(9):e609–16.
59. Koike T, Ohara S, Sekine H, Iijima K, Kato K, Shimosegawa T, Toyota T. Helicobacter pylori infection inhibits reflux esophagitis by inducing atrophic gastritis. Am J Gastroenterol. 1999;94(12):3468–72.
60. Blaser MJ. Hypothesis: the changing relationships of helicobacter pylori and humans: implications for health and disease. J Infect Dis. 1999;179(6):1523–30.
61. Chen MJ, Wu DC, Lin JM, Wu MT, Sung FC. Etiologic factors of gastric cardiac adenocarcinoma among men in Taiwan. World J Gastroenterol. 2009;15(43):5472–80.
62. Islami F, Sheikhattari P, Ren JS, Kamangar F. Gastric atrophy and risk of oesophageal cancer and gastric cardia adenocarcinoma—a systematic review and meta-analysis. Ann Oncol. 2011;22(4):754–60.
63. Huang Q, Fan X, Agoston AT, Feng A, Yu H, Lauwers G, Zhang L, Odze RD. Comparison of gastro-oesophageal junction carcinomas in Chinese versus American patients. Histopathology. 2011;59(2):188–97.
64. Csendes A, Smok G, Cerda G, Burdiles P, Mazza D, Csendes P. Prevalence of helicobacter pylori infection in 190 control subjects and in 236 patients with gastroesophageal reflux, erosive esophagitis or Barrett's esophagus. Dis Esophagus. 1997;10(1):38–42.
65. Goldblum JR, Vicari JJ, Falk GW, Rice TW, Peek RM, Easley K, et al. Inflammation and intestinal metaplasia of the gastric cardia: the role of gastroesophageal reflux and H. pylori infection. Gastroenterology. 1998;114(4):633–9.
66. Ye W, Held M, Lagergren J, Engstrand L, Blot WJ, McLaughlin JK, et al. Helicobacter pylori infection and gastric atrophy: risk of adenocarcinoma and squamous-cell carcinoma of the esophagus and adenocarcinoma of the gastric cardia. J Natl Cancer Inst. 2004;96(5):388–96.

67. Rokkas T, Pistiolas D, Sechopoulos P, Robotis I, Margantinis G. Relationship between Helicobacter pylori infection and esophageal neoplasia: a meta-analysis. Clin Gastroenterol Hepatol. 2007;5(12):1413–7, 1417.e1–2.
68. Bergman S, Geisinger KR. Esophageal aspergillosis in cytologic brushings: report of two cases associated with acute myelogenous leukemia. Diagn Cytopathol. 2004;30(5):347–9.
69. Herbrecht R, Denning DW, Patterson TF, Bennett JE, Greene RE, Oestmann JW, et al. Voriconazole versus amphotericin B for primary therapy of invasive aspergillosis. N Engl J Med. 2002;347(6):408–15.
70. Sandkovsky U, Ali KF, VanSchooneveld TC, Radio SJ, Swindells S. Disseminated histoplasmosis presenting as esophageal ulceration in an HIV-infected man. Infect Dis Clin Pract. 2013;21:383–5.
71. Kauffman CA. Histoplasmosis: a clinical and laboratory update. Clin Microbiol Rev. 2007;20(1):115–32.
72. Norder Grusell E, Dahlén G, Ruth M, Ny L, Quiding-Järbrink M, Bergquist H, et al. Bacterial flora of the human oral cavity, and the upper and lower esophagus. Dis Esophagus. 2013;26(1):84–90.
73. Yang L, Lu X, Nossa CW, Francois F, Peek RM, Pei Z. Inflammation and intestinal metaplasia of the distal esophagus are associated with alterations in the microbiome. Gastroenterology. 2009;137(2):588–97.
74. Gomes J, Antunes A, Carvalho A, Duarte R. Dysphagia as a manifestation of esophageal tuberculosis: a report of two cases. J Med Case Rep. 2011;5:447.
75. Jain SK, Jain S, Jain M, Yaduvanshi A. Esophageal tuberculosis: is it so rare? Report of 12 cases and review of the literature. Am J Gastroenterol. 2002;97(2):287–91.
76. El-Serag HB, Johnston DE. Mycobacterium avium complex esophagitis. Am J Gastroenterol. 1997;92(9):1561–3.
77. Wilcox CM. Esophageal disease in the acquired immunodeficiency syndrome: etiology, diagnosis, and management. Am J Med. 1992;92(4):412–21.
78. Paliwal M, Prasanna KS, Saraswat VA, Misra A, Krishnani N, Ghoshal UC. Varicella zoster cranial polyneuropathy presenting with dysphagia, esophagitis and gastroparesis. J Neurogastroenterol Motil. 2011;17(2):192–4.
79. Moretti F, Uberti-Foppa C, Quiros-Roldan E, Fanti L, Lillo F, Lazzarin A. Oesophagobronchial fistula caused by varicella zoster virus in a patient with AIDS: a unique case. J Clin Pathol. 2002;55(5):397–8.
80. Chen PC, Pan CC, Hsu WH, Ka HJ, Yang AH. Epstein-Barr virus-associated lymphoepithelioma-like carcinoma of the esophagus. Hum Pathol. 2003;34(4):407–11.
81. Zhang DH, Zhang QY, Hong CQ, Chen JY, Shen ZY, Zhu Y. Prevalence and association of human papillomavirus 16, Epstein-Barr virus, herpes simplex virus-1 and cytomegalovirus infection with human esophageal carcinoma: a case-control study. Oncol Rep. 2011;25(6):1731–8.
82. Sunpaweravong S, Mitarnun W, Puttawibul P. Absence of Epstein-Barr virus in esophageal squamous cell carcinoma. Dis Esophagus. 2005;18(6):398–9.
83. Cooper JS, Guo MD, Herskovic A, Macdonald JS, Martenson JA Jr, Al-Sarraf M, et al. Chemoradiotherapy of locally advanced esophageal cancer: long-term follow-up of a prospective randomized trial (RTOG 85-01). Radiation Therapy Oncology Group. JAMA. 1999;281(17):1623–7.
84. Takeuchi H, Miyata H, Ozawa S, Udagawa H, Osugi H, Matsubara H, et al. Comparison of short-term outcomes between open and minimally invasive esophagectomy for esophageal cancer using a nationwide database in Japan. Ann Surg Oncol. 2017;24(7):1821–7.
85. Boev C, Kiss E. Hospital-acquired infections: current trends and prevention. Crit Care Nurs Clin North Am. 2017;29(1):51–65.
86. Magill SS, Edwards JR, Bamberg W, Beldavs ZG, Dumyati G, Kainer MA, et al. Emerging infections program healthcare-associated infections and antimicrobial use prevalence survey team. Multistate point-prevalence survey of health care-associated infections. N Engl J Med. 2014;370(13):1198–208.

87. Kalil AC, Metersky ML, Klompas M, Muscedere J, Sweeney DA, Palmer LB, et al. Executive summary: management of adults with hospital-acquired and Ventilator-associated Pneumonia: 2016 clinical practice guidelines by the Infectious Diseases Society of America and the American Thoracic Society. Clin Infect Dis. 2016;63(5):575–82.
88. Monegro AF, Muppidi V, Regunath H. Hospital acquired infections. In: StatPearls. Treasure Island, FL: StatPearls Publishing; 2022.
89. Cillóniz C, Dominedò C, Torres A. An overview of guidelines for the management of hospital-acquired and ventilator-associated pneumonia caused by multidrug-resistant gram-negative bacteria. Curr Opin Infect Dis. 2019;32(6):656–62.
90. Sydnor ER, Perl TM. Hospital epidemiology and infection control in acute-care settings. Clin Microbiol Rev. 2011;24(1):141–73.
91. Metersky ML, Kalil AC. New guidelines for nosocomial pneumonia. Curr Opin Pulm Med. 2017;23(3):211–7.
92. Babcock HM, Zack JE, Garrison T, Trovillion E, Kollef MH, Fraser VJ. Ventilator-associated pneumonia in a multi-hospital system: differences in microbiology by location. Infect Control Hosp Epidemiol. 2003;24(11):853–8.
93. Chevallay M, Jung M, Chon SH, Takeda FR, Akiyama J, Mönig S. Esophageal cancer surgery: review of complications and their management. Ann N Y Acad Sci. 2020;1482(1):146–62.
94. Ohi M, Toiyama Y, Omura Y, Ichikawa T, Yasuda H, Okugawa Y, Fujikawa H, Okita Y, Yoshiyama S, Hiro J, Araki T, Kusunoki M. Risk factors and measures of pulmonary complications after thoracoscopic esophagectomy for esophageal cancer. Surg Today. 2019;49(2):176–86.
95. van der Sluis PC, Verhage RJ, van der Horst S, van der Wal WM, Ruurda JP, van Hillegersberg R. A new clinical scoring system to define pneumonia following esophagectomy for cancer. Dig Surg. 2014;31(2):108–16.
96. Soutome S, Hasegawa T, Yamguchi T, Aoki K, Kanamura N, Mukai T, et al. Prevention of postoperative pneumonia by perioperative oral care in patients with esophageal cancer undergoing surgery: a multicenter retrospective study of 775 patients. Support Care Cancer. 2020;28(9):4155–62.
97. Nakamura M, Iwahashi M, Nakamori M, Ishida K, Naka T, Iida T, et al. An analysis of the factors contributing to a reduction in the incidence of pulmonary complications following an esophagectomy for esophageal cancer. Langenbeck's Arch Surg. 2008;393(2):127–33.
98. Darling JD, McCallum JC, Soden PA, Korepta L, Guzman RJ, Wyers MC, et al. Results for primary bypass versus primary angioplasty/stent for lower extremity chronic limb-threatening ischemia. J Vasc Surg. 2017;66(2):466–75.
99. Li S, Su J, Sui Q, Wang G. A nomogram for predicting postoperative pulmonary infection in esophageal cancer patients. BMC Pulm Med. 2021;21(1):283.
100. D'Journo XB, Michelet P, Marin V, Diesnis I, Blayac D, Doddoli C, et al. An early inflammatory response to oesophagectomy predicts the occurrence of pulmonary complications. Eur J Cardiothorac Surg. 2010;37(5):1144–51.
101. Asaka S, Shimakawa T, Yamaguchi K, Katsube T, Usui T, Yokomizo H, Shiozawa S, Naritaka Y. Postoperative pneumonia after Esophagectomy and systemic inflammatory response syndrome. Anticancer Res. 2019;39(2):979–85.
102. Low DE, Alderson D, Cecconello I, Chang AC, Darling GE, D'Journo XB, et al. International consensus on standardization of data collection for complications associated with esophagectomy: Esophagectomy Complications Consensus Group (ECCG). Ann Surg. 2015;262(2):286–94.
103. Yin LX, Chen BM, Zhao GF, Yuan QF, Xue Q, Xu K. Scoring system to predict the risk of surgical site infection in patients with esophageal cancer after esophagectomy with cervical anastomosis. Surg Infect. 2018;19(7):696–703.
104. Young PY, Khadaroo RG. Surgical site infections. Surg Clin North Am. 2014;94(6):1245–64.
105. Raftery NB, Murphy CF, Donlon NE, Heneghan H, Donohoe CL, King S, et al. Prospective study of surgical site infections post-open esophageal cancer surgery, and the impact of care bundles. Dis Esophagus. 2021;34(12):doaa136.

106. Bell T, O'Grady NP. Prevention of central line-associated bloodstream infections. Infect Dis Clin N Am. 2017;31(3):551–9.
107. Patel AR, Patel AR, Singh S, Singh S, Khawaja I. Central line catheters and associated complications: a review. Cureus. 2019;11(5):e4717.
108. Flores-Mireles A, Hreha TN, Hunstad DA. Pathophysiology, treatment, and prevention of catheter-associated urinary tract infection. Top Spinal Cord Inj Rehabil. 2019;25(3):228–40.
109. Nickel JC, Costerton JW. Bacterial biofilms and catheters: a key to understanding bacterial strategies in catheter-associated urinary tract infection. Can J Infect Dis. 1992;3(5):261–7.
110. Dyas AR, Stuart CM, Bronsert MR, Schulick RD, McCarter MD, Meguid RA. Minimally invasive surgery is associated with decreased postoperative complications after esophagectomy. J Thorac Cardiovasc Surg. 2022;166(1):268–78.

# 35 Nutritional Support in Patients with Esophageal Cancer

Seniyye Ulgen Zengin and Beyza Betul Ozkurt

## 35.1 Nutritional Support in Patients with Esophageal Cancer

Nutritional support is important for patients with localized esophageal cancer. Many of these patients present in a nutritionally depleted state because of progressive dysphagia and in negative nitrogen balance at the time of admission [1].

Treatment has long and complicated healing process and effects postoperative nutrition in an important way. Side effects of multimodal treatment increase nutritional deficiency. Some degree of malnutrition is present in up to 80% of patients at presentation [1–3].

Malnutrition suppresses the immune system and morbidity and mortality presented high if surgery is performed on these patients. Thus, taking preoperative nutrition will eventually yield a positive nitrogen result, allowing surgery to be performed safely if needed.

## 35.2 Etiology of Malnutrition

Malnutrition has many causes in patients with esophageal cancer. Malnutrition can usually be seen as complication of local and systemic effects of malign cells and also side effects of treatment. It is important to detect causes for correct malnutrition of these patients [4, 5].

S. U. Zengin (✉) · B. B. Ozkurt
Anesthesiology and Intensive Care Department, Medical Faculty, Marmara University, İstanbul, Turkey



O. Engin (ed.), *Risk Factors and Therapy of Esophagus Cancer*,
https://doi.org/10.1007/978-3-031-47024-0_35

## 35.3 Local Effects of Tumor

In patients with locally advanced esophageal cancer, obstruction of the esophagus by tumor causes progressive dysphagia, often accompanied by weight loss. Dysphagia usually occurs when the esophageal lumen diameter is less than 13 mm (approximately 70% reduction of lumen diameter), indicating at least locally advanced disease. Weight loss results from changes in diet to accommodate dysphagia, and tumor-associated anorexia may commit. About 20% of patients experience odynophagia (painful swallowing) [4, 6].

Early signs of esophageal cancer may be mild and nonspecific. Transient solid food "sticking," easily overcome by gentle chewing and slow eating, may precede overt dysphagia. Dysphagia gradually improves as the patient switches from solids to liquids. Patients may also experience retrosternal discomfort or a burning sensation [5, 6].

## 35.4 Systemic Effects of Tumor

Cachexia is at times a hypercatabolic status and is characterized by progressive loss of skeletal muscle, partly against the background of an inflammatory response. There are many studies focusing on the mechanisms underlying the metabolic and body structure changes observed in cancer cachexia. These indicate a probably an important role for cytokine activation and for several tumor-derived and potentially cachexia-inducing substances, the point of which seems to be skeletal muscle gene products [5].

Malnutrition related to cancer cachexia can be represented as a multifactorial disorder characterized by a progressive loss of skeletal muscle mass (with or without loss of fat mass) that is not fully reversible with traditional nutritional support and leads to functional impairment. The pathophysiology is characterized as a negative protein and energy balance driven by a changing combination of reduced food intake and abnormal metabolism. Increased energy expenditure caused by systemic inflammation caused by the tumor enhances weight loss [1].

Many observations point toward cytokines, polypeptides released mainly by immune cells, as responsible for some of the metabolic disorders associated with the hypermetabolic phase that partially characterizes cancer cachexia. Because of their talent to increase resting energy consumption and induce anorexia, tumor necrosis factor (TNF) alpha, interleukin (IL) 1 beta, and IL-6 have been pointed as possible mediators of cancer cachexia. Initial studies provided conflicting data as to whether an increase in serum cytokines occurs in cancer cachexia; many studies have identified rise in peripheral blood mononuclear cell cytokine concentrations, especially TNF-alpha and IL-6, among weight-losing patients with cancer [5, 7].

Although preclinical data suggest the possibility that other mechanisms of adipose tissue loss (e.g., tumor-induced impairment of adipose tissue formation and/or lipid storage capacity) may be involved, the primary cause of fat loss in this case appears to be increased adipocyte lipolysis, not decreased lipogenesis or adipocyte cell death [8].

Although anorexia is common in advanced cancer, the dramatic weight loss experienced by patients with cachexia cannot be entirely linked to low caloric intake. Unlike simple starvation, which is characterized by a caloric deficit that can be reversed with optimal nutrition, the weight loss of cachexia cannot be adequately treated with aggressive feeding. Insufficient oral intake is superimposed on complex metabolic aberrations that cause an increase in basal energy consumption, resulting in loss of lean body mass from skeletal muscle wasting [9].

## 35.5 Effects of Treatment

Side effects of treatment have major role in malnutrition. Preoperative multimodal cancer treatments and postoperative complications effect nutritional target directly in these patients. Major complications are recurrent laryngeal nerve injury, anastomosis leak, chylothorax, and pulmonary complications [1, 2].

Vitamin D deficiency is also seen in these patients and is thought to lead to an increased inflammatory response resulting in massive epithelial damage, contributing to the development of acute lung injury (ALI) and more severe acute respiratory distress syndrome (ARDS). About 25–30% of esophagectomy patients may develop ALI and ARDS [1].

Anemia is common in the preoperative period in esophageal cancer and is a risk factor for poor clinical results as well as a strong predisposing factor for perioperative blood transfusion, which increases morbidity, mortality, and cost. Preoperative iron therapy is advisable for iron deficiency anemia [1].

Neoadjuvant patients are subject to increased nutrition risk because of the GI side effects of chemoradiotherapy (such as vomiting, diarrhea, and stomatitis) and sufficient nutrition status is important to meet the impending metabolic needs of surgical esophagectomy. Dysphagia, odynophagia, and also reflux esophagitis are most common complications after radiotherapy [1, 10].

Complications originate from the intravenous catheter in the patients are on total parenteral nutrition for 4 weeks. Catheter sepsis, thrombosis of subclavian vein are common complications [1].

## 35.6 Nutritional Assessment

Nutritional screening and evaluation should be an important part of multimodal anticancer therapy for patients with esophageal cancer. Nutritional screening should be a rapid and simple process. There is no agreement on the nutritional evaluation tool to be used, but it is critical to include dietary intake, body composition, physical activity, and exact metabolic pattern [4–7].

1. **Nutrition History of Patient**

It is important to evaluate the onset and progression rate of symptoms such as dysphagia at the first admission of patients. Knowing the previous routine of the patient gives an idea in terms of showing how much the malignancy affects nutrition. Weight loss, early satiety, solid–liquid food intake status, which foods the dysphagia first started against, alcohol consumption, smoking history, and daily total fluid intake should be questioned [5, 11, 12].

2. **Medical History and Physical Examination**

   Questioning comorbidities, observing the effects of past treatments, and localization of the tumor are important in determining the method of nutritional therapy.

3. **Anthropometric Measurements**

   It can be used to compare the patient's pretreatment values.

   (a) **Body Weight**

   Before diagnosis, 80% of all patients with esophageal cancer have over 10–15% unintentional weight loss. Weight loss is increased due to dysphagia and increased energy requirements caused by tumor-induced systemic inflammation. Severe preoperative weight loss (>10%) is associated with poor 5-year overall survival after esophagectomy, but is not associated with a higher risk of postoperative complications or length of hospital stay compared to no or limited weight loss [5, 11].

   (b) **Triceps Skin Thickness**

   Less than 10 mm in men and less than 13 mm in women are associated with malnutrition.

   (c) **Upper Arm Circumference**

   Less than 20 cm in men and less than 18 cm in women are associated with malnutrition.

   A hallmark sign of frailty is sarcopenia, the voluntary loss of skeletal muscle mass, strength, and function. Sarcopenia may be associated with an increased risk for dose-limiting toxicity during chemotherapy compared to non-sarcopenic patients with esophageal cancer and can be assessed by CT-based skeletal muscle mass measurements [5, 11, 12].

   (d) **Biochemical Parameters**

   Arginine, omega-3 fatty acids, nucleotides, and/or glutamine are specific nutrients that take part in immunonutrition. These nutrients have an important role on the immune and inflammatory responses to surgical stress as well as stimulate protein synthesis. Although low albumin is not a specific measure for determining protein deficiency, it is a marker of chronic malnutrition. Serum transferrin level is a more reliable marker in determining nutritional status because of its lower half-life than albumin. However, because of the shortest half-life of prealbumin, it gives the most reliable tissue protein measurement in determining the acute nutritional response [5, 11, 12].

   (e) **Energy Needs:**

   In cancer patients, the energy need varies depending on the increase in the basal metabolic rate. The recent ESPEN (European Society for Clinical

Nutrition and Metabolism) guidelines on nutrition in cancer patients suggest in general the following consumptions: energy 25–30 kcal/kg/day, protein 1–1.5 g/kg/day, and normal recommended dietary dose of vitamins and trace elements [5, 11, 12].

(f) **Protein Needs:**

Patients with severe dysphagia are generally in negative nitrogen balance on admission. In order to maintain a positive protein balance, it should be ensured that adequate protein intake is provided in the preoperative period [5, 11, 12].

## 35.7 Nutritional Support Therapy in Patients with Esophageal Cancer

The importance of nutritional status and dietary intake is increasingly get attention day by day and covers the whole process of esophageal cancer treatment: from the diagnostic phase to the perioperative phase to long-term support. As well as, these patients have an increased catabolism, and it should not be ignored in the calculation of the energy consumption [5, 13].

Patients with esophageal cancer present with malnutrition due to progressive dysphagia at the time of diagnosis. Swallowing difficulty should be questioned and the best tolerated nutrition program should be determined according to its severity.

Supporting selected foods with high-calorie and protein-containing oral solutions reduces the amount of food to be taken, while increasing the number of calories taken at once. Nutritional therapy should be arranged in the presence of dietitians in such a way that the patient can achieve optimum compliance. In patients with a severe nutritional risk, use of nutritional support for 10–14 days preceding major surgery is highly recommended, even if surgery delayed [13, 14].

## 35.8 Nutritional Support During Treatment

1. **Nutritional Support for Patients Receiving Radiotherapy**

   Preoperative radiotherapy potentially benefits a subgroup of patients with esophageal cancer. The use of concurrent radiation therapy frequently causes odynophagia that further aggravates preexisting dysphagia. This situation should be evaluated before radiotherapy and supportive treatment should be started. In cases where oral nutrition cannot be provided, enteral nutrition should be provided with parenteral, nasogastric tube, gastrostomy, or jejunostomy to provide nutritional support [5, 6, 13, 14].

   Radiation esophagitis is the most common and most important acute toxicity for patients whose swallowing is already compromised, manifesting as odynophagia and/or worsening of swallowing. The nasogastric tube feeding route is cumbersome, is associated with reflux esophagitis and in the setting of radiation therapy to the esophagus there is an increased incidence of disabling esophagitis.

Jejunostomy feeding requires operative placement with elemental diet support may be an optimal approach and needs to be evaluated prospectively in such a setting [13–15].

2. **Nutritional Support for Patients Receiving Chemotherapy**

   Preoperative chemotherapy potentially benefits a subgroup of patients with esophageal cancer such as radiotherapy. The ability to administer aggressive chemoradiotherapy (CRT) may depend on the initial nutritional status and the ability to sustain nutrition during therapy. Parenteral nutrition support during CRT may lead to complications that limit its usefulness and negate any potential benefit [5, 8, 13].

   Nausea, vomiting, diarrhea, and stomatitis are the most common side effects of chemotherapy. In patients receiving chemotherapy, additional medical agents may often be needed to improve oral intake [13, 14].

3. **Nutritional Support after Surgery**

   Since esophageal cancer surgery is an invasive procedure resulting in a permanent anatomical change, special focus needs to be placed on nutritional issues in both the short- and long-term postoperative period.

   For patients who need additional nutritional support, enteral nutritional support is generally seen as superior to parenteral nutrition in a patient with a functioning gut. In the postoperative period, it is associated with lower complication rates and more effective on reversal of malnutrition. At the onset, it is recommended to start enteral feeding instead of parenteral nutrition because it is regarded to decrease the number of life-threatening complications and the length of hospital stay. If there is no contraindication, enteral nutrition should be preferred because of its effects on ensuring gastrointestinal continuity, preventing intestinal villus atrophy, reducing intestinal permeability, improving local and systemic immune responses, and accelerating wound healing [5, 6, 13].

   Enteral nutrition can be administered through tube feeding or oral intake via a surgically placed jejunostomy or nasoduodenal, or jejunal tube. Both artificial routes for tube feeding entail additional costs and risks of complications such as reoperations, side-of-entry infections, side-of-entry leaks, gastrointestinal complaints (jejunostomy), and displacement (naso-post pyloric tubes) [5, 6, 13, 15].

   Since it is less invasive than other methods, nasogastric tube feeding is considered suitable for short-term feeding method. However, invasive methods should be considered in patients who are expected to receive long-term nutritional support.

   A presumed benefit to jejunostomy tube feeding is reduction of weight loss and a more rapid functional recovery. However, significant weight loss can be observed at 6 months postoperatively, despite routine application of jejunostomy tube feeding following esophagectomy. This may partly be explained by the major trauma of an esophagectomy, which inevitably leads to significant loss of peripheral tissue mass, partly by the difficulty to meet nutritional requirements orally after esophagectomy [5, 6, 13].

   Total parenteral nutrition is not usually the first choice, since esophageal cancer cells are used for nutritional purposes in the distal region of the tumor and there is a functional gastrointestinal area. However, if the patient cannot be fed enterally or it may be preferred to tolerate enteral feeding. Incidence of SIRS, sepsis, and pneumonia is lower in patients who are preferred enteral nutrition instead of total parenteral nutrition. This also means reduced ICU stays and early discharge from hospital [6, 13, 14].

Oral intake is generally thought to be contraindicated in the first postoperative days because it is assumed to increase the incidence of anastomotic leakage and aspiration causing pneumonia. Oral intake can be initiated if there is no surgical arrangement to prevent oral feeding, such as anastomotic leakage gastric distension, which is commonly used to ensure compliance with tube feeding. Tolerance is followed by starting with liquid foods first and, if tolerated, soft and small pieces of solid foods. If tolerance is good, oral intake is increased, and free regimen is started [11, 14, 15].

In cases with esophageal cancer diagnosed at an advanced stage, nutrition preference is made according to the patient [9, 10]. In patients for whom antineoplastic or surgical treatment cannot be planned, the application of invasive, aggressive, and expensive treatment methods is difficult for the patients and their relatives [11]. Therefore, the nutrition method should be planned by calculating the profit and loss ratio and considering the possible risks. In general, total parenteral nutrition can be seen as appropriate nutrition method in these patients.

4. **Nutrition in Patients Undergoing Vagotomy**

   The most common complications in vagotomy patients are gastric stasis, early satiety, distention, nausea, and vomiting. Therefore, calorie deficits and nutritional deficiencies may be seen in patients who underwent vagotomy during esophagectomy. Since gastric stasis will increase especially in fatty food intake, nutrition with low-fat foods should be preferred. It should be aimed to provide appropriate nutrition with personalized diet [5, 9].

5. **Nutrition in Patients with Colon and Jejunum Interposition**

   Although the colon and jejunum interposition method preferred after esophageal strictures and corrosive material damages, it is also a surgical method applied in esophagectomies in cases where there is not enough tissue for reanastomosis. Due to the delayed onset of peristaltic movements, oral intake begins later than in patients who underwent gastric pull-up. Food moves with the repulsive effect of swallowing and the effect of gravity. Therefore, dysphagia is a common postoperative complication in these patients. It should be recommended that patients sit upright to eat, drink fluids after each bite, and stay in a sitting position after feeding to prevent reflux [5, 13, 14].

6. **Nutrition in Patients with Esophageal Dilatation and Stenting**

   Esophageal stents are most often used for palliation in patients with inoperable tumors due to local invasion, metastatic disease, or a local recurrence after a previous resection. For patients with advanced esophageal cancer, expandable stents can provide almost immediate dysphagia relief [5, 15].

The immediate poststent replacement diet should consist of liquids, and within 24 h after stent placement, most patients are able to advance to semisolid food. One advantage of self-expanding stents over other palliative nutritional regimens is the patient's ability to quickly return to normal diet. Chemoradiotherapy, for example, only improves dysphagia if the tumor responds to treatment and can even aggravate dysphagia over the short term because of radiation induced esophagitis [5, 13, 15].

Esophageal stents are well-known tools for the palliation of esophageal cancer. The role of stents in the treatment of esophageal cancer has broadened with the use of removable stents in patients receiving neoadjuvant therapy. Self-expanding stents can effectively relieve dysphagia and increase patient quality of life with a high degree of success. Optimal nutritional outcomes occur when stent delivery is integrated with a multidisciplinary approach using nutritional counseling [5, 13, 14].

## 35.9 Conclusion

Adequate and effective nutrition is very important for patients with esophageal cancer. It is difficult to demonstrate the long-term effects of nutritional support because of short survival time. However, appropriate and adequate nutritional support in combination with mild physical activity may increase the tolerance to therapies, shortens the hospital stay, reduces morbidity and mortality, and provides a positive effect on the clinical course. For this reason, it is important that these patients are included in a well-defined multimodal program throughout the entire treatment process from the moment of diagnosis.

## References

1. Steenhagen E, van Vulpen JK, van Hillegersberg R, May AM, Siersema PD. Nutrition in peri-operative esophageal cancer management. Expert Rev Gastroenterol Hepatol. 2017;11(7):663–72. https://doi.org/10.1080/17474124.2017.1325320. Epub 2017 May 10.
2. Wang PY, Chen XK, Liu Q, et al. Application of four nutritional risk indexes in perioperative management for esophageal cancer patients. J Cancer Res Clin Oncol. 2021;147:3099–111. https://doi.org/10.1007/s00432-021-03585-8.
3. Lim ST, Choa RG, Lam KH, Wong J, Ong GB. Total parenteral nutrition versus gastrostomy in the preoperative preparation of patients with carcinoma of the oesophagus. Br J Surg. 1981;68(2):69–72. https://doi.org/10.1002/bjs.1800680202.
4. Gabor S, Renner H, Matzi V, Ratzenhofer B, Lindenmann J, Sankin O, Pinter H, Maier A, Smolle J, Smolle-Jüttner FM. Early enteral feeding compared with parenteral nutrition after oesophageal or oesophagogastric resection and reconstruction. Br J Nutr. 2005;93(4):509–13. https://doi.org/10.1079/bjn20041383.
5. Bilgin BY. Özofagus kanserli hastalarda beslenme. J Exp Clin Med. 2013;29(4S):267–72.
6. Weijs TJ, Berkelmans GH, Nieuwenhuijzen GA, Ruurda JP, van Hillegersberg R, Soeters PB, Luyer MD. Routes for early enteral nutrition after esophagectomy. A systematic review. Clin Nutr. 2015;34(1):1–6. https://doi.org/10.1016/j.clnu.2014.07.011. Epub 2014 Aug 1.
7. Nelke C, Dziewas R, Minnerup J, et al. Skeletal muscle as potential central link between sarcopenia and immune senescence. EBioMedicine. 2019;49:381–8. https://doi.org/10.1016/j.ebiom.2019.10.034.
8. Rydén M, Agustsson T, Laurencikiene J, Britton T, Sjölin E, Isaksson B, Permert J, Arner P. Lipolysis—not inflammation, cell death, or lipogenesis—is involved in adipose tissue loss in cancer cachexia. Cancer. 2008;113(7):1695–704. https://doi.org/10.1002/cncr.23802.

9. Suzuki H, Asakawa A, Amitani H, Nakamura N, Inui A. Cancer cachexia—pathophysiology and management. J Gastroenterol. 2013;48(5):574–94. https://doi.org/10.1007/s00535-013-0787-0. Epub 2013 Mar 20.
10. Sikora SS, Ribeiro U, Kane JM 3rd, Landreneau RJ, Lembersky B, Posner MC. Role of nutrition support during induction chemoradiation therapy in esophageal cancer. JPEN J Parenter Enteral Nutr. 1998;22(1):18–21. https://doi.org/10.1177/014860719802200118.
11. Kadıoğlu, P., Erişkinde nutrisyonel durumun değerlendirilmesi: Antropometrik, klinik ve biyokimyasal yöntemler. İ.Ü. Cerrahpaşa Tıp Fakültesi sürekli tıp eğitimi etkinlikleri sağlıkta ve hastalıkta beslenme sempozyum dizisi; 2004. p. 19–20.
12. Baji DB, Patel JP, Konanur Srinivasa NK, Gande A, Anusha M, Dar H. Nutrition Care in Cancer Surgery Patients: a narrative review of nutritional screening and assessment methods and nutritional considerations. Cureus. 2022;14(12):e33094. https://doi.org/10.7759/cureus.33094.
13. Jatoi A, Loprinzi CL. The role of parenteral and enteral/oral nutritional support in patients with cancer. UpToDate. 2014.
14. Muscaritoli M, Arends J, Bachmann P, Baracos V, Barthelemy N, Bertz H, et al. ESPEN practical guideline: clinical nutrition in cancer. Clin Nutr. 2021;40(5):2898–913. https://doi.org/10.1016/j.clnu.2021.02.005. Epub 2021 Mar 15.
15. Bower M, Jones W, Vessels B, Scoggins C, Martin R. Role of esophageal stents in the nutrition support of patients with esophageal malignancy. Nutr Clin Pract. 2010;25(3):244–9. https://doi.org/10.1177/0884533610368710.

# 36 Shock in Esophageal Cancer

Meliha Orhon Ergun and Ecem Guclu Ozturk

## 36.1 Definition

Shock is a condition characterized by insufficient supply of tissue oxygen demand. Often, the cause of circulatory disturbance is severe systemic hypotension. Shock states are classified according to the etiology of the circulatory disorder (Table 36.1). Cardiogenic shock may develop if there is a failure in the heart's pumping. Low cardiac output (CO) and increased systemic vascular resistance (SVR) are seen in cardiogenic shock. Bleeding due to injury to the great vessels can cause hypovolemic shock. Shock may develop due to vasodilation at the level of small vessels. This condition, which is due to a decrease in SVR, may develop due to neurogenic dysfunction such as anaphylaxis or spinal cord injury or sepsis. The mortality of all shock types and despite extensive research and aggressive management is still very high. Approximately 35–40% of patients die within 28 days of the onset of septic shock, and the mortality rate for patients with cardiogenic shock is 70–80%. Death from hypovolemic shock is highly variable and depends on the etiology, diagnosis, and speed of treatment [1].

M. Orhon Ergun (✉) · E. Guclu Ozturk
Anesthesiology and Reanimation Department, Faculty of Medicine, Marmara University, İstanbul, Turkey



O. Engin (ed.), *Risk Factors and Therapy of Esophagus Cancer*,
https://doi.org/10.1007/978-3-031-47024-0_36

**Table 36.1** Hemodynamic responses to different types of shock

| Type of shock | Cardiac index | Venous capacitance | SVR | CVP/PCWP | $SVO_2$ |
|---|---|---|---|---|---|
| Hypovolemic | ↓ | ↓ | ↑ | ↓ | ↓ |
| Septic | ↑↑ | ↑ | ↓ | ↑↓ | ↑↓ |
| Cardiogenic | ↓↓ | ↔ | ↑↑ | ↓ | ↓ |
| Neurogenic | ↑ | ↔ | ↓ | ↓ | ↓ |

*The cardiovascular responses are indicated by arrows to show an elevation* (↑), *marked elevation* (↑↑), *reduction* (↓), *marked reduction* (↓↓), *varied response* (↑↓), or *little effect* (↔). *CVP* central venous pressure; *PCWP* pulmonary capillary wedge pressure; $SVO_2$ mixed venous oxygen saturation; *SVR* systemic vascular resistance

## 36.2 Shock Types

### 36.2.1 Cardiogenic Shock

The hallmark of cardiogenic shock is primarily pumping failure. Cardiogenic shock may develop due to reasons such as pump failure due to myocardial infarction, heart failure, contusion, and cardiac laceration. Pathophysiological features are associated with decreased contractility. This condition is usually accompanied by enlargement of the cardiac chambers and venous congestion. Hypotension and respiratory failure are two symptoms of cardiogenic shock, which often develops quickly over a brief period of time [2, 3].

Determining the etiology of cardiogenic shock is extremely important, as treatment varies greatly depending on the underlying mechanism. For example, the role of β-blockers in the treatment of non-ischemic decompensated heart failure has evolved to be of increasing importance and diuresis is frequently indicated, whereas in acute ischemic ST elevation MI (STEMI) β-blockers are critical and acute diuresis has little role. In all patients presenting with heart failure, a 12-lead electrocardiogram (ECG), serum troponin measurements, B-type natriuretic peptide levels, and echocardiography should be performed to differentiate the causes of heart failure. The onset of pump failure is associated with two compensatory mechanisms: reflex vasoconstriction, which causes an increase in left ventricular (LV) workload and myocardial oxygen demand in the systemic vessels, and redistribution of blood volume toward the heart and lungs. Obstructive shock is a form of cardiogenic shock resulting from mechanical obstruction of the circulation that results in decreased cardiac output rather than primary heart failure. Etiology includes conditions such as tension pneumothorax, pericardial tamponade, or pulmonary embolism. The death rate for patients with cardiogenic shock is remains significant despite early revascularization. In situations when cardiogenic shock has occurred, multidisciplinary treatment in intensive care unit in a specialized facility is recommended [2, 4].

### 36.2.2 Septic Shock

Septic shock is a shock state in which perfusion is impaired, accompanied by infection and activation of the systemic inflammatory response. It is characterized by regional blood flow redistribution, which usually results in high CO, low SVR, hypotension, and tissue hypoperfusion [2].

In septic shock, the focus of infection is the most important factor in the deterioration of the clinic. Other noninfectious causes include acute spinal cord injury, pancreatitis, burns, fulminant liver faiure, multiple traumatic injuries, toxic shock syndrome, anaphylactic and anaphylactoid reactions, and drug or toxin reactions, including insect bites, transfusion reactions, and heavy metal poisoning. Septic shock is the most common shock syndrome, accounting for roughly two-thirds of shock patients in large intensive care populations. Physiological response in patients with systemic infections is defined in a process ranging from sepsis to severe sepsis and septic shock [5].

Cancer patients are at greater risk of severe sepsis and septic shock than the general population, possibly related to immunosuppression caused by the malignancy itself or its treatment. The incidence of severe sepsis is four times higher in cancer patients than in patients without cancer [5, 6].

The initiating event in septic shock appears to be the interaction between organism-specific ligands on pathogens and ligand-specific receptors (e.g., toll-like receptors, nucleotide-binding oligomerization domain-like receptors, and others) on cells of the innate immune system. The resulting release of immune mediators drives a complex series of events that result in altered gene expression, T-cell differentiation, complement activation, elaboration of pro-coagulation processes, and the production and release of other immunomodulatory cytokines. Together, these events produce the septic phenotype (e.g., microthrombus, endothelial dysfunction, capillary leak, vasodilation, efficacious hypovolemia, hypoperfusion, and organ failure) (Table 36.2). The effect of impaired perfusion on organ function depends on individual susceptibility to hypoxia [2, 7].

**Table 36.2** Stages of sepsis

| SIRS | Sepsis | Severe sepsis | Septic shock |
|---|---|---|---|
| • A body temperature >38 °C or <36 °C<br>• A heart rate >90 beats/min<br>• Tachypnea (respiratory rate >20/min) or hyperventilation ($PaCO_2$ < 32 mmHg)<br>• White blood cell count >12.000/mm$^3$ or <4000/mm$^3$ or >10% immature neutrophils | • Two or more SIRS criteria<br>• Documented or suspected infection | Sepsis with<br>• Hypotension (SBP < 90 mmHg) despite adequate iv fluids<br>• Lactate >4 | Severe sepsis with<br>• Persistent hypotension (SBP < 90 mmHg)<br>• End organ failure |

Septic shock can occur for many reasons. Postoperative pneumonia, fistules, and esophageal leaks are common and serious complications, which can be fatal. Recent studies have shown that pulmonary complications after esophagectomy have a negative impact on patient survival. The oral cavity is a known reservoir of pathogens that can lead to respiratory or wound infections after various types of surgeries. Aspiration of the oropharyngeal flora is the most frequent way of acquiring gram-negative pneumonia, a significant nosocomial infection [8–10].

Spontaneous perforations of the esophagus or post-surgical iatrogenic perforations can be a rapidly progressive cause of sepsis and septic shock due to leakage of gastric contents into body cavities. The absence of a serosal layer in the esophagus makes it more prone to perforation and rupture. In the event of a perforation, residual gastric contents, saliva, biliary fluid, and other secretions can infect the mediastinum, leading to chemical mediastinitis, mediastinal emphysema, inflammation, and ultimately, mediastinal necrosis. A tear in the esophageal wall can cause polymicrobial bacterial translocation and invasion to occur within a few hours. If the diagnosis is delayed or the patient does not receive adequate medical and surgical care, this can result in sepsis and ultimately death. In Surviving Sepsis Campaign, Evans L., et al. recommend administering antimicrobials as soon as possible, ideally within 1 h of detection, for adults with possible septic shock or a strong possibility of sepsis. Empirical antibiotics should be directed against the most likely pathogens (gram-negative rods, gram-positive cocci, and anaerobes). The site and type of entry of the causative microorganism may not be apparent until culture data is returned or imaging studies are complete. Once culture has resulted, antibiotic therapy should be tailored to include responsible organisms and coverage should be narrowed if appropriate. Long-term, empirical, broad-spectrum antibiotic use should be minimized as it reduces the growth of resistant organisms and causes potential complications such as fungal overgrowth and antibiotic-associated colitis from overgrowth of *Clostridium difficile* [11–13].

Nutritional support is also important in this patient population. If a duodenal leak is occurred as a cause of sepsis, careful endoscopic insertion of a fine-bore feeding tube distal to the duodenal leak is helpful for enteral feeding. A second tube, a nasogastric tube inserted into the intrathoracic stomach, will help reduce pressure in the stomach and prevent reflux of stomach contents through anastomosis [12, 14].

Total parenteral nutrition is required if feeding tube placement fails. Fibrin glue injection, placement of intraluminal stents, and clip closure of the defect are increasingly used to treat leaks; Closing the leak allows for early control of sepsis and resumption of oral feeding. Depending on the severity of the leak in the first place, the stent can be removed later. Usually 4–6 weeks will be sufficient for adequate healing [12, 15].

Mediastinal sepsis is a fatal condition when the diagnosis of esophageal perforation is delayed. Mortality was found to be 44–68% when treatment was delayed, and the most common cause was sepsis-related multiorgan failure, namely septic shock. Although the cause of anastomotic leak after esophagogastric anastomosis is thought to be multifactorial, gastric conduit ischemia undoubtedly plays an important role [15].

## 36.3 Hypovolemic/Hemorrhagic Shock

An important factor to realize is that patients with hemorrhagic shock and less than 15% blood loss have relatively few clinical symptoms. According to advanced trauma life support (ATLS), the patient may only present with anxiety. Patients with mild to moderate blood loss (15–30%) may only exhibit an increased heart rate. A heart rate greater than 100 bpm can be used as a physical sign of bleeding, but the evidentiary value is not always conclusive [16, 17].

A clinically significant drop in blood pressure is observed at the stage when patients have lost between 30 and 40% of their blood volume. For an average man weighing 75 kg (168 pounds), this equates to a loss of 2 L of blood. Recognizing blood loss is more important than compensating for blood loss [16].

Bleeding control is an essential component of resuscitation of the shocked patient. According to the trauma literature, patients with ongoing bleeding have improved survival if the time elapsed between injury and control of bleeding is shortened. Although there are no randomized controlled trials, retrospective studies provide convincing evidence in this regard [2].

Appropriate priorities in these patients are securing the airway, controlling the source of blood loss, and intravenous volume resuscitation. In trauma, identifying the body cavity that harbors active bleeding will help focus operative efforts; however, as time is of the essence, prompt treatment is essential and diagnostic laparotomy or thoracotomy may be required. Our current understanding has led to the management strategy known as damage-controlled resuscitation. This strategy begins in the emergency room and continues into the operating room and intensive care unit. Initial resuscitation is limited to maintain SBP around 80–90 mmHg. This prevents renewed bleeding from recently clotted veins [18].

Crystalloids and blood products are used to replace intravascular volume. As important as preventing severe hypotension is, excess volume resuscitation is equally dangerous. Bleeding is controlled in the operating room, multiple blood products and pharmacological agents are used both in the operating room and in the intensive care unit to warm the patients and to prevent coagulopathy [2, 18].

## 36.4 Shock Index

The shock index (SI), which uses these two variables together, was found to be more useful, as heart rate and systolic BP alone are not accurate in describing hemorrhagic shock independently, and an increase in heart rate does not always accompany a decrease in systolic blood pressure. SI is defined as heart rate divided by systolic BP. SI is known as an indicator of hemodynamic stability. However, the SI does not take into account diastolic BP and therefore a modified SI (MSI) is created. MSI is defined as heart rate divided by mean arterial pressure. A high MSI indicates a value of stroke volume and low systemic vascular resistance, which is a sign of hypodynamic circulation. In contrast, a low MSI indicates a hyperdynamic state. MSI has been considered a better predictor of mortality than SI. In addition, taking into account age, mechanism of injury, Glasgow Coma Scale (GCS) score, lactate levels, hemoglobin levels, and other physiological parameters allows us to make a statistically better prediction than a single vital sign [19].

## 36.5 Lactate and Base Deficiency

Lactate is a marker associated with injury or ischemia. It is assumed that lactate is transferred from its production site in the cytosol to neighboring cells and various organs (e.g., heart, liver, and kidney), where its oxidation continues and its metabolism continues. Lactate levels in the blood are highly dependent on the balance between production and elimination from the bloodstream. The liver is predominantly responsible for lactate clearance, and acute or chronic liver disease also affects blood lactate levels. The base deficit is the measure of millimoles of base required to correct the pH of 1 L of whole blood to 7.4. The measurement of base deficit is considered one of the most sensitive indicators of cellular resuscitation. It correlates well with lactate levels in the first 24 h after injury. When the base gap remains high, it counts as an indication of an ongoing clinical shock [19, 20].

## 36.6 Compensation Mechanisms

The body's initial response to blood loss is to create a clot at the site of hemorrhage. As bleeding continues, the earliest compensatory mechanism in response to a decrease in intravascular volume is an increase in sympathetic activity. Such an increase is mediated by pressure receptors or baroreceptors in the aortic arch, atrium, and carotid bodies. A decrease in pressure inhibits parasympathetic discharge, while norepinephrine and epinephrine are released and cause adrenergic receptors in myocardium and vascular smooth muscle to be activated. Catecholamines, antidiuretic hormones, and atrial natriuretic receptors are a few hormones and receptors that react to bleeding by constricting arterioles and muscle arteries while simultaneously raising heart rate. Blood is shifted from less critical organs (e.g., skin, skeletal muscle, and splanchnic circulation) to more critical organs (e.g., brain, liver, and kidneys). These compensatory mechanisms aim to increase cardiac output and maintain blood pressure to ensure adequate perfusion. Next, the renin–angiotensin–aldosterone system (RAAS) is activated in response to vasoconstriction and reduction in blood flow. Due to the body's attempt to maintain the volume of the circulating blood, these alterations may cause a decrease in urine production and the onset of thirst in the affected person. The release of catecholamines is thought to be responsible for the increased glucose level in hemorrhagic shock. Although the role of glucose elevation in hemorrhagic shock is not fully understood, it does not seem to affect the outcome [21, 22].

Cortisol, which is also released from the adrenal cortex, plays a major role in controlling fluid balance. In the adrenal cortex, the zona glomerulosa produces aldosterone in response to stimulation by angiotensin II. Aldosterone is a mineralocorticoid that modulates kidney function by increasing sodium recovery and potassium excretion. Angiotensin II also has a direct effect on the renal tubules: it promotes sodium reabsorption. Sodium control is the primary way the human body controls the absorption or secretion of water in the kidneys. This regulation of intravascular fluid status is also influenced by carotid baroreceptors and atrial natriuretic peptides. Signals are sent to the supraoptic and paraventricular nuclei in the brain. Antidiuretic hormone (ADH) is released from the pituitary and causes retention of free water at the kidney level. Simultaneously, volume is taken from the extravascular and cellular spaces. A water slide occurs as hydrostatic pressures decrease in the intravascular compartment. At the capillary level, hydrostatic pressures are also reduced because precapillary sphincters undergo more vasoconstriction than postcapillary sphincters [23–25].

The triad of acidosis, hypothermia, and coagulopathy is common in resuscitation patients who are bleeding or in shock from a variety of factors. Our basic knowledge is that inadequate tissue perfusion leads to lactate production and lactate production leads to acidosis. Therefore, if ATP production is insufficient to maintain body temperature, the temperature begins to drop. The resulting hypothermia impairs the activity of enzymes that work best at 37 °C. The critical issue with hypothermia for surgeons is that the enzymes of the coagulation cascade are also affected by hypothermia. If enzymes are not working optimally due to hypothermia, the coagulopathy worsens, which can contribute to uncontrolled bleeding in surgical patients from injuries or from the surgery itself [23, 26, 27].

Bleeding occurs as a result of trauma-induced coagulopathy (TIC), a dysfunctional coagulation mechanism. TIC is caused by a number of pathophysiological processes. During the resuscitative phase, tissue injury and shock cause endothelial, immune system, platelet, and coagulation activation, which is intensified by the "lethal triad" (coagulopathy, hypothermia, and acidosis). The best basic approach to shock-induced metabolic acidosis is to treat the underlying cause of the shock [26, 28, 29].

Hypothermia can be both beneficial and harmful. The beneficial aspect of hypothermia is mainly a decrease in metabolism. In trauma patients with a postoperative core temperature below 35 °C, mortality increased fourfold. It was observed that it increased seven times below 33 °C. In conclusion, hypothermia, although potentially beneficial, is harmful in trauma patients, mainly because it causes coagulopathy. After a hemorrhage, hypothermia is an indication of a poor prognosis and likely reflects metabolic dysfunction [30–32].

Tranexamic acid (TXA) is a synthetic analog of the amino acid lysine. It is an antifibrinolytic that competitively inhibits the activation of plasminogen to plasmin. Thus, it prevents the breakdown of fibrin, a protein that forms the framework of blood clots. TXA has approximately eight times the antifibrinolytic activity of its older analog, ε-aminocaproic acid. It is used to treat or prevent excessive blood loss in surgical procedures such as the heart, liver, and vascular system and in major orthopedic procedures. Its use in trauma has recently been advocated [33–35].

Cardiac output and oxygen delivery can be increased to a certain point by giving fluid during shock. The initial choice of fluid for resuscitation should be balanced crystalloids for adults with sepsis or septic shock. But if vital values cannot be achieved, an inotropic agent should be added. Norepinephrine is recommended over other vasopressors as the first-line treatment for adults with septic shock. In cases of hypovolemic shock, it is observed that regional hypoxia can continue even if the global oxygen supply is sufficient. Different organs and tissue beds are not similar in their oxygen needs or consumption. Still, one of the most effective ways to optimize oxygen delivery is to raise hemoglobin. If the hemoglobin level increases from 8.0 to 10 g/dL with blood transfusion, oxygen delivery increases by 25% [36, 37].

## 36.7 Approach

Postoperative mechanical ventilation is mandatory in sepsis patients with pulmonary dysfunction. Mechanical ventilation keeps the lung fully extended and adheres to the esophageal repair site and may provide additional support. The selective use of mechanical ventilation and positive end-expiratory pressure (PEEP) may be helpful in maintaining lung expansion [18, 38].

Patients are usually kept in NPO for a period, during which time a gastrostomy, jejunostomy, or nasojejunal tube should be used to provide enteral nutrition. If enteral access has been achieved, the decision to provide central IV access and begin parenteral nutrition depends on the surgeon's concerns about a postoperative leak (i.e., difficulty of repair and degree of contamination) as well as the patient's previous nutritional baseline. Perforation in clinically stable patients, oral intake may be initiated following contrast-enhanced imaging of the esophagus (typically a Gastrografin swallow study followed by fine barium) that fails to show leakage [19].

The most common cause of death after esophageal perforation (and repair) is multisystem organ failure because of ongoing sepsis. Mortality rates are higher for spontaneous perforations than for iatrogenic and traumatic (9–19% vs. 40%), higher for thoracic and abdominal perforations than for cervical perforations (30% vs. 6%), and higher for delayed diagnosis (>24 h) compared with early diagnosis (27% vs. 14%) [18, 19, 23].

A patient presenting with respiratory distress may require a safe airway and/or drainage of large pleural effusions secondary to a perforation. Due to the intense inflammatory response, the patient may also require treatment of septic shock with intravenous fluids and early administration of antibiotics [19, 23, 39].

## 36.8 Conditions That May Present Shock in Esophageal Cancer

### 36.8.1 Patient's Previous Status

In patients with esophageal cancer, first of all, a good anamnesis should be taken from the patient. Caution should be exercised about a possible bleeding complication in a patient with a history of bleeding tendency, a family history of coagulation disorders, or the use of anticoagulants or platelet inhibitors. Prior esophageal surgery results in increased periesophageal mediastinal fibrosis, and this is especially true after an esophagomyotomy in which the exposed submucosa tends to adhere to the anterior wall of the adjacent aorta. Mediastinal calcifications due to granulomatous disease seen on preoperative chest radiographs or CT scans usually indicate a more difficult subcarinal esophageal dissection [1, 40].

### 36.8.2 Esophageal Perforation

Esophageal perforation is a true emergency. It is a process with multiple etiologies and presentations that causes significant morbidity and mortality if not managed appropriately and aggressively. It most commonly occurs following diagnostic or therapeutic procedures. Pain is the most important finding. If subcutaneous emphysema is present, the diagnosis is almost certain [12, 41].

### 36.8.3 Spontaneous Perforation

Spontaneous perforation refers to cases without prior trauma. Perforation may be caused by a cause that disrupts the mucosal barrier, such as exposure to cancer and corrosive substances or any activity that acutely increases intraesophageal pressure. Although the majority of cases are thought to be associated with aggressive vomiting, other processes leading to this acute intraesophageal pressure may result in full-thickness disruption of the esophageal wall. Although rare, esophageal candidiasis, herpetic esophagitis, and cytomegalovirus esophagitis have been published in case reports as a source of esophageal perforation in immunosuppressive patients and those with esophageal motility disorders. Contrasting iatrogenic perforations where the stomach is empty, conservative treatment of spontaneous perforation is unlikely to be successful because of the degree of mediastinal contamination of gastrointestinal contents [12, 41, 42].

Spontaneous rupture of the esophagus is associated with a high mortality rate due to delays in diagnosis and treatment. Although there is usually a history of vomiting, in a few patients, the injury occurs silently without any previous history. When air or effusion in the pleural space is seen on a chest radiograph of a patient with esophageal perforation, the condition is often misdiagnosed as pneumothorax or pancreatitis. An elevated pleural amylase caused by the ejection of saliva from the perforation may correct the diagnosis of pancreatitis in the mind of a careless physician. If the chest X-ray is normal, a myocardial infarction or dissecting aneurysm is often mistakenly diagnosed [12, 41, 43].

A longitudinal rupture along the posterior wall of the abdominal esophagus is typical of spontaneous perforation, whereas the hypopharynx is the most damaged location in iatrogenic perforation. In the latter case, if the glottis remains closed, the pressure in the lower part of the esophagus will often equal the intragastric pressure. Cadaveric studies have shown that the esophagus is more likely to rupture when the vomit pressure exceeds 150 mmHg [44–46].

It should be kept in mind that perforations may lead to mediastinal and thoracic contamination due to the anatomy of the esophagus, as well as intra-abdominal contamination depending on the location of the perforation [2, 23].

### 36.8.4 Traumatic Perforation

Isolated esophageal injuries are rare and associated organ injuries to the vascular, pulmonary, and mediastinal structures should be expected and addressed. The possibility of esophageal perforation from blunt trauma is very rare [2, 23].

### 36.8.5 Iatrogenic Perforation

Iatrogenic perforations represent the most common etiology for esophageal perforation and can occur during an esophageal intervention such as nasogastric tube insertion or endoscopic procedures, or during a non-esophageal procedure such as incorrectly inserting an endotracheal intubation tube into the esophagus. Diagnostic flexible esophagogastroduodenoscopy (EGD) is rarely associated with esophageal perforations but predominantly occurs in the cervical esophagus and is associated with both technical and underlying anatomical problems. Intraoperative esophageal perforation can occur during any neck dissection that causes cervical esophageal injury (e.g., thyroidectomy, cervical spine treatment, carotid endarterectomy, and tracheostomy). Intrathoracic esophageal injury is most commonly associated with thoracic aortic surgery and less frequently with spinal surgery. Intra-abdominal esophageal injury is the most common and is associated with foregut or hiatus surgery [47, 48].

## 36.9 Fistulas

### 36.9.1 Carotid-Esophageal Fistulas

Carotid-esophageal fistula represents the emergency in which the perforated esophagus opens into the carotid. It usually occurs in cases of blade injury, sharp foreign body ingestion, or surgical complications [49]. Chemotherapy and radiotherapy to the neck area can also cause fistulas. The incidence of esophageal fistula in patients receiving chemoradiotherapy with esophageal cancer has been reported as 10–29% [40]. An emergency procedure is required to stop arterial bleeding. It may not be preferred, especially in patients receiving radiotherapy, since the exploration area is limited and fragile tissue increases the risk of surgery and reduces its healing ability. Instead, endovascular techniques with embolization or closed stent reconstruction have been reported to be a better alternative [50]. Sudden and pressurized blood filling into the stomach due to carotid-esophageal fistula, without adequate decompression with the nasogastric tube, it rapidly increases the pressure in the stomach and causes gastric perforation, resulting in massive perforation. Cases of hemoperitoneum and deep hypovolemic shock have been reported [51].

Compared to carotid perforation, cerebral gas embolism is a rare but clinically significant condition associated with C-E fistula. According to Bernoulli's law, gas in C-E fistula can be sucked into the carotid artery due to its high flow. The gas bubble can travel as far as the small arterioles of 30–60 μm in the intracerebral areas, break the blood–brain barrier, and cause regional brain ischemia and inflammation. Patients may exhibit headaches, limb weakness, seizures, behavioral changes, and even impaired consciousness. Hyperbaric oxygen therapy may be a treatment option if the patient's vital signs are stable [52].

Physicians must remain vigilant and perform appropriate management, including adequate decompression, fluid resuscitation, and aggressive endovascular procedures to stop bleeding [52].

### 36.9.2 Aorta-esophageal Fistulas

A patient diagnosed with cancer in the middle third of the esophagus presented with an aorto-esophageal fistula with acute upper gastrointestinal system bleeding in the follow-up after stenting with a palliative approach and radiotherapy [49, 53]. At the time of diagnosis, hypotensive, tachycardic, abdominal pain that can spread to the waist and lumbar region draws attention. Another common clinical finding is the sudden and unexplained febrile septic state resulting from direct migration of microorganisms from the intestinal lumen into the vascular system [54, 55].

Recently, more data on successful endovascular treatment has been published in the international literature. Such treatment successfully stops bleeding, but surgical correction of the gastrointestinal wall is ultimately necessary to avoid septic complications. A new method of treating thoracic aortic diseases is a minimally invasive surgical procedure called TEVAR. It is a method used in aneurysms, traumatic aortic cuts, type B dissections, ulcers, and intra-aortic intramural hematomas [56, 57].

### 36.9.3 Esophagus: Airway Fistulas

The esophagogastric anastomosis is close to the lung parenchyma and the membranous airway, which increases the risk of possible fistulation between the airway and the duct. Although such events are rare, with a reported incidence of 0.04–0.3%, they can be life-threatening and must be identified quickly [41].

Patients may initially present with mild symptoms such as coughing or more serious symptoms such as recurrent pneumonia. In the most severe cases, patients may present with mediastinitis. Clinical suspicion and early diagnosis are extremely important, as aspiration of gastric secretions into the lungs can lead to severe pneumonia and respiratory failure [4, 58].

In patients with a benign clinical presentation, conservative treatment interventions (antibiotics, not oral) may be considered; however, in severe cases where the conduit must be excised, resection is the preferred approach, and delayed reconstruction esophagostomy patient is stabilized clinically from sepsis. Malignant fistulas between the esophagus and respiratory system occur in 4.9% of patients with esophageal carcinoma worldwide [4].

Esophagorespiratory fistulas can occur spontaneously due to tumor invasion or secondary to radiation therapy, pressure necrosis caused by a previously placed plastic stent, or laser therapy. The development of aspiration symptoms in addition to dysphagia is devastating. Malignant fistulas and perforations are difficult to manage. Most untreated patients die within 1 month from malnutrition or thoracic septic shock [59–61].

## 36.10 Anastomotic Leaks and Necrosis

Necrosis and anastomotic leaks in the esophagus are among the complications that can be seen after surgery that can cause serious clinical response. If necessary, the patient should be monitored hemodynamically in the intensive care unit to follow closely for the signs of shock. Patients most commonly present with severe sepsis in the first postoperative week. Initially, there may be tachycardia or leukocytosis unexplained by rapid clinical decompensation. The most important principle in the management of such patients is high clinical suspicion [62–64].

It most commonly occurs in the thoracic esophagus but may involve the cervical and abdominal compartments. Cervical perforations are generally well tolerated because the fascia surrounding the esophagus in the neck limits the perforation. Many pharyngeal or cervical esophageal leaks resolve with antibiotics alone. If the clinical condition worsens, a neck abscess develops, or fluid enters the mediastinum, surgical treatment, including extensive drainage through a cervical incision, should be followed [62, 63, 65].

Management of intrathoracic leaks depends on the degree of sepsis. Patients with closed collections can be treated with percutaneous drainage. Patients with hemodynamic stability in the setting of sepsis should be taken to the operating room for purification and drainage. Surgical treatment in cases of uncontrolled sepsis includes debridement with possible resection in cases of necrosis and evaluation of esophageal viability. In cervical anastomosis leaks, the risk of stenosis in follow-up is high [41, 66, 67].

While the principles underlying therapy remain stable and guide decision-making, the tools in the surgeon's armory continue to evolve. The basic principles of proximal and distal closure, occlusion, externalization, or redirection of the esophageal defect, draining associated extraluminal fluid accumulations, alleviating distal esophageal obstruction, treating infection with antibiotics, and providing supportive care, including nutrition, are based on an operative, endoscopic, or noninvasive approach is followed. A treatment plan should consider not only the characteristics of the perforation, including its size and location, but also the patient's clinical status, including time from onset, extent of contamination, presence of comorbid esophageal disease, and comorbidities and performance. Whatever approach is chosen, timely and appropriate intervention clearly plays an important role in the successful resolution of this life-threatening condition [67].

The incidence of gastric conduit ischemia ranges from 0.5 to 10.4%, and this includes cases that resolve spontaneously, ranging from subclinical ischemia to overt necrosis [36]. The sequelae of conduit ischemia can be quite severe. Patients with ischemia may eventually develop a stricture or, more importantly, an anastomotic leak requiring reoperation. Conduit necrosis is the most severe degree of anastomotic leak as previously described. The mortality rate after conduit necrosis can exceed 90%, emphasizing the importance of prompt identification and treatment of this problem and prevention whenever possible [60].

## 36.11 Other Conditions That May Present with Shock

Because the esophagus is anatomically close to the trachea, heart, and descending aorta, esophageal cancer can sometimes perforate these organs or cause bleeding. In addition, metastases may bring the patient with signs of damage to various organs and tissues. In one study, a case of esophageal cancer with cervical lymph node metastasis irritated the vagus nerve, which supplies the aortic arch baroreceptors, which are closely associated with the lymph node. It caused neurogenic shock clinically accompanied by profound hypotension and bradycardia in the patient [61, 68].

## References

1. Namendys-Silva SA, González-Herrera MO, Texcocano-Becerra J, Herrera-Gómez A. Clinical characteristics, and outcomes of critically ill cancer patients with septic shock. QJM. 2011;104(6):505–11. https://doi.org/10.1093/qjmed/hcq260. Epub 2011 Jan 21
2. Brunicardi FC, et al. Chapter 5. Schwartz's principles of surgery. In: Shock. 10th ed.
3. Yoon JJ, Dreesen EB, Brownstein MR. Systemic response to trauma. In: Esther RJ, editor. Clinical foundations of musculoskeletal medicine. Cham: Springer; 2021. https://doi.org/10.1007/978-3-030-42894-5_18.
4. Mebazaa A, Combes A, van Diepen S, Hollinger A, Katz JN, Landoni G, Hajjar LA, Lassus J, Lebreton G, Montalescot G, Park JJ, Price S, Sionis A, Yannopolos D, Harjola VP, Levy B, Thiele H. Management of cardiogenic shock complicating myocardial infarction. Intensive Care Med. 2018;44(6):760–73. https://doi.org/10.1007/s00134-018-5214-9. Epub 2018 May 16.
5. Williams MD, Braun LA, Cooper LM, Johnston J, Weiss RV, Qualy RL, et al. Hospitalized cancer patients with severe sepsis. Analysis of incidence, mortality, and associated costs of care. Crit Care. 2004;8:R291–8.
6. Taccone FS, Artigas AA, Sprung CL, et al. Characteristics and outcomes of cancer patients in European ICUs. Crit Care. 2009;13:R15. https://doi.org/10.1186/cc7713.
7. Gotts JE, Matthay MA. Sepsis: pathophysiology and clinical management. BMJ. 2016;353:i1585. https://doi.org/10.1136/bmj.i1585.
8. Kinugasa S, Tachibana M, Yoshimura H, et al. Postoperative pulmonary complications are associated with worse short- and long-term outcomes after extended esophagectomy. J Surg Oncol. 2004;88:71–7.
9. Zuanazzi D, Souto R, Mattos MB, et al. Prevalence of potential bacterial respiratory pathogens in the oral cavity of hospitalised individuals. Arch Oral Biol. 2010;55:21–8.

10. Hiramatsu T, Sugiyama M, Kuwabara S, et al. Effectiveness of an outpatient preoperative care bundle in preventing postoperative pneumonia among esophageal cancer patients. Am J Infect Control. 2014;42:385–8.
11. Kassem MM, Wallen JM. Esophageal perforation and tears. In: StatPearls. Treasure Island, FL: StatPearls Publishing; 2023. https://www.ncbi.nlm.nih.gov/books/NBK532298/.
12. White RK, Morris DM. Diagnosis and management of esophageal perforations. Am Surg. 1992;58(2):112–9.
13. Evans L, Rhodes A, Alhazzani W, et al. Surviving sepsis campaign: international guidelines for management of sepsis and septic shock 2021. Intensive Care Med. 2021;47:1181–247. https://doi.org/10.1007/s00134-021-06506-y.
14. Wu JT, Mattox KL, Wall MJ Jr. Esophageal perforations: new perspectives and treatment paradigms. J Trauma Injury Infect Crit Care. 2007;63(5):1173–84. https://doi.org/10.1097/TA.0b013e31805c0dd4.
15. Salo JA, Isolauri JO, et al. Management of delayed esophageal perforation with mediastinal sepsis. Esophagectomy or primary repair? J Thorax Cardiovasc Surg. 1993;106:1088.
16. American College of Surgeons Committee on Trauma. Advanced trauma life support for doctors. 9th ed. Chicago: American College of Surgeons; 2012.
17. Subcommittee ATLS, American College of Surgeons' Committee on Trauma; International ATLS Working Group. Advanced trauma life support (ATLS®): the ninth edition. J Trauma Acute Care Surg. 2013;74(5):1363–6. https://doi.org/10.1097/TA.0b013e31828b82f5.
18. Annane D, Siami S, Jaber S, et al. Effects of fluid resuscitation with colloids vs crystalloids on mortality in critically ill patients presenting with hypovolemic shock: the CRISTAL randomized trial. JAMA. 2013;310:1809–17.
19. Dellinger RP, Levy MM, Carlet JM, et al. Surviving sepsis campaign: international guidelines for management of severe sepsis and septic shock: 2008. Crit Care Med. 2008;36:296–327.
20. Husain FA, Martin MJ, Mullenix PS, Steele SR, Elliott DC. Serum lactate and base deficit as predictors of mortality and morbidity. Am J Surg. 2003;185:485–91.
21. Gutierrez G, Reines HD, Wulf-Gutierrez ME. Clinical review: hemorrhagic shock. Crit Care. 2004;8(5):373–81. https://doi.org/10.1186/cc2851. Epub 2004 Apr 2
22. Lier H, Bernhard M, Hossfeld B. Hypovolämisch-hämorrhagischer schock. Anaesthesist. 2018;67:225–44. https://doi.org/10.1007/s00101-018-0411-z.
23. Townsend C, Beauchamp R, Evers B, Mattox K. Sabiston textbook of surgery. 20th ed.
24. Angus DC, Linde-Zwirble WT, Lidicker J, Clermont G, Carcillo J, Pinsky MR. Epidemiology of severe sepsis in the United States: analysis of incidence, outcome, and associated costs of care. Crit Care Med. 2001;29(7):1303–10.
25. Singer M, Deutschman CS, Seymour CW, et al. The third international consensus definitions for sepsis and septic shock (Sepsis-3). JAMA. 2016;315(8):801–10. https://doi.org/10.1001/jama.2016.0287.
26. Kalkwarf KJ, Cotton BA. Resuscitation for hypovolemic shock. Surg Clin North Am. 2017;97(6):1307–21. https://doi.org/10.1016/j.suc.2017.07.011.
27. Kashuk JL, et al. Postinjury life threatening coagulopathy: is 1:1 fresh frozen plasma:packed red blood cells the answer? J Trauma. 2008;65:261–70; discussion 270–271.
28. Moore EE, Moore HB, Kornblith LZ, Neal MD, Hoffman M, Mutch NJ, Schöchl H, Hunt BJ, Sauaia A. Trauma-induced coagulopathy. Nat Rev Dis Primers. 2021;7(1):30. https://doi.org/10.1038/s41572-021-00264-3. Erratum in: Nat Rev Dis Primers. 2022 Apr 22;8(1):25.
29. Hofer S, Schlimp CJ, Casu S, Grouzi E. Management of Coagulopathy in bleeding patients. J Clin Med. 2022;11(1):1. https://doi.org/10.3390/jcm11010001.
30. Inaba K, Teixeira PG, Rhee P, et al. Mortality impact of hypothermia after Cavitary explorations in trauma. World J Surg. 2009;33:864–9.
31. Kutcher ME, et al. Evolving beyond the vicious triad: differential mediation of traumatic coagulopathy by injury, shock, and resuscitation. J Trauma Acute Care Surg. 2015;78:516–23.
32. Maegele M, et al. Early coagulopathy in multiple injury: an analysis from the German trauma registry on 8724 patients. Injury. 2007;38:298–304.

33. CRASH-2 Trial Collaborators. Effects of tranexamic acid on death, vascular occlusive events, and blood transfusion in trauma patients with significant haemorrhage (CRASH-2): a randomised, placebocontrolled trial. Lancet. 2010;376:23–32.
34. Morrison JJ, Dubose JJ, Rasmussen TE, Midwinter MJ. Military application of tranexamic acid in trauma emergency resuscitation (MATTERs) study. Arch Surg. 2012;147:113–9.
35. Moore EE, et al. Rationale for the selective administration of tranexamic acid to inhibit fibrinolysis in the severely injured patient. Transfusion. 2016;56:S110–4.
36. Fleischmann-Struzek C, Mellhammar L, Rose N, et al. Incidence and mortality of hospital- and ICU-treated sepsis: results from an updated and expanded systematic review and meta-analysis. Intensive Care Med. 2020;46(8):1552–62.
37. Rhee C, Dantes R, Epstein L, et al. Incidence and trends of sepsis in US hospitals using clinical vs claims data, 2009–2014. JAMA. 2017;318(13):1241–9.
38. Gyawali B, Ramakrishna K, Dhamoon AS. Sepsis: the evolution in definition, pathophysiology, and management. SAGE Open Med. 2019;7:2050312119835043.
39. Egi M, Ogura H, Yatabe T, Atagi K, Inoue S, Iba T, Kakihana Y, et al. The Japanese clinical practice guidelines for management of sepsis and septic shock 2020 (J-SSCG 2020). J Intensive Care. 2021;9(1):1–144.
40. Kawakami T, Tsushima T, Omae K, et al. Risk factors for esophageal fistula in thoracic esophageal squamous cell carcinoma invading adjacent organs treated with definitive chemoradiotherapy: a monocentric case-control study. BMC Cancer. 2018;18:e573. https://doi.org/10.1186/s12885-018-4486-3.
41. Lerut T, Coosemans W, Decker G, et al. Anastomotic complications after esophagectomy. Dig Surg. 2002;19:92–8.
42. Hardwick RH. Oesophageal emergencies. Medicine. 2015;43(3):157–60. https://doi.org/10.1016/j.mpmed.2014.12.001.
43. Blencowe NS, Strong S, Hollowood AD. Spontaneous oesophageal rupture." BMJ. 2013:346.
44. Kassem MM, Wallen JM. Esophageal perforation, rupture, and tears. In: StatPearls. Treasure Island, FL: StatPearls Publishing; 2019.
45. Yeo CJ. Shackelford's surgery of the alimentary tract, 2 volume set. 8th ed. Philadelphia: Elsevier; 2018.
46. Bryant AS, Cerfolio RJ. Esophageal trauma. Thorac Surg Clin. 2007;17(1):63–72.
47. Kaman L, Iqbal J, Kundil B, Kochhar R. Management of Esophageal Perforation in adults. Gastroenterology Res. 2010;3(6):235–44. https://doi.org/10.4021/gr263w. Epub 2010 Nov 20
48. Brinster CJ, Singhal S, Lee L, Marshall MB, Kaiser LR, Kucharczuk JC. Evolving options in the management of esophageal perforation. Ann Thorac Surg. 2004;77:1465–83.
49. Hollander JE, Quick G. Aortoesophageal fistula: a comprehensive review of the literature. Am J Med. 1991;91:279–87. https://doi.org/10.1016/0002-9343(91)90129-l.
50. Wormald JCR, Dindyal S, Thomas R, Peters CJ, Sritharan K. Aorto-esophageal fistula: the multi-disciplinary team approach to management. Clin Case Rep. 2016;4:800–2. https://doi.org/10.1002/ccr3.631.
51. Guerrero I, et al. Hemorrhagic shock secondary to aortoesophageal fistula as a complication of esophageal cancer. Cureus. 2020;12(2):e7146. https://doi.org/10.7759/cureus.7146.
52. Sivaraman SK, Drummond R. Radiation-induced aortoesophageal fistula: an unusual case of massive upper gastrointestinal bleeding. J Emerg Med. 2002;23:175–8. https://doi.org/10.1016/s0736-4679(02)00488-2.
53. Ćeranić D, Nikolić S, Lučev J, et al. Fatal bleeding due to an aorto-esophageal fistula: a case report and literature review. World J Clin Cases. 2022;10(31):11493–9.
54. Cendan JC, Thomas JB 4th, Seeger JM. Twenty-one cases of aortoenteric fistula: lessons for the general surgeon. Am Surg. 2004;70:583-7; discussion 587.
55. Hsu WF, Lin CC, Chang KM, Lee TH. Primary aortoesophageal fistula: a rare but fatal cause of upper gastrointestinal bleeding. J Dig Dis. 2013;14:676–8. https://doi.org/10.1111/1751-2980.12070.
56. Lee S, Srinivasa N, R, A Rigberg D, Yanagawa J, Benharash P, M Moriarty J. Aortoesophageal fistula involving the central aortic arch salvaged with emergent percutaneous TEVAR, great

vessel coverage and in vivo graft fenestration. Diagn Interv Radiol. 2021;27:122–5. https://doi.org/10.5152/dir.2020.20033.
57. Ćeranić D, Nikolić S, Lučev J, Slanič A, Bujas T, Ocepek A, Skok P. Fatal bleeding due to an aorto-esophageal fistula: a case report and literature review. World J Clin Cases. 2022;10(31):11493.
58. Tsuchihashi K, Yoshihiro T, Aikawa T, et al. Metastatic esophageal cancer presenting as shock by injury of vagus nerve mimicking baroreceptor reflex. Medicine (Baltimore). 2017;96(49):e8987.
59. Wright CD, Mathisen DJ, Wain JC. Reinforced primary repair of thoracic esophageal perforation. Ann Thorac Surg. 1995;60:245–8.
60. Martini N, Goodner JL, D'Angio GJ, Beattie EJ. Tracheoesophageal fistula due to cancer. J Cardiovasc Sung. 1970;59:319–24.
61. Burt M, Diehl W, Martini N, et al. Malignant esophagorespiratory fistula: management options and survival. Ann Thorac Surg. 1991;52:1222–9.
62. Cassivi SD. Leaks, strictures, and necrosis: a review of anastomotic complications following esophagectomy. Semin Thorac Cardiovasc Surg. 2004;16:124–32.
63. Messager M, Warlaumont M, Renaud F, et al. Recent improvements in management of esophageal anastomotic leak after surgery for cancer. Eur J Surg Oncol. 2017;43:258–69.
64. Freeman RK, Ascioti AJ, Giannini T, Mahidhara RJ. Analysis of unsuccessful esophageal stent placements for esophageal perforation, fistula, or anastomotic leak. Ann Thorac Surg. 2012;94(3):959–65.
65. Minnich DJ, Yu P, Bryant AS, Jarrar D, Cerfolio RJ. Management of thoracic esophageal perforations. Eur J Cardiothorac Surg. 2011;40:931–7.
66. Dickinson KJ, Blackmon SH. Management of conduit necrosis following esophagectomy. Thorac Surg Clin. 2015;25:461–70.
67. Meyerson SL, Mehta CK. Managing complications II: conduit failure and conduit airway fistulas. J Thorac Dis. 2014;6:S364–71.
68. Han J, Wang Z, Liu C. Survival and complications after neoadjuvant chemotherapy or chemoradiotherapy for esophageal cancer: a meta-analysis. Future Oncol. 2021;17(17):2257–74. https://doi.org/10.2217/fon-2021-0021. Epub 2021 Mar 19.

# 37 Histopathology of Esophageal Carcinoma

Pinar Atasoy and Sibel Sensu

Squamous cell carcinoma is the most common esophageal carcinoma worldwide. The remaining group mostly consists of adenocarcinomas, the numbers of which have been increasing in the last few decades. Rarely, adenosquamous carcinomas and small cell carcinomas of the esophagus may also develop [1].

In this section, the histopathological features of preneoplastic and neoplastic epithelial tumors of the esophagus will be explained. The two main preneoplastic (precursor) lesions of the esophagus are Barret's dysplasia and squamous dysplasia. In the last decade, there has been a transition from surgery to ablation in the management of Barrett's esophagus cases with high-grade dysplasia [2]. In cases with low-grade dysplasia, there is still no consensus on the treatment. Therefore, Barret's dysplasia is currently classified into two groups as low grade and high grade. Today, we have a lot of information about the molecular pathways of Barret's esophagus and its precursor lesions and their pathological characteristics in carcinogenesis. There is much more knowledge about the pathological and clinical features and biological behaviors of the most frequently detected Barret dysplasias (intestinal and foveolar type) than in the past decade. Unfortunately, it is still difficult to distinguish Barret's esophagus with dysplasia from non-neoplastic regenerative lesions [2].

There is no definite consensus on the definition of Barret's esophagus. Namely, while the condition of goblet cells is required for diagnosis in the United States, this condition is not required in Asian and European countries. Adenocarcinomas of the esophagus and the esophagogastric junction are evaluated together in the new WHO classification) (Table 37.1) [2]. The reason is the similarities in etiologial, histological, and biological characteristics of these tumors [2].

P. Atasoy (✉) · S. Sensu
Pathology Department, Medicine Faculty, Istinye University, İstanbul, Turkey
e-mail: pinar.atasoy@istinye.edu.tr; sibel.sensu@istinye.edu.tr


O. Engin (ed.), *Risk Factors and Therapy of Esophagus Cancer*,
https://doi.org/10.1007/978-3-031-47024-0_37

**Table 37.1** WHO classification of tumors of the esophagus

| | |
|---|---|
| **Benign epithelial tumors and precursors** | |
| 8052/0 | Squamous cell papilloma NOS |
| 8060/0 | Squamous cell papillomatosis |
| 8148/0 | Esophageal glandular dysplasia (intraepithelial neoplasia), low grade |
| 8148/2 | Esophageal glandular dysplasia (intraepithelial neoplasia), high grade |
| 8077/0 | Esophageal squamous intraepithelial neoplasia (dysplasia), low grade |
| 8077/2 | Esophageal squamous intraepithelial neoplasia (dysplasia), high grade |
| **Malignant epithelial tumors** | |
| 8140/3 | Adenocarcinoma NOS |
| 8200/3 | Adenoid cystic ca |
| 8430/3 | Mucoepidermoid ca |
| 8070/3 | Squamous cell carcinoma NOS |
| 8051/3 | Verrucous SCC |
| 8074/3 | SCC, spindle cell |
| 8083/3 | Basaloid SCC |
| 8020/3 | Carcinoma, undifferentiated NOS |
| 8082/3 | Lymphoepithelioma-like ca |
| 8240/3 | Neuroendocrine tumor NOS |
| 8240/3 | NET, Grade 1 |
| 8249/3 | NET, Grade 2 |
| 8249/3 | NET, Grade 3 |
| 8246/3 | Neuroendocrine carcinoma NOS |
| 8013/3 | Large-cell NEC |
| 8041/3 | Small-cell NEC |
| 8154/3 | MiNEN |
| 8045/3 | Combined small-cell adenocarcinoma |
| 8045/3 | Combined small-cell SCC |

*SCC* squamous cell carcinoma; *MiNEN* mixed nonneuroendocrine-neuroendocrine tumor; *NEC* neuroendocrine carcinoma, *NET* neuroendocrine tumor; *ca* carcinoma

## 37.1 Precursor Lesions

### 37.1.1 Barret's Esophagus and Dysplasias

Barret's esophagus is the most important risk factor in the development of adenocarcinoma. Esophageal adenocarcinomas may rarely develop from heterotopic gastric mucosa or submucosal glands [1]. The morphology of these tumors is indistinguishable from adenocarcinomas in Barrett's background.

Barret's esophagus is defined as the transformation of normal esophageal epithelium to metaplastic columnar epithelium [1–3]. This metaplastic transformation usually occurs in response to reflux of acidic gastric contents. It is still controversial whether Barret's esophagus is congenital or acquired because the precise definition of the gastro-esophageal junction is unclear, and there are microscopic variations. However, many clinical and experimental studies support that this change is an acquired pathology that results from the re-epithelialization of the ulcerated mucosa due to the acid effect [4].

The squamous epithelium first transforms into cardiac-type columnar epithelium that does not contain goblet cells. Although the origin of columnar cells is not known for certain, there are various theories. These cells may have migrated to the metaplastic area from the gastric mucosa, may have developed from the stem cells found here, or may have originated from the submucosal gland [5–7]. This process is followed by goblet cell metaplasia and ends with the development of dysplasia. Intestinal metaplasia containing goblet cells is important for the development of adenocarcinoma [1]. However, it has been reported that both dysplasia and invasive carcinomas can develop from cell clones that do not contain goblet cells and that this change may even occur in cases of short-segment columnar metaplasia. The accumulation of multiple genetic and epigenetic changes is extremely important in the development and progression of dysplasia [8, 9].

In the definition of "The American College of Gastroenterology," a mucosal change consistent with Barrett detected on endoscopy should also be confirmed in endoscopic biopsy [10]. According to the British school, intestinal metaplasia is not required for the diagnosis of Barrett's esophagus. In this school, it is thought that the esophageal mucosa lined with columnar epithelium should be evaluated in favor of Barret's esophagus on the support of endoscopic findings, since intestinal-type epithelium may not be found in all biopsies depending on sampling [11]. Another finding supporting this view is the presence of immunophenotypic and flow cytometric abnormalities similar to those in intestinal metaplasia in columnar cells without goblet [12].

Another controversial issue is "intestinal metaplasia at the gastroesophageal junction". While researchers suggest that all intestinal metaplasia in this region should be considered as Barrett's esophagus [13, 14], others state that these lesions may have a multifactorial origin, therefore they should be considered as "intestinal metaplasia of the junction" [15]. Although immunohistochemical markers (CDX2, Das1, CK7/20) were defined to distinguish whether intestinal metaplasia in this region is from the esophagus or the proximal stomach, none of them were found to be sufficiently sensitive and specific [15]. The presence of glandular structures showing intestinal metaplasia under the squamous epithelium, the presence of hybrid glands, and esophageal glands/ducts may be a clue in the differentiation of the two entities [16]. Another interesting feature detected in Barret's esophagus is the presence of a newly developed muscle layer on the surface of the muscularis mucosa. This finding, also called "re-duplication," causes the lamina propria to appear to be divided into two layers, superficial and deep [17, 18]. This finding has clinical significance. Tumor invasions in the area of re-duplication can be confused with invasion of the deeper muscularis propria, leading to over-reporting of tumor stage.

Barrett's esophagus is also divided into two groups, the long segment (the classical form and describes endoscopic changes covering an area of at least 3 cm) and the short segment (changes occupying less than 3 cm). Similar follow-up is applied in both groups [3].

About 5% of patients with esophageal mucosa lined with columnar epithelium may develop low- or high-grade dysplasia. Low-grade dysplasia may remain the same, regress, or develop into high-grade dysplasia or adenocarcinoma. High-grade dysplasia may also regress to low-grade dysplasia, but 30–50% of cases transform into invasive carcinoma within an average of 4 years [19–21]. In some cases, it is almost impossible to distinguish reactive atypia due to inflammation from true dysplasia. These cases are included in the "indefinite for dysplasia" group in the Vienna classification used in dysplasia grading [1, 22].

### 37.1.2 Macroscopy

The columnar epithelium in the esophagus is velvety red. Columnar epithelium may surround the mucosa or may appear as finger-like islands. Dysplastic epithelium is usually endoscopically normal, although granularity, plaques, or erosions may sometimes be present [1].

### 37.1.3 Microscopy

#### 37.1.3.1 Diagnostic Criteria in Barret's Esophagus

Most of the cases diagnosed with Barret's esophagus do not have dysplasia, but when it does occur, it is an important risk factor for adenocarcinoma [23]. The criteria for the Vienna classification were determined for the first time in 1988 and revised by Montgomery et al. in 2001 (Table 37.2) [3].

1. **Negative for Dysplasia**

   The mucosal roof is preserved. The shape-size difference is not evident in the nuclei and is localized at the base. The nucleo-cytoplasmic ratio is not increased, the nuclear contours are regular, and the nucleoli are not prominent. Focal nuclear layering is acceptable, and dystrophic goblet cells not in contact with the

**Table 37.2** Vienna classification for the grading of dysplasia

| |
|---|
| Negative for neoplasia or dysplasia |
| Indefinite for neoplasia or dysplasia |
| Noninvasive low-grade neoplasia (low-grade adenoma or dysplasia) |
| Noninvasive high-grade neoplasia |
| High-grade adenoma or dysplasia |
| Noninvasive ca (carcinoma in situ) |
| Suspicion for invasive ca |
| Invasive neoplasia |
| Intramucosal ca |
| Submucosal ca or deeper |

*ca* carcinoma

lumen can be found in the apical region (Fig. 37.1). If there are signs of inflammation, ulceration, and erosion, some nuclear atypia can be accepted [3].

2. **"Indefinite for Dysplasia"**

   The mucosal roof is moderately impaired. Nuclear abnormalities are not as pronounced as dysplasia. Excess dystrophic goblet cells, diffuse nuclear stratification, decreased/absent mucin production, increased cytoplasmic basophilia, and increased mitotic activity are the main morphological features. This diagnosis should be kept as limited as possible; should be used in patients with insufficient evidence for the diagnosis of dysplasia, if possible [3].

3. **Dysplasia (Low and High Grade)**

   Structural changes in the dysplastic epithelium are villus-like structure formation on the surface, crowding, or budding in the glands. Foveolar (gastric/non-intestinal type) and intestinal-type dysplasia are the two most common dysplasias [24]. Coexistence of these two types is also not uncommon. Although the grading system suggested by Reid can be used, the grading system preferred by pathologists today is the Vienna classification [22, 25].

   (a) *Intestinal Dysplasia*

      In intestinal dysplasia, goblet cells, and enterocyte-like cells and columnar cells coexist.

      - Low-grade intestinal dysplasia may have cytological atypia but no or minimal structural abnormality. Elongation, nuclear growth, hyperchromasia, and stratification are seen in epithelial cells. Stratification is limited to the basal region of the cytoplasm. The number of goblet cells is variable and decreases as the degree of dysplasia increases (Fig. 37.2) [2].
      - Cytological atypia is more common in high-grade intestinal dysplasia and is accompanied by structural abnormalities. The nuclei are three to four times larger than the normal lymphocyte and are stratified from the basal to the surface, covering the entire layer. Nuclei have significant pleomorphism, irregular contours, and loss of polarity. Mitotic activity is increased in the surface epithelium and atypical mitoses are common. Shape/size variation, budding, back-to-back glands, and cribriform appearance are not uncommon in crypts (Fig. 37.3). The presence of either high-grade

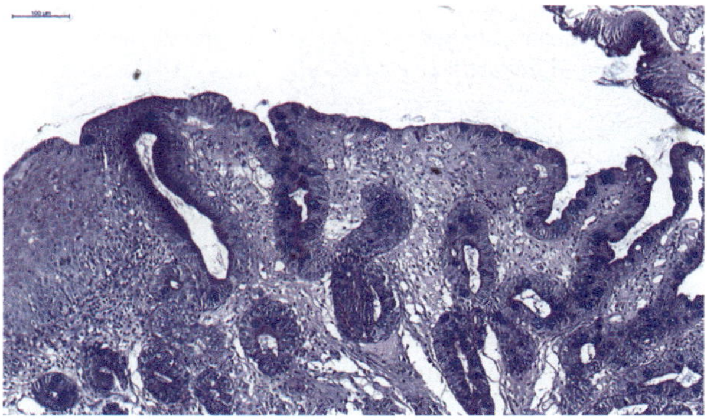

**Fig. 37.1** Barret's esophagus: Goblet cells are observed between columnar epithelial cells (D-PAS/AB; ×100)

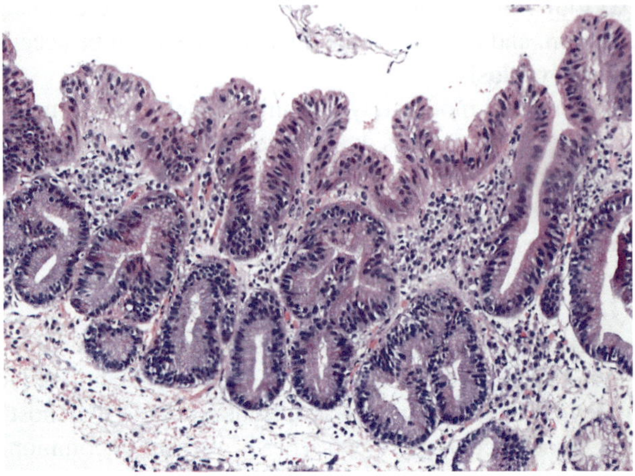

**Fig. 37.2** Low-grade, intestinal-type dysplasia: Single glands that have elongated, enlarged, hyperchromatic cells with mild proliferation. Mitotic activity is increased and superficial maturation is lost (H-E; ×100)

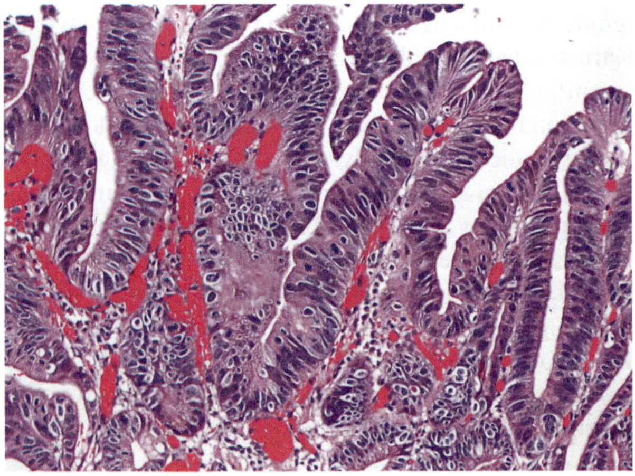

**Fig. 37.3** High-grade, intestinal-type dysplasia. Highly enlarged, compact glands lined by cells with oval-elongated hyperchromatic nuclei, prominent nucleoli. Full-thickness cellular stratification, increased mitotic activity, loss of polarity, and pleomorphism are observed (H-E; ×100)

cytological or structural findings is sufficient for the diagnosis of high-grade dysplasia, but usually both are combined [2, 3].

(b) *Foveolar (non-intestinal) dysplasia:*

- *In low-grade foveolar dysplasia*, the number of goblet cells is low, but a distinctive mucinous appearance in the cytoplasm is the characteristic finding. Usually single-row, fairly uniform columnar cells are present. Cells are small or slightly enlarged, round-oval and localized basally. No increase in stratification or pleomorphism is observed. In most cases,

cytological atypia is low grade, but rarely, high-grade cytological changes can be detected [2].
- *In high-grade foveolar dysplasia*, the nucleocytoplasmic ratio is markedly increased, the nuclear contours are irregular, the chromatin pattern is clear, and there are prominent nucleoli and increased mitotic activity [19]. Foveolar dysplasia may develop in metaplastic columnar mucosa that does not contain goblet cells. When dysplasia is found to be limited to the crypt baseline at an early stage, it can also be called "crypt dysplasia" [26].

4. **Intramucosal Adenocarcinoma**

**This definition is used for carcinomas that exceed the gland basement membrane and infiltrate the lamina propria or penetrate the muscularis mucosa. In mucosal biopsies, mostly submucosal invasion cannot be evaluated properly. Glands back to back without leaving any stroma, infiltration of individual or small tumor cell groups in the lamina propria, and the presence of atypical glands containing luminal necrosis can be evaluated as strong clues in terms of invasion [3].**

## 37.2 Squamous Dysplasia of the Esophagus

Neoplastic changes in the squamous epithelium of the esophagus without invasion is called esophageal squamous dysplasia. It is observed that the frequency of this diagnosis increases in regions where the incidence of esophageal squamous cell carcinoma is high [3, 27]. While squamous dysplasia can be encountered alone in the esophagus, the lesion is seen adjacent to an invasive carcinoma in approximately one third of the cases. It has been reported that the incidence is higher in patients who have not received radiotherapy before and whose main lesion is superficial [28]. Sometimes it is seen that the dysplastic lesion is anatomically separate from the main tumor. It has been found that the dysplastic change can progress toward the submucosal gland ducts, extend to the submucosal glands, and in some cases, the dysplastic cells show a pagetoid spread pattern [3]. Studies on pathogenesis have reported p53 overexpression and CDKN2A (P16INK4a) hypermethylation in some cases [29].

The terms intramucosal carcinoma (in cases where the carcinoma cells do not extend beyond the muscularis mucosa), superficial (or microinvasive) carcinoma, (in cases where the invasive squamous tumor does not exceed the submucosa), and superficial spreading carcinoma (in the presence of a tumor with a lateral intramucosal spread up to at least 2 cm beyond the invasive lesion) are also used [3, 30].

In ICD-0 coding; it is named as esophageal squamous intraepithelial dysplasia (as low/high grade). In ICD-11 coding; esophageal squamous dysplasia is separated as esophageal squamous intraepithelial neoplasia (dysplasia) (low grade) and esophageal carcinoma in situ and esophageal squamous intraepithelial neoplasia (dysplasia) (high grade) [27].

### 37.2.1 Macroscopy

Squamous dysplasia can be seen anywhere in the esophagus as a small, superficial, erythematous area or as a flat or nodular lesion, and sometimes the mucosa appears completely normal [1, 26].

Superficial carcinomas can be divided into squamous, rough, verrucous, polypoid, and ulcerated infiltrating patterns. Those who are more polypoid are more likely to invade the submucosa and metastasize to the lymph node. While lymph node metastasis is not expected in intramucosal carcinomas, lymph node involvement was detected in 20–50% of cases with submucosal invasion. There is a relationship between the depth of submucosal invasion and the risk of nodal metastasis [3, 31–33].

### 37.2.2 Microscopy

Cellular and architectural changes are found in cases of squamous dysplasia. At the cellular level, enlargement of nuclei, increase in nucleus/cytoplasm ratio, pleomorphism, hyperchromasia, loss of polarity, and overlapping of cells are remarkable. The presence of abnormal epithelial maturation is an indicator of architectural atypia [1, 27, 34] (Fig. 37.4).

Grade determination in squamous dysplasia is a controversial issue, and two grading systems are currently recommended. In the triple system, cases are graded as mild, moderate, and severe. On the other hand, in the WHO Tumor Classification, it is recommended to use the dual system in which cases are divided into low and high grade. Accordingly, regardless of the extent of epithelial involvement, cases involving the lower one-half of the esophageal epithelium and showing mild cytological atypia are considered low grade, while cases involving more than one-half of the epithelium and severe cytological atypia are considered high grade [27, 35]. High-grade dysplasia cases also include cases called "carcinoma in situ" in Japan and some Asian countries [54]. Balloon cytology and brush cytology methods of the

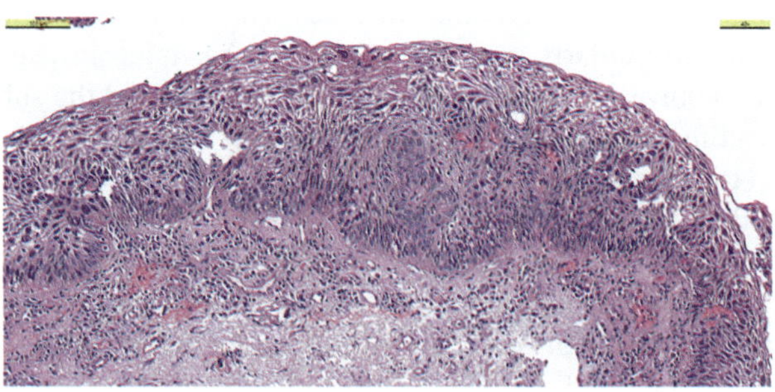

**Fig. 37.4** Intraepithelial squamous dysplasia; polarity loss and overlapping in squamous epithelium. Nucleomegaly, increase in nuclear/cytoplasmic ratio, pleomorphism, and hyperchromasia are seen in cells (H-E; ×40)

esophagus are recommended for the early detection of squamous dysplasia. During this cytological examination, the size of squamous cell nuclei is taken into account [27, 36].

It can be difficult to distinguish squamous dysplasia from a variety of benign reactive squamous lesions. In the esophagus, the normal squamous epithelium consists of regularly maturing stratified squamous cells with extensive clear eosinophilic cytoplasm. As in cases of reflux esophagitis, changes such as basal cell hyperplasia, thickening of the basal zone, and elongation of the lamina propria papillae are noted in reactive changes [35].

## 37.3 Malignant Epithelial Tumors of Esophagus

### 37.3.1 Invasive Adenocarcinoma

The majority of invasive cancers arising from the Barrett esophageal floor are adenocarcinomas. Findings suggesting that these tumors develop from Barret's mucosa are the presence of goblet cells adjacent to the neoplasia and the tumor center being on the esophageal side of the gastro-esophageal junction. These tumors may be multicentric and are usually in advanced stages at the time of diagnosis. They have infiltrated the stomach wall and invaded the lymph nodes. Tumors developing in this region are structurally and immunohistochemically similar to intestinal-type adenocarcinomas seen in the stomach. Signet ring cell carcinomas are rare in this region, but they are more aggressive than those in the stomach [1–3].

#### 37.3.1.1 Pathogenesis

In response to the damaging effect of acid or bile reflux, stem cells located at the base of the gastroesophageal epithelium are reprogrammed into columnar cells and are called "columnar cell change" [37, 38]. Over time, this epithelium can evolve in two different directions. In the first pathway, there may be differentiation in the direction of parietal or principal cells in the proximal gastric mucosa. In the second pathway, there may be transformation into goblet and Paneth cells [38]. Barret's esophagus develops from the intestinal tract containing goblet cells. Recent studies have shown that intestinal metaplasia is always present in the early stages of Barret's neoplasia [39]. Genetic and epigenetic changes in Barret's esophagus lead to dysplasia on metaplastic background. It is also important in the transformation from dysplasia to adenocarcinoma [40–42]. Currently, there is no defined specific biomarker to detect dysplasia and predict the progression of dysplasia to carcinoma.

#### 37.3.1.2 Macroscopy

It may be in the form of a small nodular lesion in the early stage and may not be detected endoscopically in this period. Pale salmon colored mucosa with irregular tongue extension adjacent to carcinoma represents Barret's esophagus. The majority of invasive adenocarcinomas are usually diagnosed in advanced stages as ulcerated and infiltrative lesions. Only 10–15% of cases exhibit exophytic growth.

Papillary carcinomas or diffuse infiltrating adenocarcinomas like linitis plastica can also be seen rarely [2, 43].

Adenocarcinomas, which are usually diagnosed in advanced stages, may show different macroscopic features. These are in the form of stricture formation, polypoid development, ulcerative or diffuse infiltrative growth pattern [44]. The cut surface is gray-white and there are masses that infiltrate a part of the muscular layer, and some invade the surrounding soft tissues and trachea. Tumors with predominant intraluminal growth may obstruct the lumen, leading to total obstruction. Tumors localized distally usually infiltrate the stomach [45].

#### 37.3.1.3 Microscopy

These features of esophageal adenocarcinomas, which may be of gastric, intestinal, or hybrid origin, are also shown morphologically and immunohistochemically [46, 47]. Barret's dysplasia can be detected in the mucosa adjacent to adenocarcinoma. There are subtypes of esophageal adenocarcinomas that have no clinical significance: tubular, papillary, mucinous, and signet ring cell. These subtypes may coexist at different rates in tumors. The most common proliferation pattern is tubular type [2].

Adenocarcinomas are graded according to the triple grading system according to the AJCC (American Joint Committee on Cancer) classification. If more than 95% of the tumor is formed of well-developed glands, it is grade 1 (well-differentiated), and if 50% to 95% of the tumor is glandular, it is grade 2 (moderately differentiated). If the gland formation rate is below 50%, it is considered as grade 3 (poorly differentiated) [48]. (Fig. 37.5). If large extracellular mucin pools are formed in the tumor, it is called "mucinous adenocarcinoma". Signet ring cell carcinomas are rare and very difficult to detect in frozen sections and macroscopically. Helpful clues to distinguish signet ring tumor cells from histiocytes and lymphocytes are tumor cells forming nests, cytoplasmic mucin vacuoles, and nuclear hyperchromasia [49] (Fig. 37.6).

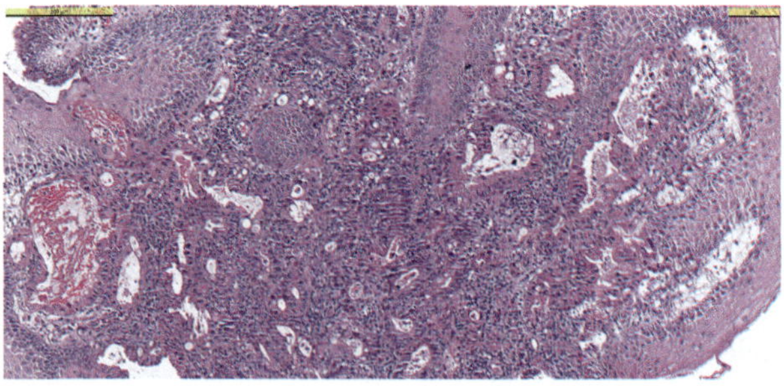

**Fig. 37.5** Moderately differentiated adenocarcinoma forming focal gland-like structures under the squamous epithelium of the esophagus (H-E; ×40)

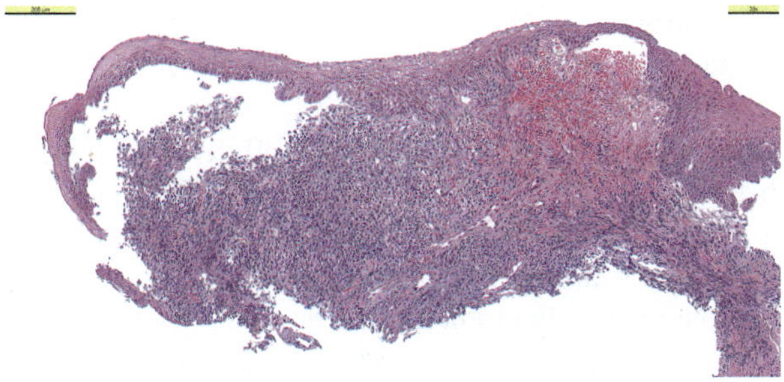

**Fig. 37.6** Signet ring cell carcinoma; Single malignant cell infiltration without forming any organization under the squamous epithelium (H-E; ×20)

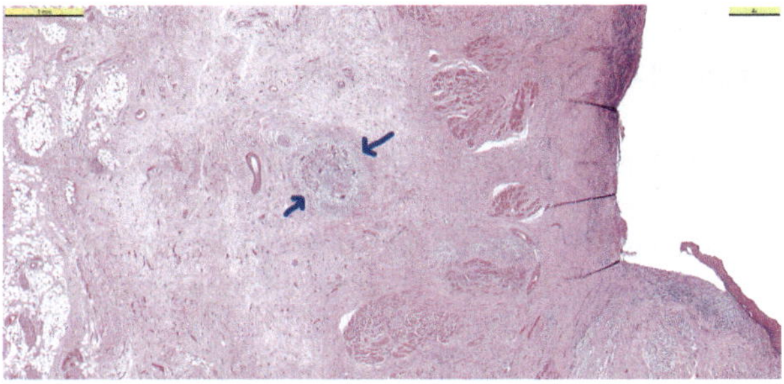

**Fig. 37.7** Due to the treatment effect, ulceration on the surface, fibrosis surrounding the muscle fibers in the deep tissues and foreign body reaction in a focal focus are observed (H-E; ×4). Blue arrows: Foreign body reactions

### 37.3.1.4 Prognosis

The most important parameter determining the prognosis in esophageal adenocarcinomas is the pathological stage. Other pathological factors are various histological parameters such as tumor size, grade, lymphovascular invasion, perineural invasion and tumor budding, and tumor subtype. Treatment-related parameters are the type of resection and the condition of the surgical margins. Another parameter that has become very important today is the response of the tumor to neoadjuvant therapy. As a result of the widespread use of chemoradiotherapy before surgery in many patients, the therapeutic effect is frequently observed in resection specimens [1]. Pathological findings observed in response to treatment are ulceration, inflammation, fibrosis, and calcifications (Fig. 37.7). Viable tumor cells may persist in small groups and may even have significant atypia due to the treatment effect. Sometimes, it may be necessary to perform immunohistochemical examination to detect viable tumor cells. In a regressed squamous cell carcinoma, only keratinous material containing foreign body reactions can be seen. In a treated adenocarcinoma, mucin pools can be observed in large areas [1]. "tumor regression grade" (TRG) is frequently used to determine the response of the tumor to treatment [50]. Basically, the Mandard system is used, which analyzes the ratio of residual tumor to fibrosis by dividing it into five groups [51, 52] (Table 37.3). In addition, the Beckery system, which evaluates changes in four stages in terms of ease of use, is also preferred by some pathologists [51].

Adenocarcinomas developing on the basis of Barret's esophagus have a poor prognosis, with a 5-year survival rate of less than 20% [55]. As in many tumors, the most important prognostic parameter is the tumor stage (Table 37.4) [2]. Depth of invasion and lymph node involvement are particularly important [53–57]. Tumor regression after neoadjuvant chemotherapy is also a strong prognostic marker [58].

Other potential prognostic parameters are lymphatic density increase, extracapsular lymph node involvement, HER2 amplification, and abnormal β-catenin expression [59]. There may be intraepithelial spread through submucosal glands or ducts, such as breast tumors [60].

## 37.4 Differential Diagnosis

One of the most important differential diagnoses, especially in mucosal biopsies, is "atypical regenerative atypia" [61]. In some squamous cell carcinomas, intercellular acantholysis is prominent and may mimic adenocarcinoma. True glandular and/or mucus-producing component can also be detected in approximately 20% of cases and are called adenosquamous carcinomas [62].

It may be difficult to differentiate the esphageal adenocarcinomas from the gastric adenocarcinomas. If the center of the tumor is more than 2 cm from the junction and does not involve the junction, it should be considered as a gastric tumor [49].

### 37.4.1 Squamous Cell Carcinoma NOS

Squamous cell carcinoma of the esophagus (SCC) is a malignant epithelial neoplasia with squamous cell differentiation. Approximately 50–60% of cases are located in the middle third of the esophagus. About 30% are in the lower third and 10–20% are in the upper third of the esophagus. SCCs are classified as superficial (early) and advanced tumors, and the cases diagnosed in the superficial stage are increasing thanks to screening programs in high-risk populations. Although most of the

**Table 37.3** Mandard and Becker system for tumor regression rate [53, 54]

| Mandard system | Becker system |
|---|---|
| TRG 1: Residual cancer is absent; fibrosis is extending through various layers of the esophageal wall (complete regression) | TRG 1a: No cancer is present |
| TRG 2: Rare residual cancer is present which is scattered through the fibrosis | TRG 1b: Less than 10% cancer is present |
| TRG 3: An increase is present in the number of residual cancer cells; both fibrosis is still dominant | TRG 2: 10–50% cancer is present |
| TRG 4: Residual cancer is more than fibrosis | TRG 3: More than 50% cancer is present |
| TRG 5: Regressive changes are absent | |

**Table 37.4** TNM staging for esophagus tumors

| | |
|---|---|
| **T: Primary tumor** | |
| Tx | Can not be assessed |
| T0 | No evidence of primary tumor |
| Tis | High grade dysplasia (malignant cells are confined to the basement membrane) |
| T1 | Invasion of the lamina propria, muscularis mucosa, or submucosa |
| T1a | Invasion of the lamina propria/muscularis mucosa |
| T1b | Invasion of the submucosa |
| T2 | Invasion of the muscularis propria |
| T3 | Invasion of the adventitia |
| T4 | Invasion of the adjacent structures |
| T4a | Invasion of the pleura, pericardium, diaphragm, azygos vein, or peritoneum |
| T4b | Invasion of the other adjacent structures (aorta, trachea, vertebral body, etc.) |
| **N: Regional lymph nodes** | |
| NX | Cannot be assessed |
| N0 | No metastasis |
| N1 | Metastasis in 1 or 2 lymph nodes |
| N2 | Metastasis in 3–6 lymph nodes |
| N3 | Metastasis in ≥7 lymph nodes |
| **M: Distant metastasis** | |
| M0 | None |
| M1 | Distant metastasis |

Note: pM0 and pMX are not valid categories

esophageal SCCs belong to the NOS group, there are also subtypes such as verrucous carcinoma, spindle cell SCC, and basaloid SCC [3].

#### 37.4.1.1 Pathogenesis

Histologically, SCC of the esophagus develops as a gradual transformation of a normal squamous mucosa, first into low-grade and then high-grade intraepithelial neoplasia, and finally, the emergence of invasive SCC in this area. The TP53 mutation is thought to be the main driver of mutation in this transformation [27]. During the period of intraepithelial neoplasia, aneuploidy, copy-number changes, amplification of genes such as EGFR and silencing due to hypermethylation in genes such as CDKN2A draw attention [27, 34]. The necessary mutations for neoplasia to acquire an invasive character are unknown. EIF5A2 amplification is thought to be related to the epithelial-mesenchymal transition and its association with invasion and migration capacity [63].

#### 37.4.1.2 Macroscopy

Cases of superficial SCC may be plaque-like, polypoid, depressed, or occult. Tumors detected in advanced stages appear as an exophytic (60%), ulcerated (25%), or infiltrative (15%) mass. These patterns can also be seen together. The classification of the Japanese Esophageal Society is useful in macroscopic classification (Fig. 37.8) [1, 27, 64].

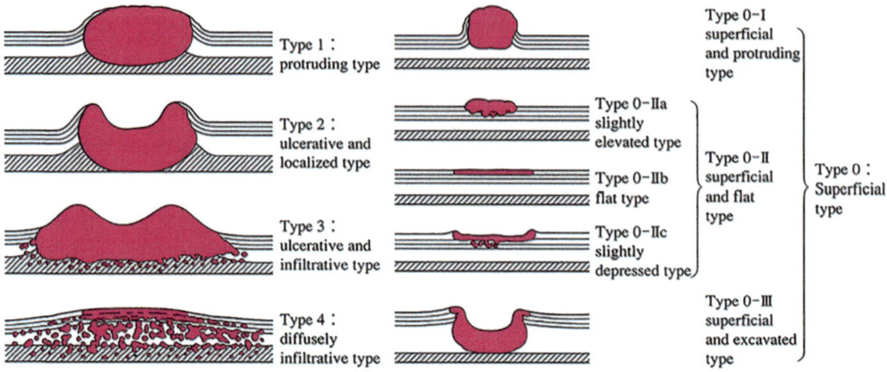


**Fig. 37.8** Japanese classification of esophageal cancer

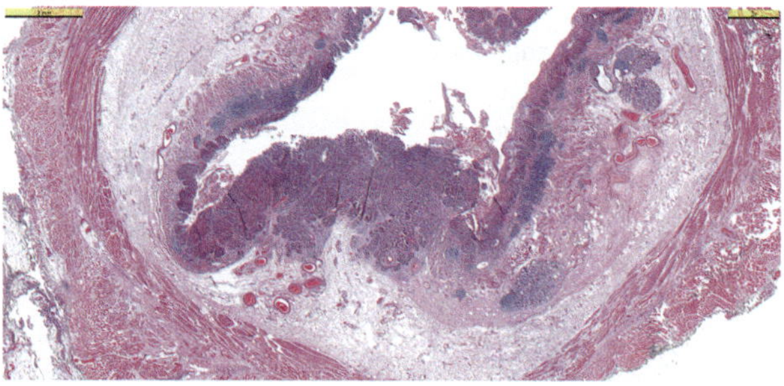

**Fig. 37.9** A moderately differentiated squamous cell carcinoma with solid cell islands in the circularly sampled full thickness esophageal wall (H-E; ×2)

The tumor is gray-white on the cross-sectional surface and may invade the muscular wall, and it can spread to the surrounding soft tissues and trachea. Tumors that grow intraluminal and obstruct the lumen are also present. Esophageal SCCs located distally may invade the stomach. In some cases, there may be submucosal extension 5 cm or even more from the gross margins of the tumor. Spread along the submucosal glands and ducts may also be seen. Vascular invasion is present in most of the cases [4]. The presence of tumor nodules in the esophagus or stomach wall away from the main mass due to intratumoral lymphatic spread (presence of intramural metastases) has been reported in 11–16% of the cases. More than one primary tumor focus was found in 14–31% of the cases [1, 3].

### 37.4.1.3 Microscopy

In esophageal SCC, as in other anatomical areas, nuclear atypia features as well as abnormal keratinization, abnormal maturation, and keratin pearls help the diagnosis [3, 65] (Fig. 37.9).

In SCC, neoplastic cells spread both horizontally and vertically in the subepithelial space. In grading, cytological atypia, mitotic activity, presence of intercellular bridges (bridging), and keratinization are taken into account. A triple grading system (Grades 1, 2, and 3) is often used. However, due to the high inter-observer variation between Grades 1 and 2, some prefer the dual system (Grades 1–2 and Grade 3).

Grade 1 (well differentiated): Enlarged cells with large eosinophilic cytoplasm are seen, intercellular bridges and keratin pearls are prominent. Cytological atypia is rare. Mitotic rate is low. Boundaries of invasion are repulsive. Cells show regular order.

Grade 2 (moderately differentiated): Cytological atypia is evident and cellular polarity is impaired. Mitotic rate is increased. Although parakeratosis is seen on the surface, keratin pearls are few in number.

Grade 3 (poorly differentiated): As the grade of the tumor increases, the proportion of basaloid cells also increases. In Grade 3, basaloid cells forming nests predominate. Necrosis is noticeable in the middle of these cell populations. Parakeratosis and keratinized cells are very rare.

Focal glandular or focal neuroendocrine differentiation can be found in 20–30% of SCC cases [3, 56]. Rarely, an intraepithelial tumor component resembling Paget's disease has been reported. However, most of these cases were associated with underlying adenocarcinoma [1, 3, 66].

#### 37.4.1.4 Subtypes

**Verrucous SCC** is a neoplasia that usually develops in the background of chronic irritation, esophagitis, or previous esophageal injury. Most of the cases are in the form of a raised mucosal lesion in the lower 1/3 of the esophagus. In some cases, association with HPV1 and HPV11 has been demonstrated. This slow-growing tumor, which is not expected to metastasize, consists of highly differentiated squamous cells with minimal cytological atypia and mitotic activity and papillary protrusions toward the surface. Although the granular cell layer cannot be seen in between, pronounced keratinization draws attention. There are also keratin accumulations in the basal parts of the papillary structures. Wide bulbous areas are seen to progress and invade in a repulsive manner [1, 67]. (Fig. 37.10).

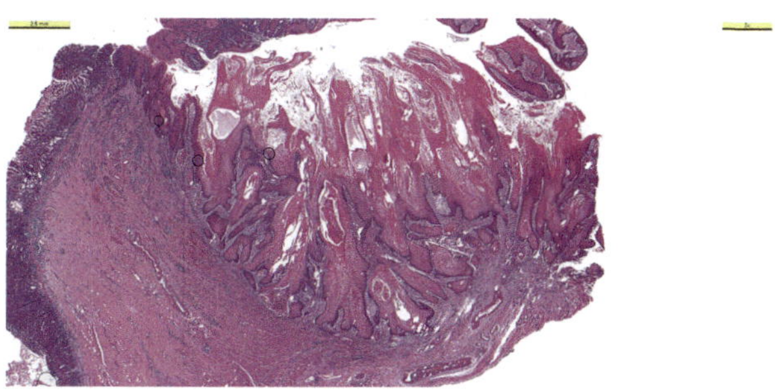

**Fig. 37.10** Verrucous carcinoma; tumor growth with bulbous and repulsive infiltrates with prominent papillomatosis and keratinization on the surface (H-E; ×2)

**Spindle cell SCC (carcinosarcoma, sarcomatoid carcinoma)** constitute approximately 2% of all esophageal carcinomas. It is a neoplasia with a polypoid growth pattern, usually in the middle or lower 1/3 esophagus. Histologically, a biphasic cell population consisting of neoplastic squamous cells and spindle cells is seen. Squamous cells are well-moderately differentiated. Sometimes only carcinoma in situ is seen. The spindle cells are high-grade and show osseous, cartilaginous, or muscular differentiation. Intraluminal growth of the tumor, rather than deep invasion, is a possible reason for its better prognosis compared to an SCC NOS of the same size [1, 3, 27, 68].

**Basaloid SCC** is a subtype that is more common in males and accounts for approximately 5% of all esophageal carcinomas. Unlike oropharyngeal basaloid SCCs, it is not associated with HPV. Central comedonecrosis can be seen in the tumor formed by basaloid cells forming solid layers or nests. Rarely, pseudoglandular or cribriform areas may be detected, which may require differential diagnosis with adenoid cystic carcinoma. It may also need to be differentiated from high-grade neuroendocrine carcinoma by immunohistochemical analysis. This very aggressive tumor is thought to have a worse prognosis than SCC NOS [1, 27, 69, 70].

## 37.5 Differential Diagnosis

These entities should be considered in differential diagnosis:

- In some cases, it may be difficult to distinguish reactive atypia due to inflammation from atypia observed in dysplasia or invasive carcinoma [1, 71].
- Reactive stromal cells in ulceration areas may be confused with malignancy [1, 71].
- Chemoradiotherapy may cause epithelial atypia, making differential diagnosis difficult (Fig. 37.11) [1, 3, 72].
- Pseudoepitheliomatous hyperplasia is distinguished by the presence of squamous proliferation but absence of cytological atypia and invasion [35, 71].
- SCC can be confused with squamous papilloma, which is usually a small and incidental lesion. This lesion is characterized by papillary proliferation of squamous cells without cytological atypia. It often shows less inflammation and/or parakeratosis compared to SCC [35, 71].
- In small biopsies, it may be difficult to distinguish SCC NOS from SCC subtypes, undifferentiated carcinoma, or adenocarcinoma. In these cases, clinical data and morphological features as well as immunohistochemical studies can be helpful. CK7 positivity and negative squamous cell markers such as CK5/6, p63, and p40 are in favor of adenocarcinoma. The positivity of neuroendocrine markers such as synaptophysin, chromogranin, and CD56 is in favor of NE carcinoma [27, 35].
- Sarcomas and spindle cell melanoma might be difficult to differentiate. Primary sarcomas of the esophagus are very rare. S100 is used in the differential diagnosis

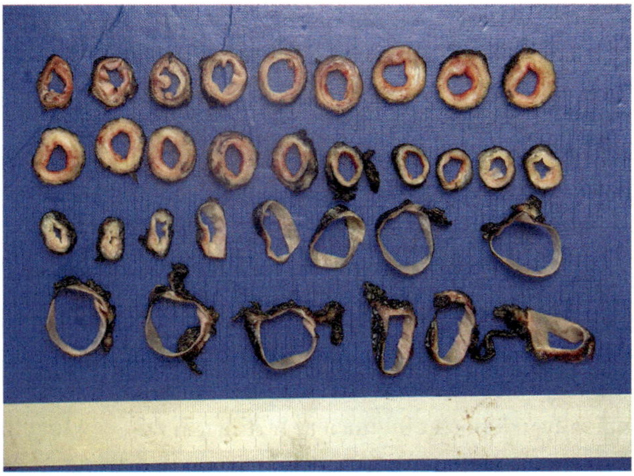


**Fig. 37.11** In the fully sampled esophageal specimen in posttreatment surgery, macroscopically complete tumor regression findings are observed

of melanoma, and CD117 is used in the differential diagnosis of gastrointestinal stromal tumor (GIST). It should be kept in mind that GIST is very rare in the esophagus, and C117 may also be positive in melanoma [1, 27].

- SCC from other primary sites: It is not possible to distinguish an SCC that can spread directly from the lung, only by morphological features. In this case, it is necessary to benefit from imaging methods and clinical examinations [27].

Cytological examination may also be useful in the diagnosis of esophageal squamous cell carcinoma. It is thought that squamous neoplasia can be recognized more easily in the early stage in cytological samples taken by direct mucosal brushing or blind sampling with techniques such as the Cytosponge procedure [27, 36]. It has been reported that these methods are cost effective for screening populations at risk.

Due to the rich lymphatic drainage of the esophagus, SCC frequently spreads to the lymph nodes in the periesophageal area. Also, tumors may spread in the submucosal space of the stomach, possibly via the submucosal lymphatic plexus. Metastases to distant organs, liver, lung, and adrenal glands are also common [3].

### 37.5.1 Adenosquamous Carcinoma

Adenosquamous carcinoma of the esophagus consists of distinct malignant squamous and glandular components [27, 73]. Adenosquamous carcinoma usually originates in the middle part of the esophagus. In recent years, it has been frequently encountered in the lower esophagus section. Its clinical features are similar to adenocarcinoma of the esophagus and squamous cell carcinoma (SCC) [27, 73].

The origin of adenosquamous carcinoma is not well known. There is an opinion that the esophageal duct originates from stem cells showing biphasic differentiation. Another opinion is that a subpopulation of primary SCC shows glandular differentiation, or squamous differentiation occurs in an adenocarcinoma. There is also a hypothesis that it can be formed by the fusion of two different tumors (collision tumor). Due to the common embryological origin of the esophageal and salivary glands, it seems likely to originate from the esophageal submucosal glands [27, 73].

## 37.6 Macroscopy and Microscopy

The macroscopic appearance of adenosquamous carcinoma is similar to SCC. Microscopically, adenocarcinoma and SCC areas are seen together. According to the Japanese Classification of Esophageal Cancer, 20% or more of each component is required for diagnosis. Otherwise, the tumor is named according to the dominant histological character. If the differentiation of the tumor is good, keratinization and intercellular bridges can be seen in squamous areas, while the presence of glandular structures and intra/extracellular mucin in adenocarcinoma areas is remarkable. The squamous and glandular areas can be intertwined or stand separately. In general, squamous areas are localized more superficially, and glandular areas are more deeply localized. In cytological examinations, malignant squamous and glandular cells can also be detected [3, 27, 74].

### 37.6.1 Mucoepidermoid Carcinoma of the Esophagus

Adenosquamous and mucoepidermoid carcinoma of the esophagus are tumors that contain both squamous and adenoid component, but the content of these two components is different from each other. Adenosquamous carcinoma is composed of separate malignant squamous and glandular components. However, mucoepidermoid carcinoma is an esophageal neoplasm that is composed of an admixture of malignant epidermoid, intermediate, and mucous cells. Just like adenosquamous carcinoma, mucoepidermoid carcinoma also arises most commonly in the middle esophagus [75, 76], although a predominance of lower oesophageal cases was observed in one recent series [77, 78].

The clinical features are due to mass effect and obstruction, which are similar to those of conventional carcinomas of the esophagus. These are rare tumors. They are common in in fifth and sixth decades and more common in males than in females [75–78].

The risk factors are not different from conventional squamous cell carcinoma. Pathogenesis of these carcinomas of the esophagus is of uncertain origin. The best evidence is for an origin from a stem cell [75, 79], probably from the esophageal duct, giving rise to biphasic differentiation [80]. According to another theory, these tumors are simply primary squamous cell carcinomas from which a subpopulation has undergone diverging glandular differentiation [81], or primary adenocarcinomas showing squamous differentiation [79, 82, 83]. Another possibility is the existence of a collision tumor of two separate primary carcinomas (one glandular and one squamous). The origin of these tumors is esophageal submucosal glands, supported by the common embryology of esophageal and salivary glands, but further evidence is needed. Mucoepidermoid carcinomas have defined molecular characteristics that include translocations resulting in fusion genes detected in salivary gland tumors, which are not found in adenosquamous carcinomas [84]. Macroscopic appearance is indistinguishable from squamous cell carcinoma.

In histopathological examination of mucoepidermoid carcinomas, the main pattern is glands and nests of both malignant squamoid cells and admixed mucin-containing epithelial cells. Exceptionally, the tumors may have prominent sclerosis with lymphoid tissue and eosinophils [85].

The cytology of these lesions may be tricky according to the sampled localization. A mixture of cytologically malignant squamous and glandular cells should make pathologist to consider the diagnosis of adenosquamous or mucoepidermoid carcinoma [84].

Essential diagnostic criteria for mucoepidermoid carcinoma are to detect not only intermediate cells but also mixed glandular and squamous cells that may show true glandular or mucous cell differentiation [84].

Staging of these rare tumors is not clear. There is not enough evidence of whether the staging of these tumors should follow that of squamous cell carcinoma or adenocarcinoma. Although some studies suggest that adenosquamous and mucoepidermoid carcinomas may be more aggressive than conventional squamous cell carcinoma, the studies are sufficient to determine the prognosis of these carcinomas compared with more common esophageal carcinomas [77, 83, 86, 87].

### 37.6.2 Adenoid Cystic Carcinoma of the Esophagus

Adenoid cystic carcinoma of the esophagus is a malignant esophageal epithelial tumor of glandular differentiation with epithelial and myoepithelial cells that form glandular and pseudoglandular lumina, which are arranged as cribriform, tubular, or solid architecture [84].

The anatomic localization of adenoid cystic carcinomas is generally the middle third of the esophagus [88, 89]. The most common symptom is dysphagia according to the mass effect. Endoscopy and EUS may be used to confirm the diagnosis and determine the invasion of the tumor. In endoscopic examination, the tumor appears as a protruding/elevated or ulcerative lesion. Radiological examination with CT, MRI, or PET is important in the clinical staging of the carcinoma [84].

Esophageal adenoid cystic carcinoma is a very rare tumor, and nearly 100 cases are reported in the literature [88, 89]. It is more common in Asian population [88, 89]. This tumor constitutes about 0.1% of all esophageal malignancies, and it is more common in men than in women, and it most often occurs in the seventh decade of life [88, 89].

Macroscopically, adenoid cystic carcinoma causes a protruding solid mass in the esophageal wall which can present with ulceration [88–90]. It originates from the submucosa; therefore, in early stages, the mucosa is still intact. Mean size is approximately of 56 mm, but the dimensions can be highly variable in size [91–93]. Histopathology adenoid cystic carcinoma consists of a mixture of epithelial and myoepithelial cells that form cribriform, tubular (glandular), or solid patterns. In the cribriform pattern, tumor cells form cystic lumina, which contain either basophilic glycosaminoglycans that are Alcian blue positive (true glands) or hyalinized basal lamina material that is PASD-positive (pseudoglands). In the cribriform and tubular patterns, the glands are lined by inner epithelial and outer myoepithelial cells, whereas the solid pattern shows no lumina. Perineural infiltration and lymphovascular permeation are typical and often just like adenoid cystic carcinomas in other localizations [88]. This malignancy may be detected with squamous cell carcinoma or with dysplasia/carcinoma in situ [94].

Adenoid cystic carcinoma is positive for myoepithelial cell markers such as p63, S100, SMA, and calponin. The epithelial cells are positive for cytokeratin, CEA, and KIT (CD117) [89, 95]. It has differential diagnosis with basaloid squamous cell carcinoma because it often has a pseudoglandular pattern similar to that of adenoid cystic carcinoma [70]. Lack of squamous cell differentiation markers, central necrosis, prominent mitotic figures, and immunoreactivity with myoepithelial markers are used in differential diagnosis [84].

In most instances, diagnosis is made by typical histological pattern described above. Staging of this tumor is same as esophageal adenocarcinoma. Prognosis depends on the pathological stage. As endoscopic examination is very common in Japan, half of the cases consisted of cancer limited to the submucosal layer, with only rare lymph node metastasis [88]. In other populations, there is high incidence of metastasis to lymph nodes, liver, lung, and brain. The prognosis is poor, with a 1-year survival rate of 23% [96].

### 37.6.3 Neuroendocrine Neoplasias of the Esophagus

In the latest WHO classification, there is a distinction between well-differentiated neuroendocrine tumors (NET) of the GIS and poorly differentiated neuroendocrine carcinomas (NEC), previously called carcinoids. These two tumor groups, which were previously evaluated in the same group due to their positive neuroendocrine markers, are now accepted as separate entities. Neuroendocrine neoplasms (NEN) are divided into two main groups as NET and NEC. NETs are clinically slower-growing tumors. In these tumors in which the triple grading system is used, the mitotic index and Ki-67 proliferation index are based on the grade determination (Table 37.5) [2]. Tumor grade may progress both in the primary tumor and in metastases. The risk of metastasis is low after complete resection in early stage and small NETs. It is more common in high-grade and large tumors. However, long-term survival is possible even in advanced-stage and treatment-resistant cases. Grading is mainly based on mitotic activity and Ki-67 proliferation index [97]. The number of

**Table 37.5** Classification and grading of neuroendocrine neoplasms (NENs)

| Terminology | Differentiation | Grade |
|---|---|---|
| NET, G1 | Well differentiated | Low |
| NET, G2 | | Intermediate |
| NET, G3 | | High |
| NEC, small cell type (SCNEC) | Poorly differentiated | High* |
| NEC, large-cell type (LCNEC) | | |
| MiNEN | Well or poorly differentiated | Variable |

*NET* neuroendocrine tumor; *NEC* neuroendocrine carcinoma; *MiNEN* mixed neuroendocrine-nonneuroendocrine neoplasm

*Poorly differentiated NECs are not formally graded but are considered high-grade

mitoses per 2 $mm^2$ is important in mitotic activity (the number of mitosis at 10 BBA at 40X magnification). Another important parameter is the evaluation of the Ki-67 proliferation index. If there is a mismatch in the mitotic index and Ki-67 index, the higher grade is taken as the basis [97].

NECs are high-grade tumors by definition. They constitute more than 90% of esophageal neuroendocrine tumors [98]. In previous classifications, grade 3 neuroendocrine tumors were considered synonymous with poorly differentiated neuroendocrine carcinomas, but today these two tumors are accepted as separate entities [2, 3].

#### 37.6.3.1 Macroscopy

NETs are usually small lesions. In a study of 19 cases, the mean tumor diameter was reported as 2.4 cm [99]. NECs are exophytic or ulcerated, large-volume tumors. Infiltration into deep tissues is the characteristic finding [100].

#### 37.6.3.2 Microscopy

Insular or cribriform growth pattern is essential in NETs [3]. Tumor cells are medium in size, with ample cytoplasm, fairly uniform, and have a low nucleocytoplasmic ratio. The oval nucleus with a fine granular pattern may contain a small nucleolus. Tumor stroma is well vascularized, and necrosis is usually absent. Neuroendocrine differentiation needs to be verified by expression of chromogranin A and synaptophysin. Immunohistochemically, other neuroendocrine markers such as serotonin, (entero)glucagon, PP, gastrin, and calcitonin may also be positive [101–103].

NECs are poorly differentiated epithelial tumors that show neuroendocrine differentiation morphologically and immunohistochemically. The typical neuroendocrine structure is not evident in NECs. It has two subtypes, small cell NEC (SCNEC) and large cell NEC (LCNEC). Esophageal large-cell neuroendocrine carcinomas (LCNEC) usually develop in a solid pattern. Rosette-like or palisatic patterns may be seen. Extensive and widespread necrosis is characteristic. NECs have high mitotic activity (>20 at 2 $mm^2$). The Ki-67 proliferation index should also be greater than 20%. Especially since the Ki-67 index may change after treatment, it would not be healthy to use the Ki-67 index alone to differentiate NEC from grade 3 NET [2].

SCNECs are small to medium sized; It consists of cells with a high nucleocytoplasmic ratio and narrow cytoplasm. The nucleus is elongated and has a finely scattered chromatin pattern. The nucleus is usually not observed. Neuroendocrine differentiation should also be proven in this group. Synaptophysin expression is stable, whereas chromogranin A expression shows focal and pale staining in only 60% of cases [104].

## 37.7 Mixed Neuroendocrine Neoplasias

### 37.7.1 MiNENs (Mixed Neuroendocrine Nonneuroendocrine Neoplasms)

They are mixed tumors with neuroendocrine and non-neuroendocrine components. The term "MiNEN" is used as an abbreviation of the term "Mixed neuroendocrine nonneuroendocrine neoplasm". In the neuroendocrine component, neuroendocrine differentiation must also be proven by the positivity of synaptophysin and/or chromogranin A. Both components should be shown in separate foci in at least 30% of the tumor, both morphologically and immunohistochemically (Table 37.6). it usually has the characteristics of poorly differentiated NEC, poorly differentiated squamous cell carcinoma, or adenocarcinoma [105]. The cases that received neoadjuvant therapy should not be reported as MiNEN if this diagnosis was not given before treatment. In these cases, neuroendocrine morphology has no prognosis as in cases with de novo diagnosis [106, 107]. Although "30%" is an important criterion in terms of diagnosis, the presence of focal (<30%) "small cell NEC" should be stated in the report as it will negatively affect the prognosis. Although it is recommended to grade both components separately, it is known that the neuroendocrine component is more important in determining the prognosis [108].

#### 37.7.1.1 Collision" Tumors

Collision tumors may rarely develop in the esophagus in the form of well-differentiated neuroendocrine tumor and adenocarcinoma [109]. These tumors do not meet the criteria for the MiNEN group.

#### 37.7.1.2 Staging

There is no specific staging system for esophageal NENs. Staging is the same as for other esophageal carcinomas.

**Table 37.6** Mixed neuroendocrine-nonneuroendocrine neoplasms (MİNENs) of the esophagus

| Esophagus and esophagogastric junction |
|---|
| • Mixed squamous cell carcinoma-NEC (SCNEC/LCNEC) |
| • Mixed adenocarcinoma-NEC (SCNEC/LCNEC) |
| • Mixed adenocarcinoma-NET |

*NET* neuroendocrine tumor; *NEC* neuroendocrine carcinoma; *SCNEC* small cell neuroendocrine carcinoma; *LCNEC* large-cell neuroendocrine carcinoma

#### 37.7.1.3 Prognosis

The prognosis is also generally good in NETs. Tumor size and extent are the most important parameters in prognosis. Metastatic extension is rare in the NET group [110]. On the other hand, the prognosis is very poor in NECs. Metastases are usually present at the time of diagnosis. Presence of distant metastases is the strongest prognostic parameter [111]. There is no significant difference in prognosis between LCNEC and SCNEC [111]. The most important predictor in prognosis is the Ki-67 proliferation index [69]. MiNENs have a better prognosis than pure NECs, and the average life expectancy reaches 20 months [111] The most important parameter determining the prognosis is the Ki-67 proliferation index in the NEC component [108].

In differential diagnosis, basaloid squamous cell carcinoma should be taken into account. Discrimination is possible by immunohistochemical demonstration of squamous differentiation.

**Acknowledgement** We would like to thank Prof. Dr. Süha Göksel for contributing to our chapter with macroscopic and microscopic photographs that she had the kindness to share with us.

## References

1. Deere HMR. Chapter 2. Pathology of esophageal cancer. In: Reznek RH, Husband JE, editors. Carcinoma of the esophagus. Cambridge University Press; 2008.
2. Lam AK, Ochiai A, Odze RD. Tumours of the oesophagus. In: WHO classification of digestive system tumours. 5th ed. 2019.
3. Goldblum JR. Chapter 13. Esophagus. In: Goldblum JR, editor. Rosai and Ackerman's surgical pathology. 11th ed. Philadelphia: Elsevier; 2018. p. 501–27.
4. Spechler SJ, Souza RF. Barrett's esophagus. N Engl J Med. 2014;371(9):836–45.
5. Dunbar KB, Spechler SJ. Controversies in Barrett esophagus. Mayo Clin Proc. 2014;89(7):973–84.
6. Chandrasoma PT, Der R, Dalton P, et al. Distribution and significance of epithelial types in columnar-lined esophagus. Am J Surg Pathol. 2001;25(9):1188–93.
7. Suo Z, Nesland JM. Barrett's esophagus: intestinal metaplasia or phenotypic shift of undifferentiated elements in the stem cells. Ultrastruct Pathol. 2002;26(2):53–4.
8. Weaver JMJ, Ross Innes CS, Shannon N, et al. Ordering of mutations in preinvasive disease stages of esophageal carcinogenesis. Nat Genet. 2014;46(8):837–43.
9. Stelow EB, Murad FM, Debol SM, et al. A limited immunocytochemical panel for the distinction of subepithelial gastrointestinal mesenchymal neoplasms sampled by endoscopic ultrasound-guided fine-needle aspiration. Am J Clin Pathol. 2008;129(2):219–25.
10. Sampliner RE. Practice guidelines on the diagnosis, surveillance and therapy of Barrett's esophagus. Am J Gastroenterol. 1998;93:1028–31.
11. Shepherd NA, Biddlestone LR. The histopathology and cytopathology of Barrett's oesophagus. In: Manek S, editor. CPD bulletin cellular pathology, vol. 1. London: Rila Publications; 1999. p. 39–44.
12. Liu W, Hahn H, Odze RD, Goyal RK. Metaplastic esophageal columnar epithelium without goblet cells shows DNA content abnormalities similar to goblet cell-containing epithelium. Am J Gastroenterol. 2009;104(4):816–24.
13. Chandrasoma P. Controversies of the cardiac mucosa and Barrett's oesophagus. Histopathology. 2005;46(4):361–73.

14. DeMeester SR, Wickramasinghe KS, Lord RVN, et al. Cytokeratin and DAS-1 immunostaining reveal similarities among cardiac mucosa, CIM, and Barrett's esophagus. Am J Gastroenterol. 2002;97(10):2514–23.
15. Goldblum JR. The significance and etiology of intestinal metaplasia of the esophagogastric junction. Ann Diagn Pathol. 2002;6(1):67–73.
16. Srivastava A, Odze RD, Lauwers GY, et al. Morphologic features are useful in distinguishing Barrett esophagus from carditis with intestinal metaplasia. Am J Surg Pathol. 2007;31(11):1733–41.
17. Hahn HP, Shahsafaei A, Odze RD. Vascular and lymphatic properties of the superficial and deep lamina propria in Barrett esophagus. Am J Surg Pathol. 2008;32(10):1454–61.
18. Lewis JT, Wang KK, Abraham SC. Muscularis mucosae duplication and the musculo-fibrous anomaly in endoscopic mucosal resections for Barrett esophagus: implications for staging of adenocarcinoma. Am J Surg Pathol. 2008;32(4):566–71.
19. Altorki NK, Sunagawa M, Little AG, Skinner DB. High-grade dysplasia in the columnar lined esophagus. Am J Surg. 1991;161:97–9.
20. Pera M, Trastek VF, Carpenter HA, et al. Barrett's esophagus with high-grade dysplasia: an indication for esophagectomy? Ann Thorac Surg. 1992;54:199–204.
21. Tseng EE, Wu TT, Yeo CJ, Heitmiller RF. Barrett's esophagus with high grade dysplasia: surgical results and long-term outcome—an update. J Gastrointest Surg. 2003;7:164–70.
22. Reid BJ, Haggitt RC, Rubin CE, et al. Observer variation in the diagnosis of dysplasia in Barrett's esophagus. Hum Pathol. 1988;19(2):166–78.
23. Lagergren J, Bergström R, Lindgren A, Nyrén O. Symptomatic gastroesophageal reflux as a risk factor for esophageal adenocarcinoma. N Engl J Med. 1999;340(11):825–31.
24. Bita VN, Souza RF, Odze FD. Barrett's esophagus: a comprehensive and contemporary review for pathologists. Am J Surg Pathol. 2016;40(5):e45–66.
25. Schlemper RJ, Riddell RH, Kato Y, et al. The Vienna classification of gastrointestinal epithelial neoplasia. Gut. 2000;47(2):251–5.
26. Lomo LC, Blount PL, Sanchez CA, et al. Crypt dysplasia with surface maturation: a clinical, pathologic, and molecular study of a Barrett's esophagus cohort. Am J Surg Pathol. 2006;30(4):423–35.
27. Tabuko K, Fujii S. Oesophageal squamous dysplasia in WHO classification of digestive system tumours. WHO Classification of Tumours Editorial Board. 5th ed. 2019.
28. Taylor PR, Abnet CC, Dawsey SM. Squamous dysplasia—the precursor lesion for esophageal squamous cell carcinoma. Cancer Epidemiol Biomarkers Prev. 2013;22(4):540–52.
29. Poosari A, Nutravong T, Namwat W, Wasenang W, Sa-Ngiamwibool P, Ungareewittaya P. The relationship between $P16^{INK4A}$ and TP53 promoter methylation and the risk and prognosis in patients with oesophageal cancer in Thailand. Sci Rep. 2022;12(1):10337.
30. Rubio CA, Liu FS, Zhao HZ. Histological classification of intraepithelial neoplasias and microinvasive squamous carcinoma of the esophagus. Am J Surg Pathol. 1989;13(8):685–90.
31. Araki K, Ohno S, Egashira A, et al. Pathologic features of superficial esophageal squamous cell carcinoma with lymph node and distal metastasis. Cancer. 2002;94(2):570–5.
32. Moon JY, Kim GH, Kim JH, et al. Clinicopathologic factors predicting lymph node metastasis in superficial esophageal squamous cell carcinoma. Scand J Gastroenterol. 2014;49(5):589–94.
33. Li B, Chen H, Xiang J, et al. Prevalence of lymph node metastases in superficial esophageal squamous cell carcinoma. J Thorac Cardiovasc Surg. 2013;146(5):1198–203.
34. Businello G, Parente P, Mastracci L, Pennelli G, Traverso G, Milione M, Bellan E, Michelotto M, Kotsafti A, Grillo F, Fassan M. The pathologic and molecular landscape of esophageal squamous cell carcinogenesis. Cancers (Basel). 2020;12(8):2160.
35. Savant D, Zhang Q, Yang Z. Squamous neoplasia in the esophagus. Arch Pathol Lab Med. 2021;145(5):554–61.
36. Pan QJ, Roth MJ, Guo HQ, et al. Cytologic detection of esophageal squamous cell carcinoma and its precursor lesions using balloon samplers and liquid-based cytology in asymptomatic adults in Llinxian, China. Acta Cytol. 2008;52(1):14–23.

37. Zhang W, Wang DH. Origins of metaplasia in Barrett's esophagus: is this an esophageal stem or progenitor cell disease? Dig Dis Sci. 2018;63(8):2005–12.
38. Quante M, Graham TA, Jansen M. insights into the pathophysiology of esophageal adenocarcinoma. Gastroenterology. 2018;154(2):406–20.
39. Allanson BM, Bonavita J, Mirzai B. Early Barrett esophagus-related neoplasia in segments 1 cm or longer is always associated with intestinal metaplasia. Mod Pathol. 2017;30(8):1170–6.
40. Islam F, Tang JC, Gopalan V, Lam AK. Epigenetics: DNA methylation analysis in esophageal adenocarcinoma. Methods Mol Biol. 2018.
41. Lee KTW, Gopalan V, Lam AK. Somatic DNA copy-number alterations detection for esophageal adenocarcinoma using digital polymerase chain reaction. Methods Mol Biol. 2018;1756:195–212.
42. Lee KTW, Smith RA, Gopalan V, Lam AK. Targeted Single Gene Mutation In Esophageal Adenocarcinoma. Methods Mol Biol. 2018;1756:213–29.
43. Giovannini M, Seitz JF, Monges G, et al. Fine-needle aspiration cytology guided by endoscopic ultrasonography: results in 141 patients. Endoscopy. 1995;27:171–7.
44. Oda I, Abe S, Kusano C, et al. Correlation between endoscopic macroscopic type and invasion depth for early esophagogastric junction adenocarcinomas. Gastric Cancer. 2011;14(1):22–7.
45. Amano T, Matsumoto T, Hayashi T, et al. Subepithelial extension of squamous cell carcinoma in the esophagus: histopathological study using D2-40 immunostaining for 108 superficial carcinomas. Pathol Int. 2007;57(12):759–64.
46. Khor TS, Alfaro EE, Ooi EMM. Divergent expression of MUC5AC, MUC6, MUC2, CD10, and CDX-2 in dysplasia and intramucosal adenocarcinomas with intestinal and foveolar morphology: is this evidence of distinct gastric and intestinal pathways to carcinogenesis in Barrett esophagus? Am J Surg Pathol. 2012;36(3):331–42.
47. Brown IS, Whiteman DC, Lauwers GY. Foveolar type dysplasia in Barrett esophagus. Mod Pathol. 2010;23(6):834–43.
48. Lam AK. Application of pathological staging in esophageal adenocarcinoma. Methods Mol Biol. 2018;1756:93–103.
49. https://app.expertpath.com/document/adenocarcinoma-esophagus/71de2bf9-38b4-4898-abf6-7be318e4e274?searchTerm=esoph. Accessed 2 Apr 2023.
50. Noble F, Nolan L, Bateman AC. Refining pathological evaluation of neoadjuvant therapy for adenocarcinoma of the esophagus. World J Astroenterol. 2013;19(48):9282–93.
51. Langer R, Becker K. Tumor regression grading of gastrointestinal cancers after neoadjuvant therapy. Virchows Arch. 2018;472(2):175–86.
52. Noble F, Lloyd MA, Turkington R, et al. Multicentre cohort study to define and validate pathological assessment of response to neoadjuvant therapy in oesophagogastric adenocarcinoma. Br J Surg. 2017;104(13):1816–28.
53. Hosokawa Y, Kinoshita T, Konishi M, et al. Clinicopathological features and prognostic factors of adenocarcinoma of the esophagogastric junction according to Siewert classification: experiences at a single institution in Japan. Ann Surg Oncol. 2012;19(2):677–83.
54. Torres C, Turner JR, Wang HH, et al. Pathologic prognostic factors in Barrett's associated adenocarcinoma: a follow-up study of 96 patients. Cancer. 1999;85(3):520–8.
55. Rice TW, Blackstone EH, Adelstein DJ, et al. Role of clinically determined depth of tumor invasion in the treatment of esophageal carcinoma. J Thorac Cardiovasc Surg. 2003;125(5):1091–102.
56. Rice TW, Zuccaro G, Adelstein DJ, et al. Esophageal carcinoma: depth of tumor invasion is predictive of regional lymph node status. Ann Thorac Surg. 1998;65(3):787–92.
57. Yoon HH, Khan M, Shi Q, et al. The prognostic value of clinical and pathologic factors in esophageal adenocarcinoma: a mayo cohort of 796 patients with extended follow-up after surgical resection. Mayo Clin Proc. 2010;85(12):1080–9.
58. Hölscher AH, Drebber U, Schmidt H, Bollschweiler E. Prognostic classification of histopathologic response to neoadjuvant therapy in esophageal adenocarcinoma. Ann Surg. 2014;260(5):779–84; discussion 784–785.

59. Pozdnyakova O, Hoang MMP, Dresser KA, Mahalingam M. Prognostic value of E-cadherin, beta-catenin, CD44v6, and HER2/neu in metastatic cutaneous adenocarcinoma. Arch Pathol Lab Med. 2009;133(8):1285–90.
60. Takubo K, Takai A, Takayama S, et al. Intraductal spread of esophageal squamous cell carcinoma. Cancer. 1987;59(10):1751–7.
61. Arista-Nasr J, Rivera I, Martinez-Benitez B, et al. Atypical regenerative hyperplasia of the esophagus in endoscopic biopsy: a mimicker of squamous esophagic carcinoma. Arch Pathol Lab Med. 2005;129(7):899–904.
62. Zhang HD, Chen CG, Gao YY, et al. Primary esophageal adenosquamous carcinoma: a retrospective analysis of 24 cases. Dis Esophagus. 2014;27(8):783–9.
63. Li Y, Fu L, Li JB, et al. Increased expression of EIF5A2, via hypoxia or gene amplification, contributes to metastasis and angiogenesis of esophageal squamous cell carcinoma. Gastroenterology. 2014;146(7):1701–13.e9.
64. Japan Esophageal Society. Japanese classification of esophageal cancer, 11th edition: part I. Esophagus. 2017;14(1):1–36.
65. Lam AK. Histopathological assessment for esophageal squamous cell carcinoma. Methods Mol Biol. 2020;2129:7–18.
66. Abraham SC, Wang H, Wang KK, Wu T-T. Paget cells in the esophagus: assessment of their histopathologic features and near-universal association with underlying esophageal adenocarcinoma. Am J Surg Pathol. 2008;32(7):1068–74.
67. Tabuchi S, Koyanagi K, Nagata K, Ozawa S, Kawachi S. Verrucous carcinoma of the esophagus: a case report and literature review. Surg Case Rep. 2020;6(1):35.
68. Zhang B, Xiao Q, Yang D, Li X, Hu J, Wang Y, Wang W. Spindle cell carcinoma of the esophagus: a multicenter analysis in comparison with typical squamous cell carcinoma. Medicine (Baltimore). 2016;95(37):e4768.
69. Song H, Tetangco E, Ton L, Barrett A, Yap JEL. Beyond squamous cell carcinoma: basaloid squamous cell carcinoma of the esophagus. Cureus. 2021;13(1):e12619.
70. Li TJ, Zhang YX, Wen J, Cowan DF, Hart J, Xiao SY. Basaloid squamous cell carcinoma of the esophagus with or without adenoid cystic features. Arch Pathol Lab Med. 2004;128(10):1124–30.
71. Tsai SJ, Lin CC, Chang CW, Hung CY, Shieh TY, Wang HY, Shih SC, Chen MJ. Benign esophageal lesions: endoscopic and pathologic features. World J Gastroenterol. 2015;21(4):1091–8.
72. Yamamoto M, Doki Y, Shiozaki H, et al. Evaluation of the histologic effect of chemoradiation therapy for squamous cell carcinomas of the esophagus by assessing morphologic features of surgical specimens. Dis Esophagus. 2000;13(4):293–300.
73. Fukai H, Koide N, Yanagisawa N, Koyama Y, Kitagawa N, Ogihara Y, Ohya M. A case report of adenosquamous carcinoma of the esophagogastric junction. Surg Case Rep. 2022;8(1):82.
74. Chen SB, Liu DT, Chen YP. Surgical resection for esophageal adenosquamous carcinoma: an analysis of 56 cases. World J Surg Oncol. 2022;20(1):143.
75. Chen SB, Weng HR, Wang G, Yang JS, Yang WP, Liu DT, Chen YP, Zhang H. Primary adenosquamous carcinoma of the esophagus. World J Gastroenterol. 2013;19(45):8382–90.
76. Ni PZ, Yang YS, Hu WP, Wang WP, Yuan Y, Chen LQ. Primary adenosquamous carcinoma of the esophagus: an analysis of 39 cases. J Thorac Dis. 2016;8(10):2689–96.
77. Yendamuri S, Malhotra U, Hennon M, Miller A, Groman A, Halloon A, Reid ME. Clinical characteristics of adenosquamous esophageal carcinoma. J Gastrointest Oncol. 2017;8(1):89–95.
78. Chen S, Chen Y, Yang J, Yang W, Weng H, Li H, Liu D. Primary mucoepidermoid carcinoma of the esophagus. J Thorac Oncol. 2011;6(8):1426–31.
79. Lam KY, Loke SL, Ma LT. Histochemistry of mucin secreting components in mucoepidermoid and adenosquamous carcinoma of the oesophagus. J Clin Pathol. 1993;46(11):1011–5.
80. van Rees BP, Rouse RW, de Wit MJ, van Noesel CJ, Tytgat GN, van Lanschot JJ, Offerhaus GJ. Molecular evidence for the same clonal origin of both components of an adenosquamous Barrett carcinoma. Gastroenterology. 2002;122(3):784–8.
81. Zhao S, Xue Q, Ye B, Lu H, He J, Zhao H. Synchronous primary carcinosarcoma and adenosquamous carcinoma of the esophagus. Ann Thorac Surg. 2011;91(3):926–8.

82. Pandilla R, Kotapalli V, Gowrishankar S, et al. Distinct genetic aberrations in oesophageal adeno and squamous carcinoma. Eur J Clin Investig. 2013;43(12):1233–9.
83. Lam KY, Dickens P, Loke SL, Fok M, Ma L, Wong J. Squamous cell carcinoma of the oesophagus with mucin-secreting component (muco-epidermoid carcinoma and adenosquamous carcinoma): a clinicopathologic study and a review of literature. Eur J Surg Oncol. 1994;20(1):25–31.
84. Odze RD. Tumors of oesophagus. In: Odze RD, editor. WHO classification of tumors digestive system tumours. Lyon, France: World Health Organisation; 2019. p. 23–59.
85. Mewa Kinoo S, Maharaj K, Singh B, Govender M, Ramdial PK. Primary esophageal sclerosing mucoepidermoid carcinoma with "tissue eosinophilia". World J Gastroenterol. 2014;20(22):7055–60.
86. Hagiwara N, Tajiri T, Tajiri T, Miyashita M, Sasajima K, Makino H, Matsutani T, Tsuchiya Y, Takubo K, Yamashita K. Biological behavior of mucoepidermoid carcinoma of the esophagus. J Nippon Med Sch. 2003;70(5):401–7.
87. Evans M, Liu Y, Chen C, Steuer C, et al. Adenosquamous carcinoma ofthe esophagus: an NCDB-based investigation on comparative features and overall survival in a rare tumor. Oncology. 2017;93(5):336–42.
88. Sawada G, Moon J, Saito A, Odagiri K, Kimura Y, Takahashi G, Yamashita S, Inoue M, Irei T, Nakahira S, Shimizu Y, Tominaga H, Kuraoka K, Taniyama K, Hatanaka N. A case of adenoid cystic carcinoma of the esophagus. Surg Case Rep. 2015;1(1):119.
89. Zhou Y, Zang Y, Xiang J, Tang F, Chen Z. Adenoid cystic carcinoma of the cardia: report of a rare case and review of the Chinese literature. Oncol Lett. 2014;8(2):726–30.
90. Guo XF, Mao T, Gu ZT, Fang WT, Chen WH, Shao JC. Adenoid cystic carcinoma of the esophagus: report of two cases and review of the Chinese literature. Diagn Pathol. 2012;7:179.
91. Epstein JI, Sears DL, Tucker RS, Eagan JW Jr. Carcinoma of the esophagus with adenoid cystic differentiation. Cancer. 1984;53(5):1131–6.
92. Yoshikawa K, Kinoshita A, Hirose Y, et al. Endoscopic submucosal dissection in a patient with esophageal adenoid cystic carcinoma. World J Gastroenterol. 2017;23(45):8097–103.
93. Matsumoto M, Nomiyama T, Nakae J, Nishikawa H. Combination chemotherapy for a senile patient with adenoid cystic carcinoma of the esophagus: a case report. Jpn J Clin Oncol. 1993;23(4):258–62.
94. Cerar A, Jutersek A, Vidmar S. Adenoid cystic carcinoma of the esophagus. A clinicopathologic study of three cases. Cancer. 1991;67(8):2159–64.
95. Terada T. Primary combined adenoid cystic carcinoma, basaloid squamous cell carcinoma, and squamous cell carcinoma of the esophagus. Endoscopy. 2012;44(Suppl 2 UCTN):E102–3.
96. Petursson SR. Adenoid cystic carcinoma of the esophagus. Complete response to combination chemotherapy. Cancer. 1986;57(8):1464–7.
97. van Velthuysen ML, Groen EJ, van der Noort V, et al. Grading of neuroendocrine neoplasms: mitoses and Ki-67 are both essential. Neuroendocrinology. 2014;100(2–3):221–7.
98. McCall CM, Shi C, Cornish TC, Klimstra DS, Tang LH, et al. Grading of well-differentiated pancreatic neuroendocrine tumors is improved by the inclusion of both Ki67 proliferative index and mitotic rate. Am J Surg Pathol. 2013;37(11):1671–7.
99. Estrozi B, Bacchi CE. Neuroendocrine tumors involving the gastroenteropancreatic tract: a clinicopathological evaluation of 773 cases. Clinics (Sao Paulo). 2011;66(10):1671–5.
100. Ramezani M, Sadeghi M. Carcinoid tumour of the oesophagus: a systematic review. Prz Gastroenterol. 2018;13(3):196–9.
101. Huang Q, Wu H, Nie L, et al. Primary high-grade neuroendocrine carcinoma of the esophagus: a clinicopathologic and immunohistochemical study of 42 resection cases. Am J Surg Pathol. 2013;37(4):467–83.
102. Hoang MP, Hobbs CM, Leslie H. Carcinoid tumor of the esophagus: a clinicopathologic study of four cases. Am J Surg Pathol. 2002;26(4):517–22.
103. Alperstein A, Fertig RM, Feldman M, et al. Septic thrombophlebitis of the internal jugular vein, a case of Lemierre's syndrome. Intractable Rare Dis Res. 2017;6(2):137–40.

104. Saw EC, Yu GS, Wagner G, Heng Y. Synchronous primary neuroendocrine carcinoma and adenocarcinoma in Barrett's esophagus. J Clin Gastroenterol. 1997;24(2):116–9.
105. Tustumi F, Takeda FR, Uema RH, et al. Primary neuroendocrine neoplasm of the esophagus—report of 14 cases from a single institute and review of the literature. Arq Gastroenterol. 2017;54(1):4–10.
106. Shia J, Tickoo SK, Guillem JG, et al. Increased endocrine cells in treated rectal adenocarcinomas: a possible reflection of endocrine differentiation in tumor cells induced by chemotherapy and radiotherapy. Am J Surg Pathol. 2002;26(7):863–72.
107. Shia J, Guillem JG, Moore HG, et al. Patterns of morphologic alteration in residual rectal carcinoma following preoperative chemoradiation and their association with long-term outcome. Am J Surg Pathol. 2004;28(2):215–23.
108. Milione M, Maisonneuve P, Pellegrinelli A, et al. Ki67 proliferative index of the neuroendocrine component drives MANEC prognosis. Endocr Relat Cancer. 2018;25(5):583–93.
109. Chuah SK, Hu TH, Kuo CM, et al. Upper gastrointestinal carcinoid tumors incidentally found by endoscopic examinations. World J Gastroenterol. 2005;11(44):7028–32.
110. Shaheen NJ, Falk GW, Iyer PG, et al. ACG clinical guideline: diagnosis and management of Barrett's esophagus. Am J Gastroenterol. 2016;111(1):30–50.
111. Milione M, Maisonneuve P, Spada F, Pellegrinelli A, et al. The clinicopathologic heterogeneity of grade 3 gastroenteropancreatic neuroendocrine neoplasms: morphological differentiation and proliferation identify different prognostic categories. Neuroendocrinology. 2017;104(1):85–93.

# Immunohistochemical and Molecular Pathologic Features of Esophagus Carcinomas

38

Yesim Gurbuz and Nusret Erdogan

Immunohistochemical and molecular pathologic features of esophagus carcinoma are a complex subject. At first, as we know the major two groups of esophagus carcinomas are adenoid and squamous type. Origins and precancerous lesions of these two groups are completely different from each other. There are also other rare types of carcinomas such as adenoid cystic, neuroendocrine carcinoma esophagus which have totally different origins. The immunohistochemical and molecular pathologic changes of these subgroups are totally different from each other [1].

Immunohistochemistry is used generally for differential diagnosis of poorly differentiated esophagus carcinoma subgroups or other primary neoplasms. Hematogenous metastasis of other malignancies is very rare, but the esophagus has very close neighborhoods with some organs that produce malignancy. The part of the proximal esophagus in the neck region and tumor originates from neighboring organs may make a direct invasion. The great part of distal esophagus is neighboring mediastinum. As a result, tumors from mediastinum and respiratory tract can make invasion by neighboring. When the tumor is poorly differentiated and in advanced stage, it may be difficult to find the origin and make the right diagnosis. Immunohistochemistry can be too beneficial to identify the origin and type of the tumor. Immunohistochemical expression of some proteins may be also beneficial to establish the treatment protocol. But it is not as popular as breast, colon, and stomach. Also, immunohistochemistry is beneficial in predicting the precancerous potential of some lesions [1, 2].

Genetic alterations are also very important in the carcinogenetic pathway of both adenocarcinoma and squamous carcinoma. But it has only limited value to choose the targeted therapy of adenocarcinoma of the esophagus.

Y. Gurbuz (✉) · N. Erdogan
Pathology Department, Medicine Faculty, Istinye University, Istanbul, Turkey
e-mail: yesim.gurbuz@istinye.edu.tr; nusret.erdogan@istinye.edu.tr



O. Engin (ed.), *Risk Factors and Therapy of Esophagus Cancer*,
https://doi.org/10.1007/978-3-031-47024-0_38

## 38.1 Immunohistochemical Features of Esophagus Carcinomas and Their Precancerous Lesions

### 38.1.1 Squamous Cell Carcinoma

Esophageal squamous cell carcinomas are immunoreactive for pancytokeratin, particularly high-molecular-weight cytokeratin (CK5/6), which is specific to squamous epithelium. Another highly sensitive marker of squamous cell carcinoma is p63. CK5/6 and p63 are used in distinguishing squamous cell carcinoma from adenocarcinoma in routine practice. Human chorionic gonadotrophin (hCG) immunoreactivity can be observed in some poorly differentiated carcinomas without histopathological trophoblastic differentiation. Basement membrane components, such as laminin and type IV collagen synthesis, also can be detected [1, 3].

When we look at the subgroups of squamous cell carcinoma, sarcomatoid carcinoma has differential diagnostic problems with sarcomas. We observe cytokeratin immunoreactivity in the epithelial-appearing component and also in some of the sarcoma-like component in this tumor. Markers such as CK5/6, p63, and p40 can be extremely helpful in the diagnosis of sarcomatoid squamous cell carcinomas. They are also very helpful in highlighting the squamous component of an adenosquamous cell carcinoma (Fig. 38.1). The epithelial component may exhibit focal neuroendocrine features as an additional sign of multidirectional differentiation. There is a specific immunohistochemical staining pattern in basaloid squamous cell carcinoma, the cells express CK5/6 as well as keratins 14 and 19 at the periphery of the basaloid nests [1, 4].

### 38.1.2 Barret's Dysplasia

Barret's esophagus is the glandular metaplasia of squamous epithelium of esophagus against gastroesophageal reflux. Barret's dysplasia is a precancerous lesion for adenocarcinoma of the esophagogastric junction. Immunohistochemistry of p53, AMACR, and IMP3 is sometimes useful for differentiating between non-dysplastic and dysplastic epithelium [2]. Dysplasia shows an increased Ki-67 proliferation

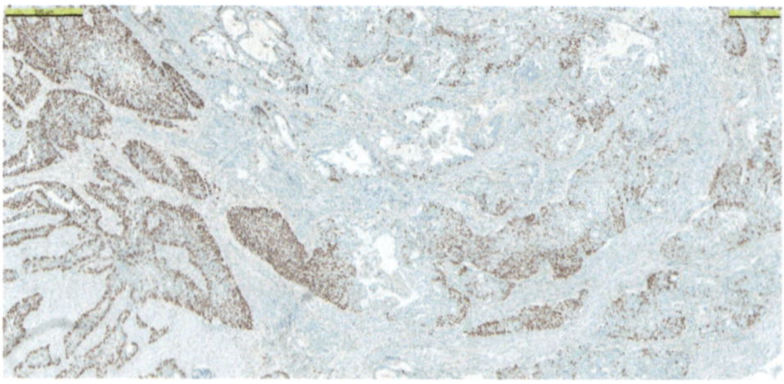

**Fig. 38.1** p40 immunostaining highlights the squamoid component in an adenosquamous cell carcinoma (p40; ×10)

index, which can also be detected in the surface epithelium in high-grade dysplasia [3] (Fig. 38.2).

### 38.1.3 Adenocarcinoma of the Esophagus and Esophagogastric Junction NOS

If the tumor is poorly differentiated, it can be difficult to distinguish a poorly differentiated adenocarcinoma from a poorly differentiated squamous cell carcinoma in a biopsy of a distal esophageal tumor. It is very important as treatment protocols of these two malignancies are totally different from each other. Squamous cell carcinomas are strongly positive for CK5/6, and p40, but adenocarcinomas are strongly positive for CK7 and negative for squamous markers. If the tumor does not stain with both types of differentiation markers and not morphologically identifiable squamous or glandular features, the diagnosis of undifferentiated carcinoma must be used. Some poorly differentiated adenocarcinomas may have neuroendocrine differentiation [4]; such cases are more resistant to therapy. Preoperative chemoradiation may also cause diagnostic pitfalls. It may be difficult to find malignant tumor cells in acellular mucin pools after neoadjuvant chemoradiotherapy [5]. Cytokeratin immunohistochemistry may be helpful to identify the carcinoma cells. Treatment-associated changes of non-neoplastic epithelia may include atypia and pleomorphism that mimic changes in carcinoma cells. Atrophic and metaplastic glands may also cause false overdiagnosis [6].

### 38.1.4 Esophageal Adenoid Cystic Carcinoma

Esophageal adenoid cystic carcinoma is of myoepithelial origin and positive for myoepithel markers such as p63, S100, SMA, and calponin. The epithelial cells are positive for cytokeratin, CEA, and KIT (CD117) [7, 8]. Basaloid squamous cell carcinoma may be considered in the differential diagnosis because it often has a pseudoglandular pattern similar to that of adenoid cystic carcinoma [9]. Immunohistochemistry helps differential diagnosis with myoepithelial markers.

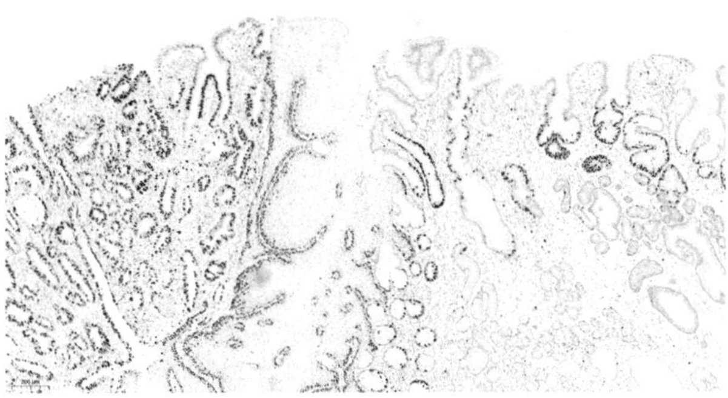

**Fig. 38.2** On the left side of the picture, a significant increase in Ki-67 index is observed in the dysplastic epithelium of Barret's esophagus (Ki-67; ×5)

### 38.1.5 Esophageal Undifferentiated Carcinoma

Lymphoepithelioma-like carcinoma [10] is considered to be a distinct subtype of undifferentiated carcinoma. This tumor is only occasionally positive for EBV [10–12]. When present, cytokeratin positivity may help exclude nonepithelial neoplasms such as melanoma, lymphoma, and sarcoma. In the differential diagnosis of undifferentiated carcinoma from neuroendocrine carcinoma NEC; chromogranin A, synaptophysin, and CD56 can be used. Esophageal undifferentiated carcinoma may be differentiated from poorly differentiated squamous cell carcinoma with p63 and p40 immunopositivity. Immunohistochemical detection of mucins helps in the differential diagnosis of poorly differentiated adenocarcinoma [3].

### 38.1.6 Neuroendocrine Carcinoma of Esophagus

Neuroendocrine differentiation should be confirmed by immunohistochemistry. Neuroendocrine differentiation is confirmed by the expression of chromogranin A and synaptophysin. Synaptophysin expression is a consistent feature, whereas chromogranin A expression, present in about 60% of cases, is usually focal and faint [13] Various hormones have been detected by immunohistochemistry, including serotonin, (entero)glucagon, PP, gastrin, and calcitonin [14–16]. VMAT2 expression, suggestive of an enterochromaffin-like (ECL) cell-like phenotype, has been described in some cases [17, 18]. TTF1 immunoreactivity is also observed in most of the cases [13]. The main differential diagnosis is basaloid squamous cell carcinoma, which usually shows immunohistochemical evidence of squamous cell differentiation, including expression of p63, p40, and CK5/6 (618); and lack of immunoreactivity with neuroendocrine markers [13].

Prognosis of the tumor is directly relevant to grading that depends on the Ki-67 proliferation index [19]. Mixed neuroendocrine non-neuroendocrine neoplasms (MiNENs) might have a better prognosis than pure NECs, the median survival time is about 20 months [20], and prognosis is based on the Ki-67 proliferation index of the NEC component [21].

## 38.2 Molecular Pathologic Changes in Esophageal Carcinomas

### 38.2.1 Barret's Dysplasia

If we summarize Barret's esophagus, there are irritant effects of acid/biliary reflux of gastric and intestinal contents and dysbiosis (microbial imbalance). This causes the reprogramming of progenitor cells in the basal portion of squamous epithelium of esophagus into columnar cell lineage [22, 23]. The reparative epithelium follows one of two lines of differentiation: either a gastric pathway (parietal and chief cells) or an intestinal pathway (goblet and Paneth cells) [23]. Barret's esophagus is characterized by intestinal pathway, with goblet cells, and we know that early Barret's neoplasia is always associated with intestinal metaplasia [24]. Barret's esophagus may progress through dysplasia to adenocarcinoma. Underlying molecular events, related to early changes, are alterations of the cell-cycle regulatory genes, apoptosis, cell signaling, and adhesion pathways [25, 26]. Late changes in Barret's esophagus-associated neoplasia include common genomic abnormalities, losses and gains in chromosome function, and (most importantly) DNA instability characterized by an increased 4N (tetraploid) cell fraction and aneuploidy. Also mutations in PONA, CCND1. TP53, IGF2BP3, and AMACR are detected in Barret's dysplasia [26–29].

### 38.2.2 Adenocarcinoma of the Esophagus and Esophagogastric Junction NOS

The genetic and epigenetic changes of progression from Barret's esophagus is a matter of study for many years [30–32]. Mutations of some genes such as TP53 and SMAD4 are restricted to high-grade dysplasia and adenocarcinoma [25, 33]. Recently, next-generation sequencing techniques have given rise to global projects involving whole-genome sequencing of esophageal adenocarcinoma [34]. These projects showed genetic pathways and mutations that take place in pathogenesis [35, 36] and identified novel genes [26, 37]. Currently, there are no clinical applications for these comprehensive but complex data. It seems likely that clinically relevant and diagnostically useful prognostic and predictive markers will be used in the near future. It is emphasized in the data from The Cancer Genome Atlas (TCGA) that there is similar chromosomal instability in esophageal adenocarcinoma and gastric carcinoma [3].

Molecular changes in adenocarcinoma of the esophagus is directly related to outcome and treatment protocol. Trastuzumab, an antibody targeting the human EGFR family member ERBB2 (HER2), is accepted to be used in the targeted therapy of advanced or metastatic adenocarcinoma of the esophagogastric junction in combination with other chemotherapy. Indication of this therapy is detection of ERBB2 gene by immunohistochemical and molecular pathologic techniques. Amplification of the ERBB2 gene demonstrated by in situ hybridization and the overexpression of the ERBB2 (HER2) protein demonstrated by immunohistochemistry in esophageal adenocarcinoma are predictive of response to ERBB2-targeted therapy. Various testing protocols are used in different centers. Some recommend performing both immunohistochemistry and in situ hybridization, whereas many others recommend in situ hybridization only in the event of equivocal (2+) immunohistochemical findings. The ERBB2 immunscore is defined as 0, 1+ (faint), 2+ (weak to moderate), or 3+ (strong) on the basis of membrane staining [38]. Esophagogastric adenocarcinomas that are positive for ERBB2 often show basolateral or lateral membrane staining just like gastric carcinomas and unlike breast carcinomas, which often show complete membrane staining [39]. The immuno-oncology agent pembrolizumab has shown promising early results for the treatment of advanced and metastatic esophagogastric junction adenocarcinoma [40, 41]. High microsatellite instability and PDL1 overexpression are good predictive factors for the response of esophageal adenocarcinoma to immunotherapy [42].

### 38.2.3 Esophageal Squamous Cell Carcinoma NOS

Squamous carcinoma of the esophagus is the most common tumor of this organ. Esophageal squamous cell carcinoma develops step-by-step progression, with accumulating genetic abnormalities driving progression from histologically normal squamous mucosa to low-grade intraepithelial neoplasia (dysplasia) to high-grade intraepithelial neoplasia and finally to invasive squamous cell carcinoma. These molecular pathologic changes consist of accumulation of somatic mutations and epigenetic changes in oncogenes, tumor suppressor genes, and cell adhesion molecules [1].

TP53 mutation is the earliest and initiator mutation [43]. Aneuploidy, copy-number alterations, changes related to the amplification of genes, such as EGFR, and the silencing of genes such as CDKN2A due to promoter hypermethylation are the genetic changes identified at the intraepithelial neoplasia [44]. The specific mutations required for the invasion which is characteristic of invasive squamous cell carcinoma are still not clear and are important. EIF5A2 amplification has been shown to be a factor related to the acquisition of invasive and migratory capability via epithelial-mesenchymal transition may be an important molecular pathologic change [44].

Genetic abnormalities are very common in esophageal squamous cell carcinoma. Concerning the cell cycle regulatory genes such as p53 gene, mutations that occur in chromosome 17 might be detected in intraepithelial squamous neoplasia. TP53 mutation is detected in different frequencies and types in different geographic regions. This data led us to think that some TP53 mutations may be the result of exposure to exogenous irritant factors. However, TP53 does not share the same tobacco-associated mutations as in lung cancers [45]. Amplification of cyclin D1 (11q13) occurs in 20–40% of squamous cell carcinomas and exists in cancers that retain expression of the Rb protein, suggesting that these two factors cooperate within the same pathway [46].

Inactivation of CDKN2A, with homozygous deletion or de nova methylation, is related to advanced cancer. Transcriptional inactivation of the FHIT gene (fragile histidine triad), which is known as a probable tumor suppressor on 3p14, and deletion of the TOG gene on 17q25 are other important genetic changes [47, 48]. Mutations in other cell-cycle regulatory genes, such as RB1, NFE2L2, CHEK1, CHEK2, CCND1, CDK4, CDK6, and MDM2, have also been identified [49–51].

NOTCH 1 and NOTCH3 genes control cell differentiation. Mutations of these genes are detected in as many as 28% of cases [51].

EGFR (HER1) signaling pathway is also important just like in other adenocarcinomas. EGFR overexpression, reported in 59.6—76% of cases, is an adverse prognostic factor [52].

Mutations and/or amplifications in oncogens such as **RAS** and **AKT** family oncogenes are seen in at least 75% of cases [49].

Epigenetic factors including DNA methylation, chromatin modification. RNA editing, and loss of genomic imprinting are relatively common in esophageal squamous cell carcinoma [43, 52]. Promoter hypermethylation-related silencing of CDKN2A leads to overexpression of p53 [53].

Inherited diseases may also cause genetic alteration. Tylosis, an autosomal dominant disorder, caused by a missense mutation in RHBDF2. results in overactivation of the EGFR signaling pathway [54]. Likewise, Fanconi anemia, an autosomal recessive disorder, which has a mutation that actives in DNA repair [55].

Also, loss of heterozygosity (LOH) is frequently observed in the analyses of clones on 3p21.3 and 9q32 in esophageal cancer (WHO 2152). This causes identification of the novel genes DLEC1 (deleted in lung and esophageal cancer-1) and DEC1 (deleted in esophageal cancer-1) [56–59]. The function of these genes needs to be more detected. Reverse-transcriptase-polymerase chain reaction (RT-PCR) experiments indicate that 33–53% of primary esophageal cancers lack functional transcripts of DLEC 1 or DEC1 cDNA into cancer cell lines that suppress cell growth. In primary esophageal cancers, silencing mutations of LRP1 B (low-density lipoprotein receptor-related protein 1 B) and CRABP1 (cellular retinoic acid binding protein 1) expression is detected by genetic and/or epigenetic mechanisms are observed frequently [60, 61].

Amplification of several proto-oncogenes has also been reported: FGF4 (HST1), FGF6 (HST2), EGFR, MYC [45]. Analyses of genome-wide gene expression profiles and proteomic approaches have identified candidate tumor suppressor genes, oncogenes, and cancer-related microRNAs [62–65]. The mechanisms by which these various genetic events correlate with phenotypical changes, but the sequence of events are not fully understood.

Chromosome aneuploidy (in particular, gains in chromosomes 3, 10, 12, and 20) is common in oesophageal squamous cell carcinoma [3]. DNA studies have shown that two-thirds to three-fourths of the cases have an aneuploid pattern, which correlates with a higher grade and a higher incidence of nodal metastases. Heterogeneity in DNA ploidy, whether comparing the primary tumor with its metastasis or comparing different areas of the primary tumor, is common [1].

Other genetic abnormalities in squamous carcinoma are single nucleotide polymorphisms, including **TP53 polymorphisms** [49], which have been detected in patients with esophageal squamous cell carcinoma. A common somatic mutation signature in esophageal squamous cell carcinoma is **G:C-»AT transitions**, interestingly, which is a typical mutation signature induced by acetaldehyde [52].

### 38.2.4 Esophageal Neuroendocrine Neoplasms

A recent study [66] showed a high rate of inactivating mutations in TP53 and RB1 NOTCH1, FAT1, and FBXW7. TP53- and RB1-inactivating mutations are similar to small-cell NEC (SCNEC). PDE3A, PTPRM, and CBLN2 recurrent mutations were reported in esophageal or neuroendocrine tumorigenesis [20].

**Acknowledgement** We would like to thank Prof. Dr. Süha Göksel for contributing to our chapter with macroscopic and microscopic photographs that she had the kindness to share with us.

## References

1. John GR. Esophagus. In: Goldblum JR, Lamps LW, McKenney JK, Myers JL, editors. Rosai and Ackerman's surgical pathology. 11th ed. Philadelphia: Elsevier; 2018. p. 502–20.
2. Michopoulos S. Critical appraisal of guidelines for screening and surveillance of Barret's esophagus. Ann Transl Med. 2018;6(13):259.
3. Odze RD. Tumors of oesophagus. In: Odze RD, editor. WHO classification of tumors digestive system tumours. Lyon, France: World Health Organisation; 2009. p. 23–59.
4. Wang KL, Yang Q, Cleary KR, Swisher SG, Correa AM, Komaki R, Ajani JA, Rashid A, Hamilton SR, Wu TT. The significance of neuroendocrine differentiation in adenocarcinoma of the esophagus and esophagogastric junction after preoperative chemoradiation. Cancer. 2006;107(7):467–74.
5. Chirieac LR, Swisher SG, Ajani JA, Komaki RR, Correa AM, Morris JS, Roth JA, Rashid A, Hamilton SR, Wu TT. Posttherapy pathologic stage predicts survival in patients with esophageal carcinoma receiving preoperative chemoradiation. Cancer. 2005;103(7):1347–55.
6. Langer R, Becker K. Tumor regression grading of gastrointestinal cancers after neoadjuvant therapy. Virchows Arch. 2018;472(2):175–86.
7. Zhou Y, Zang Y, Xiang J, Tang F, Chen Z. Adenoid cystic carcinoma of the cardia: report of a rare case and review of the Chinese literature. Oncol Lett. 2014;8(2):726–30.
8. Terada T. Primary combined adenoid cystic carcinoma, basaloid squamous cell carcinoma, and squamous cell carcinoma of the esophagus. Endoscopy. 2012;44 Suppl 2 UCTN:E102–3.
9. Li TJ, Zhang YX, Wen J, Cowan DF, Hart J, Xiao SY. Basaloid squamous cell carcinoma of the esophagus with or without adenoid cystic features. Arch Pathol Lab Med. 2004;128(10):1124–30.
10. Terada T. Epstein-Barr virus associated lymphoepithelial carcinoma of the esophagus. Int J Clin Exp Med. 2013;6(3):219–26. Epub 2013 Mar 21.
11. Nakasono M, Hirokawa M, Suzuki M, Takizawa H, Okitsu H, Okamura S, Muguruma N, Ito S, Sano T. Lymphoepithelioma-like carcinoma of the esophagus: report of a case with non-progressive behavior. J Gastroenterol Hepatol. 2007;22(12):2344–7.
12. Chino O, Kijima H, Shimada H, Mizutani K, Nishi T, Tanaka H, Tanaka M, Serizawa A, Tajima T, Makuuchi H. Esophageal squamous cell carcinoma with lymphoid stroma: report of 3 cases with immunohistochemical analyses. Gastrointest Endosc. 2001;54(4):513–7.
13. Huang Q, Wu H, Nie L, Shi J, Lebenthal A, Chen J, Sun Q, Yang J, Huang L, Ye Q. Primary high-grade neuroendocrine carcinoma of the esophagus: a clinicopathologic and immunohistochemical study of 42 resection cases. Am J Surg Pathol. 2013;37(4):467–83.
14. Hoang MP, Hobbs CM, Sobin LH, Albores-Saavedra J. Carcinoid tumor of the esophagus: a clinicopathologic study of four cases. Am J Surg Pathol. 2002;26(4):517–22.
15. Fertig RM, Alperstein A, Diaz C, Klingbeil KD, Vangara SS, Misawa R, Reed J, Gaudi S. Metastatic neuroendocrine tumor of the esophagus with features of medullary thyroid carcinoma. Intractable Rare Dis Res. 2017;6(3):224–9.
16. Saw EC, Yu GS, Wagner G, Heng Y. Synchronous primary neuroendocrine carcinoma and adenocarcinoma in Barret's esophagus. J Clin Gastroenterol. 1997;24(2):116–9.
17. Cary NR, Barron DJ, McGoldrick JP, Wells FC. Combined oesophageal adenocarcinoma and carcinoid in Barret's oesophagitis: potential role of enterochromaffin-like cells in oesophageal malignancy. Thorax. 1993;48(4):404–5.

18. Klöppel G, Rindi G, Anlauf M, Perren A, Komminoth P. Site-specific biology and pathology of gastroenteropancreatic neuroendocrine tumors. Virchows Arch. 2007;451(Suppl 1):S9–27.
19. Milione M, Maisonneuve P, Spada F, Pellegrinelli A, Spaggiari P, Albarello L, Pisa E, Barberis M, Vanoli A, Buzzoni R, Pusceddu S, Concas L, Sessa F, Solcia E, Capella C, Fazio N, La Rosa S. The clinicopathologic heterogeneity of grade 3 gastroenteropancreatic neuroendocrine neoplasms: morphological differentiation and proliferation identify different prognostic categories. Neuroendocrinology. 2017;104(1):85–93.
20. Maruf DM, Khurana H, Rashid A, Correa AM, Anandasabapathy S, Krishnan S, Komaki R, Ajani JA, Swisher SG, Hofstetter WL. Retrospective study of clinicopathologic features and prognosis of high-grade neuroendocrine carcinoma of the esophagus. Am J Surg Pathol. 2008;32(9):1404–11.
21. Milione M, Maisonneuve P, Pellegrinelli A, Grillo F, Albarello L, Spaggiari P, Vanoli A, Tagliabue G, Pisa E, Messerini L, Centonze G, Inzani F, Scarpa A, Papotti M, Volante M, Sessa F, Fazio N, Pruneri G, Rindi G, Solcia E, Rosa L, et al. Ki67 proliferative index of the neuroendocrine component drives MANEC prognosis. Endocr Relat Cancer. 2018;25(5):583–93.
22. Zhang W, Wang DH. Origins of metaplasia in Barret's esophagus: is this an esophageal stem or progenitor cell disease? Dig Dis Sci. 2018;63(8):2005–12.
23. Quante M, Graham TA, Jansen M. Insights into the pathophysiology of esophageal adenocarcinoma. Gastroenterology. 2018;154(2):406–20.
24. Allanson BM, Bonavita J, Mirzai B, Khor TS, Raftopoulos SC, de Boer WB, Brown IS, Kumarasinghe MP. Early Barret esophagus-related neoplasia in segments 1 cm or longer is always associated with intestinal metaplasia. Mod Pathol. 2017;30(8):1170–6.
25. Weaver JMJ, Ross-Innes CS, Shannon N, Lynch AG, Forshew T, Barbera M, Murtaza M, Ong CJ, Lao-Sirieix P, Dunning MJ, Smith L, Smith ML, Anderson CL, Carvalho B, O'Donovan M, Underwood TJ, May AP, Grehan N, Hardwick R, Davies J, Oloumi A, et al. OCCAMS consortium. Ordering of mutations in preinvasive disease stages of esophageal carcinogenesis. Nat Genet. 2014;46(8):837–43.
26. Dulak AM, Stojanov P, Peng S, Lawrence MS, Fox C, Stewart C, Bandla S, Imamura Y, Schumacher SE, Shefler E, McKenna A, Carter SL, Cibulskis K, Sivachenko A, Saksena G, Voet D, Ramos AH, Auclair D, et al. Exome and whole-genome sequencing of esophageal adenocarcinoma identifies recurrent driver events and mutational complexity. Nat Genet. 2013;45(5):478–86.
27. Stachler MD, Taylor-Weiner A, Peng S, McKenna A, Agoston AT, Odze RD, Davison JM, Nason KS, Loda M, Leshchiner I, Stewart C, Stojanov P, Seepo S, Lawrence MS, Ferrer-Torres D, Lin J, Chang AC, Gabriel SB, Lander ES, Beer DG, Getz G, et al. Paired exome analysis of Barret's esophagus and adenocarcinoma. Nat Genet. 2015;47(9):1047–55. https://doi.org/10.1038/ng.3343. Epub 2015 Jul 20.
28. Varghese S, Lao-Sirieix P, Fitzgerald RC. Identification and clinical implementation of biomarkers for Barret's esophagus. Gastroenterology. 2012;142(3):435–41.
29. Zeki S, Fitzgerald RC. The use of molecular markers in predicting dysplasia and guiding treatment. Best Pract Res Clin Gastroenterol. 2015;29(1):113–24.
30. Islam F, Gopalan V, Law S, Tang JC, Chan KW, Lam AK. MiR-498 in esophageal squamous cell carcinoma: clinicopathological impacts and functional interactions. Hum Pathol. 2017;62:141–51.
31. Lee KTW, Smith RA, Gopalan V, Lam AK. Targeted single gene mutation in esophageal adenocarcinoma. Methods Mol Biol. 2018;1756:213–29.
32. Lee KTW, Gopalan V, Lam AK. Somatic DNA copy-number alterations detection for esophageal adenocarcinoma using digital polymerase chain reaction. Methods Mol Biol. 2018;1756:195–212.
33. Ross-Innes CS, Becq J, Warren A, Cheetham RK, Northen H, O'Donovan M, Malhotra S, di Pietro M, Ivakhno S, He M, Weaver JMJ, Lynch AG, Kingsbury Z, Ross M, Humphray S, Bentley D, Fitzgerald RC. Whole-genome sequencing provides new insights into the clonal architecture of Barret's esophagus and esophageal adenocarcinoma. Nat Genet. 2015;47(9):1038–46.

34. Pillai S, Gopalan V, Lam AK. DNA genome sequencing in esophageal adenocarcinoma. Methods Mol Biol. 2018;1756:231–46.
35. Secrier M, Li X, de Silva N, Eldridge MD, Contino G, Bornschein J, MacRae S, Grehan N, O'Donovan M, Miremadi A, Yang TP, Bower L, Chettouh H, Crawte J, Galeano-Dalmau N, Grabowska A, Saunders J, Underwood T, Waddell N, Barbour AP, et al. Mutational signatures in esophageal adenocarcinoma define etiologically distinct subgroups with therapeutic relevance. Nat Genet. 2016;48(10):1131–41.
36. Fels Elliott DR, Perner J, Li X, Symmons MF, Verstak B, Eldridge M, Bower L, O'Donovan M, Gay NJ, OCCAMS Consortium; Fitzgerald RC. Impact of mutations in toll-like receptor pathway genes on esophageal carcinogenesis. PLoS Genet. 2017;13(5):e1006808.
37. Noorani A, Bornschein J, Lynch AG, Secrier M, Achilleos A, Eldridge M, Bower L, Weaver JMJ, Crawte J, Ong CA, Shannon N, MacRae S, Grehan N, Nutzinger B, O'Donovan M, Hardwick R, Tavaré S, Fitzgerald RC, Oesophageal Cancer Clinical and Molecular Stratification (OCCAMS) Consortium. A comparative analysis of whole genome sequencing of esophageal adenocarcinoma pre- and post-chemotherapy. Genome Res. 2017;27(6):902–12.
38. Koopman T, Louwen M, Hage M, Smits MM, Imholz AL. Pathologic diagnostics of HER2 positivity in gastroesophageal adenocarcinoma. Am J Clin Pathol. 2015;143(2):257–64.
39. Grillo F, Fassan M, Sarocchi F, Fiocca R, Mastracci L. HER2 heterogeneity in gastric/gastroesophageal cancers: from benchside to practice. World J Gastroenterol. 2016;22(26):5879–87.
40. Piro G, Carbone C, Santoro R, Tortora G, Melisi D. Predictive biomarkers for the treatment of resectable esophageal and esophago-gastric junction adenocarcinoma: from hypothesis generation to clinical validation. Expert Rev Mol Diagn. 2018;18(4):357–70.
41. Weinberg BA, Xiu J, Hwang JJ, Shields AF, Salem ME, Marshall JL. Immuno-oncology biomarkers for gastric and gastroesophageal junction adenocarcinoma: why PD-L1 testing May not be enough. Oncologist. 2018;23(10):1171–7.
42. Shaib WL, Nammour JP, Gill H, Mody M, Saba NF. The future prospects of immune therapy in gastric and esophageal adenocarcinoma. J Clin Med. 2016;5(11):100.
43. Lin DC, Wang MR, Koeffler HP. Genomic and epigenomic aberrations in esophageal squamous cell carcinoma and implications for patients. Gastroenterology. 2018;154(2):374–89.
44. Li Y, Fu L, Li JB, Qin Y, Zeng TT, Zhou J, Zeng ZL, Chen J, Cao TT, Ban X, Qian C, Cai Z, Xie D, Huang P, Guan XY. Increased expression of EIF5A2, via hypoxia or gene amplification, contributes to metastasis and angiogenesis of esophageal squamous cell carcinoma. Gastroenterology. 2014;146(7):1701–13.e9.
45. Montesano R, Hollstein M, Hainaut P. Genetic alterations in esophageal cancer and their relevance to etiology and pathogenesis: a review. Int J Cancer. 1996;69(3):225–35.
46. Jiang W, Zhang YJ, Kahn SM, Hollstein MC, Santella RM, Lu SH, Harris CC, Montesano R, Weinstein IB. Altered expression of the cyclin D1 and retinoblastoma genes in human esophageal cancer. Proc Natl Acad Sci USA. 1993;90(19):9026–30.
47. Montesano R, Hainaut P. Molecular precursor lesions in oesophageal cancer. Cancer Surv. 1998;32:53–68.
48. von Brevern M, Hollstein MC, Risk JM, Garde J, Bennett WP, Harris CC, Muehlbauer KR, Field JK. Loss of heterozygosity in sporadic oesophageal tumors in the tylosis oesophageal cancer (TOC) gene region of chromosome 17q. Oncogene. 1998;17(16):2101–5.
49. Song Y, Li L, Ou Y, Gao Z, Li E, Li X, Zhang W, Wang J, Xu L, Zhou Y, Ma X, Liu L, Zhao Z, Huang X, Fan J, Dong L, Chen G, Ma L, Yang J, Chen L, et al. Identification of genomic alterations in oesophageal squamous cell cancer. Nature. 2014;509(7498):91–5.
50. Lin DC, Hao JJ, Nagata Y, Xu L, Shang L, Meng X, Sato Y, Okuno Y, Varela AM, Ding LW, Garg M, Liu LZ, Yang H, Yin D, Shi ZZ, Jiang YY, Gu WY, Gong T, Zhang Y, Xu X, et al. Genomic and molecular characterization of esophageal squamous cell carcinoma. Nat Genet. 2014;46(5):467–73.
51. Gao YB, Chen ZL, Li JG, Hu XD, Shi XJ, Sun ZM, Zhang F, Zhao ZR, Li ZT, Liu ZY, Zhao YD, Sun J, Zhou CC, Yao R, Wang SY, Wang P, Sun N, Zhang BH, Dong JS, Yu Y, et al. Genetic landscape of esophageal squamous cell carcinoma. Nat Genet. 2014;46(10):1097–102.

52. Ohashi S, Miyamoto S, Kikuchi O, Goto T, Amanuma Y, Muto M. Recent advances from basic and clinical studies of esophageal squamous cell carcinoma. Gastroenterology. 2015;149(7):1700–15.
53. Taghavi N, Biramijamal F, Sotoudeh M, Khademi H, Malekzadeh R, Moaven O, Memar B, A'rabi A, Abbaszadegan MR. p16INK4a hypermethylation and p53, p16 and MDM2 protein expression in esophageal squamous cell carcinoma. BMC Cancer. 2010;10:138.
54. Blaydon DC, Etheridge SL, Risk JM, Hennies HC, Gay LJ, Carroll R, Plagnol V, McRonald FE, Stevens HP, Spurr NK, Bishop DT, Ellis A, Jankowski J, Field JK, Leigh IM, South AP, Kelsell DP. RHBDF2 mutations are associated with tylosis, a familial esophageal cancer syndrome. Am J Hum Genet. 2012;90(2):340–6.
55. Moldovan GL, D'Andrea AD. How the fanconi anemia pathway guards the genome. Annu Rev Genet. 2009;43:223–49.
56. Daigo Y, Nishiwaki T, Kawasoe T, Tamari M, Tsuchiya E, Nakamura Y. Molecular cloning of a candidate tumor suppressor gene, DLC1, from chromosome 3p21.3. Cancer Res. 1999;59(8):1966–72.
57. Leung AC, Wong VC, Yang LC, Chan PL, Daigo Y, Nakamura Y, Qi RZ, Miller LD, Liu ET, Wang LD, Li JL, Law S, Tsao SW, Lung ML. Frequent decreased expression of candidate tumor suppressor gene, DEC1, and its anchorage-independent growth properties and impact on global gene expression in esophageal carcinoma. Int J Cancer. 2008;122(3):587–94.
58. Nishiwaki T, Daigo Y, Kawasoe T, Nagasawa Y, Ishiguro H, Fujita M, Furukawa Y, Nakamura Y. Isolation and characterization of a human cDNA homologous to the Xenopus laevis XCAP-C gene belonging to the structural maintenance of chromosomes (SMC) family. J Hum Genet. 1999;44(3):197–202.
59. Yang L, Leung AC, Ko JM, Lo PH, Tang JC, Srivastava G, Oshimura M, Stanbridge EJ, Daigo Y, Nakamura Y, Tang CM, Lau KW, Law S, Lung ML. Tumor suppressive role of a 2.4 Mb 9q33-q34 critical region and DEC1 in esophageal squamous cell carcinoma. Oncogene. 2005;24(4):697–705.
60. Sonoda I, Imoto I, Inoue J, Shibata T, Shimada Y, Chin K, Imamura M, Amagasa T, Gray JW, Hirohashi S, Inazawa J. Frequent silencing of low density lipoprotein receptor-related protein 1B (LRP1B) expression by genetic and epigenetic mechanisms in esophageal squamous cell carcinoma. Cancer Res. 2004;64(11):3741–7.
61. Tanaka K, Imoto I, Inoue J, Kozaki K, Tsuda H, Shimada Y, Aiko S, Yoshizumi Y, Iwai T, Kawano T, Inazawa J. Frequent methylation-associated silencing of a candidate tumor-suppressor, CRABP1, in esophageal squamous-cell carcinoma. Oncogene. 2007;26(44):6456–68.
62. Daigo Y, Nakamura Y. From cancer genomics to thoracic oncology: discovery of new biomarkers and therapeutic targets for lung and esophageal carcinoma. Gen Thorac Cardiovasc Surg. 2008;56(2):43–53.
63. Guo Y, Chen Z, Zhang L, Zhou F, Shi S, Feng X, Li B, Meng X, Ma X, Luo M, Shao K, Li N, Qiu B, Mitchelson K, Cheng J, He J. Distinctive microRNA profiles relating to patient survival in esophageal squamous cell carcinoma. Cancer Res. 2008;68(1):26–33.
64. Qi Y, Chiu JF, Wang L, Kwong DL, He QY. Comparative proteomic analysis of esophageal squamous cell carcinoma. Proteomics. 2005;5(11):2960–71.
65. Yamabuki T, Daigo Y, Kato T, Hayama S, Tsunoda T, Miyamoto M, Ito T, Fujita M, Hosokawa M, Kondo S, Nakamura Y. Genome-wide gene expression profile analysis of esophageal squamous cell carcinomas. Int J Oncol. 2006;28(6):1375–84.
66. Wang F, Liu DB, Zhao Q, Chen G, Liu XM, Wang YN, Su H, Qin YR, He YF, Zou QF, Liu YH, Lin YE, Liu ZX, Bei JX, Xu RH. The genomic landscape of small cell carcinoma of the esophagus. Cell Res. 2018;28(7):771–4.

# 39 Bone Metastasis and Treatment in Esophageal Cancer

Ugur Onur Kasman, Ozgur Korkmaz, Seyit Ali Gumustas, and Gultekin Sitki Cecen

## 39.1 Esophageal Cancer

### 39.1.1 Etiology and Pathology

The 5-year survival rate of esophageal cancers is 15–25%. It is the sixth most common type of cancer that causes death [1]. Approximately 70% of esophageal cancers occur in men, and there is a two- to fivefold difference in incidence and mortality rates in terms of gender [2]. Alcohol, smoking, and abdominal obesity are likely to contribute to its higher prevalence in men [3, 4].

Squamous cell carcinoma, adenocarcinoma, sarcomas, small-cell carcinomas, lymphomas, and melanomas are the histological subtypes of esophageal cancer [5]. Adeno and epidermoid cancers, which are among the histological types of esophageal cancers, are more common than other histological subgroups [6]. Alcohol and tobacco use, Howel–Ewans syndrome, Plummer–Wilson syndrome, peptic esophagitis, human papilloma virus infections, and excessive heat consumption are reported to be predisposing factors in the etiology of epidermoid cancers. In adenocarcinomas, Barrett's esophagus and reflux are indicated as predisposing factors [7].

U. O. Kasman · O. Korkmaz
Department of Orthopedics and Traumatology, Faculty of Medicine, Bahceşehir University, Istanbul, Turkey

S. A. Gumustas
Orthopedics and Traumatology Clinic, Acibadem Fulya Hospital, Istanbul, Turkey

G. S. Cecen (✉)
Department of Orthopedics and Traumatology, Faculty of Medicine, Istinye University, Istanbul, Turkey



O. Engin (ed.), *Risk Factors and Therapy of Esophagus Cancer*,
https://doi.org/10.1007/978-3-031-47024-0_39

Epidermoid cancers are more common in the upper and middle esophagus, whereas adenocarcinomas are more common in the distal esophagus. Approximately half of the patients with esophageal cancer develop distant metastases within 5 years [8]. No association has been identified between *Helicobacter pylori* infection and squamous cell esophageal cancer [9].

### 39.1.2 Diagnosis

Dysphagia is the most common clinical symptom among patients with esophageal cancer. Swallowing difficulties are seen primarily with solid foods and then with liquid foods. Physical examination may reveal hepatomegaly and supraclavicular lymphadenopathy on palpation. Endoscopy-guided biopsy is important in diagnosis [7].

### 39.1.3 Treatment

The main approach for treatment is surgery. Even in patients who have undergone complete surgical resection, 5-year survival rates are low. Esophageal stents can be implanted for palliative treatment. A combination of surgery, radiotherapy, and chemotherapy has better outcomes for treating esophagal cancer more successful than single treatment methods. Radiotherapy applications are performed before and after surgery. 5FU/leucovorin/oxaliplatin and docetaxel are used in chemotherapy [10]. Surgical treatments include total gastrectomy with distal esophagectomy or esophagectomy with transhiatal or transthoracic approach [11]. Recently, minimally invasive transthoracic esophagectomy has become a preferred approach [12].

## 39.2 Bone Metastases

Metastasis means displacement and localization. Primary tumor cells metastasize in three ways, via neighborhood, lymphatic, and hematogenous routes [13]. Metastasis caused via the hematogenous route is more common than metastasis via the neighborhood and lymphatic route. In the hematogenous metastasis type, venous metastasis is more common than arterial metastasis. Bones are anatomical structures to which malignancies frequently metastasize due to their dense vascular structure. After the lung and liver, bones are the third most common anatomical structure to be metastasized [14]. Detection and early treatment of bone metastases are important for patient survival and quality of life. Bone sialoprotein and osteopontin exhibit multiple activities known to promote malignant cell proliferation, differentiation, invasion, and metastasis of several osteotropic cancers [15]. Calcium ($Ca^{2+}$) is known to be effective in cancer cell proliferation, migration, and invasion. The $Ca^{2+}$

signaling pathway has been identified as critical to bone metastasis and mediates the differentiation of osteoclasts and osteoblasts [16].

Experimental research has shown that up to 80% of cells released from the primary tumor manage to pass the first steps of extravasation, approximately 2–4% initiate the development of micrometastases, and less than 0.01% survive and form metastatic foci leading to macrometastases [17, 18].

Bone metastases are most frequently observed in the vertebrae, in the pelvic bones, and in the extremities, respectively. Metastasis in the proximal parts of the extremities (proximal femur and humerus) is detected more frequently than in the distal bones [19].

Following metastasis to the bone, osteolytic lesions develop if bone destruction occurs, but osteoblastic lesions develop if the new bone is regenerated. Both osteoblastic and osteolytic lesions may occur together and are called mixed types. Bone metastases are lytic with a rate of 75%, osteoblastic with 15%, and mixed with 10% [19].

### 39.2.1 Osteolytic Metastases

It causes cortical destruction in osteolytic bone metastases (Fig. 39.1). Pathologic fractures can be seen after cortical destruction (Fig. 39.2). Multiple myeloma, renal

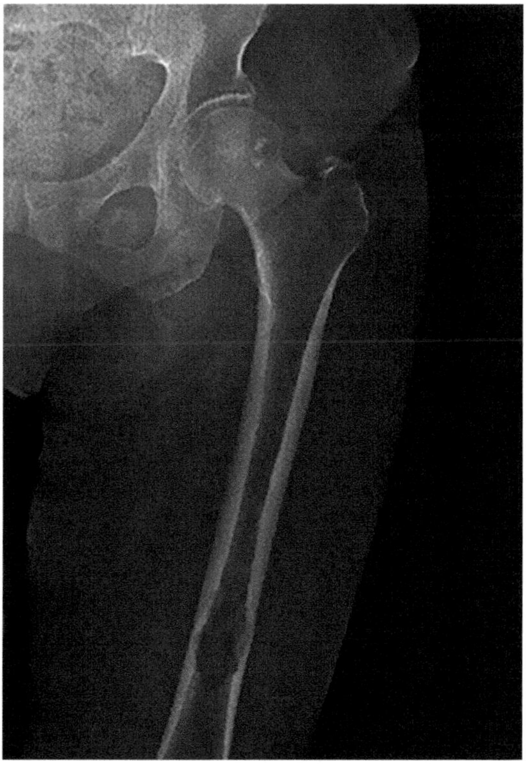

**Fig. 39.1** Bone lesion after osteolytic metastasis in the femoral diaphysis

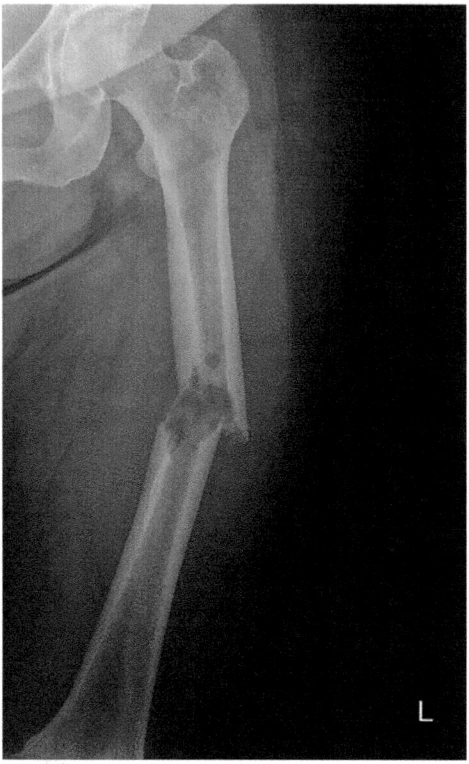


**Fig. 39.2** Pathological femur fracture after metastasis in the femoral diaphysis

cell carcinoma, nonsmall-cell lung cancer, lymphoma, and thyroid cancer are the main malignancies that cause osteolytic metastasis. Parathyroid hormone-related peptides have been implicated in osteolytic metastases [20]. The receptor activator of nuclear factor-kappaB ligand has an important role in osteoclast activity [21].

### 39.2.2 Osteoblastic Metastases

These metastases occur with new bone formation (Fig. 39.3). Transforming growth factor, bone morphogenic protein, and endothelin-1 have been found to cause osteoblast formation in osteoblastic metastases. It is observed in prostate cancer and small-cell lung cancer metastases [22].

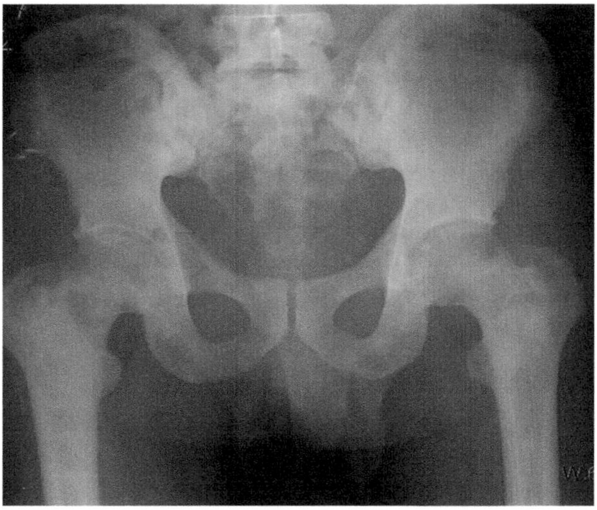

**Fig. 39.3** Osteoblastic metastasis. Osteoblastic metastases in the vertebrae, pelvis, and both proximal femurs

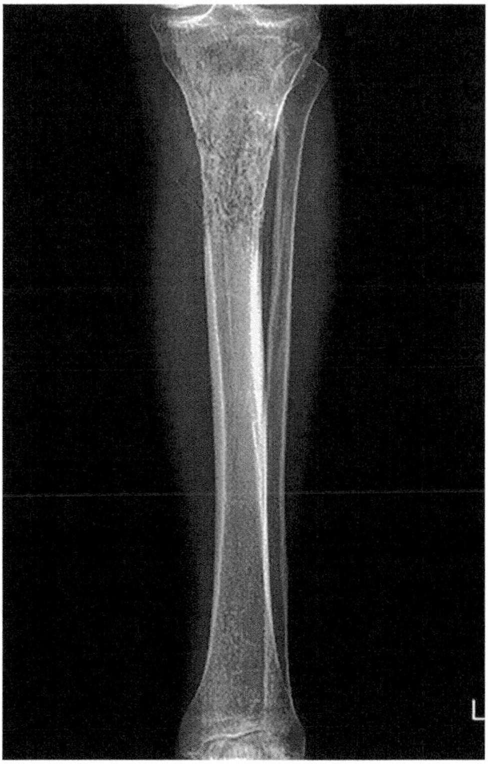


**Fig. 39.4** Mixed-type metastasis. Areas of osteoblastic and lytic metastases are observed and pathologic fracture of the right collum femoris is observed

## 39.2.3 Mixed-Type Metastases

Both osteolytic and osteoblastic patterns are present in this type of metastasis (Fig. 39.4). Gastrointestinal and breast cancer metastases are usually mixed [19].

### 39.2.4 Clinical Presentation

The clinical presentation of patients with bone metastasis varies. It may be detected incidentally during radiologic imaging, and these patients may not have any clinical symptoms. Patients may present with complaints of pain due to metastasis. The pain may be persistent, and pain during nighttime may be observed in patients. Various cytokines and mediators secreted by tumor cells and the mechanical pressure created in the surrounding tissues by the volume effect of the metastatic mass are responsible for the pain [23, 24]. The patient may present in the emergency room with a pathologic fracture. Metastasis should be considered first in radiologically detected bone lesions, particularly in elderly patients. Vertebral metastases may cause neurologic deficits in patients [19]. Patients may consult a physician for various complaints, such as mild numbness and tingling to complete paralysis.

In the physical examination of the patients, a neurovascular evaluation of the affected extremity is performed. The lymphatic system evaluation should be performed. Lymphadenopathies should be evaluated in the axillary region for the upper extremities and in the inguinal region for the lower extremities. Tenderness, firmness, and mobility should be assessed in the presence of a mass. Hypercalcemia and hypertrophic pulmonary osteoarthropathy may be observed in bone metastases. Metastases may cause hypercalcemia secondary to rapid bone destruction. Lethargy, anorexia, nausea, dehydration, confusion, and coma may be observed because of hypercalcemia. In hypertrophic pulmonary osteoarthropathy, periosteal thickening of short and long bones occurs, and swollen joints can be seen [25].

Bone metastases may be solitary or multifocal. In solitary lesions, primary tumors should be considered in the differential diagnosis [26].

## 39.3 Radiology

The primary imaging modality for bone metastases is direct radiography. Direct radiography can determine whether the metastatic lesion is lytic, blastic, or mixed. Conventional bone scintigraphy is the standard imaging modality for radiologic screening of bone metastases. However, due to the limited sensitivity of scintigraphy in detecting vertebral lesions, imaging modalities such as single photon emission computed tomography, magnetic resonance imaging (MRI), and positron emission tomography-computed tomography (PET-CT) should be used in patients with a high probability of bone metastases [27]. Radiologic examination of the area of involvement detected with scintigraphy should be performed with direct radiography. The metastatic site can then be examined in further detail using three-dimensional imaging techniques such as MRI and CT [26]. In particular, CT allows the assessment of the risk of pathologic fractures and the identification of cortical damage. MRI is the best imaging method for differentiating pathologic tissues from normal tissues [28].

## 39.4 Biopsy

In metastatic bone lesions, fine-needle biopsy and incisional biopsy can be performed. Diagnostic rates are higher when fine-needle biopsy is performed under radiological imaging [29].

### 39.4.1 Treatment of Bone Metastases

The treatment of metastatic bone lesions involves a combination of pharmacotherapy, radiotherapy, and surgery [30]. The life expectancy of patients is also important in determining the treatment [31]. Fewer surgical options are available for patients with bone metastases whose life expectancy is less than 12 months [32].

Our primary objective for treating metastatic bone lesions includes preventing pathologic fractures, enabling the patient to use their extremities for daily activities, and pain management.

One of the antiresorptive drugs, bisphosphonates, can be used to prevent the decrease in bone density that occurs when osteoclastic activity is increased. Additionally, tumor-related hypercalcemia is treated with bisphosphonates [33]. Studies have shown that bisphosphonates cause apoptosis in osteoclasts and in tumor cells [34, 35]. Bisphosphonates and denosumab are two commonly used therapeutic agents in the pharmacotherapy of bone metastases [36]. Fluorouracil, capecitabine, and the platinum drugs cisplatin and oxaliplatin are used in the initial chemotherapy regimen for metastatic lesions. Docetaxel and epirubicin are also used [37].

Palliative radiotherapy can be performed to reduce the pain caused by metastatic bone lesions. Embolization can be performed in metastatic tumors rich in vascular structure [38].

The aim of the surgical treatment of bone metastases is to prevent pathologic fractures or to fix the fracture after it has occurred. In surgical fixation, bone cement can be used with internal fixation materials to increase stability. If there is a metastasis close to the joint, segmental bone resection and prosthesis replacement can be performed [39]. In cases of widespread spread of metastatic lesions, limb amputation may be performed. Decompression and instrumentation can be performed in vertebral metastases [19].

The risk of pathologic fracture of metastatic lesions is an important indication for the decision of surgical treatment. If the rate of defective area formed in the bone cortex is 50%, the strength of the bone decreases by 60–90% [40]. If there is no risk of pathologic fracture in bone metastases, radiologic follow-up can be performed. Although the risk of fracture is lower in osteoblastic lesions, the risk of fracture is higher in osteolytic lesions. Therefore, more caution should be exercised in the follow-up of osteolytic lesions. In prophylactic surgeries that are performed to reduce the risk of fracture after detection of metastatic bone lesions, lower extremity surgeries can be performed if the life expectancy is more than 6 months. If the life expectancy is 3 months, surgical treatments for the vertebrae can be performed. In patients with a life expectancy of more than 3 months, prophylactic surgical treatments for the upper extremities can be performed. It has been reported that prophylactic surgeries are more effective when they are performed before the general condition of patients with bone metastases deteriorates [41].

In pathologic fractures secondary to metastatic bone lesions, osteosynthesis is performed with intramedullary nails and plates (Fig. 39.5). These methods provide additional support for osteosynthesis with bone cementum during surgical fixation. If extensive bone resections are performed during surgeries, intercalary prostheses can be used [26] (Fig. 39.6).

Surgical treatment of metastatic femoral proximal end lesions is of primary importance. Improving the patient's quality of life, pain palliation, and remobilization bring surgical treatment to the forefront. Internal fixation and reconstruction with endoprosthesis are two important surgical treatment alternatives. Although internal fixation is primarily planned, the lower postoperative complication rate in endoprosthesis applications is an important advantage [42, 43].

Recently, many new palliative treatment options for bone metastases have emerged, including stereotactic body radiation therapy, embolization, thermal ablation techniques, electrochemotherapy, and high-intensity focused ultrasound. These

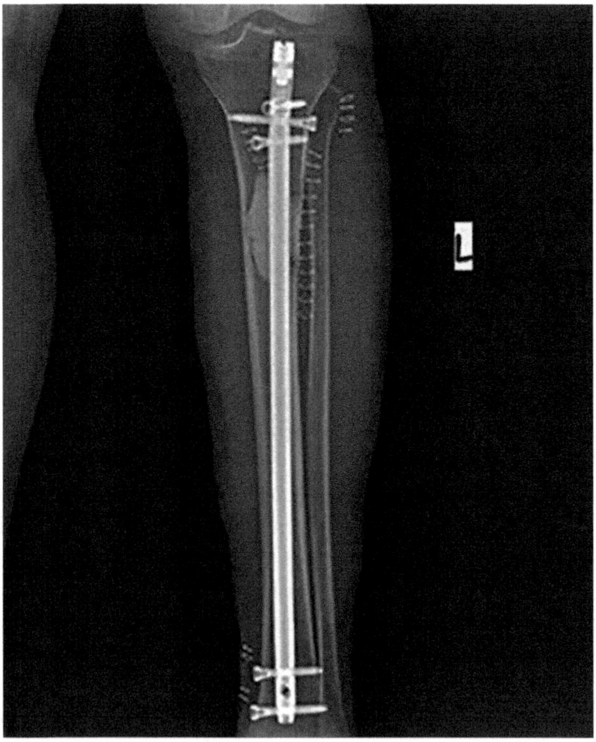

**Fig. 39.5** Fixation with bone cement and intramedullary nail in tibial bone metastasis

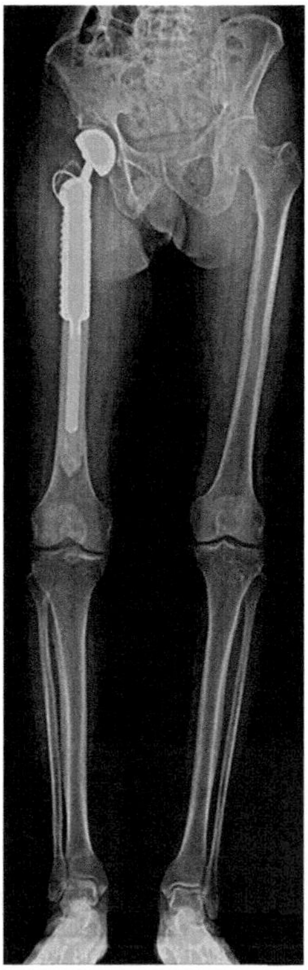

**Fig. 39.6** Resection prosthesis for metastatic lesion of the proximal end of the femur

techniques are useful for patients who may not benefit from surgery or radiotherapy [44–46]. Electrochemotherapy treatment has reduced the pain and improved the quality of life of patients [47].

### 39.4.2 Bone Metastases and Treatment of Esophageal Cancers

Due to the rarity and low life expectancy of esophageal cancers, there are no large series of studies on the treatment of bone metastases of esophageal cancers. Approximately half of the patients diagnosed with esophageal cancer have distant metastases at the time of diagnosis. Distant metastases occur in more than one-third of patients in the treatment phase after diagnosis [48]. Because bone metastases of esophageal cancers are seen in the advanced stages, they are not frequently detected [49].

The average survival of patients with esophageal cancer patients with distant metastasis has been reported to be 5 months [50, 51]. One-year survival has been reported to be 25.3%. Patients with bone metastases have a poor prognosis, but patients who received chemotherapy have better survival. Not receiving chemotherapy and having elevated serum carcinoembryonic antigen have been identified as risk factors that shorten the survival of patients [52]. In another study, bone metastases were detected in 462 patients (5.2%) out of 8916 esophageal cancer patients, and the mean survival in patients with bone metastases was 5 months. Independent risk factors for bone metastases in esophageal cancers were determined as being under 65 years of age, being a male, having a T1 stage, advanced N stage, and non-bone organ metastases [53]. After examining 1470 patients with adeno and epidermoid esophageal cancers, it was found that the most common distant metastasis was to the liver, whereas the rate of bone metastases was 15.3%. Distant lymph node and bone metastases in adeno and epidermoid esophageal cancers are not related to the histologic type of cancer. No association has been identified between bone metastases and any risk factors [54]. Ai et al. found that adenoids had a higher rate of metastasis to bone than epidermoid cancers [55]. Male gender without lung and liver metastases has been found to be a major and independent risk factor for bone metastasis in middle esophageal cancers [56].

According to the results of a study involving 58 patients with bone metastases due to esophageal cancer, multiple bone metastases were detected in 38 patients. Thoracic vertebral metastases were detected in 31 patients (53.4%), lumbar vertebral metastases in 18 patients (31.0%), and pelvic bone metastases in 16 patients (27.6%). It was found that the metastases were osteolytic in 52 patients (89.7%), mixed in two patients (3.4%), and intertrabecular in four patients (6.9%). No bone metastasis of osteoblastic character was detected [52].

Small-cell carcinoma of the esophagus is rare [57]. Multiple metastases can be seen in small-cell carcinomas of the esophagus, and metastases in bones have been detected [58]. Since there are limited number of studies on small-cell carcinomas of the esophagus in the literature, there are no large series of studies on bone metastases and their treatments.

In esophageal cancer patients with bone metastases, the mean survival time was found to be longer with combined radiotherapy and chemotherapy than with single chemotherapy or single radiotherapy [53].

Pathologic fractures, spinal cord compressions, and hypercalcemia may be seen due to bone metastases of esophageal cancer. Radiotherapy and surgical treatments may be needed to treat these complications [59].

According to the radiotherapy treatment results of bone metastases seen after esophageal cancer surgery, radiotherapy was reported to be effective in reducing metastatic mass and pain palliation [60].

The rarity and short survival of esophageal cancers is the main reason for the scarcity of literature on the detection and treatment of bone metastases. In the diagnosis, follow-up, and treatment of bone metastases in esophageal cancers, it is recommended to apply the diagnosis and treatment protocols of bone metastases of other cancers (Figs. 39.7, 39.8, 39.9, and 39.10).

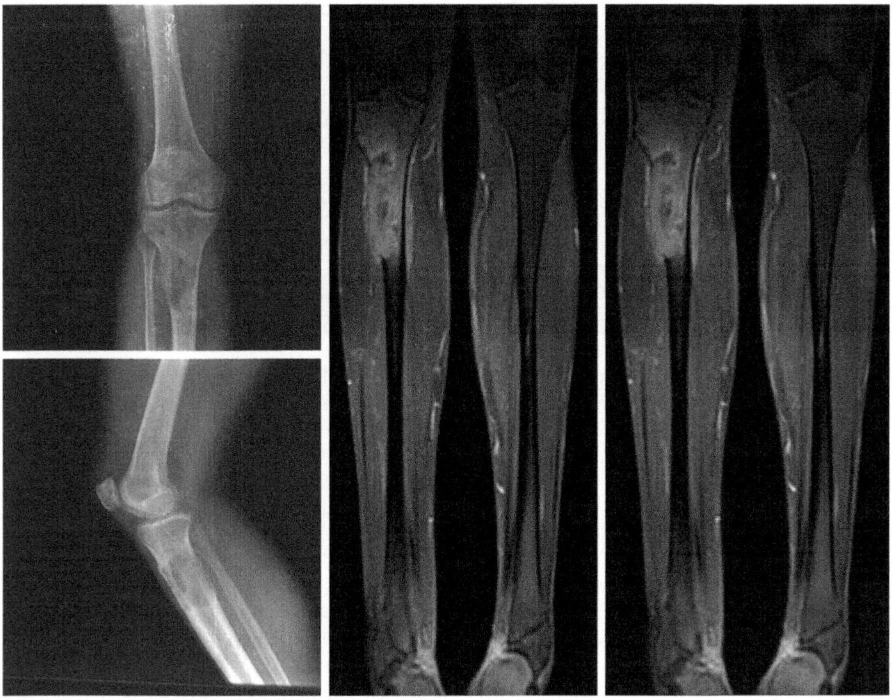

**Fig. 39.7** Preoperative radiographs and magnetic resonance imaging (MRI) images of esophageal cancer tibia proximal end metastasis

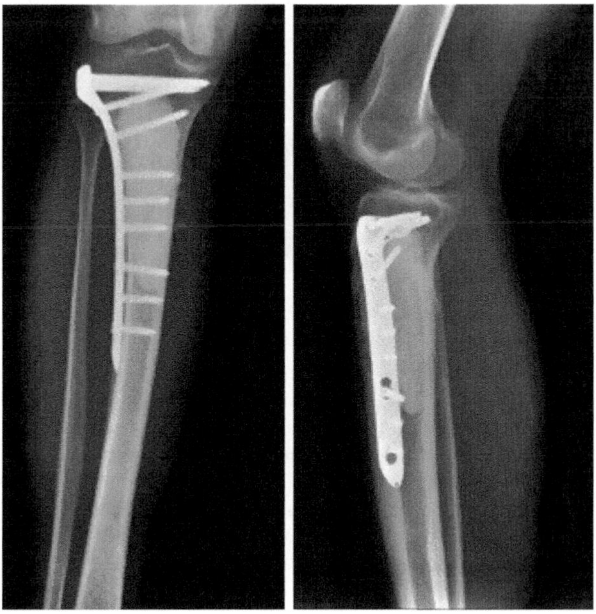

**Fig. 39.8** In order to prevent pathologic fracture, osteosynthesis was performed with plate screws after curettage and additional mechanical support was provided with bone cement

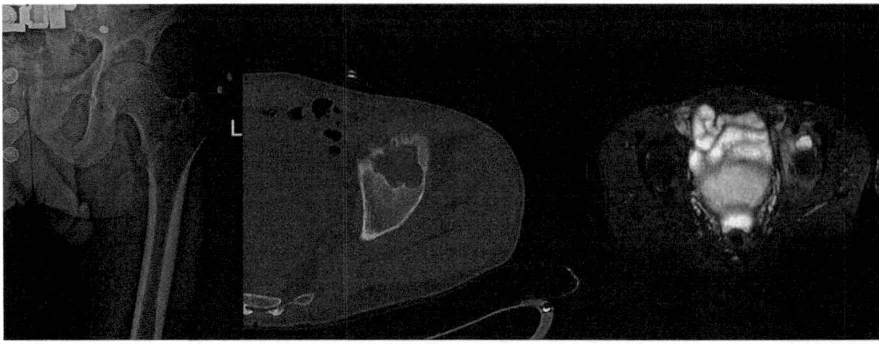


**Fig. 39.9** Preoperative radiograph, computed tomography (CT), and magnetic resonance imaging (MRI) images of esophageal cancer metastasis to the left acetabular region

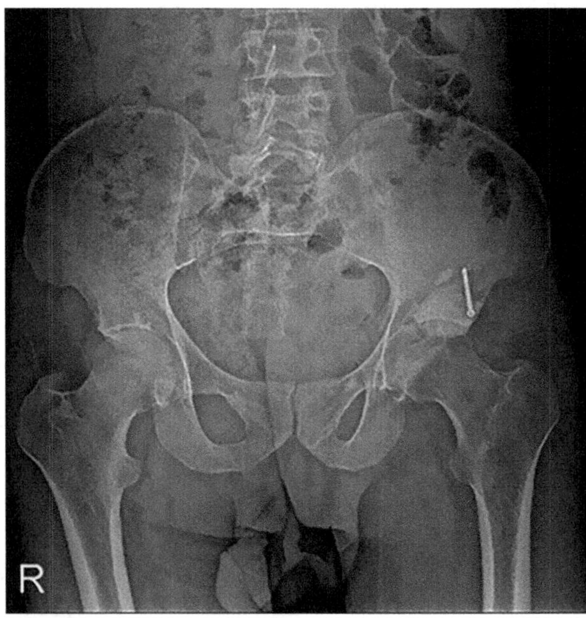


**Fig. 39.10** In the postoperative radiograph, the metastatic lesion in the left acetabular region was curated, filled with bone cement, and fixed with screws

## References


1. Pennathur A, Gibson MK, Jobe BA, Luketich JD. Oesophageal carcinoma. Lancet. 2013;381(9864):400–12.
2. Collaborators GBDOC. The global, regional, and national burden of oesophageal cancer and its attributable risk factors in 195 countries and territories, 1990–2017: a systematic analysis for the global burden of disease study 2017. Lancet Gastroenterol Hepatol. 2020;5(6):582–97.
3. Choi YJ, Lee DH, Han KD, Kim HS, Yoon H, Shin CM, et al. The relationship between drinking alcohol and esophageal, gastric or colorectal cancer: a nationwide population-based cohort study of South Korea. PLoS One. 2017;12(10):e0185778.

4. Chen Q, Zhuang H, Liu Y. The association between obesity factor and esophageal caner. J Gastrointest Oncol. 2012;3(3):226–31.
5. Zhang Y. Epidemiology of esophageal cancer. World J Gastroenterol. 2013;19(34):5598–606.
6. Huang FL, Yu SJ. Esophageal cancer: risk factors, genetic association, and treatment. Asian J Surg. 2018;41(3):210–5.
7. Demir G. Gastrointestinal sistem kanserleri. Yazıcı H, Hamuryudan V, Sonsuz A. Cerrahpaşa İç Hastalıkları. İstanbul. İstanbul medikal yayıncılık. 2005. p. 98–104.
8. Hoeppner J, Kulemann B. Circulating tumor cells in esophageal cancer. Oncol Res Treat. 2017;40(7–8):417–22.
9. Gao H, Li L, Zhang C, Tu J, Geng X, Wang J, Zhou X, Jing J, Pan W. Systematic review with meta-analysis: association of *Helicobacter pylori* infection with esophageal cancer. Gastroenterol Res Pract. 2019;2019:1953497.
10. Grizzi G, Petrelli F, Di Bartolomeo M, Viti M, Texeira Moraes M, Luciani A, Passalacqua R, Ghidini M, Tomasello G, Baiocchi GL, Celotti A. Preferred neoadjuvant therapy for gastric and gastroesophageal junction adenocarcinoma: a systematic review and network meta-analysis. Gastric Cancer. 2022;25(5):982–7.
11. Schlottmann F, Casas MA, Molena D. Evidence-based approach to the treatment of esophagogastric junction tumors. World J Clin Oncol. 2022;13(3):159–67.
12. de Groot EM, Goense L, Kingma BF, Haverkamp L, Ruurda JP, van Hillegersberg R. Trends in surgical techniques for the treatment of esophageal and gastroesophageal junction cancer: the 2022 update. Dis Esophagus. 2023;36:doac099.
13. Briganti A, Suardi N, Gallina A, Abdollah F, Novara G, Ficarra V, Montorsi F. Predicting the risk of bone metastasis in prostate cancer. Cancer Treat Rev. 2014;40(1):3–11.
14. Hage WD, Aboulafia AJ, Aboulafia DM. Incidence, location, and diagnostic evaluation of metastatic bone disease. Orthop Clin North Am. 2000;31(4):515–28.
15. Kruger TE, Miller AH, Godwin AK, Wang J. Bone sialoprotein and osteopontin in bone metastasis of osteotropic cancers. Crit Rev Oncol Hematol. 2014;89(2):330–41.
16. Xie T, Chen S, Hao J, Wu P, Gu X, Wei H, Li Z, Xiao J. Roles of calcium signaling in cancer metastasis to bone. Explor Target Antitumor Ther. 2022;3(4):445–62.
17. Luzzi KJ, MacDonald IC, Schmidt EE, Kerkvliet N, Morris VL, Chambers AF, Groom AC. Multistep nature of metastatic inefficiency: dormancy of solitary cells after successful extravasation and limited survival of early micrometastases. Am J Pathol. 1998;153(3):865–73.
18. Fidler IJ. Metastasis: quantitative analysis of distribution and fate of tumor emboli labeled with 125 I-5-iodo-2′-deoxyuridine. J Natl Cancer Inst. 1970;45(4):773–82.
19. Campanacci M, Enneking WF. Bone and soft tissue tumors. Metastatic bone disease. Wien, New York: Springer-Verlag; 1999. p. 755–80.
20. Southby J, Kissin MW, Danks JA, Hayman JA, Moseley JM, Henderson MA, Bennett RC, Martin TJ. Immunohistochemical localization of parathyroid hormone-related protein in human breast cancer. Cancer Res. 1990;50(23):7710–6.
21. Dougall WC, Glaccum M, Charrier K, Rohrbach K, Brasel K, De Smedt T, Daro E, Smith J, Tometsko ME, Maliszewski CR, Armstrong A, Shen V, Bain S, Cosman D, Anderson D, Morrissey PJ, Peschon JJ, Schuh J. RANK is essential for osteoclast and lymph node development. Genes Dev. 1999;13(18):2412–24.
22. Keller ET, Zhang J, Cooper CR, Smith PC, McCauley LK, Pienta KJ, Taichman RS. Prostate carcinoma skeletal metastases: cross-talk between tumor and bone. Cancer Metastasis Rev. 2001;20(3–4):333–49.
23. Selvaggi G, Scagliotti GV. Management of bone metastases in cancer: a review. Crit Rev Oncol Hematol. 2005;56(3):365–78.
24. Clohisy DR, Mantyh PW. Bone cancer pain. Cancer. 2003;97(3 Suppl):866–73.
25. Mirra JM. Metastases. In: Mirra JM, Picci P, Gold RH, editors. Bone tumors. Lea and Febiger; 1989. p. 1495–518.
26. Dabak N, Göçer H, Çıraklı A. İskelet sistemi metastazlarına yaklaşım. Dabak N. Multidisipliner yaklaşımla kemik ve yumuşak doku tümörleri. Ankara BAYT Bilimsel Araştırmalar Basın Yayın ve Tanıtım. p. 405–15.

27. Schirrmeister H, Arslandemir C. Diagnosis of skeletal metastases in malignant extraskeletal cancers. In: Heymann D, editor. Bone cancer progression and therapeutic approaches. Elsevier; 2010. p. 283–94.
28. Evans AJ, Robertson JF. Magnetic resonance imaging versus radionuclide scintigraphy for screening in bone metastases. Clin Radiol. 2000;55(8):653–4.
29. Rougraff BT, Kneisl JS, Simon MA. Skeletal metastases of unknown origin. A prospective study of a diagnostic strategy. J Bone Joint Surg Am. 1993;75(9):1276–81.
30. Errani C, Mavrogenis AF, Cevolani L, Spinelli S, Piccioli A, Maccauro G, Baldini N, Donati D. Treatment for long bone metastases based on a systematic literature review. Eur J Orthop Surg Traumatol. 2017;27(2):205–11.
31. Errani C, Cosentino M, Ciani G, Ferra L, Alfaro PA, Bordini B, Donati DM. C-reactive protein and tumour diagnosis predict survival in patients treated surgically for long bone metastases. Int Orthop. 2021;45(5):1337–46.
32. Errani C, Bazzocchi A, Spinnato P, Facchini G, Campanacci L, Rossi G, Mavrogenis AF. What's new in management of bone metastases? Eur J Orthop Surg Traumatol. 2019;29(7):1367–75.
33. Body JJ, Coleman RE, Piccart M. Use of bisphosphonates in cancer patients. Cancer Treat Rev. 1996;22(4):265–87.
34. Selvaggi G, Scagliotti G. Management of bone metastases in cancer: a review. Clin Rev Oncol Hematol. 2005;56(3):365–78.
35. Rogers M, Watts D, Russel R. Overview of bisphosphonates. Cancer. 1997;80:1652–60.
36. Mollica V, Nuvola G, Tassinari E, Nigro MC, Marchetti A, Rosellini M, Rizzo A, Errani C, Massari F. Bone targeting agents in patients with prostate cancer: general toxicities and osteonecrosis of the jaw. Curr Oncol. 2022;29(3):1709–22.
37. Al-Batran SE, Hartmann JT, Probst S, Schmalenberg H, Hollerbach S, Hofheinz R, Rethwisch V, Seipelt G, Homann N, Wilhelm G, et al. Phase III trial in metastatic gastroesopha-geal adenocarcinoma with fluorouracil, leucovorin plus either oxaliplatin or cisplatin: a study of the Arbeitsgemeinschaft Internistische Onkologie. J Clin Oncol. 2008;26(9):1435–42.
38. Janjan N. Radiation of bone metastases: conventional techniques and the role of systemic radiopharmaceuticals. Cancer. 1997;80:1628–45.
39. Axelrod D, Gazendam AM, Ghert M. The surgical management of proximal femoral metastases: a narrative review. Curr Oncol. 2021;28(5):3748–57.
40. Hipp JA, Springfield DS, Hayes WC. Predicting pathologic fracture risk in the management of metastatic bone defects. Clin Orthop Relat Res. 1995;312:120–35.
41. Bouthors C, Laumonerie P, Crenn V, Prost S, Blondel B, Fuentes S, Court C, Mazel C, Charles YP, Sailhan F, Bonnevialle P, Members of the SoFCOT. Surgical treatment of bone metastasis from osteophilic cancer. Results in 401 peripheral and spinal locations. Orthop Traumatol Surg Res. 2022;108(4):103193.
42. Forsberg JA, Wedin R, Bauer H. Which implant is best after failed treatment for pathologic femur fractures? Clin Orthop Relat Res. 2013;471(3):735–40.
43. Steensma M, Boland PJ, Morris CD, Athanasian E, Healey JH. Endoprosthetic treatment is more durable for pathologic proximal femur fractures. Clin Orthop Relat Res. 2012;470(3):920–6.
44. Tsukamoto S, Kido A, Tanaka Y, Facchini G, Peta G, Rossi G, Mavrogenis AF. Current overview of treatment for metastatic bone disease. Curr Oncol. 2021;28(5):3347–72.
45. Fini M, Salamanna F, Parrilli A, Martini L, Cadossi M, Maglio M, Borsari V. Electrochemotherapy is effective in the treatment of rat bone metastases. Clin Exp Metastasis. 2013;30(8):1033–45.
46. Bianchi G, Campanacci L, Ronchetti M, Donati D. Electrochemotherapy in the treatment of bone metastases: a phase II trial. World J Surg. 2016;40(12):3088–94.
47. Campanacci L, Cevolani L, De Terlizzi F, Saenz L, Alì N, Bianchi G, Donati DM. Electrochemotherapy is effective in the treatment of bone metastases. Curr Oncol. 2022;29(3):1672–82.
48. Rustgi AK, El-Serag HB. Esophageal carcinoma. N Engl J Med. 2014;371(26):2499–509.
49. Enzinger PC, Mayer RJ. Esophageal cancer. N Engl J Med. 2003;349(23):2241–52.

50. Shiozaki H, Sudo K, Xiao L, Wadhwa R, Elimova E, Hofstetter WL, Skinner HD, Lee JH, Weston B, Bhutani MS, Blum MA, Maru DM, Ajani JA. Distribution and timing of distant metastasis after local therapy in a large cohort of patients with esophageal and esophagogastric junction cancer. Oncology. 2014;86(5–6):336–9.
51. Robb WB, Messager M, Dahan L, Mornex F, Maillard E, D'Journo XB, Triboulet JP, Bedenne L, Seitz JF, Mariette C, Fédération Francophone de Cancérologie Digestive; Société Française de Radiothérapie Oncologique; Union des Centres de Lutte Contre le Cancer; Groupe Coopérateur Multidisciplinaire en Oncologie; French EsoGAstric Tumour Working Group - Fédération de Recherche En Chirurgie. Patterns of recurrence in early-stage oesophageal cancer after chemoradiotherapy and surgery compared with surgery alone. Br J Surg. 2016;103(1):117–25.
52. Imura Y, Yamamoto S, Wakamatsu T, Tanaka T, Tamiya H, Sugimura K, Miyata H, Ishihara R, Yano M, Naka N. Clinical features and prognostic factors in patients with esophageal cancer with bone metastasis. Oncol Lett. 2020;19(1):717–24.
53. Wang RC, Liu XL, Qi C, Chen H, Liu YY, Li DM, Song HZ, Yi J. Bone metastasis of esophageal carcinoma diagnosed as a first primary tumor: a population-based study. Transl Cancer Res. 2022;11(1):113–23.
54. Wu SG, Zhang WW, Sun JY, Li FY, Lin Q, He ZY. Patterns of distant metastasis between histological types in esophageal cancer. Front Oncol. 2018;8:302.
55. Ai D, Zhu H, Ren W, Chen Y, Liu Q, Deng J, Ye J, Fan J, Zhao K. Patterns of distant organ metastases in esophageal cancer: a population-based study. J Thorac Dis. 2017;9(9):3023–30.
56. Qin Y, Mao J, Liang X, Wang N, Yuan M, Zhu J, Wu D, Wang Q. Bone metastasis in esophageal adenocarcinoma and squamous cell carcinoma: a SEER-based study. Gen Thorac Cardiovasc Surg. 2022;70(5):479–90.
57. Pantvaidya GH, Pramesh CS, Deshpande MS, Jambhekar NA, Sharma S, Deshpande RK. Small cell carcinoma of the esophagus: the Tata Memorial Hospital experience. Ann Thorac Surg. 2002;74(6):1924–7.
58. Wu Z, Ma JY, Yang JJ, Zhao YF, Zhang SF. Primary small cell carcinoma of esophagus: report of 9 cases and review of literature. World J Gastroenterol. 2004;10(24):3680–2.
59. Berenson JR, Rosen LS, Howell A, Porter L, Coleman RE, Morley W, Dreicer R, Kuross SA, Lipton A, Seaman JJ. Zoledronic acid reduces skeletal-related events in patients with osteolytic metastases. Cancer. 2001;91(7):1191–200.
60. Nakaya S, Ishiguro H, Fujihata S, Samoto Y, Okubo T, Sagawa H, Tanaka T, Ogawa R, Takahashi H, Matsuo Y, Takiguchi S. [Radiotherapy for bone metastasis after esophageal cancer surgery]. Gan To Kagaku Ryoho. 2019;46(1):91–3.

# Neurological Manifestations in Metastases of Esophageal Cancer

# 40

Sevgi Ferik and Hacer Erdem Tilki

Esophageal cancer has a poor prognosis, usually with high mortality and morbidity. Esophageal cancer is the 11th cause of cancer worldwide. In addition, it ranks sixth in cancer-related deaths [1].

Esophageal cancer is histologically divided into two main categories: adenocarcinoma and squamous cell carcinoma [2]. There are significant racial differences in the histological types of esophageal cancer. Chasala et al. reported that squamous cell carcinoma is common in black patients and adenocarcinoma in white patients [3].

Clinical signs and symptoms in esophageal cancer occur depending on the size, location, distant metastasis, and invasion of the tumors.

Central nervous system (CNS) metastases are the secondary spread of primary systemic cancers originating from tissues other than the CNS to the CNS. Usually seen in breast, lung, and melanoma patients, CNS metastases are associated with poor prognostic outcomes and pose distinct clinical challenges [4].

CNS metastases from esophageal carcinoma are rare, but their incidence is increasing. It is thought that the development of treatment methods, the prolongation of survival, and the application of advanced imaging methods are associated with the increased frequency of neurological involvement in these patients [5].

## 40.1 Brain Metastases

The most common sites for the spread of esophageal cancer metastases are lymph nodes, bones, liver, adrenal glands, lungs, and brain [6].

S. Ferik (✉) · H. E. Tilki
Departments of Neurology and Clinical Neurophysiology, School of Medicine, Ondokuz Mayis University, Samsun, Turkey
e-mail: sevgi.ferik@omu.edu.tr



O. Engin (ed.), *Risk Factors and Therapy of Esophagus Cancer*,
https://doi.org/10.1007/978-3-031-47024-0_40

Brain metastases in esophageal cancer were first reported in 1932 [5]. Although a limited number of cases were reported in the first years, it is seen that the number of cases and case series reported in the literature has increased with the progress in imaging methods. The incidence of brain metastases of esophageal cancer is approximately 0.6–1.5% [7].

Metastases are thought to occur by local invasion and hematogenous spread, but brain metastases in esophageal cancers are thought to occur especially by hematogenous spread [7]. Patients with esophageal cancer and brain metastases rarely have lung metastases. Due to the anatomical location of the Batson venous plexus and the absence of valves, it is thought that there is a way for the lesion to spread to the brain without spreading to the lungs [8, 9].

In case series reported from different countries, it has been reported that brain metastases can be seen in all histopathological types of esophageal cancers [5]. In addition, although brain metastases are seen especially in the advanced stages, there are cases where they are seen in the early stages. In some individual case reports, brain metastasis was found before the primary cancer of the esophagus was detected [5].

It is thought that the risk of brain metastasis increases significantly in cases with lymph node metastasis and local invasion [9]. In addition, the authors reported an increased risk of brain metastases in patients with large primary tumors [8, 9].

Common symptoms and signs in patients with esophageal carcinoma with brain metastases are weakness, headache, seizures, and cerebellar dysfunction [8].

Enhancement of thin-walled cystic lesions on computed tomography (CT) images has been described as a primary feature of brain metastases in esophageal cancer. Therefore, more research investigating the imaging properties is needed [10].

Brain metastases are frequently reported in the cerebral hemisphere [5]. However, spontaneous metastases that spread to uncommon areas other than the cerebral hemispheres are also increasingly reported and ultimately affect the diagnosis, staging, and treatment plan [11]. Cerebellum metastases in esophageal cancers are rare and unexpected [11].

A case of esophageal cancer with cerebellum metastasis has been reported from Turkey. The patient is a 54-year-old woman presenting with a complaint of headache, and histopathological examination of the lesion, in this case, revealed esophageal adenocarcinoma metastasis [12].

Primary pineal tumors are rare, accounting for less than 1% of all CNS tumors, and metastases to the pineal region are rare. In addition, pineal region metastases are rarely seen in esophageal cancers. In our literature review, only three cases of esophageal cancer with pineal region metastases cases were described in the literature. The histology of these three cases was consistent with adenocarcinoma, presenting progressive changes in mental status, dizziness, and diplopia [13, 14].

## 40.2 Leptomeningeal Metastases

Leptomeningeal carcinomatosis describes the cerebrospinal fluid involvement of cancer. Leptomeningeal carcinomatosis associated with esophageal cancer is considered a rare form of metastatic spread of this tumor. The most common symptoms in leptomeningeal metastases are mental status changes and headaches. Diplopia, sensory or motor abnormalities, and seizures may also occur [15].

Our knowledge of leptomeningeal metastases of esophageal cancers is limited to the reported cases and case series. Although adenocarcinoma is the most common histology in these cases, according to the literature, other histologies have also been reported [16, 17].

Imaging studies are the first and most frequently used method in diagnosing leptomeningeal metastases, but the gold standard diagnosis method is made by demonstrating malignant cells. Therefore, if CNS imaging studies of a patient with esophageal cancer with any neurological symptoms are regular, leptomeningeal metastases should be suspected [17].

## 40.3 Spine Metastasis

Metastasis to the vertebral column can be seen in approximately 3–5% of all cancers. However, it has rarely been reported in esophageal cancers. Furthermore, intradural lesions constitute only 6% of malignant lesions detected in the vertebral column. This further highlights the rarity of intradural metastatic pathology in general [18].

For example, a case of cauda equina syndrome with *impaired perineal sensation* and limb weakness has been reported in the literature. Histopathological findings of this case were consistent with esophageal adenocarcinoma [18].

Recently, a 68-year-old male patient was reported intramedullary spinal cord (ISCM) metastasis from esophageal squamous cell carcinoma (ESCC). Similarly, to our knowledge, this is the sixth case of ISCM from esophageal cancer reported. He has been diagnosed with weakness on his right side, although he had pain in his neck for 2 years after his ESCC diagnosis. The gadolinium-enhanced magnetic resonance imaging (MRI) of the cervical spine revealed a mixed-intense intramedullary tumoral lesion in the C4-C5 level. In addition, the lesion has a more intense thin rim of peripheral enhancement. This case highlighted the importance of gadolinium-enhanced MRI for early diagnosis and treatment in ISCM [19].

## 40.4 Recurrent Laryngeal Nerve Metastasis

An advanced thoracic ESCC can be presented as hoarseness due to recurrent laryngeal nerve palsy. It could have resulted from primary tumors or nodal metastasis along the recurrent laryngeal nerve. It has already been shown in 15 patients with ESCC that esophagectomy might be used for treatment. This is especially the right option for young patients with cT1/T2 tumors. It could also be helpful for patients with an excellent response to neoadjuvant treatments. However, most of the postoperative complications of ESCC esophagectomy have also been found to be related to pulmonary tissue [20].

An 81-year-old male patient has recently been reported with a complaint of hoarseness. First, he had superficial esophageal cancer 1 year before this complaint. After he underwent endoscopic submucosal dissection (ESD), he followed up with an idiopathic vocal cord paralysis diagnosis since CT could not reveal any abnormality. During follow-up, 2 months after the ESD operation, he had hoarseness, and 10 months after the ESD, a CT scan showed mediastinal lymph node swelling. The histopathological examination was suitable for squamous cell carcinoma of the lymph node. It was similar to the primary esophageal tumor. This finding might approve that laryngeal nerve paralysis presenting with hoarseness is caused by lymph node metastasis of superficial esophageal cancer [21].

## 40.5 Glossopharyngeal Neuralgia-Asystole Syndrome

Reflex cardiovascular syndromes induced by cervical malignant tumors are classified into glossopharyngeal neuralgia-asystole syndrome, carotid sinus syndrome, and parapharyngeal space lesions syncope syndrome. Until now, two mechanisms have been suggested to explain the reason for syncope in neck carcinoma. One of them, the tumor, can directly invade and stimulate the glossopharyngeal nerve or at least the peripheral branches of it. Therefore, via afferent glossopharyngeal stimulation, the caudal nucleus of the solitary tract in the brainstem could be stimulated. In addition, this stimulation leads to the activation of the efferent fibers, activating the parasympathetic systems. This might be an apparent reason for the bradycardia and even asystole. The other one might be again afferent glossopharyngeal stimulation. At this option, this stimulation might activate the brainstem area in the spinal nucleus of the trigeminus. Furthermore, this stimulation could be an inhibitory effect on vasomotor areas. Therefore, this might cause peripheral vasodilation with severe hypotension. Therefore, a physician has to be aware that syncope can also be caused by glossopharyngeal neuralgia [22–24].

Recently, a patient has been reported with glossopharyngeal neuralgia and repeated syncope related to the recurrence of ESCC. A 78-year-old Japanese male was first referred to a hospital due to repeated syncopal attacks. The patient diagnosed with early ESCC was treated with ESD 3 years before syncopal attacks. However, the patient noticed a left cervical mass 3 years after the ESD, and then he experienced repeated syncopal attacks at the same time. The laboratory tests, echocardiography, electrocardiogram, and brain CT revealed no abnormal result explaining repeated syncope. Interestingly, the patient has always experienced pharyngeal pain before syncope. Therefore, this case was considered to belong to the glossopharyngeal neuralgia-asystole syndrome category. This should be due to the spread of neck cancer or lymphoma around the glossopharyngeal nerve. It might also be due to vascular/stylohyoid ligament compression of the glossopharyngeal nerve by the tumor. Although glossopharyngeal neuralgia might be a clue for the glossopharyngeal neuralgia-asystole syndrome, this diagnosis can be pretty challenging since its rarity. The paroxysmal, electric shock-like, stabbing pain in the pharynx and the base of the tongue should be alerted by the physician about glossopharyngeal neuralgia. These complaints increase while simultaneously talking. In this case, repeated syncope resulted from the glossopharyngeal neuralgia due to the recurrence of esophageal carcinoma. It might be approved that the tumor size got smaller after simultaneous chemoradiation therapy. Moreover, his symptoms wholly resolved [25].

## 40.6 Penile Corpus Cavernosum Metastasis

Penile corpus cavernosum metastases due to ESCC are rare but also fatal. Recently, an 84-year-old male patient was reported. He was a smoker and had curative resection of ESCC a year ago. He had severe penile pain and dysuria for a month. Finally, by biopsy, he was diagnosed with metastatic ESCC. It has been delivered primarily from the esophagus. Although his symptoms were partially relieved by radiotherapy and nonsteroidal anti-inflammatory drugs, the disease aggressively progressed. The patient died due to cancer cachexia and multiple metastases quickly. Because cancer is disseminated in 4 months, this will probably be explained in the future via more research about the underlying mechanism of metastasis [26].

## 40.7 Dermatomyositis

Dermatomyositis is an idiopathic inflammatory myopathy. In these patients, underlying malignancy is frequently found. Dermatomyositis cannot be counted among the metastases, but there are a few cases of dermatomyositis in patients with esophageal cancer in the literature. Since the main subject of this section is metastases, this subject will not be explained in detail. Still, it should be considered when diagnosing metastases in patients with esophageal cancer presenting with neurological findings [27].

## References

1. Global Burden of Disease Cancer Collaboration. Global, regional, and national cancer incidence, mortality, years of life lost, years lived with disability, and disability-adjusted life-years for 29 cancer groups, 1990 to 2017: a systematic analysis for the global burden of disease study. JAMA Oncol. 2019;5(12):1749–68.
2. Harada K, Rogers JE, Iwatsuki M, Yamashita K, et al. Recent advances in treating oesophageal cancer. F1000Res. 2020;9:F1000. Faculty Rev-1189.

3. Chalasani N, Wo JM, Waring JP. Racial differences in the histology, location, and risk factors of esophageal cancer. J Clin Gastroenterol. 1998;26(1):11–3.
4. Boire A, Brastianos PK, Garzia L, Valiente M. Brain metastasis. Nat Rev Cancer. 2020;20(1):4–11.
5. Feng W, Zhang P, Zheng X, Chen M, et al. Incidence and treatment of brain metastasis in patients with esophageal carcinoma. World J Gastroenterol. 2015;21(19):5805–12.
6. Viaro AL, Roballo CA, de Campos PT, Teixeira CO, et al. Occult esophageal squamous cell carcinoma with metastases to the spine and central nervous system. Autops Case Rep. 2015;5(1):33–7.
7. Yamamoto T, Kuroda J, Takezaki T, Shinojima N, et al. Characteristics of brain metastases from esophageal carcinoma. Surg Neurol Int. 2014;5:137.
8. Ogawa K, Toita T, Sueyama H, Fuwa N, et al. Brain metastases from esophageal carcinoma: natural history, prognostic factors, and outcome. Cancer. 2002;94(3):759–64.
9. Weinberg JS, Suki D, Hanbali F, Cohen ZR, et al. Metastasis of esophageal carcinoma to the brain. Cancer. 2003;98(9):1925–33.
10. Takeshima H, Kuratsu J, Nishi T, Soyama N, et al. Metastatic brain tumours from oesophageal carcinoma: neuro-imaging and clinicopathological characteristics in Japanese patients. Acta Neurochir. 2001;143(1):31–5; discussion 35–6.
11. Shaheen O, Ghibour A, Alsaid B. Esophageal cancer metastases to unexpected sites: a systematic review. Gastroenterol Res Pract. 2017;2017:1657310.
12. Tuna H, Bozkurt M, Sarilar C, et al. Esophageal carcinoma metastasis to cerebellum: a case report. Turk Neurosurg. 2008;18(1):65–9.
13. Flanagan ME, Williams JR, Emerson SN, et al. Clinicopathologic characteristics of metastatic esophageal carcinoma isolated to the pineal region: a case report and review of the literature. Exp Mol Pathol. 2017;102(2):247–50.
14. Schuster JM, Rostomily RC, Hahn C, et al. Two cases of esophageal carcinoma metastatic to the pineal region with a review of the literature. Surg Neurol. 1998;49(1):100–2; discussion 102–3.
15. Chamberlain MC. Neoplastic meningitis. Oncologist. 2008;13(9):967–77.
16. Lukas RV, Mata-Machado NA, Nicholas MK, et al. Leptomeningeal carcinomatosis in esophageal cancer: a case series and systematic review of the literature. Dis Esophagus. 2015;28(8):772–81.
17. Aulakh AS, Buttar A, Piperdi B. Leptomeningeal Carcinomatosis in esophageal cancer: case report and review of literature. J Gastrointest Cancer. 2012;43(Suppl 1):84–8.
18. Land CF, Bowden BD, Morpeth BG, et al. Intradural extramedullary metastasis: a review of literature and case report. Spinal Cord Ser Cases. 2019;5:41.
19. Shen B, Ba Z, Huang Y, et al. Intramedullary spinal cord metastasis from esophageal squamous cell carcinoma: case report and literature review. BMC Neurol. 2023;23(1):100.
20. Ozaki A, Mine S, Yoshino K, et al. Outcomes of esophagectomy for patients with esophageal squamous cell carcinoma accompanied by recurrent laryngeal nerve palsy at diagnosis. Esophagus. 2022;19(2):233–9.
21. Takayama H, Komura T, Yoshio T, et al. Case report of a patient with recurrence after endoscopic submucosal dissection for superficial esophageal cancer, diagnosed with mediastinal lymph node endoscopic ultrasound-fine needle aspiration based on the symptom of hoarseness. Nihon Shokakibyo Gakkai Zasshi. 2021;118(3):264–71.
22. Cicogna R, Bonomi FG, Curnis A, Mascioli G, et al. Parapharyngeal space lesions syncope-syndrome. A newly proposed reflexogenic cardiovascular syndrome. Eur Heart J. 1993;14(11):1476–83.
23. Cocci A, Hakenberg OW, Cai T, Nesi G, et al. Prognosis of men with penile metastasis and malignant priapism: a systematic review. Oncotarget. 2017;9(2):2923–30.
24. Numakura K, Tadachi K, Shimoda J. A case of metastatic tumor of penis from esophageal carcinoma. Hinyokika Kiyo. 2008;54(12):795–7.

25. Nagata K, Tajiri K, Ueda A, Okuda Y, et al. Glossopharyngeal neuralgia with syncope caused by recurrence of esophageal squamous cell carcinoma. Intern Med. 2019;58(7):933–6.
26. Song L, Wang Y, Weng G. Metastasis in penile corpus cavernosum from esophageal squamous carcinoma after curative resection: a case report. BMC Cancer. 2019;19(1):162.
27. Karp SJ. Acute dermatomyositis associated with squamous carcinoma of the oesophagus. J R Soc Med. 1985;78(9):770–1.

# Surgical Treatment of Brain Metastases of Esophageal Cancer

# 41

Mehmetzeki Yildiz, Emre Zorlu, and Ahmet Colak

## 41.1 Introduction

The most common brain tumor types in adults are metastases. Brain metastases account for approximately 25–35% of malignancies. However, brain metastasis sourced from esophageal tumors is quite rare. In Western countries, adenocarcinomas are more commonly associated with brain metastases, while in some Asian countries, squamous cell carcinomas are more common. The frequency of esophageal tumors ranges from 1.4 to 5%. The increasing incidence of metastases in recent years may be attributed to more sensitive imaging methods or longer overall survival. Smith et al. reported that brain metastases had developed in 13% of 53 patients with esophageal cancer, during follow-up. Nevertheless, in another study conducted in 2021, the incidence of brain metastases in 19, 225 patients diagnosed with squamous cell carcinoma was only 0.34%. Main reasons for this variability are limited available information, small case series, and death from other causes before the detection of brain metastases. Even with autopsy series conducted in the past and brain scans performed at the time of diagnosis, the rate does not exceed 5% [1–4].

## 41.2 Symptomatology

Brain metastases often develop in specific areas of the brain and therefore the symptoms may vary depending on the affected areas. For instance, metastases in frontal part of the brain may cause symptoms such as changes in behavior and personality, memory loss, and low motivation. Metastases in the middle part of the brain may cause symptoms such as difficulty in coordinating movement, imbalance, difficulty in walking, and abdominal pain. Metastases in the posterior of the brain may cause

M. Yildiz (✉) · E. Zorlu · A. Colak
Department of Neurosurgery, Faculty of Medicine, Bahcesehir University, Istanbul, Turkey



O. Engin (ed.), *Risk Factors and Therapy of Esophagus Cancer*,
https://doi.org/10.1007/978-3-031-47024-0_41

symptoms such as visual and hearing impairments, dizziness, nausea, vomiting, and coordination problems. However, brain metastases may not always be symptomatic on their own. An increase in intracranial pressure due to metastasis may cause nausea and vomiting, which can be mistakenly attributed to the primary tumor in the esophagus. Metastases from esophageal tumors may also be asymptomatic, especially in the early stages, and the symptoms may only become apparent in advanced stages. This causes to late diagnosis of brain metastasis [5, 6].

## 41.3 Risk Factors

It is difficult to determine which patients are at risk of brain metastasis due to the limited number of patients in most studies. It is known that more than 70–80% of brain metastases from esophageal cancer are at stage III or IV. A significant difference in tumor size has been found between patients with and without brain metastases. The average tumor size was shown to be larger in patients with brain metastases (8.63 cm) compared to those without (less than 5.12 cm). Song et al. also found the average tumor size to be 6 cm in patients with brain metastasis [6–8].

According to some population-based studies, brain metastasis is detected in 6.2% of patients diagnosed with esophageal adenocarcinoma cancer and only in 2.1% of patients with squamous cell carcinoma. Based on these findings, it can be suggested that the rate of brain metastasis in adenocarcinoma is higher than in squamous cell carcinoma. However, the histology of the tumor is not considered an independent risk factor for brain metastasis in esophageal cancer [9].

Taking into account the current studies, it is observed that brain metastases can occur independently of the histology of esophageal cancer. Smith and colleagues observed that particularly for the adenocarcinoma patients, the brain lesions were the first site of metastasis. However, Stuart and colleagues found that isolated brain metastases mostly occurred in squamous cell carcinoma patients. A study covering 1760 patients, which is one of the largest studies, showed that histological type did not affect the risk of brain metastasis. This study also found that diabetes was the only independent risk factor associated with brain metastases, and the response to treatment was strongly associated with isolated brain recurrence. On the other hand, effective chemoradiotherapy treatments have also been observed to be associated with brain metastases in previous studies. Neoadjuvant chemoradiation followed by surgery (trimodality therapy [TMT]) can control esophageal cancer somehow to a degree, but may not be able to reach all tumor cells circulating beyond the blood-brain barrier. In addition, it has been noted that Human Epidermal Growth Factor Receptor 2 (HER2), which is overexpressed in 15–25% of invasive breast cancers and is a prognostic marker that determines the aggressive behavior of the tumor, is a common pathway that triggers the potential of esophageal cancer to metastasize to the brain [10–14].

According to one of the recent analyses, the presence of bone and lung metastasis, patients age being younger than 65 years old, American Indian/Alaska Native race (compared to White race), upper esophageal involvement, adenocarcinoma histologic subtype of esophagus, higher N stage, and liver metastases are positively associated with the development of brain metastasis. These studies suggest that in elderly patients, capillary sclerosis may prevent metastasis spread. Additionally, the higher rate of adenocarcinoma metastasis has been attributed to HER2 gene overexpression. However, there are also studies with opposing views on this topic [15, 16].

There is no common lymphatic or vascular drainage for the brain and esophagus. Therefore, two different pathways have been identified for metastasis:

1. Brain metastasis from esophageal cancer may be due to lung metastasis and subsequent secondary lung tumor metastasis. However, lung metastases are only detected in 15–30% of patients with brain metastasis, which may be due to the presence of undetected micrometastases in the lungs in routine examinations.
2. Metastatic spread of esophageal cancer to the brain may occur vascularly between the esophagus and brain through Batson's vertebral venous plexus. Both of these pathways are hypothetically accepted and yet have not been proven [1, 8].

## 41.4 Imaging

Diagnosis can be made with brain CT, MRI, or PET. Routine brain scans are not performed due to the low incidence of metastasis, but imaging should be done as soon as the patient shows neurological symptoms and if the size of the primary tumor is large. When symptoms appear, tumor sizes are generally noticed to have increased. Takeshima et al. claimed that a cystic tumor with a thin peripheral contrast enhancement in brain MRI of patients diagnosed with esophageal tumors, especially in a high-risk population, could be a metastatic brain tumor from esophageal tumors. In addition, in this study, it was stated that lesions smaller than 1 cm were seen as cystic lesions with a thin peripheral halo in contrast-enhanced brain CT. Brain metastatic tumors can generally be characterized by diffusion-weighted MRI. Depending on their histology and cellularity, these tumors can exhibit different signal intensities in brain diffusion MRI. Well-differentiated adenocarcinomas are hypointense, while small- and large-cell neuroendocrine tumors are hyperintense [17, 18].

MRI imaging effectively reveals accurate anatomical information of brain metastasis. MRI has advantages over CT in detecting pathological changes in normal tissue components with higher sensitivity, and in diagnosing intracranial parenchymal tumors, providing more detailed and accurate descriptions of tumor size and associated abnormalities. In recent years, advanced MRI methods such as MR spectroscopy, perfusion-weighted imaging, and diffusion-weighted imaging have provided more valuable information about tumor biology. Additionally, due to its better scanning resolution, MRI can detect smaller lesions (5 mm in diameter) compared to PET-CT (10 mm in diameter) [3].

## 41.5 Treatment

Due to the rarity of brain metastases originating from esophageal carcinoma, there is no definitive method for treatment. Two strategies can be considered including supportive or definitive treatment. Supportive treatment aims to manage the complications caused by the brain lesion. Definitive treatment aims to treat the malignancy, improve the patient's survival, and restore neurological function. Treatment options may include WBRT or stereotactic radiosurgery (SRS), chemotherapy or surgery, and radiotherapy. Metastatic brain tumors can occur as single or multiple forms, and the number of lesions does not have a significant impact on survival. However, patients who have a single metastatic brain lesion and who continue to receive long-term chemotherapy after the appearance of metastases may be expected to achieve long-term survival. Studies have shown that SRS or radiotherapy provides effective treatment options for controlling neurological symptoms and tumor control. Surgical removal of metastases can be performed for both single and multiple lesions. If other metastases are under control and the patient's Karnofsky Performance Status is good, surgical options may be recommended [5, 6, 19].

Some studies have shown that surgery combined with radiotherapy leads to better survival rates. Yoshida's study showed an average survival time of 26.2 months in patients who underwent SR while Weinberg's study only indicated a 3.9-month survival time. The majority of patients with brain metastases die due to systemic reasons. This indicates that treating brain metastases of systemic diseases, such as esophageal cancer, does not significantly improve the average survival time. First, these conflicting results suggest that surgical treatment of brain metastases in cancer types with high mortality rates, such as esophageal cancer, may not significantly increase survival rates. However, surgical treatment may play an important role in reducing symptoms. Second, it is known that there is an improvement in the neurological condition of patients after surgical treatment of brain metastases. This is important for improving the quality of life of these patients. Finally, it has been shown that the rate of surgical complications falls within the previously reported range [8, 20, 21].

The aim of SR in metastatic disease is to locally control the disease, to improve neurological symptoms, to improve survival, and to confirm histological diagnosis. Studies have shown that SR is the optimal treatment for patients with solitary metastasis. Tumor size and location can also affect the decision for surgical treatment. In patients with multiple brain metastases, if there is a large and symptomatic lesion, it should be resected to improve neurological symptoms. However, patients with multiple lesions are generally not suitable for surgical resection. In patients with high disease stages and low survival rates, SR should not be considered. The addition of WBRT to surgery has been shown to increase survival rates compared to the use of WBRT alone. Adding surgery to WBRT reduces recurrences, decreases neurological deaths, and preserves functional independence [5, 6, 22].

It has been a primary treatment method for brain metastasis for a long time. Compared to supportive treatment alone, WBRT can improve patients' symptoms and median survival time. In addition, WBRT can control the emergence of new metastatic lesions, reduce neurological defects and the need for salvage therapy, and control micro-metastatic lesions not detected by MRI. Patients must have a Karnofsky performance score (KPS) of 70 or higher and must be able to independently care for themselves to be suitable for WBRT. After WBRT, increases in survival, local control of metastases, improvement in neurological function, and control of undiagnosed micrometastases have been observed. However, when compared to combined treatments such as SRS and surgery, there is a decrease in survival and an increase in neurological deaths. Therefore, if the patient's condition allows, WBRT is no longer a standalone treatment option [6, 20, 23, 24].

The role of chemotherapy in patients with brain metastases is controversial. Most current chemotherapeutic agents are unable to reach the brain due to the blood–brain barrier. Temozolomide (TMZ) has shown promising results as an effective drug in recent trials. Case series have shown that chemotherapy, when given in combination with SR and WBRT, significantly improves survival rates. Clinical reports suggest that TMZ may improve progression-free survival or enhance radiation response [25, 26].

Surgical resection of metastases has been a standard treatment for solitary metastatic lesions, especially in patients with good performance status and limited extracranial disease. However, many patients with metastases in other organs are not suitable for surgery. The combination of SR and WBRT has shown good survival rates in patients with isolated brain metastases from esophageal cancer. Conflicting results have been reported regarding the combination of SR and SRS. Some studies have reported that SRS effectively controls brain metastases after surgical resection, while other studies indicate similar success rates for these therapeutic methods. Adjuvant WBRT after SRS or surgery has been found to be effective in controlling recurrences in patients with one to three brain metastases [20, 27].

Rades et al. have shown that 1-year survival and local tumor control after WBRT + SRS appear to be as effective as surgery + WBRT. In their study, the recursive partitioning analysis (RPA) class I and II patients with 1–3 brain metastases treated with SRS alone (18–25 Gy) showed improvement in local control and brain control compared to WBRT (30–40 gray). RPA class is strongly associated with survival and it is believed that RPA class I and II patients with controlled primary disease and a limited number of brain lesions may benefit from aggressive treatment. Aoyama et al. found a significant difference in local tumor recurrence 1-year after SRS and WBRT compared to SRS alone; however, there was no statistically significant difference in 1-year overall survival. Muacevic et al., did not find a significant difference in tumor control between SRS alone and WBRT and surgery in patients with a single metastasis smaller than 3 cm, although the second group had fewer metastases in other parts. In summary, there is no difference in survival outcomes when using SRS or WBRT alone or in combination for multiple brain metastases. However, it may help reduce recurrence and control micrometastases [28–30].

Additionally, recent studies have shown that SRS can stimulate the release of certain antigens in the central nervous system and can also have an effect on some immunosuppressive processes. Therefore, it is recommended to treat patients with brain metastases with a combination of radiation and immune checkpoint inhibitors

(ICI) due to their potential synergy. A meta-analysis including 17 studies, which involved 534 patients with brain metastases treated with SRS/ICI, showed that the use of ICI in combination with SRS significantly increased the one-year survival rates compared to the use of SRS alone (64.6% vs. 51.6%, $P = 0.00027$). Xiao and colleagues also found that combining ICI with SRS could reduce the incidence of new brain metastases and provide positive survival outcomes. In this study, a patient received 16 cycles of ICI and survived for 16 months after being diagnosed with asymptomatic brain metastases on July 26, 2019. At the last follow-up, brain lesions had disappeared. The efficacy of ICI in patients with brain metastases should be further explored and confirmed [2, 31].

In a study conducted by Smith et al., the data of 85 patients who took part in a chemoradiotherapy trial were analyzed, and it was found that brain disease recurrence was detected as the first site in 7% of patients after esophagectomy. The average disease-free period is only 5.4 months. This study reports one of the highest rates of brain metastasis in esophageal cancer recurrence. In another study by Stuart et al., isolated recurrent disease in the brain was observed in 4.4% of patients who underwent neoadjuvant chemoradiotherapy and minimally invasive esophagectomy. This study confirms previous studies that most patients with brain metastases have recurrence only in the brain. The detection of brain metastases was based on new neurological symptoms in all patients. It is noted that in most patients with brain metastases, symptoms were present before the diagnosis, and brain imaging is not part of the current follow-up strategy, but is recommended especially within 2 years based on the risk of recurrent brain metastases, particularly for high-risk patients [10, 14].

Based on the current cumulative evidence, there is a difficulty in determining the most appropriate treatment for managing these patients due to insufficient research on their treatment. To select the best therapeutic strategy, the patient's overall condition, disease stage, histology, age, KPS, number, size, and location of metastases should be taken into consideration. Patients with a solitary brain lesion larger than 3 cm are treated with resection and, if necessary, WBRT. SRS is recommended for solitary lesions smaller than 3 cm. Conversely, patients with multiple lesions may not be suitable candidates for SR alone. In patients with one to three metastatic lesions, SR followed by WBRT has significantly improved survival rates, while in patients with four or more metastases, SR before SRS has been found to provide significant improvement in survival rates. If possible, the combination of WBRT with SRS and the addition of chemotherapy to the treatment have also been recommended for patients with multiple brain metastases [5].

## 41.6 Prognosis

The prognosis for esophageal cancer with brain metastasis is generally poor. The time between diagnosis of primary esophageal cancer and brain metastasis ranges from 5.6 to 30 months. After diagnosis of brain metastasis, the reported average survival time is 3.8 months. Various classifications have been made to determine prognostic factors, but no significant results have been obtained. Age and KPS are the most important prognostic factors. RPA classification includes KPS, control of primary tumor, presence or absence of extracranial metastases, and age criteria. Class I patients with the best survival rate are defined as younger than 65 years of age, KPS higher than or equal to 70, and no extracranial metastasis; class III patients with the worst survival rate have KPS lower than 70, and all other patients are class II. RPA classification can help evaluating the benefit of aggressive treatments for patients with better prognosis (RPA class I or II) [28, 32].

In addition, the average survival time after brain metastasis treatment is approximately 7 months in other studies. The absence of extracranial metastasis, solitary brain lesions, and KPS higher than 90 have been found to be associated with better survival rates in up to 14% of patients. Prognosis is also affected by the type of primary tumor, the time interval between the diagnosis of primary tumor and brain metastasis, the formation of brain metastasis, and the presence of other systemic metastasis [1, 5, 33].

Recently, evidence supporting the concept of oligometastatic esophageal cancer has emerged, showing a good response to local consolidative therapy. This is similar to what is known in oligometastatic lung, colorectal, or breast cancer. Kroese and colleagues' recent study demonstrated that local consolidative therapy with metastasectomy or stereotactic radiation in addition to systemic therapy was associated with a favorable prognosis in aggressively treating oligometastatic esophagogastric cancer (median survival of 35 and 16 months, respectively). Regarding isolated brain metastases, Stuart and colleagues' study showed that most patients with brain disease recurrence could be treated with a combination of surgery, SRS, or both. The survival rate in this group reached 44%, 2 years after the detection of brain disease recurrence. Similarly, Nobel and colleagues' earlier study reported the largest group of 38 patients for the treatment of brain metastases, including surgery (79%), or whole-brain radiation (71%), and SRS (18%), with a median survival time of 12 months [11, 14, 34].

## References


1. Go PH, Klaassen Z, Meadows MC, Chamberlain RS. Gastrointestinal cancer and brain metastasis: a rare and ominous sign. Cancer. 2011;117(16):3630–40.
2. Xiao L, Mowery YM, Czito BG, Wu Y, Gao G, Zhai C, et al. Brain metastases from esophageal squamous cell carcinoma: clinical characteristics and prognosis. Front Oncol. 2021;11:652509.
3. Wei X, Luo P, Chen X, Wang Z, Xu L, Xie H, et al. Is it necessary for patients with potentially resectable esophageal squamous cell cancer to receive routine preoperative brain MRI/CT? Thoracic Cancer. 2022;13:3304.
4. Smith RS, Miller RC. Incidence of brain metastasis in patients with esophageal carcinoma. World J Gastroenterol: WJG. 2011;17(19):2407.
5. Esmaeilzadeh M, Majlesara A, Faridar A, Hafezi M, Hong B, Esmaeilnia-Shirvani H, et al. Brain metastasis from gastrointestinal cancers: a systematic review. Int J Clin Pract. 2014;68(7):890–9.
6. Song Z, Lin B, Shao L, Zhang Y. Brain metastases from esophageal cancer: clinical review of 26 cases. World Neurosurg. 2014;81(1):131–5.

7. Ogawa K, Toita T, Sueyama H, Fuwa N, Kakinohana Y, Kamata M, et al. Brain metastases from esophageal carcinoma: natural history, prognostic factors, and outcome. Cancer. 2002;94(3):759–64.
8. Weinberg JS, Suki D, Hanbali F, Cohen ZR, Lenzi R, Sawaya R. Metastasis of esophageal carcinoma to the brain. Cancer. 2003;98(9):1925–33.
9. Cheng S, Yang L, Dai X, Wang J, Han X. The risk and prognostic factors for brain metastases in esophageal cancer patients: an analysis of the SEER database. BMC Cancer. 2021;21(1):1–12.
10. Smith RS, Foster NR, Jatoi A, Thomé SD, Miller RC. Incidence of brain metastasis as first event in patients with esophageal carcinoma: a report from three prospective alliance clinical trials. J Gastrointest Cancer. 2022:1–9.
11. Nobel TB, Dave N, Eljalby M, Xing X, Barbetta A, Hsu M, et al. Incidence and risk factors for isolated esophageal cancer recurrence to the brain. Ann Thorac Surg. 2020;109(2):329–36.
12. Rice TW, Khuntia D, Rybicki LA, Adelstein DJ, Vogelbaum MA, Mason DP, et al. Brain metastases from esophageal cancer: a phenomenon of adjuvant therapy? Ann Thorac Surg. 2006;82(6):2042–2049.e2.
13. Cleary JM, Mamon HJ, Szymonifka J, Bueno R, Choi N, Donahue DM, et al. Neoadjuvant irinotecan, cisplatin, and concurrent radiation therapy with celecoxib for patients with locally advanced esophageal cancer. BMC Cancer. 2016;16(1):1–9.
14. Stuart SK, Kuypers TJ, Martijnse IS, Heisterkamp J, Matthijsen RA. Patients with isolated brain metastases from esophageal carcinoma after minimally invasive esophagectomy may not have a dismal prognosis. J Gastrointest Cancer. 2022;34:1–5.
15. Mitra D, Clark JW, Shih HA, Oh KS, Brastianos PK, Wo JY, et al. Enrichment of HER2 amplification in brain metastases from primary gastrointestinal malignancies. Oncologist. 2019;24(2):193–201.
16. Feilchenfeldt J, Varga Z, Siano M, Grabsch H, Held U, Schuknecht B, et al. Brain metastases in gastro-oesophageal adenocarcinoma: insights into the role of the human epidermal growth factor receptor 2 (HER2). Br J Cancer. 2015;113(5):716–21.
17. Hayashida Y, Hirai T, Morishita S, Kitajima M, Murakami R, Korogi Y, et al. Diffusion-weighted imaging of metastatic brain tumors: comparison with histologic type and tumor cellularity. Am J Neuroradiol. 2006;27(7):1419–25.
18. Takeshima H, Kuratsu J, Nishi T, Soyama N, Miura M, Masumitsu T, et al. Metastatic brain tumours from oesophageal carcinoma: neuro-imaging and clinicopathological characteristics in Japanese patients. Acta Neurochir. 2001;143(1):31–6.
19. Domeki Y, Nakajima M, Takahashi M, Kikuchi M, Yokoyama H, Ogata H, et al. Treatment strategy for brain metastases from esophageal cancer. Tumori J. 2020;106(2):109–14.
20. Yoshida S. Brain metastasis in patients with esophageal carcinoma. Surg Neurol. 2007;67(3):288–90.
21. Stavrinou P, Plambeck L, Proescholdt M, Ghadimi M, Goldbrunner R, Grau S. Brain metastases from esophageal cancer: a retrospective analysis of the outcome after surgical resection followed by radiotherapy. Medicine. 2019;98(34):e16653.
22. Black PM, Johnson MD. Surgical resection for patients with solid brain metastases: current status. J Neuro-Oncol. 2004;69(1):119–24.
23. Andrews DW, Scott CB, Sperduto PW, Flanders AE, Gaspar LE, Schell MC, et al. Whole brain radiation therapy with or without stereotactic radiosurgery boost for patients with one to three brain metastases: phase III results of the RTOG 9508 randomised trial. Lancet. 2004;363(9422):1665–72.
24. Kondziolka D, Lunsford L, Flickinger J. Controversies in the management of multiple brain metastases: the roles of radiosurgery and radiation therapy. 2001. p. 47–58.
25. Zhang P, Yao L, Chen M, Feng W. Prognostic factors affecting long-term outcomes in patients with brain metastasis from esophageal carcinoma. Chin J Cancer Res. 2020;32(6):768.
26. Qie S, Ran Y, Yang H, Cui G, Liu M, Sun X, et al. Brain metastases from esophageal cancer: a case report. Medicine. 2020;99(24):e20223.

27. Kocher M, Soffietti R, Abacioglu U, Villa S, Fauchon F, Baumert BG, et al. Adjuvant whole-brain radiotherapy versus observation after radiosurgery or surgical resection of one to three cerebral metastases: results of the EORTC 22952-26001 study. J Clin Oncol. 2011;29(2):134.
28. Rades D, Dziggel L, Bartscht T, Gliemroth J. Predicting overall survival in patients with brain metastases from esophageal cancer. Anticancer Res. 2014;34(11):6763–5.
29. Aoyama H, Shirato H, Tago M, Nakagawa K, Toyoda T, Hatano K, et al. Stereotactic radiosurgery plus whole-brain radiation therapy vs stereotactic radiosurgery alone for treatment of brain metastases: a randomized controlled trial. JAMA. 2006;295(21):2483–91.
30. Muacevic A, Wowra B, Siefert A, Tonn JC, Steiger HJ, Kreth FW. Microsurgery plus whole brain irradiation versus gamma knife surgery alone for treatment of single metastases to the brain: a randomized controlled multicentre phase III trial. J Neuro-Oncol. 2008;87(3):299–307.
31. Lehrer EJ, Peterson J, Brown PD, Sheehan JP, Quiñones-Hinojosa A, Zaorsky NG, et al. Treatment of brain metastases with stereotactic radiosurgery and immune checkpoint inhibitors: an international meta-analysis of individual patient data. Radiother Oncol. 2019;130:104–12.
32. Gaspar LE, Scott C, Murray K, Curran W. Validation of the RTOG recursive partitioning analysis (RPA) classification for brain metastases. Int J Radiat Oncol Biol Phys. 2000;47(4):1001–6.
33. Venur VA, Ahluwalia MS. Prognostic scores for brain metastasis patients: use in clinical practice and trial design. Chin Clin Oncol. 2015;4(2).
34. Kroese TE, van Laarhoven HW, Nilsson M, Lordick F, Guckenberger M, Ruurda JP, et al. Definition of oligometastatic esophagogastric cancer and impact of local oligometastasis-directed treatment: a systematic review and meta-analysis. Eur J Cancer. 2022;166:254–69.

# 42 Surgical Treatment of Lung Metastasis in Metastatic Esophageal Cancer

Nezih Onur Ermerak and Bedrettin Yildizeli

## 42.1 Epidemiology of Esophageal Cancer

Cancer is a major problem worldwide even though there have been ongoing advances in both conservative and surgical treatment. Although it is relatively rare compared to other malignancies of the digestive system, esophageal cancer is one of the most aggressive malignancies by having a 20% 5-year survival for all stages. Moreover, it is the eighth most common cause of cancer worldwide along with being the sixth most common cause of cancer-related mortality. The incidence of esophageal cancer is 5.9 per 100,000 population. Most of the patients are male with a significant difference in the mortality between sexes. There are two main histological types: esophageal adenocarcinoma and esophageal squamous cell carcinoma; however, the majority of all esophageal cancer patients have esophageal squamous cell histopathology worldwide. Although squamous cell carcinoma is still the most common subtype, the number of esophageal adenocarcinoma patients has been increasing every day. While the risk factors for adenocarcinoma mainly can be listed as obesity, smoking, and gastroesophageal reflux disease, the risk factors attributed to squamous cells are smoking and alcohol consumption. In addition to that, the incidence of the histological type may differ according to geographic region, lifestyle, and race. Moreover, recent studies suggested the genetic component in the development of the disease [1–9].

N. O. Ermerak (✉) · B. Yildizeli
Department of Thoracic Surgery, Faculty of Medicine, Marmara University, Istanbul, Turkey
e-mail: onur.ermerak@marmara.edu.tr; byildizeli@marmara.edu.tr


O. Engin (ed.), *Risk Factors and Therapy of Esophagus Cancer*,
https://doi.org/10.1007/978-3-031-47024-0_42

## 42.2 Diagnosis and Staging

Most of the patients have a diagnosis in the late stages due to the insidious nature of the disease. The most common complaints are progressive dysphagia and weight loss. Additionally, chest pain and odynophagia can accompany the clinical presentation, especially when there is an ulceration in the tumor or invasion of the lesion to the mediastinum. On the other hand, some patients may get a diagnosis following other incidental findings such as anemia, mediastinal lymphadenopathies, or hoarseness due to recurrent laryngeal nerve involvement. Obstruction of the esophageal lumen with the tumor also can be the first presentation in some of the later-staged patients. Dysphagia being the most common symptom, most patients are first evaluated with a barium esophagram demonstrating a dilated esophagus proximal to the obstruction and narrowing of the lumen distal to the lesion. Upper gastrointestinal endoscopy is the gold standard diagnostic tool in the management of highly suspicious patients by providing an opportunity for both detection of the tumor and tissue sampling. It is important to describe the endoscopic findings including the proximal and distal margins and size of the tumor meticulously in the endoscopy report for surgical planning, stent placement, or post-treatment evaluation in the future [5, 10, 11].

Clinical staging plays an important role in decision-making for the treatment plan. Due to the complexity of the disease, it is useful to use multiple diagnostic modalities. Most of the physicians prefer to start evaluation with a computed tomography (CT) scan of the chest and abdomen with intravenous contrast for the visualization of the lymph nodes and metastatic lesions. It is recommended to use fluorodeoxyglucose-positron emission tomography/computed tomography (FDG-PET/CT) for clinical staging. FDG-PET/CT not only yields better information about detecting the metastatic lesions, but it is also useful for surveillance following treatment for further planning. Investigation with endoscopic ultrasound (EUS) is important for loco-regional staging, if there is suspicion of regional lymph node involvement or tumor invasion. Eighth edition American Joint Committee on Cancer (AJCC) Cancer Staging Manual is used for staging esophageal cancer. This classification includes three different groups which are clinical (cTNM), pathological (pTNM), and post neoadjuvant (ypTNM) stage groups. Additionally, the grade of the tumor (cG) plays an important role in the staging of early-stage cancers [12–15].

## 42.3 Treatment Options

Treatment of esophageal cancer depends on variable factors and should be discussed with a multidisciplinary approach [16, 17].

## 42.4 Early-Stage Esophageal Cancer

This group includes the stages of cT1-T2N0M0 patients. Endoscopic resection (ER) can be the treatment of choice when it is indicated. Indications for ER can be listed as: histopathology of high-grade intraepithelial neoplasia or mucosal carcinoma, no lymph node invasion, no vascular invasion, no ulcerations, and well or moderately differentiated grade. There are some studies that compare ER with surgery. Zheng and colleagues reported that despite the effectiveness of ER in early-stage esophageal cancer, esophagectomy has better long-term survival. On the other hand, Chu et al. found out that esophagectomy yielded more unadjusted life years than endoscopic therapy but fewer quality-adjusted life years. Thus, treatment options must be chosen according to the patient [18, 19].

## 42.5 Locally Advanced Esophageal Cancer

### 42.5.1 Neoadjuvant Chemoradiotherapy

Neoadjuvant chemoradiation is the treatment of choice in patients with a locally advanced disease who are candidates for surgery. Data from multiple trials about the locally advanced esophageal cancer confirmed that surgery following preoperative chemoradiation provides better survival and R0 resections compared to esophagectomy alone [20–23].

### 42.5.2 Neoadjuvant Chemotherapy

Although there are studies presenting the advantages of neoadjuvant chemotherapy, data about its effectiveness is not as much as neoadjuvant chemoradiotherapy. Ando and friends compared the use of chemotherapy neoadjuvant versus adjuvant and reported a better survival in favor of neoadjuvant chemotherapy. On the other hand, another study advocated the inferiority of neoadjuvant chemotherapy in overall survival when compared to neoadjuvant chemoradiotherapy [24, 25].

### 42.5.3 Squamous Cell Carcinoma

There are several studies and trials defining trimodality treatment as the standard of care for resectable esophageal cancer patients. CROSS trial treated 363 resectable esophageal cancer patients with preoperative chemoradiotherapy plus surgery and they reported a significant increase in R0 resection rates along with a better median overall survival. In addition to this study, NEOCRTEC study reported their findings about 451 patients who received neoadjuvant chemoradiotherapy. They reported better 5-year overall and disease-free survivals. Additionally, they had a higher R0 resection rate [26, 27].

### 42.5.4 Adenocarcinoma

Neoadjuvant chemoradiotherapy is the accepted standard option for the treatment of locally advanced esophageal adenocarcinoma. The benefit of neoadjuvant chemoradiotherapy was proven by various meta-analyses and randomized clinical trials. The higher pathological response and increased R0 resection rates are well documented. It is still controversial whether surgical resection is needed or not after a complete pathological response following neoadjuvant treatment. Additionally, some studies exist reporting the inferiority of neoadjuvant treatment without surgical resection in esophageal adenocarcinoma patients [26, 27].

## 42.6 Treatment of Metastatic Esophageal Cancer

Patients with metastatic disease have a poor prognosis. They have a 1 year of median overall survival when they receive treatment as chemotherapy only. Even though they differ in biology and immunology, they receive similar chemotherapy regimens. Cisplatin or oxaliplatin and a fluoropyrimidine 5-fluorouracil or capecitabine are the mainstay agents for the standard treatment protocols. In addition to classical treatment options, advances in immunotherapy provided promising data in recent years. Phase III Keynote-590 trial demonstrated better overall survival in 749 randomized squamous cell esophageal cancer patients who either received pembrolizumab plus 5-fluorouracil and cisplatin or placebo plus 5-fluorouracil and cisplatin. In addition to that, the CheckMate 648 trial included 970 squamous cell esophageal cancer patients. Patients were randomized into three separate groups: nivolumab plus ipilimumab, nivolumab plus cisplatin, and fluorouracil, or chemotherapy alone. Improved overall survival was detected in patients receiving nivolumab and chemotherapy, especially in patients with tumor cells PD-L1 (TPS) $\geq$ 1%. Some phase III studies showed an improvement in OS with the combination of chemotherapy and anti-PD1 chemotherapy. In the KEYNOTE-590 trial, 201 patients (13%) had CPS $\geq$ 10 adenocarcinoma demonstrating favorable results by adding pembrolizumab to chemotherapy. 1581 patients with gastroesophageal junction and esophageal adenocarcinoma were randomized to receive nivolumab plus ipilimumab, nivolumab plus oxaliplatin, and fluorouracil or chemotherapy alone in Check Mate 649 trial. They reported better overall survival in the nivolumab plus chemotherapy group [28, 29].

## 42.7 Surgical Management of Pulmonary Metastasis of Esophageal Carcinoma

Although there have been major advances in the treatment of esophageal cancer, it is still one of the most fatal malignancies. The most common sites of distant hematogenous metastasis can be listed as the lung, liver, bone, and brain. When we compare the survival rates between locoregional recurrence and hematogenous metastasis, it is obvious that patients with hematogenous metastasis have poorer survival. Although pulmonary metastasectomy is a standard method of treatment for patients whose primary cancer is controlled, systemic chemotherapy is mostly preferred due to the occurrence of pulmonary metastasis in combination with extrapulmonary metastatic lesions [30, 31].

The incidence of pulmonary metastasis of esophageal carcinoma can vary between 17.5% and 41.4%. Although there are various studies about the role of metastasectomy in colorectal carcinoma, germ cell tumors, and sarcomas and data supporting the acceptance of metastasectomy, few studies exist about the evaluation and treatment plan for the pulmonary metastasis of esophageal cancer. It is still controversial whether to perform pulmonary metastasectomy or not, for the metastasis of esophageal carcinoma due to the lack of outcomes after the surgery. Kanamori and friends published their results after pulmonary metastasectomy of esophageal cancer. Their study included 33 patients with a 5% operative morbidity rate without any 30-day mortality. They achieved complete resection in 30 patients. They reported their 1-, 3-, and 5-year survival rates as 79.4%, 47.8%, and 43%, respectively, with a 17.9-month median survival time. Additionally, they reported disease-free survival of less than 16 months. Similarly, Ichikawa et al. published their experience on pulmonary metastasectomy of esophageal carcinoma including 23 patients. They had no perioperative morbidity or mortality. They reported 1-, 3-, and 5-year survival rates of 73.9%, 43.5%, and 43.5%, respectively. The median disease-free survival of their series was 15.5 months. They also reported recurrence in 14 (66.7%) of the patients with median of 5-month median time to recurrence after metastasectomy. In another study from Japan, Dr. Shiono and colleagues presented their data regarding the outcomes of pulmonary metastasectomy of esophageal cancer. They reported data of 49 patients which is the largest series in the literature so far. They had no perioperative mortality. Their median survival time was 18 months. They experienced recurrence in 16 patients (33%). They reported an overall 5-year survival of 29.6%. They highlighted the impact of disease-free intervals on prognosis. They found out that patients having a disease-free interval of less than 12 months had significantly worse prognosis compared to patients with disease-free interval of more than 12 months [32–35].

## 42.8 Patient Selection

The criterion for patient selection can be summarized as:

- Locally controlled primary cancer
- No extrapulmonary metastasis
- Tolerable margin of safety
- Feasible complete resection
- Tolerable pulmonary function capacity
- WHO/ECOG performance status 0 or 1

## 42.9 Type of the Surgery

The main goal of pulmonary metastasectomy is to achieve complete resection of the metastatic lesions along with maximal preservation of the healthy lung tissue. Thus, the type of resection can vary from wedge resection and segmentectomy to lobectomy and bilobectomy according to the location and margins of the lesions. Although there is data regarding systemic mediastinal lymph node sampling/dissection during metastasectomy for other malignancies, no data exists regarding the role of systemic mediastinal lymph node sampling/dissection in pulmonary metastasectomy for esophageal cancer. Minimally invasive surgery has become the preferred surgical technique in the last decade compared to open technique-thoracotomy due to having less traumatic impact on patients. Video-assisted thoracoscopic surgery (VATS) and robotic-assisted thoracoscopic surgery (RATS) are the preferred surgical techniques today. The preference for surgical technique depends on the experience of the surgeon and the characteristics of the metastatic lesions [36, 37].

## 42.10 Conclusions

Esophageal cancer is an aggressive cancer with poor prognosis, but there has been an ongoing improvement in the management and treatment of the disease. Although we need more data to establish a guideline for describing the absolute benefit of pulmonary metastasectomy, this treatment modality should be taken into consideration when complete resection is feasible in patients who can tolerate surgery.

## References


1. Fitzmaurice C, et al. Global burden of disease cancer collaboration global, regional, and national cancer incidence, mortality, years of life lost, years lived with disability, and disability-adjusted life-years for 32 cancer groups, 1990 to 2015: a systematic analysis for the global burden of disease study. JAMA Oncol. 2017;3(4):524–48.
2. Siegel RL, et al. Cancer statistics, 2022. CA Cancer J Clin. 2022;72(1):7–33.
3. Uhlenhopp DJ, et al. Epidemiology of esophageal cancer: update in global trends, etiology and risk factors. Clin J Gastroenterol. 2020;13(6):1010–21.
4. Liu C-Q, et al. Epidemiology of esophageal cancer in 2020 and projections to 2030 and 2040. Thoracic Cancer. 2023;14(1):3–11.
5. Waters JK, Reznik SI. Update on management of squamous cell esophageal cancer. Curr Oncol Rep. 2022;24(3):375–85.
6. Lindkvist B, et al. Metabolic risk factors for esophageal squamous cell carcinoma and adenocarcinoma: a prospective study of 580 000 subjects within the me-can project. BMC Cancer. 2014;14(1):1–12.
7. Holmes RS, Vaughan TL. Epidemiology and pathogenesis of esophageal cancer. In: Seminars in radiation oncology, vol. 17. WB Saunders; 2007.
8. Hongo M, Nagasaki Y, Shoji T. Epidemiology of esophageal cancer: orient to occident. Effects of chronology, geography and ethnicity. J Gastroenterol Hepatol. 2009;24(5):729–35.
9. Yang J, et al. Understanding esophageal cancer: the challenges and opportunities for the next decade. Front Oncol. 2020;10:1727.

10. Alsop BR, Sharma P. Esophageal cancer. Gastroenterol Clin. 2016;45(3):399–412.
11. Daly JM, et al. Esophageal cancer: results of an American College of Surgeons patient care evaluation study. J Am Coll Surg. 2000;190(5):562–72.
12. Bajaj SS, et al. Early vs delayed surgery for esophageal cancer during the COVID-19 pandemic. J Am Coll Surg. 2022;235(2):174–84.
13. Choi Y, et al. Trimodality therapy for locally advanced esophageal squamous cell carcinoma: the role of volume-based PET/CT in patient management and prognostication. Eur J Nucl Med Mol Imaging. 2022:1–12.
14. Radlinski M, Shami VM. Role of endoscopic ultrasound in esophageal cancer. World J Gastrointest Endoscopy. 2022;14(4):205.
15. Byrd DR, et al. AJCC cancer staging manual. In: Amin MB, Edge SB, Frederick L, editors. Greene, vol. 1024. New York: Springer; 2017.
16. Watanabe M, et al. Recent progress in multidisciplinary treatment for patients with esophageal cancer. Surg Today. 2020;50:12–20.
17. Egyud MR, Tseng JF, Suzuki K. Multidisciplinary therapy of esophageal cancer. Surg Clin. 2019;99(3):419–37.
18. Saeki H, et al. Role of surgery in multidisciplinary treatment strategies for locally advanced esophageal squamous cell carcinoma. Ann Gastroenterol Surg. 2020;4(5):490–7.
19. Zheng H, Kang N, Huang Y, Zhao Y, Zhang R. Endoscopic resection versus esophagectomy for early esophageal cancer: a meta-analysis. Transl Cancer Res. 2021;10(6):2653–62. https://doi.org/10.21037/tcr-21-182.
20. Chu JN, Choi J, Tramontano A, Morse C, Forcione D, Nishioka NS, Abrams JA, Rubenstein JH, Kong CY, Inadomi JM, Hur C. Surgical vs endoscopic management of T1 esophageal adenocarcinoma: a modeling decision analysis. Clin Gastroenterol Hepatol. 2018;16(3):392–400.e7. https://doi.org/10.1016/j.cgh.2017.10.024. Epub 2017 Nov 24.
21. van Heijl M, et al. Neoadjuvant chemoradiation followed by surgery versus surgery alone for patients with adenocarcinoma or squamous cell carcinoma of the esophagus (CROSS). BMC Surg. 8.
22. Shapiro J, et al. Neoadjuvant chemoradiotherapy plus surgery versus surgery alone for oesophageal or junctional cancer (CROSS): long-term results of a randomised controlled trial. Lancet Oncol. 2015;16(9):1090–8.
23. Pasquali S, et al. Survival after neoadjuvant and adjuvant treatments compared to surgery alone for resectable esophageal carcinoma. Ann Surg. 2017;265(3):481–91.
24. Goense L, et al. Role of neoadjuvant chemoradiotherapy in clinical T2N0M0 esophageal cancer: a population-based cohort study. Eur J Surg Oncol. 2018;44(5):620–5.
25. Ando N, Kato H, Igaki H, Shinoda M, Ozawa S, Shimizu H, et al. A randomized trial comparing postoperative adjuvant chemotherapy with cisplatin and 5-fluorouracil versus preoperative chemotherapy for localized advanced squamous cell carcinoma of the thoracic esophagus (JCOG9907). Ann Surg Oncol. 2012;19(1):68–74.
26. Burmeister BH, Thomas JM, Burmeister EA, Walpole ET, Harvey JA, Thomson DB, et al. Is concurrent radiation therapy required in patients receiving preoperative chemotherapy for adenocarcinoma of the oesophagus? A randomised phase II trial. Eur J Cancer. 2011;47(3):354–60.
27. Eyck BM, van Lanschot JJB, Hulshof M, van der Wilk BJ, Shapiro J, van Hagen P, et al. Ten-year outcome of neoadjuvant chemoradiotherapy plus surgery for esophageal cancer: the randomized controlled CROSS trial. J Clin Oncol. 2021;39(18):1995–2004.
28. Yang H, Liu H, Chen Y, Zhu C, Fang W, Yu Z, et al. Long-term efficacy of neoadjuvant chemoradiotherapy plus surgery for the treatment of locally advanced esophageal squamous cell carcinoma: the NEOCRTEC5010 randomized clinical trial. JAMA Surg. 2021;156(8):721–9.
29. Sun JMSL, Manish AS, et al. Pembrolizumab plus chemotherapy versus chemotherapy alone for first-line treatment of advanced oesophageal cancer (KEYNOTE-590): a randomised, placebo-controlled, phase 3 study. Lancet. 2021;398(10302):759–71.
30. Yamauchi Y, et al. Survival after lung Metastasectomy from esophageal cancer: results from a multi-institutional database. Cancers. 2023;15(5):1472.

31. Lo C-M, et al. Long-term survival after pulmonary metastasectomy in patients with esophageal squamous cell carcinoma with lung metastasis. J Cardiothorac Surg. 2022;17(1):1–7.
32. Doki Y, Ajani JA, Kato K, Xu J, Wyrwicz L, Motoyama S, et al. Nivolumab combination therapy in advanced esophageal squamous-cell carcinoma. N Engl J Med. 2022;386(5):449–62.
33. Malhotra GK, et al. Global trends in esophageal cancer. J Surg Oncol. 2017;115(5):564–79.
34. Kanamori J, et al. The role of pulmonary resection in tumors metastatic from esophageal carcinoma. Jpn J Clin Oncol. 2017;47(1):25–31.
35. Ichikawa H, et al. Operative treatment for metachronous pulmonary metastasis from esophageal carcinoma. Surgery. 2011;149(2):164–70.
36. Shiono S, et al. Disease-free interval length correlates to prognosis of patients who underwent metastasectomy for esophageal lung metastases. J Thorac Oncol. 2008;3(9):1046–9.
37. Lim E, et al. Video-assisted thoracoscopic or open lobectomy in early-stage lung cancer. NEJM Evidence. 2022;1(3):EVIDoa2100016.

# Follow-Up of Patients with Surgical Esophageal Cancer Resection

# 43

Semra Demirli Atici and Aras Emre Canda

Esophageal cancer is the sixth most common cause of cancer-related deaths and the eighth most common malignancy worldwide [1, 2]. Esophageal cancer has a one-quarter overall survival rate in 5-year period despite advances in multimodal therapy, increasing imaging modalities, and early detection [3–5]. One of the reasons for this poor prognosis is that the disease has a recurrence rate of 80–85%, despite curative treatment methods [6–8]. Therefore, early detection of recurrence after surgery has an important role in the prognosis, oncologic outcomes of the disease, and health-related quality of life of the patient [9].

The aim of follow-up after treatment of esophageal cancer is to early detect and treat recurrence of the disease which includes lymph nodes, local, organ- disseminated or mixed [10]. There is no consensus on the follow-up interval and follow-up methods (endoscopic, imaging, and laboratory findings) on how patients should be monitored for recurrence after curative surgical esophagectomy [6, 11]. Therefore, routine imaging modalities and procedures may vary as part of postoperative follow-up [12].

Different studies have reported the use of computed tomography (CT) scan, positron emission tomography (PET)/CT scan, upper endoscopy, and serum carcinoembryonic antigen levels for surveillance of the disease [13–19]. Although endoscopic ultrasound (EUS) has been shown to be more sensitive than upper gastrointestinal endoscopy alone for the detection of loco-regional recurrences of the disease, it has not been used for the surveillance of asymptomatic patients.

S. D. Atici (✉)
Department of General Surgery, Acibadem Kent Hospital, Izmir, Turkey

KRC Private Center for Colorectal Surgery and Peritoneal Surface Malignancies, Izmir, Turkey

A. E. Canda
KRC Private Center for Colorectal Surgery and Peritoneal Surface Malignancies, Izmir, Turkey


O. Engin (ed.), *Risk Factors and Therapy of Esophagus Cancer*,
https://doi.org/10.1007/978-3-031-47024-0_43

Earlier detection of recurrence followed by curative surgical treatment might result in prolonged tumor-free survival. Takeuchi et al. [11] investigated the differences in oncological outcomes in patients with relapse detected by routine imaging examinations after surgical esophagectomy, according to the relapse detection method and follow-up interval. In total, 527 patients who underwent R0 resection were evaluated in the outpatient clinic every 3 months, thoracoabdominal computerized tomography (CT) was performed every 4–6 months, and esophagogastroduodenoscopy every 6 months. They reported that among patients diagnosed with relapse at follow-up after surgical resection, patients with pStage IV disease had a better survival rate with imaging surveillance by thoracoabdominal CT ≤5 months apart than those with 6-month intervals in this retrospective study [11]. However, they also reported that this different follow-up interval did not show a significant difference in survival in patients with pStage I-III disease.

The guideline published by European Society For Medical Oncology (ESMO) in 2022; recommends that patients be followed up regularly by the same multidisciplinary team after surgery [12]. The vast majority (90%) of recurrences develop within the first 2 years after surgical treatment for esophageal cancer [12, 20, 21]. For this reason, it was stated that especially newly developing symptoms (abdominal or chest pain, weight loss, vomiting, dysphagia to solid or liquids, progressive hoarseness of voice), nutritional status, and psychosocial support should be kept in mind during the 3-month follow-up periods of the patients in the postoperative first 2 years [12].

Chinese guidelines recommend follow-up every 3 months for the first 2 years, every 6 months for the third and fifth years, and annually thereafter in patients with esophageal cancer who have undergone curative surgery [22]. During these intermittent follow-up periods, PET-CT, magnetic resonance imaging (MRI), and bone scanning are not recommended unless the patient has a suspicion of newly developing metastases [22].

Although ESMO and Delphi consensus about following up esophageal cancer recommends close monitoring of symptoms during routine follow-ups, retrospective studies have reported that recurrent disease may occur in patients before symptoms develop [22, 23]. Different studies have also supported that symptoms mostly occur after the disease has relapsed or metastasized [24, 25].

Surveillance endoscopy has a limited role in detecting asymptomatic local recurrence [11, 25]. Because most physicians think that further evaluation with endoscopic or radiological examinations should be encouraged when signs and symptoms suggestive of disease recurrence occur [24, 26].

The Canadian Society of Thoracic Surgeons recommends follow-up at 3, 6, 12, 18, and 24 months for the first 2 years after surgery and then annually [27]. However, they strongly recommend cessation of smoking and an unscheduled interim evaluation if the patient has become symptomatic. The Canadian Society of Thoracic Surgeons recommends a follow-up period based on disease stage, unlike ESMO and Chinese guidelines [22, 23, 27–29]. Clinical and physical examination is recommended for all patients with different stages of esophageal cancer. The duration of frequency varies between different community recommendations, depending on the stage of the disease.

Routine postoperative surveillance can detect recurrent disease earlier than symptom-triggered surveillance [2, 6, 30]. Toh et al. [28] conducted a national survey of surgeons experienced in esophageal surgery from 77 different hospitals. A questionnaire study was conducted about the approaches, follow-up periods, and methods of the surgeons to the patients they followed up for curative esophagectomy- and/or complete response to chemoradiotherapy for esophageal cancer. This study reported that most of the experienced surgeons had their patients undergo upper gastrointestinal endoscopy at least once a year for following for 5 years after surgery. However, the rate and frequency of upper gastrointestinal endoscopy were higher in patients with esophageal cancer who responded fully to chemoradiotherapy than in patients with esophageal cancer who had undergone surgery. It was also stated that the number and frequency of upper gastrointestinal endoscopies in patient follow-ups were higher than other imaging methods such as FDG-PET/CT and abdominal ultrasonography (USG) [28, 29]. Surgeons stated that they followed their patients for a minimum of 5 years after curative esophagectomy, and they followed patients with outpatient follow-up and physical examination, usually more than four times a year during the first 2 years of these follow-up periods like Japanese guidelines recommend [31]. Seventy-five percent of the participating hospitals in this survey study reported that they continued their patient follow-up until the seventh year, and 40% until the tenth postoperative year [28]. However, Lou et al. [25] reported that the detection value of local or metastatic disease in follow-up scans performed after the sixth year postoperatively decreased significantly, thus screening after the sixth year was unnecessary.

In conclusion, it should not be forgotten that recurrent or metastatic disease that develops in approximately half of the patients who underwent curative surgery for esophageal cancer can provide long-term survival with early diagnosis and early treatment. Prospective studies investigating the use, frequency, duration, and method of surveillance after esophageal surgery have not been conducted. Although there are local guidelines, a common consensus and follow-up system based on it should be established and the effectiveness of the follow-up interval should be verified. Contrast-enhanced thoracoabdominal CT and annual upper gastrointestinal endoscopy are recommended as follow-up examinations, with a physical examination every 3 or 6 months.

## References

1. Siegel RL, Miller KD, Jemal A. Cancer statistics, 2019. CA Cancer J Clin. 2019;69:7–34. https://doi.org/10.3322/caac.21551.
2. Mukkamalla SKR, Recio-Boiles A, Babiker HM. Esophageal cancer. In: StatPearls. Treasure Island, FL: StatPearls Publishing; 2023.
3. Arnold M, Ferlay J, Van Berge Henegouwen MI, Soerjomataram I. Global burden of oesophageal and gastric cancer by histology and subsite in 2018. Gut. 2020;69(9):1564–71.

4. Kamangar F, Nasrollahzadeh D, Safiri S, et al. The global, regional, and national burden of oesophageal cancer and its attributable risk factors in 195 countries and territories, 1990-2017: a systematic analysis for the global burden of disease study 2017. Lancet Gastroenterol Hepatol. 2020;5(6):582–97.
5. Moyes LH, Anderson JE, Forshaw MJ. Proposed follow up programme after curative resection for lower third oesophageal cancer. World J Surg Oncol. 2010;8:75. https://doi.org/10.1186/1477-7819-8-75.
6. Chidambaram S, Sounderajah V, Maynard N, et al. Evaluation of post-operative surveillance strategies for esophageal and gastric cancers: a systematic review and meta-analysis. Dis Esophagus. 2022;35:doac034. https://doi.org/10.1093/dote/doac034.
7. Dobashi A, Li DK, Mavrogenis G, Visrodia KH, Bazerbachi F. Endoscopic Management of Esophageal Cancer. Thorac Surg Clin. 2022;32(4):479–95. https://doi.org/10.1016/j.thorsurg.2022.07.005.
8. Waters JK, Reznik SI. Update on management of squamous cell esophageal cancer. Curr Oncol Rep. 2022;24(3):375–85. https://doi.org/10.1007/s11912-021-01153-4.
9. Elliott JA, Markar SR, Klevebro F, Johar A, Goense L, Lagergren P, Zaninotto G, van Hillegersberg R, van Berge Henegouwen MI, Nilsson M, Hanna GB, Reynolds JV, ENSURE Study Group. An international multicenter study exploring whether surveillance after esophageal cancer surgery impacts oncological and quality of life outcomes (ENSURE). Ann Surg. 2022;277:e1035. https://doi.org/10.1097/SLA.0000000000005378.
10. Sugiyama M, Morita M, Yoshida R, et al. Patterns and time of recurrence after complete resection of esophageal cancer. Surg Today. 2012;42:752–8.
11. Takeuchi M, Kawakubo H, Matsuda S, Fukuda K, Nakamura R, Kitagawa Y. The usability of intensive imaging surveillance after esophagectomy in patients with esophageal cancer. Ann Surg Oncol. 2023;30(4):2190–7. https://doi.org/10.1245/s10434-022-12739-y.
12. Obermannová R, Alsina M, Cervantes A, Leong T, Lordick F, Nilsson M, van Grieken NCT, Vogel A, Smyth EC, ESMO Guidelines Committee. Oesophageal cancer: ESMO clinical practice guideline for diagnosis, treatment and follow-up. Ann Oncol. 2022;33(10):992–1004. https://doi.org/10.1016/j.annonc.2022.07.003.
13. Mariette C, Balon JM, Piessen G, Fabre S, Van Seuningen I, Triboulet JP. Pattern of recurrence following complete resection of esophageal carcinoma and factors predictive of recurrent disease. Cancer. 2003;97(7):1616–23. https://doi.org/10.1002/cncr.11228.
14. Pande SS, Purandare N, Puranik A, Shah S, Agrawal A, et al. Role of 18F-FDG PET/CT in restaging of esophageal cancer after curative-intent surgical resection. Nucl Med Commun. 2020;41(9):959–64. https://doi.org/10.1097/MNM.0000000000001229.
15. Liu H, Hu Z, Yang X, Dai T, Chen Y. Comparison of [$^{68}$Ga]Ga-DOTA-FAPI-04 and [$^{18}$F]FDG uptake in esophageal cancer. Front Oncol. 2022;12:875081. https://doi.org/10.3389/fonc.2022.875081.
16. Lightdale CJ. Endoscopic ultrasonography in the diagnosis, staging and follow-up of esophageal and gastric cancer. Endoscopy. 1992;24(Suppl 1):297–303. https://doi.org/10.1055/s-2007-1010487.
17. Jing JX, Wang Y, Xu XQ, Sun T, Tian BG, Du LL, Zhao XW, Han CZ. Tumor markers for diagnosis, monitoring of recurrence and prognosis in patients with upper gastrointestinal tract cancer. Asian Pac J Cancer Prev. 2014;15(23):10267–72. https://doi.org/10.7314/apjcp.2014.15.23.10267.
18. Cosgrove ND, Mullady DK. Endoscopic evaluation of the esophageal cancer patient after chemoradiotherapy for persistent/recurrent cancer. Dis Esophagus. 2018;31(7). https://doi.org/10.1093/dote/doy023.
19. Kudou M, Shiozaki A, Fujiwara H, Konishi H, Arita T, Kosuga T, Morimura R, Murayama Y, Komatsu S, Kuriu Y, Ikoma H, Nakanishi M, Ichikawa D, Okamoto K, Otsuji E. Efficacy of PET-CT in the diagnosis and treatment of recurrence after esophageal cancer surgery. Anticancer Res. 2016;36(10):5473–80. https://doi.org/10.21873/anticanres.11128.

20. Rodríguez-Camacho E, Pita-Fernández S, Pértega-Díaz S, López-Calviño B, Seoane-Pillado T. Characteristics and pattern of recurrence after curative surgery in oesophageal cancer. Rev Esp Enferm Dig. 2015;107(9):539–46. https://doi.org/10.17235/reed.2015.3748/2015.
21. Parry K, Visser E, van Rossum PS, Mohammad NH, Ruurda JP, van Hillegersberg R. Prognosis and treatment after diagnosis of recurrent esophageal carcinoma following esophagectomy with curative intent. Ann Surg Oncol. 2015;22(Suppl 3):S1292–300. https://doi.org/10.1245/s10434-015-4840-5.
22. National Health Commission of the People's Republic of China. Chinese guidelines for diagnosis and treatment of esophageal carcinoma 2018 (English version). Chin. J Cancer Res. 2019;31(2):223–58. https://doi.org/10.21147/j.issn.1000-9604.2019.02.01.
23. Abate E, DeMeester SR, Zehetner J, Oezcelik A, Ayazi S, Costales J, Banki F, Lipham JC, Hagen JA, DeMeester TR. Recurrence after esophagectomy for adenocarcinoma: defining optimal follow-up intervals and testing. J Am Coll Surg. 2010;210(4):428–35. https://doi.org/10.1016/j.jamcollsurg.2010.01.006.
24. Chidambaram S, Patel NM, Sounderajah V, Alfieri R, Bonavina L, Cheong E, et al. Identifying a core symptom set triggering radiological and endoscopic investigations for suspected recurrent esophago-gastric cancer: a modified Delphi consensus process. Dis Esophagus. 2022;36(1):doac038. https://doi.org/10.1093/dote/doac038.
25. Lou F, Sima CS, Adusumilli PS, Bains MS, Sarkaria IS, Rusch VW, Rizk NP. Esophageal cancer recurrence patterns and implications for surveillance. J Thorac Oncol. 2013;8(12):1558–62. https://doi.org/10.1097/01.JTO.0000437420.38972.fb.
26. Blom RL, Nieuwkerk PT, van Heijl M, et al. Patient preferences in screening for recurrent disease after potentially curative esophagectomy. Dig Surg. 2012;29(3):206–12.
27. https://www.canadianthoracicsurgeons.ca/2020/09/21/follow-up-and-surveillance-of-esophageal-cancer-treated-with-curative-intent/.
28. Toh Y, Kitagawa Y, Kuwano H, et al. A nation-wide survey of follow-up strategies for esophageal cancer patients after a curative esophagectomy or a complete response by definitive chemoradiotherapy in Japan. Esophagus. 2016;13:173–81. https://doi.org/10.1007/s10388-015-0511-7.
29. Kitagawa Y, Uno T, Oyama T, Kato K, Kato H, Kawakubo H, Kawamura O, Kusano M, Kuwano H, Takeuchi H, Toh Y, Doki Y, Naomoto Y, Nemoto K, Booka E, Matsubara H, Miyazaki T, Muto M, Yanagisawa A, Yoshida M. Esophageal cancer practice guidelines 2017 edited by the Japan esophageal society: part 2. Esophagus. 2019;16(1):25–43. https://doi.org/10.1007/s10388-018-0642-8.
30. Haveman JW. Intensive surveillance after Esophagectomy in patients with esophageal cancer: when, why, and how often? Ann Surg Oncol. 2023;30(4):1948–9. https://doi.org/10.1245/s10434-022-12767-8.
31. Toh Y, Oki E, Minami K, et al. Follow–up and recurrence after a curative esophagectomy for patients with esophageal cancer: the frst indicators for recurrence and their prognostic values. Esophagus. 2010;7:37–43.

# Evaluation of Childhood Events as Risk Factors for the Development of Esophageal Cancer in the Future

44

Selami Sozubir

## 44.1 Childhood Esophageal Cancer

The prevalence of esophageal cancer (squamous cell carcinoma, adenocarcinoma) peaks between the ages of 35 and 64, and it is the sixth most common cancer-related cause of death worldwide. Smoking, drinking alcohol, achalasia, consuming hot beverages, deficiency in zinc, vitamins C and E, folates, intake of red meat, socio-economic position, and genetic factors are among the risk factors for esophageal squamous cell carcinoma (SCC). Reflux esophagitis, Barrett's esophagus, obesity, and drinking alcohol are all risk factors for developing esophageal adenocarcinoma (AC) [1].

However, esophageal cancers are scarcely seen in the pediatric age group, and most of the literature about the esophageal tumors in children consists of case reports. The Surveillance, Epidemiology, and End Results (SEER) investigation found just nine malignant esophageal cancers in patients younger than 20 between 1973 and 2008. One of the largest series was presented by Kumar et al. with four cases of SCC and three of AC with the oldest patient being 19 years of age. As malignant esophageal tumors in children, the majority of cases reported in the literature consist of SCC and AC. Other malignant esophageal tumors that have been documented in childhood include lymphoma, melanoma, and synovial cell sarcoma [2–15].

Although the causes behind the onset of esophageal cancers in younger age groups are not certain, chronic irritation from a variety of known environmental carcinogens and gastric contents in chronic reflux cause esophageal epithelial cancers. It is very clear that most of the cases have been mainly described in association with Barrett's esophagus (BE), which is considered the precursor lesion of esophageal cancer. In childhood, approximately 31.6% of patients with esophageal cancers

S. Sozubir (✉)
Pediatric Surgery Department, Medicine Faculty, Istinye University, Istanbul, Turkey



O. Engin (ed.), *Risk Factors and Therapy of Esophagus Cancer*,
https://doi.org/10.1007/978-3-031-47024-0_44

were diagnosed with BE, and 63.2% had preexisting conditions like spinal palsy, esophageal atresia repair in infancy, history of caustic ingestion, obesity, and low birth weight, all of which can be associated with gastroesophageal reflux disease (GERD), a risk factor for BE [16–19].

The percentage of BE in children with esophageal cancer is lower when compared with the adults. This may also be due to more patients undergoing upper endoscopy studies in adult age group and the duration of the irritation in esophagus. BE mainly develops as a result of severe and chronic GERD. However, factors that increase the severity and chronicity of childhood-specific GERD should be considered in terms of both childhood esophageal cancer and future esophageal cancer. Therefore, the main clinical priority in the pediatric population is also to stop GERD-affected children from getting BE and to identify GERD-affected children who are at risk of developing BE [18, 20, 21].

When evaluated in general, there is no significant difference between childhood esophageal cancers and adult esophageal cancers in terms of etiology, symptoms, management, and types. Like adults, dysphagia with significant weight loss, anemia, dehydration, and presence of a mass in the distal esophagus are the most frequent findings at the initial diagnosis of esophageal cancers in children.

## 44.2 Gastroesophageal Reflux, Gastroesophageal Reflux Disease, and Barrett's Esophagus in Childhood

BE is characterized by the replacement of squamous epithelium by columnar epithelium of the intestinal type in the distal esophagus. Despite the lack of information regarding BE in children, the prevalence of BE in children seems to increase as the severity and chronicity of GER increase resulting with GERD (Fig. 44.1a and b) [22, 23].

Pediatric patients have frequent GER, which affects 100% of newborns under 3 months old, 40% of infants under 6 months old, and up to 20% of infants under 12 months old. In 1.5-year-old children, GERD occurs in 7–20%. In the adult population with GERD, BE is prevalent at a rate of 6–12%. Children with GERD had a BE prevalence that ranged from 0.3 to 4.8%, and in the population of children with GERD that is severe enough to require surgery, BE was found in 7.3% (Fig. 44.1c and d) [22, 24–30].

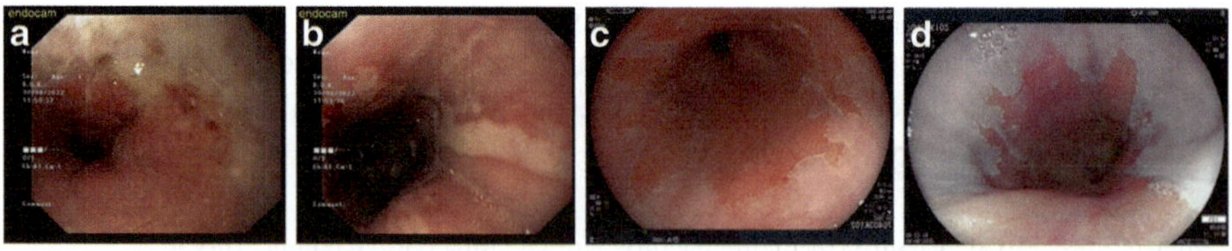


**Fig. 44.1** (**a** and **b**) show the chronic and severe esophagitis with GERD in a child. Images (**c** and **d**) are the typical appearance of Barrett's esophagus

The length of reflux symptoms has been hypothesized to be a risk factor for BE, with a threefold increased risk of BE when symptoms last for more than 5 years and even a sixfold increased risk when symptoms last for more than 10 years in adults. BE may develop in children with reflux symptoms after a mean period of 5.3 years. Age at diagnosis of BE and the mean interval between the onset of reflux symptoms and diagnosis of BE in children are not so clear and detectable. However, the duration of GERD symptoms is not the only possible risk factor for developing BE in the adult population; male gender, presence of a hiatal hernia, age above 50 years, and alcohol consumption are also some risk factors. In the pediatric population, the latter two risk factors are not applicable. On the other hand, it may be possible that some specific risk factors for severe GERD in children are existing, such as neurological impairment, pediatric chronic lung disease, genetic disorders, caustic injuries, and some congenital abnormalities [31–34].

In 38% of individuals with BE who were being followed up, endoscopy or histology could no longer detect the Barrett's segment. This could well imply that metaplasia can be reversed and that progression to dysplasia and cancer can be prevented. Furthermore, BE may contribute to the emergence of esophageal adenocarcinoma, indicating that this phenomenon may also potentially affect children [22, 35, 36].

The passage of time, which plays a significant role in the progression of some esophageal cancers, highlights the necessity of close monitoring of children who have risk factors. Due to the increased lifetime risk for esophageal adenocarcinoma, endoscopic monitoring in children may be desirable when BE is discovered at a young age. BE in children should, like in adults, be diagnosed with multiple biopsies showing the presence of columnar epithelium, including intestinal metaplasia. Therefore, the recommendation is long-term follow-up to identify specific risk factors for BE, both long-segment BE and short-segment BE, and to establish if endoscopic screening and/or surveillance is necessary in childhood, in which case it should be started, and in which patient population [22].

## 44.3 Risk Factors Predisposing Barrett's Esophagus in Children

There are certain underlying disorders that predispose pediatric patients to the severe and chronic GERD and its complications like BE apart from genetic predisposition. These are caustic injuries, esophageal atresia, chronic lung disease especially cystic fibrosis, neurologic impairment, obesity, low birth weight, and other rare inflammatory problems of esophagus.

## 44.4 Caustic Ingestion

Caustic ingestion remains a complex and important public health problem worldwide, in adults and children. Ingesting a caustic substance (acids and alkalis) damages tissue and can cause harm to the mouth, pharynx, hypopharynx, esophagus, stomach, duodenum, and even the jejunum. 20 to 60% of people may get concurrent stomach and intestinal damage [37, 38].

These compounds injure the esophagus in many ways, and the end result is the advancement of the organ's stenosis and fibrosis. Dysphagia is the most prevalent symptom, and its severity is correlated with the degree of stenosis. Moreover, odynophagia is present. Due to the substantial weight loss, the damage to nutritional status is obvious [39–41].

Caustic ingestion of acidic or alkaline agents or strong irritants can induce severe esophageal corrosive injury and increase esophageal cancer risk, mainly squamous cell carcinoma, with an interval from one to three decades after ingestion. Approximately 1–4% of all patients with esophageal cancer have a history of caustic ingestion. Estimates of the prevalence of esophageal cancer in patients with a history of ingestion of a corrosive agent have ranged from 2 to 16% [15, 42].

Cancer is most commonly observed at the areas of anatomic narrowing and may be related to increased exposure to the caustic substance. Diagnosing corrosive esophageal cancer is more difficult than diagnosing de novo esophageal cancer because of preexisting symptoms of dysphagia. Furthermore, endoscopic evaluation and surveillance have limited roles in these cases because of severe esophageal luminal narrowing. Endoscopic screening is recommended for patients following caustic ingestion. Therefore, the necessity of radiological studies as well as endoscopic one in the follow-up of these cases should be emphasized [42–46].

## 44.5 Esophageal Atresia

Another predisposing condition to severe GERD includes those patients with esophageal atresia (EA), in which most of the cases of esophageal adenocarcinoma have been described.

EA is a rare congenital malformation that needs surgical correction soon after birth, with a worldwide prevalence of 2.43/10,000 births. Improved surgical and critical care methods have raised survival rates up to 93% in specialized centers over the past 40 years; as a result, more of these children have reached adulthood [47, 48].

Many EA patients suffer from GER, with a reported prevalence of 32.8–54.2% in infancy/childhood and 5.9–66.7% in adolescence/adulthood. Chronic GER may cause damage to the mucosa lining of the esophagus, which can develop in esophagitis, gastric metaplasia, or intestinal metaplasia, also known as BE [49, 50].

Children with esophageal atresia followed for a mean of 36 years show a prevalence of BE of 11% [1–7]. The prevalence of BE is fourfold higher in young adults with esophageal atresia, and the prevalence of esophageal squamous cell carcinoma is 108-fold higher than in the general population. The estimated incidence rate of BE, which predisposes to esophageal adenocarcinoma, is 0.5% per year of follow-up analysis [51–53].

This result may have significant effects on how young individuals transition from pediatric to adult gastroenterology treatment and undergo ongoing endoscopic follow-up testing to help with the early detection of pertinent lesions. Therefore, children with EA need to have very close follow-up.

Additionally, children with EA have a lot of diagnostic imaging, which exposes them to radiation and may raise their risk of developing cancer later in life [54].

## 44.6 Cystic Fibrosis (CF)

The overall cancer risk in the cystic fibrosis population has been shown to be approximately the same as in the general population. However, CF patients have an increased risk for developing gastrointestinal malignancies. In a 10-year study, CF patients developed significantly more gastrointestinal cancers than expected with a standardized incidence ratio (SIR) of 5.1. More specifically, there was an increased risk of cancers of the small intestine (SIR 24.8), colon (SIR 7.4), biliary tract (SIR 39.0), liver (SIR 4.1), esophagus (SIR 5.4), and pancreas (SIR 2.6) [55, 56].

Children with chronic lung disease, in particular patients with cystic fibrosis, have also been shown to have a higher prevalence of severe GERD and BE. It has been suggested that the standardized incidence ratio of esophageal adenocarcinoma in those patients is significantly higher. Just like children with EA, children with chronic lung disease and cystic fibrosis should be followed closely [20, 55, 56].

## 44.7 Neurologic Impairment

One of the frequent related factors that predispose to severe GERD in children is neurologic impairment. In institutionalized people, it was discovered that GERD was more common and severe in patients with scoliosis, cerebral palsy, and use of anticonvulsant drugs or other benzodiazepines or who had an IQ below 3. 10–25% of institutionalized intellectually disabled people have symptoms of vomiting, regurgitation, or rumination. Of those patients that had an endoscopy, BE was found in 18 (14.0%) and peptic strictures in five (3.9%) [20, 21].

In children with iron-deficiency anemia with neurologic impairment, columnar metaplasia of the esophagus given the associated risk of malignant transformation may be present, even if without overt gastrointestinal symptoms. Therefore, early endoscopic evaluation should also be considered in this specific patient population [57].

## 44.8 Obesity

The recent obesity epidemic has been associated with an increased incidence of GERD both in adults and children. It is unclear how it will affect the prevalence of BE in children, but pediatric cross-sectional studies have already demonstrated that moderately and extremely obese kids are more likely than normal-weight kids to be diagnosed with GERD (OR 1.16, 95% CI: 1.02–1.32 and 1.32, 95% CI: 1.13–1.56, respectively) [33, 58].

## 44.9 Eosinophilic Esophagitis

Eosinophilic esophagitis (EoE) is an allergy-mediated esophageal inflammation that produces severe esophagitis. Uncertainty exists regarding the connection between BE and esophageal neoplasms and a chronic inflammatory illness like EoE. Long-term follow-up of these patients will be required to determine if BE will occur more frequently in those patients given the rising frequency of EoE [20].

## References

1. Short MW, Burgers KG, Fry VT. Esophageal cancer. Am Fam Physician. 2017;95(1):22–8.
2. Zhuge Y, Cheung MC, Yang R, et al. Pediatric intestinal foregut and small bowel solid tumors: a review of 105 cases. J Surg Res. 2009;156:95–102.
3. Kumar A, Shukla NK, Mishra MC, et al. Primary esophageal carcinoma in teens. J Surg Oncol. 1992;50:254–7.
4. Theilen TM, Chou AJ, et al. Esophageal adenocarcinoma and squamous cell carcinoma in children and adolescents: report of 3 cases and comprehensive literature review. Pediatr Surg Case Rep. 2016;5:23–9. https://doi.org/10.1016/j.epsc.2015.12.008.
5. Issaivanan M, Redner A, Weinstein T, et al. Esophageal carcinoma in children and adolescents. J Pediatr Hematol Oncol. 2012;34:63–7.
6. Basque GJ, Boline JE, Holyoke JB. Malignant melanoma of the esophagus: first reported case in a child. Am J Clin Pathol. 1970;53:609–11.
7. Oberiter V, Fabecic-Sabadi V, Bajakic D. [Esophageal carcinoma in a 12-year-old girl (author's transl)]. Lijec Vjesn. 1976;98:422–4.
8. Soni NK, Chatterji P. Carcinoma of the oesophagus in an eight-year-old child. J Laryngol Otol. 1980;94:327–9.
9. Inayat F, Munir A, Wahab A, Younus F, Zafar F, Ullah W. Primary esophageal diffuse large B-cell lymphoma: a comparative review of 15 cases. J Investig Med High Impact Case Rep. 2018;6:2324709618820887. https://doi.org/10.1177/2324709618820887.
10. Karwasra RK, Yadav V, Bansal AR. Esophageal carcinoma in a 17-year-old man. Am J Gastroenterol. 1999;94:1122–3.
11. Allam AR, Fazili FM, Khawaja FI, et al. Esophageal carcinoma in a 15-year-old girl: a case report and review of the literature. Ann Saudi Med. 2000;20:261–4.
12. Anton-Pacheco J, Cano I, Cuadros J, et al. Synovial sarcoma of the esophagus. J Pediatr Surg. 1996;31:1703–5.
13. Haghighi P, Mohallatee EA, Nasr K, et al. Childhood cancer in southern Iran. Cancer. 1974;34:1842–8.
14. Tampi C, Pai S, Doctor VM, et al. HPV-associated carcinoma of esophagus in the young: a case report and review of literature. Int J Gastrointest Cancer. 2005;35:135–42.
15. Dewar JM, Courtney JT, Byrne MJ, et al. Esophageal cancer in a young woman after treatment for osteosarcoma. Med Pediatr Oncol. 1988;16:287–9.
16. Ronkainen J, Aro P, Storskrubb T, et al. Prevalence of Barrett's esophagus in the general population: an endoscopic study. Gastroenterology. 2005;129:1825–31.
17. Adzick NS, Fisher JH, Winter HS, et al. Esophageal adenocarcinoma 20 years after esophageal atresia repair. J Pediatr Surg. 1989;24:741–4.

18. Hassall E, Dimmick JE, Magee JF. Adenocarcinoma in childhood Barrett's esophagus: case documentation and the need for surveillance in children. Am J Gastroenterol. 1993;88:282–8.
19. Kaijser M, Akre O, Cnattingius S, et al. Preterm birth, low birth weight, and risk for esophageal adenocarcinoma. Gastroenterology. 2005;128:607–9.
20. Jadcherla SR, Nurko S. Esophageal disease in pediatrics. Ann N Y Acad Sci. 2011;1232:401–4. https://doi.org/10.1111/j.1749-6632.2011.06060.x.
21. Sherman PM, Hassall E, Fagundes-Neto U, et al. A global, evidence-based consensus on the definition of gastroesophageal reflux disease in the pediatric population. Am J Gastroenterol. 2009;104:1278–95.
22. Jeurnink SM, van Herwaarden-Lindeboom MY, Siersema PD, Fischer K, Houwen RH, van der Zee DC. Barrett's esophagus in children: does it need more attention? Dig Liver Dis. 2011;43(9):682–7. https://doi.org/10.1016/j.dld.2011.02.003.
23. Orenstein SR, Izadnia F, Khan S. Gastroesophageal reflux disease in children. Gastroenterol Clin N Am. 1999;28:947–69.
24. Nelson SP, Chen EH, Syniar GM, et al. Prevalence of symptoms of gastroesophageal reflux during infancy. A pediatric practice-based survey. Pediatric Practice Research Group. Arch Pediatr Adolesc Med. 1997;151:569–72.
25. Jolley SG, Lorenz ML, Hendrickson M, et al. Esophageal pH monitoring abnormalities and gastroesophageal reflux disease in infants with intestinal malrotation. Arch Surg. 1999;134:747–52.
26. Campos GM, Peters JH, DeMeester TR, et al. The pattern of esophageal acid exposure in gastroesophageal reflux disease influences the severity of the disease. Arch Surg. 1999;134:882–7.
27. Treem WR, Davis PM, Hyams JS. Gastroesophageal reflux in the older child: presentation, response to treatment and long-term follow-up. Clin Pediatr (Phila). 1991;30:435–40.
28. Hassall E, Kerr W, El-Serag HB. Characteristics of children receiving proton pump inhibitors continuously for up to 11 years duration. J Pediatr. 2007;150(262–7):267.
29. El-Serag HB, Bailey NR, Gilger M, et al. Endoscopic manifestations of gastroesophageal reflux disease in patients between 18 months and 25 years without neurological deficits. Am J Gastroenterol. 2002;97:1635–9.
30. El-Serag HB, Gilger MA, Shub MD, et al. The prevalence of suspected Barrett's esophagus in children and adolescents: a multicenter endoscopic study. Gastrointest Endosc. 2006;64:671–5.
31. Gatenby PA, Ramus JR, Caygill CP, et al. The influence of symptom type and duration on the fate of the metaplastic columnar-lined Barrett's oesophagus. Aliment Pharmacol Ther. 2009;29:1096–105.
32. Shaheen N, Ransohoff DF. Gastroesophageal reflux, Barrett esophagus, and esophageal cancer: scientific review. JAMA. 2002;287:1972–81.
33. Veugelers PJ, Porter GA, Guernsey DL, et al. Obesity and lifestyle risk factors forgastroesophageal reflux disease. Barrett esophagus and esophageal adenocarcinoma. Dis Esophagus. 2006;19:321–8.
34. Kerkhof M, Steyerberg EW, Kusters JG, et al. Predicting presence of intestinal metaplasia and dysplasia in columnar-lined esophagus: a multivariate analysis. Endoscopy. 2007;39:772–8.
35. Peters FT, Ganesh S, Kuipers EJ, et al. Endoscopic regression of Barrett's oesophagus during omeprazole treatment; a randomised double blind study. Gut. 1999;45:489–94.
36. Cheu HW, Grosfeld JL, Heifetz SA, et al. Persistence of Barrett's esophagus in children after antireflux surgery: influence on follow-up care. J Pediatr Surg. 1992;27:260–4.
37. Contini S, Scarpignato C. Caustic injury of the upper gastrointestinal tract: a comprehensive review. World J Gastroenterol. 2013;19(25):3918–30. https://doi.org/10.3748/wjg.v19.i25.3918.
38. De Lusong MAA, Timbol ABG, Tuazon DJS. Management of esophageal caustic injury. World J Gastrointest Pharmacol Ther. 2017;8(2):90–8. https://doi.org/10.4292/wjgpt.v8.i2.90.
39. Andreollo NA, Lopes LR, Inogutti R, Brandalise NA, Leonardi LS. Conservative treatment of benign esophageal strictures using dilation. Analysis of 500 cases. Rev Assoc Med Bras. 2001;47(3):236–43. https://doi.org/10.1590/s0104-42302001000300036.

40. Chirica M, Kelly MD, Siboni S, Aiolfi A, Riva CG, Asti E, et al. Esophageal emergencies: WSES guidelines. World J Emerg Surg. 2019;14:26. https://doi.org/10.1186/s13017-019-0245-2.
41. Zargar SA, Kochhar R, Mehta S, Mehta SK. The role offiberoptic endoscopy in the management of corrosive ingestion and modified endoscopic classification of burns. Gastrointest Endosc. 1991;37(2):165–9. https://doi.org/10.1016/s0016-5107(91)70678-0.
42. Noh SY, Kim HJ, Lee HJ, Park SH, Lee JS, Kim AY, Ha HK. Corrosive-induced carcinoma of esophagus: esophagographic and CT findings. AJR Am J Roentgenol. 2017;208(6):1237–43. https://doi.org/10.2214/AJR.16.17138.
43. Bigger IA, Vinson PP. Carcinoma secondary to burn of the esophagus from ingestion of lye; report of a case. Surgery. 1950;28:887–9.
44. Bigelow NH. Carcinoma of the esophagus developing at the site of lye stricture. Cancer. 1953;6:1159–64.
45. Kiviranta UK. Corrosion carcinoma of the esophagus: 381 cases of corrosion and nine cases of corrosion carcinoma. Acta Otolaryngol. 1952;42:89–95.
46. Hopkins RA, Postlethwait RW. Caustic burns and carcinoma of the esophagus. Ann Surg. 1981;194:146–8.
47. Pedersen RN, Calzolari E, Husby S, et al. Oesophageal atresia: prevalence, prenatal diagnosis and associated anomalies in 23 European regions. Arch Dis Child. 2012;97:227–32.
48. Wang B, Tashiro J, Allan BJ, et al. A nationwide analysis of clinical outcomes among newborns with esophageal atresia and tracheoesophageal fistulas in the United States. J Surg Res. 2014;190:604–12.
49. Wang KK, Sampliner RE. Practice Parameters Committee of the American College of Gastroenterology. Updated guidelines 2008 for the diagnosis, surveillance and therapy of Barrett's esophagus. Am J Gastroenterol. 2008;103:788–97.
50. Vergouwe FWT, Ijsselstijn H, Biermann K, et al. High prevalence of Barrett's esophagus and esophageal squamous cell carcinoma after repair of esophageal atresia. Clin Gastroenterol Hepatol. 2018;16(4):513–521.e6. https://doi.org/10.1016/j.cgh.2017.11.008.
51. Tovar JA, Fragoso AC. Gastroesophageal reflux after repair of esophageal atresia. Eur J Pediatr Surg. 2013;23(3):175–81. https://doi.org/10.1055/s-0033-1347911.
52. Vergouwe FW, Ijsselstijn H, Wijnen RM, et al. Screening and surveillance in esophageal atresia patients: current knowledge and future perspectives. Eur J Pediatr Surg. 2015;25(4):345–52. https://doi.org/10.1055/s-0035-1559817.
53. Sistonen SJ, Koivusalo A, Lindahl H. Cancer after repair of esophageal atresia: population-based long-term follow-up. J Pediatr Surg. 2008;43(4):602–5. https://doi.org/10.1016/j.jpedsurg.2007.12.002.
54. Yousef Y, Baird R. Radiation exposure and attributable cancer risk in patients with esophageal atresia. J Pediatr Gastroenterol Nutr. 2018;66(2):234–8. https://doi.org/10.1097/MPG.0000000000001701.
55. Neglia JP, FitzSimmons SC, Maisonneuve P, Schöni MH, Schöni-Affolter F, Corey M, Lowenfels AB. The risk of cancer among patients with cystic fibrosis. Cystic Fibrosis and Cancer Study Group. N Engl J Med. 1995;332(8):494–9. https://doi.org/10.1056/NEJM199502233320803.
56. Alexander CL, Urbanski SJ, Hilsden R, et al. The risk of gastrointestinal malignancies in cystic fibrosis: case report of a patient with a near obstructing villous adenoma found on colon cancer screening and Barrett's esophagus. J Cyst Fibros. 2008;7:1–6.
57. Van Arsdall MR, Nair S, Moye LM, Nguyen TT, Saleh ZM, Rhoads JM. Columnar metaplasia of the esophagus presenting as iron deficiency anemia in children with neurologic impairment or congenital esophageal atresia. Am J Case Rep. 2022;23:e937255. https://doi.org/10.12659/AJCR.937255.
58. Koebnick C, Getahun D, Smith N, et al. Extreme childhood obesity is associated with increased risk for gastroesophageal reflux disease in a large population-based study. Int J Pediatr Obes. 2011;6:e257–63.

# Systemic Treatment of Esophageal Cancer

# 45

Sema Turker

## 45.1 Introduction

Esophageal cancer is the seventh most common type of cancer and the sixth most common cause of mortality due to cancer, based on GLOBOCAN 2020 data [1]. Esophageal cancer has two histologic subtypes: squamous cell carcinoma (SCC) and adenocarcinoma (AC). SCC is the most common type worldwide. Smoking and alcohol are major risk factors for SCC, while Barret's esophageal metaplasia (a complication of gastroesophageal reflux disease [GERD]), obesity, and smoking are risk factors for adenocarcinoma [2].

Progressive dysphagia and weight loss are common in patients with esophageal cancer. Endoscopic biopsy is usually used to diagnose esophageal or esophagogastric junction (EGJ) cancer. In esophageal cancer, staging is important in determining prognosis and treatment. The American Joint Committee on Cancer (AJCC) and Union for International Cancer Control (UICC) tumor, node, and metastasis (TNM) staging system is widely used for esophageal cancer [3]. Endoscopic biopsy and endoscopic ultrasonography are recommended in locoregional staging (T and N). FDG-PET/CT is more sensitive than contrast-enhanced CT for the detection of metastases and is now widely used for the detection of occult metastases when metastases are not seen on initial staging CT scans [4].

Clinical staging, tumor subtype, and tumor location determine the treatment of esophageal cancer. Before curative treatment, the patient's nutrition should be regulated. Enteral nutrition is regulated by jejunostomy or nasogastric tube. Endoscopic stent placement is not recommended as it may harm prognosis [5].

S. Turker (✉)
Department of Internal Medicine, Faculty of Medicine, Bahcesehir University, Istanbul, Turkey
e-mail: sema.turker@med.bau.edu.tr



O. Engin (ed.), *Risk Factors and Therapy of Esophagus Cancer*,
https://doi.org/10.1007/978-3-031-47024-0_45

For patients with T1N0 esophageal or esophagogastric junction AC or SCC, surgical or endoscopic resection is the treatment of choice [6]. The most appropriate approach for clinical T2N0 disease remains controversial. There are different guidelines from different expert groups regarding the indications for neoadjuvant therapy as compared to the indications for initial resection [7, 8].

## 45.2 Neoadjuvant and Adjuvant Treatment

The multimodal approach to the curative management of locally advanced esophageal cancers varies worldwide and includes preoperative chemoradiotherapy, preoperative, and perioperative chemotherapy depending on tumor histology and anatomical location.

The CROSS trial is an assessment of current practice regarding surgery after neoadjuvant chemoradiotherapy. The participants consisted of 275 patients (75%) with adenocarcinoma and 84 patients (23%) with squamous cell carcinoma. Carboplatin and paclitaxel were given weekly in combination with radiation at a dose of 41.4 Gy. Patients receiving neoadjuvant chemoradiotherapy with carboplatin and paclitaxel had significantly better overall survival and disease-free survival [9]. This study demonstrated that triple combination therapy increased both the R0 resection rate from 69 to 92% and the median survival from 24 to 49.4 months compared to surgery alone, setting a new standard [10].

Neoadjuvant chemotherapy is the other treatment option for patients with esophageal cancer. In the MAGIC trial, three cycles of epirubicin-cisplatin-5-FU (ECF) before and after surgery were superior to surgery alone in terms of R0 resection rate and overall survival [11]. The FLOT4 study aims to evaluate perioperative treatments in patients with resectable gastric or GEJ adenocarcinoma. Docetaxel-based triple FLOT is compared with anthracycline-based triple ECF/ECX. FLOT was associated with a significant reduction in mortality compared to ECF/ECX, hazard ratio (HR) = 0.77–95%, and confidence interval (CI) = 0.63–0.94. Median overall survival was 50 months in the FLOT group and 35 months in ECF/ECX group [12]. Therefore, for patients with resectable GEJ or gastric AC, FLOT represents a new treatment option.

We have only limited data available for a head-to-head comparison of chemotherapy with chemoradiotherapy. In 2021, an abstract of the phase 3 Neo-AEGIS trial was presented. Neo-AEGIS compared two standard regimens in the perioperative period, CRT (CROSS regimen) or perioperative chemotherapy (ECF regimen or FLOT in the MAGIC trial). In total, 178 patients (CROSS) and 184 patients (MAGIC/FLOT) were enrolled and received preoperative treatment. A higher rate of tumor regression and pathologic complete response was seen with CRT, according to preliminary results [13]. However, most patients on CT were treated with the old ECF regimen rather than the FLOT regimen. A higher rate of efficacy and perioperative response is expected with the FLOT regimen. Data comparing the CROSS-CRT regimen with FLOT are expected from the Phase III ESOPEC trial [14].

For esophageal cancer, adjuvant treatment after neoadjuvant chemoradiotherapy and surgery has not been established. In the CheckMate 577 study of patients at high risk for recurrence, median disease-free survival was 22.4 months among 532 patients receiving adjuvant nivolumab compared to 11.0 months among 262 patients in the placebo arm ($P < 0.001$). With the results of this study, the use of nivolumab has started to be recommended for patients who have received chemoradiotherapy before surgery and have residual disease in postoperative pathological evaluation [15]. Adjuvant nivolumab is recommended regardless of PD-L1 level.

Definitive chemoradiotherapy is another treatment option for nonmetastatic esophageal cancer. The standard regimen for conventional definitive CRT is four cycles of cisplatin, 5-FU (or capecitabine) in 28 fractions at 50.4 Gy with RT (or 50 Gy in 25 fractions) [16]. Alternatively, cycles of folinic acid, 5-FU, and oxaliplatin (FOLFOX) may be given [17]. Definitive CRT may be recommended for patients with SCC or esophageal adenocarcinoma that cannot be resected or who do not wish to undergo surgery.

## 45.3 Metastatic Esophageal Cancer Treatment

The goals of chemotherapy in patients with advanced esophagogastric cancer are relief of symptoms, improvement in quality of life, and prolongation of survival. The survival benefit of palliative systemic chemotherapy in patients with advanced esophageal cancer has been demonstrated in several controlled trials and meta-analyses [18]. For both ESCC and EAC, infusional cisplatin and 5-fluorouracil chemotherapy have traditionally been the standard first-line treatment option for patients with metastatic disease [19]. Oxaliplatin and capecitabine are not inferior to cisplatin and 5-fluorouracil, respectively.

As with other cancers, targeted therapies and immunotherapies have improved overall survival in patients with esophageal cancer in recent years. KEYNOTE 590 study investigated the addition of cisplatin and 5 fluorouracil to pembrolizumab treatment in patients with previously untreated, locally advanced or metastatic esophageal SCC, esophageal adenocarcinoma, or EGJ adenocarcinoma. Adding pembrolizumab to chemotherapy significantly prolonged both OS and PFS compared to chemotherapy alone. In this study, the highest overall survival rate was observed in patients diagnosed with SCC and patients with PDL-1 CPS values above 10% [20].

The CHECKMATE-648 study evaluated patients with previously untreated advanced esophageal squamous cell carcinoma. The study included a chemotherapy arm, a chemotherapy + nivolumab arm, and a nivolumab + ipilimumab arm. The results of the CHECKMATE-648 study showed that patients receiving nivolumab survived statistically longer than those receiving chemotherapy alone. Median overall survival was 13.2 months in the nivolumab, fluorouracil, and cisplatin arm; 12.8 months in the nivolumab and ipilimumab arm; and 10.7 months in the chemotherapy-only arm [21, 22].

Phase III randomized open-label ATTRACTION-3 study compared nivolumab with paclitaxel or docetaxel monotherapy for the second-line treatment of esophageal squamous cell cancer. PDL-1 level was not included in this study. The primary endpoint of overall survival was 10.5 months in the nivolumab group and 8.0 months in the chemotherapy group. Nivolumab is recommended for patients with previously treated advanced esophageal squamous cell carcinoma as it shows a significant improvement in overall survival and a favorable safety profile compared to chemotherapy [23].

The KEYNOTE 181 study evaluated 628 patients with advanced/metastatic squamous cell carcinoma or esophageal adenocarcinoma progressing after chemotherapy. The patients who were treated with second-line chemotherapy were compared with patients who received pembrolizumab. OS was longer with pembrolizumab in patients with CPS $\geq$ 10 (median, 9.3 vs. 6.7 months) [24].

Paclitaxel, irinotecan, and docetaxel regimens can be given to patients who cannot receive immunotherapy as second-line treatment in metastatic esophageal cancer. For MSI-H/dMMR or TMB-H tumors, pembrolizumab is treatment option for second-line or subsequent therapy in patients with metastatic disease if it was not administered for front-line therapy [25].

The management of metastatic esophageal adenocarcinoma is like that of metastatic gastric adenocarcinoma. Tumor tissue should be tested for HER2 overexpression and/or amplification before trastuzumab treatment in all patients with advanced gastroesophageal adenocarcinoma who are considered good candidates for combination therapy with trastuzumab. As a result of the TOGA trial, trastuzumab in combination with chemotherapy has become the standard of care for patients with HER2-positive advanced stomach or gastroesophageal junction cancer [26]. A single-arm, open-label Phase II study in 37 previously untreated patients with HER2-positive esophageal, gastric, or EGJ cancer demonstrated the safety and efficacy of combining the immune checkpoint inhibitor pembrolizumab with first-line trastuzumab plus platinum-containing chemotherapy [27].

The open-label, randomized, phase II DESTINY-Gastric-01 study demonstrated the benefit of fam-trastuzumab deruxtecan in previously treated HER2-positive gastric cancer. Patients were randomly assigned to receive fam-trastuzumab deruxtecan or the physician's preferred chemotherapy (irinotecan [89%] or paclitaxel [11%]) while receiving two prior lines of treatment, including trastuzumab. The fam-trastuzumab-deruxtecan group had a significantly higher objective response rate (51% vs. 14%) and significantly longer median overall survival (12.5 vs. 8.4 months) and median PFS (5.6 vs. 3.5 months) [28].

Ramucirumab is a targeted anti-angiogenic monoclonal antibody. It works through the inhibition of the VEGFR-2 protein. Phase III RAINBOW trial compared weekly paclitaxel (80 mg/m$^2$ on days 1, 8, and 15 of each 28-day cycle) plus ramucirumab (8 mg/kg IV every other day). Ramucirumab significantly improved median overall survival (9.6 vs. 7.4 months), PFS (4.4 vs. 2.9 months), and objective response rate (28 vs. 16%) [29].

In a study of patients with metastatic gastric or gastroesophageal cancer who had previously received two lines of treatment, trifluridine tripacil was compared with placebo. Median overall survival was 5.7 months in the trifluridine-tipiracil group and 3.6 months in the placebo arm. For patients with adequate performance status, trifluridine-tipiracil is a reasonable option at or beyond third-line treatment [30].

Comprehensive genomic profiling through a validated NGS assay should be offered to patients with metastatic esophageal cancer. Patients with esophageal and EGJ cancer should be encouraged to participate in well-designed clinical trials investigating novel therapeutic strategies to further advance the management of these diseases [31].

## References

1. Sung H, Ferlay J, Siegel RL, Laversanne M, et al. Global cancer statistics 2020: GLOBOCAN estimates of incidence and mortality worldwide for 36 cancers in 185 countries. CA Cancer J Clin. 2021;71(3):209–49.
2. Engel LS, Chow WH, Vaughan TL, Gammon M, et al. Population attributable risks of esophageal and gastric cancers. J Natl Cancer Inst. 2003;95(18):1404–13.
3. Rice TW, Patil DT, Blackstone EH. 8th edition AJCC/UICC staging of cancers of the esophagus and esophagogastric junction: application to clinical practice. Ann Cardiothorac Surg. 2017;6(2):119–30.
4. Obermannová R, Alsina M, Cervantes A, Leong T, et al. Oesophageal cancer: ESMO clinical practice guideline for diagnosis, treatment, and follow-up. Ann Oncol. 2022;33(10):992–04.
5. Mariette C, Gronnier C, Duhamel A, Mabrut JY, et al. Expanding covered metallic stent as a bridge to surgery in esophageal cancer: impact on oncologic outcomes. J Am Coll Surg. 2015;220(3):287–96.
6. Cen P, Hofstetter WL, Lee JH, Ross WA, et al. Value of endoscopic ultrasound staging in conjunction with the evaluation of lymphovascular invasion in identifying low-risk esophageal carcinoma. Cancer. 2008;112(3):503–10.
7. Mariette C, Dahan L, Mornex F, Maillard E, et al. Surgery alone versus chemoradiotherapy followed by surgery for stage I and II esophageal cancer: final analysis of randomized controlled phase III trial FFCD 9901. J Clin Oncol. 2014;32(23):2416–22.
8. NCCN clinical practice guidelines in oncology: esophageal and esophagogastric junction cancers. National Comprehensive Cancer Network. 2023. https://www.nccn.org/professionals/physician_gls/f_guidelines.asp#esophageal.
9. Van Hagen P, Hulshof MC, van Lanschot JJ, Steyerberg EW, et al. Preoperative chemoradiotherapy for esophageal or junctional cancer. N Engl J Med. 2012;366:2074–84.
10. Eyck BM, van Lanschot JJB, Hulshof MC, van der Wilk BJ, et al. Ten-year outcome of neoadjuvant chemoradiotherapy plus surgery for esophageal cancer: the randomized controlled CROSS trial. J Clin Oncol. 2021;39(18):1995–04.
11. Cunningham D, Allum WH, Stenning SP, Thompson JN, et al. Perioperative chemotherapy versus surgery alone for resectable gastroesophageal cancer. N Engl J Med. 2006;355(1):11–20.
12. Al-Batran SE, Homann N, Schmalenberg H, Kopp HG, et al. Perioperative chemotherapy with docetaxel, oxaliplatin, and fluorouracil/leucovorin (FLOT) versus epirubicin, cisplatin, and fluorouracil or capecitabine(ECF/ECX) for resectable gastric or gastroesophageal junction (GEJ) adenocarcinoma (FLOT4-AIO):a multicenter, randomized phase 3 trial. J Clin Oncol. 2017;35:4004.
13. Reynolds JV, Preston SR, O'Neill B, Lowery MA, et al. Neo-AEGIS (neoadjuvant trial in adenocarcinoma of the esophagus and Esophagogastric Junction international study): preliminary results of phase III RCT of CROSS versus perioperative chemotherapy (modified MAGIC or FLOT protocol). J Clin Oncol. 2021;39(15):4004.

14. Van der Wilk BJ, Eyck BM, Lagarde SM, van der Gaast A, et al. The optimal neoadjuvant treatment of locally advanced esophageal cancer. J Thorac Dis. 2019;11(5):621.
15. Kelly RJ, Ajani JA, Kuzdzal J, Zander T, et al. Adjuvant nivolumab in resected esophageal or gastroesophageal junction cancer N. Engl J Med. 2021;384(13):1191–03.
16. Conroy T, Galais MP, Raoul JL, Bouché O, et al. Definitive chemoradiotherapy with FOLFOX versus fluorouracil and cisplatin in patients with oesophageal cancer (PRODIGE5/ ACCORD17): final results of a randomized, phase 2/3 trial. Lancet Oncol. 2014;15(3):305–14.
17. Cunningham D, Allum WH, Stenning SP, et al. Perioperative chemotherapy versus surgery alone for resectable gastroesophageal cancer. N Engl J Med. 2006;355(1):11–20.
18. Janmaat VT, Steyerberg EW, van der Gaast A, Mathijssen RH, et al. Palliative chemotherapy and targeted therapies for esophageal and gastroesophageal junction cancer. Cochrane Database Syst Rev. 2017;11:CD004063.
19. Shah MA. Update on metastatic gastric and esophageal cancers. J Clin Oncol. 2015;33(16):1760–9.
20. Shah MA, Altorki N, Patel P, Harrison S, et al. Improving outcomes in patients with oesophageal cancer. Nat Rev Clin Oncol. 2023;1-18:390.
21. Sun JM, Shen L, Shah MA, Enzinger P, et al. Pembrolizumab plus chemotherapy versus chemotherapy alone for first-line treatment of advanced oesophageal cancer (KEYNOTE-590): a randomised, placebo-controlled, phase 3 study. Lancet Oncol. 2021;398:759–71.
22. Doki Y, Ajani JA, Kato K, Xu J, et al. Nivolumab combination therapy in advanced esophageal squamous cell carcinoma. N Engl J Med. 2022;386(5):449–62.
23. Kato K, Cho BC, Takahashi M, et al. Nivolumab versus chemotherapy in patients with advanced oesophageal squamous cell carcinoma refractory or intolerant to previous chemotherapy (ATTRACTION-3): a multicentre, randomized, open-label, phase 3 trial. Lancet Oncol. 2019;20(11):1506–17.
24. Kojima T, Shah MA, Muro K, Francois E, et al. Randomized phase III KEYNOTE-181 study of pembrolizumab versus chemotherapy in advanced esophageal cancer. J Clin Oncol. 2020;38(35):4138–48.
25. Marabelle A, Le DT, Ascierto PA, Di Giacomo AM, et al. Efficacy of pembrolizumab in patients with noncolorectal high microsatellite instability/mismatch repair–deficient cancer: results from the phase II KEYNOTE-158 study. J Clin Oncol. 2020;38(1):1–10.
26. Bang YJ, Van Cutsem E, Feyereislova A, Chung HC, et al. Trastuzumab in combination with chemotherapy versus chemotherapy alone for treatment of HER2-positive advanced gastric or gastro-oesophageal junction cancer (ToGA): a phase 3, open-label, randomized controlled trial. Lancet Oncol. 2010;376(9742):687–97.
27. Janjigian YY, Maron SB, Chatila WK, Millang B, et al. First-line pembrolizumab and trastuzumab in HER2-positive oesophageal, gastric, or gastro-oesophageal junction cancer: an open-label, single-arm, phase 2 trial. Lancet Oncol. 2020;21(6):821–31.
28. Shitara K, Bang YJ, Iwasa S, Sugimoto N, et al. Trastuzumab deruxtecan in previously treated HER2-positive gastric cancer. N Engl J Med. 2020;382:2419–30.
29. Wilke H, Muro K, Van Cutsem E, Oh SC, et al. Ramucirumab plus paclitaxel versus placebo plus paclitaxel in patients with previously treated advanced gastric or gastro-oesophageal junction adenocarcinoma (RAINBOW): a double-blind, randomized phase 3 trial. Lancet Oncol. 2014;15(11):1224–35.
30. Shitara K, Doi T, Dvorkin M, Mansoor W, et al. Trifluridine/tipiracil versus placebo in patients with heavily pretreated metastatic gastric cancer (TAGS): a randomized, double-blind, placebo-controlled, phase 3 trial. Lancet Oncol. 2018;19(11):1437-48.
31. Cai H, Li M, Deng R, Wang M, et al. Advances in molecular biomarkers research and clinical application progress for gastric cancer immunotherapy. Biomark Res. 2022;10(1):67.

# The Role of Radiation Therapy in the Management of Esophageal Cancer

46

Cengiz Gemici

## 46.1 General Information

Esophageal cancer is composed of two different histopathologic types: squamous cell carcinoma and adenocarcinoma. Although they differ in their etiologies, geographic distribution, the part of the organ where they develop, and response to treatment, they are mostly considered as a single entity.

Esophagus is an organ that has parts in the neck, thorax, and abdomen. Esophagus has been divided in to four sections [1, 2].

1. The cervical esophagus extends from upper esophageal sphincter (the cricopharyngeus muscle) to the thoracic inlet, approximately 15–20 cm from the incisors.
2. The upper thoracic esophagus extends from the thoracic inlet to the lower border of the azygos vein, approximately 20–25 cm from the incisors.
3. The middle thoracic esophagus extends from the lower border of azygos vein to the inferior pulmonary veins, approximately 25–30 cm from the incisors.
4. The lower thoracic esophagus extends from the inferior pulmonary veins to the stomach, approximately 30–40 cm from the incisors.

While squamous cell carcinoma is the predominant histology in the cervical and the upper third of the esophagus, the adenocarcinoma predominates in the lower (distal) part of the organ. Management of the tumors originating from the distal part of the esophagus is determined by the position of the tumor with respect to the gastroesophageal junction (GEJ). Siewert divided GEJ into three parts [3].

C. Gemici (✉)
Medical Park Hospital Group, Istanbul, Turkey





O. Engin (ed.), *Risk Factors and Therapy of Esophagus Cancer*,
https://doi.org/10.1007/978-3-031-47024-0_46

While tumors in the upper part of the GEJ (Type I) are considered as esophageal cancer, tumors in the middle and lower parts of the GEJ (Types II and III) are considered as gastric cancer [3]. However, in the recent American Joint Committee on Cancer (AJCC) staging manual, while Siewert Type I and II tumors are included under the esophageal cancer staging classification, Siewert Type III tumors are included under the gastric cancer staging classification [4].

Majority of the esophageal cancer patients present with locally advanced or metastatic disease at presentation. The lack of serosal envelope and the rich submucosal lymphatic network of the esophagus lead to extensive local infiltration and lymph node involvement [5, 6].

The pattern of lymphatic drainage of the esophagus depends on the location of the tumor in the organ. Tumors of the cervical and upper third of the thoracic esophagus mostly involve the cervical and the superior mediastinal lymph nodes. Tumors of the middle third of the esophagus may disseminate craniocaudally involving lymph nodes in the paratracheal, hilar, subcarinal, periesophageal, and pericardial nodal basins. Tumors in the distal esophagus primarily drain to lymph nodes in the lower mediastinum and celiac axis regions. Because of the extensive lymphatic network within the wall of the esophagus, skip lymph node metastases are common. While tumors in the upper third of the organ may spread to nodal basins of the celiac axis, tumors in the distal esophagus may spread to the cervical lymph nodes [1, 2].

Extensive, longitudinal interconnecting system of lymphatics facilitates not only early lymphatic spread of the tumors but also potential risk for lymphatic involvement longitudinally throughout the entire length of the organ [7]. Even superficial esophageal tumors can spread to the lymph nodes. While the incidence of nodal involvement is around 14–21% in T1 tumors, this rate rises to 60% in T2 tumors [8–12]. Autopsy studies showed that 60% of the patients had residual or recurrent tumors after curative surgery. In these studies, local recurrence was observed in 25.6% of the cases, while lymph node metastases were observed in 41.9% of the cases [13].

High locoregional failures are expected after surgical resection due to the anatomical difficulty of completely removing the tumor and the lymph nodes [13]. A striking and unknown detail about the involved lymph nodes in esophageal cancer is their microscopic involvement in most of the cases. Nodal involvement in majority of the patients cannot be identified radiologically or clinically. Involved lymph nodes are radiologically identifiable in only 1/3rd of the cases [8–10]. Therefore, it is not appropriate to rely on different imaging methods to determine the spread of the disease. Spread pattern of lymph node metastases in defining target volumes will be more valuable in radiotherapy planning and field design [14].

Median survival after esophagectomy for localized disease is 15–18 months and 5-year survival rate is around 20–25% [13, 15–17]. While locoregional recurrences are predominant in squamous cell carcinoma histology, distant recurrences are common in adenocarcinoma histology [5, 13].

## 46.2 Staging of Esophageal Cancer

The eighth edition of AJCC for staging of esophageal cancer is the current staging system [4]. The most important change in the eighth edition is the separation of staging by histologic classification. Squamous cell carcinoma and adenocarcinoma of the esophagus are now classified separately.

Cancers involving the GEJ with an epicenter within 2 cm of the proximal cardia (Siewert-type I-II tumors) are classified as esophageal cancer. Siewert type III tumors are classified as gastric cancer. The new staging system does not specify the number of lymph nodes to be removed but suggests that as many lymph nodes as possible should be resected [4].

## 46.3 Treatment Strategies

Surgery was the major treatment approach in esophageal cancer. However, the risk of both local and distant metastases has resulted in multimodality treatment strategies. Randomized clinical trials demonstrated the benefit of neoadjuvant treatment strategies like chemotherapy, chemoradiotherapy with respect to surgery alone. Some clinical trials have also questioned the role of surgery especially in squamous cell carcinoma of the esophagus where there is only local control but not a survival benefit with the addition of surgery [1, 2].

## 46.4 Surgery

Early esophageal tumors (Tis, T1N0) can be treated with surgery alone. Advances in endoscopic resection techniques have replaced surgery in selected early-stage tumors with no risk factors (low histologic grade and no lymphovascular invasion) [1, 2].

The major goal of surgery is R0 resection and appropriate lymph node removal with minimal morbidity and mortality. Mortality rates have decreased from above 20% to 3–4% in high-volume centers with the advances in anesthesia, surgical techniques, critical care, and the management of complications postoperatively [16, 17].

Survival rates for surgery alone for esophageal cancer historically were about 20% at 5 years. The most contemporary CROSS trial demonstrated 33% 5-year survival in a locally advanced cohort treated with surgery alone. (Most of the patients had pathological T3 disease and were pathologically node positive.) [18, 19].

Another contemporary French study also achieved a 5-year survival rate of 33% after surgery alone in a study limited only to clinical stages I and II patients 39% of patients were upstaged to stage III pathologically after surgery [20].

Low survival rates due to the high risk of locoregional and distant recurrences after surgery alone necessitated new treatment approaches.

## 46.5 Preoperative Chemotherapy

There are several potential advantages of induction chemotherapy before surgery. They may include downstaging of the disease and facilitation of surgical resection, improvement in local control, immediate relief of dysphagia in patients responding to induction chemotherapy, and most importantly the potential eradication of micrometastatic disease and thus prevention of distant metastases [1, 2].

Besides these advantages, there may be disadvantages of preoperative chemotherapy like potential development of chemotherapy resistance, delay in definitive treatment with the risk of further spread of the disease. These are major concerns as approximately 50% of patients do not respond to chemotherapy. Further deterioration in the patient's already marginal nutritional status and delay in local disease control are also a concern when surgery is not the first treatment. Controversy continues as to whether preoperative chemotherapy alone is sufficient to achieve high R0 curative resection rates in esophagectomy and whether concurrent chemotherapy and radiotherapy are superior to chemotherapy alone [1, 2].

Trials evaluating the use of induction chemotherapy followed by surgery for the treatment of esophageal cancer have been conducted since 1970s. This treatment approach was evaluated in parallel with concurrent chemotherapy and radiotherapy followed by surgery or concurrent chemotherapy and radiotherapy as definitive treatment [1, 2].

Earlier trials included mostly patients with squamous cell carcinoma, [21] but the recent trials with the predominance of adenocarcinoma in the west, included mostly adenocarcinoma [22–27]. In some trials, gastric cancer patients treated together with adenocarcinoma of the distal esophagus or gastroesophageal junction [22–24].

There are two major randomized trials comparing preoperative chemotherapy and surgery with surgery alone.

In the Medical Research Council OEO2 trial, 802 patients with resectable esophageal cancer were randomly assigned to receive either two cycles of preoperative fluorouracil and cisplatin followed by surgery or surgery alone [28]. Although the long-term follow-up of this study confirmed the survival benefit of preoperative chemotherapy with fluorouracil and cisplatin, with a 23% 5-year survival rate in the preoperative chemotherapy group compared to 17.1% in the surgery alone group ($P = 0.03$), the INT-113 trial, another large, randomized trial failed to demonstrate a survival advantage for the same approach [29]. There was no difference in median survival in the INT-133 trial (14.9 vs. 16.1 months; $p = 0.53$).

Pathologic complete responses after preoperative chemotherapy were rare and reported in only 4% of the patients. R0 resection rates and distant metastases rates were similar in both surgery alone arm and preoperative chemotherapy and surgery arm with no difference in patterns of failure in both arms. It is unclear how the preoperative chemotherapy increases the survival rate in esophageal cancer treatment. After these two controversial trials, a positive trial has been reported by Cunningham et al. in 2006 (MAGIC Trial) [22]. The trial included mostly gastric cancer patients while 26% of the patients treated had tumors in the GEJ and lower esophagus. 503

patients were randomized either to three cycles of preoperative and three cycles of postoperative Epirubicin/Cisplatin/5-FU chemotherapy or surgery alone. Perioperative chemotherapy resulted in 13% improvement in 5-year overall survival (23–36%). However, there were no major pathologic complete responses, and no improvement in distant metastases rates and no improvement in the rate of reported complete resection in patients treated with preoperative chemotherapy compared with surgery alone (66–69%). Although the result of the MAGIC trial was magic, this trial became worldwide the new standard in the treatment of resectable gastric cancer together with distal esophageal cancer.

Recent results of the FLOT4 trial from Germany have challenged the MAGIC trial in the preoperative treatment of gastroesophageal adenocarcinoma [27]. Preoperative chemotherapy with either the ECF or ECX regimen was compared to the FLOT regimen, 24-h infusion of 5-FU administered with leucovorin and oxaliplatin, docetaxel combination. Of the 716 patients included in the trial, 66% had type 1–3 GEJ cancers, and 34% had distal gastric cancers. All end points including median progression-free survival (30 months vs. 18 months), median overall survival (50 months vs. 35 months, HR 0.77, $P = 0.012$), and projected 5-year overall survival (45% vs. 36%) favored the FLOT regimen over ECF/ECX. Rates of R0 resection were higher with FLOT (84% vs. 77%). More patients treated with FLOT had ≤ T1 disease (25% vs. 10%) and node negative disease at surgery (49% vs. 41%).

Based on the result of the FLOT4 trial, the three-drug chemotherapy regimen containing docetaxel (FLOT protocol) has emerged as the new standard preoperative chemotherapy regimen for adenocarcinoma of distal esophagus and GEJ. This approach; however, has not been adopted for squamous cell carcinoma of the esophagus given the negative results of INT-0113 trial and the marginal benefits for preoperative chemotherapy reported in OEO2 trial. Neoadjuvant chemoradiotherapy is still the preferred treatment approach in patients with squamous cell carcinoma of the esophagus [28–30].

## 46.6 Preoperative Chemoradiotherapy

High locoregional recurrence rates and difficulty to achieve high R0 resection rates after surgery were the major reasons for the integration of radiotherapy to the treatment of this dismal disease.

Early trials with integration of preoperative and postoperative radiotherapy without chemotherapy to surgery have failed to yield any benefit over surgery alone. However, preoperative radiotherapy concomitant with chemotherapy has the potential to downstage the disease, increase complete resection rate with negative circumferential margins, eradicate micrometastatic disease, and thus reduce the risk of both local and distant disease recurrence. The combined use of concurrent chemotherapy and radiation therapy trials began in the late 80s, early 90s. Surgery which was the principal treatment in those days was insufficient treatment with high local and distant failure rates. As in the surgery control arm of the INT-0113 trial, R0 resection rate was possible in 59% of the patients with a 31% local failure rate [29].

Early randomized trials failed to demonstrate a sustained survival advantage with preoperative chemoradiotherapy due to methodological problems either related to radiation treatment parameters in radiotherapy arm or surgery-related parameters in surgery alone arm of the trials [31–34]. Hypofractionated radiotherapy with high toxicity and split-course radiation treatments with breaks during radiotherapy were the major drawbacks of the radiotherapy in these trials.

A recent meta-analysis pooling randomized trials of preoperative chemoradiotherapy and preoperative chemotherapy followed by surgery versus surgery alone for resectable esophageal cancer demonstrated a better survival advantage with the preoperative chemoradiotherapy [30]. This meta-analysis included 1854 patients enrolled in 12 randomized trials. Preoperative chemoradiotherapy was associated with a reduction in the risk of death (HR, 0.78, 95% CI, 0.70–0.88; $p < 0.001$) compared with surgery alone. In this analysis, similar effects were seen in patients both with squamous cell carcinoma (HR, 0.80; 95% CI, 0.68–0.93) and adenocarcinoma (HR, 0.75; 95% CI, 0.59–0.95).

The greatest advantage of preoperative chemoradiotherapy in resectable esophageal cancer is the increase in R0 resection rates and, as a result, decrease in locoregional recurrences [30]. The recent Dutch CROSS phase III randomized trial which provides the strongest data for the role of preoperative chemoradiotherapy demonstrated not only better locoregional control rates with this treatment but also better distant disease control rates [18, 19]. In this study, 368 patients with resectable esophageal cancer (majority adenocarcinoma, 75%) were randomized to preoperative irradiation (41.4 Gy in 23 fractions) with concurrent weekly carboplatin and paclitaxel followed by surgery or randomized to surgery alone. This protocol was well tolerated, with 92% of patients completed radiotherapy and 91% of patients completed the planned 5 cycles of chemotherapy. While R0 resection was possible in 92% of the patients in the chemoradiotherapy arm, it was possible in only 69% of the patients who were operated directly ($p < 0.001$). A high pathological complete response (pCR) was achieved with preoperative chemoradiotherapy. Pathologic complete response rate was 29% for whole group. While the pCR rate was 23% for adenocarcinoma, it was 49% for squamous cell carcinoma, and the difference was significant, $p = 0.008$. While pathologic lymph node positivity was observed in only 31% of the patients who underwent preoperative chemoradiotherapy, it was observed in 75% of the patients who were treated with surgery-alone ($p < 0.001$) [18, 19, 30].

Another important finding in this study was similar postoperative complications and in hospital mortality rates between the two groups. With a median follow-up of 7 years, preoperative chemoradiotherapy provided significant improvement in overall survival (HR, 0.68; 95% CI, 0.53–0.88; $p = 0.003$). While median survival was 48.6 months for the group treated with preoperative chemoradiotherapy, it was 24 months for the surgery-alone group; 5-year survival was 47% versus 33%, respectively. Although the survival difference was statistically significant in both the adenocarcinoma and squamous cell carcinoma subgroups, the survival benefit seemed to be greater in the squamous cell carcinoma subgroup (squamous cell carcinoma: HR, 0.45; 95% CI, 0.24–0.84; adenocarcinoma: HR, 0.73; 95% CI, 0.52–0.99) [18, 19].

In summary, CROSS Trial demonstrated that preoperative chemoradiotherapy not only decreases locoregional recurrences but also decreases distant metastases. No reduction in distant metastases rates was observed in preoperative chemotherapy trials published up to the CROSS Trial in patients with resectable esophageal cancer. Preoperative chemoradiotherapy and surgery in resectable esophageal cancer have the highest level of evidence with respect to preoperative chemotherapy both in squamous cell carcinoma and adenocarcinoma [18, 19].

## 46.7 Preoperative Chemotherapy vs. Preoperative Chemoradiotherapy

Several preliminary randomized trials have compared preoperative chemotherapy to preoperative chemoradiotherapy [35–37]. All these preliminary randomized trials were in favor of preoperative chemoradiotherapy with respect to pCR rates, lymph node downstaging, and R0 resection rates. Unfortunately, none of the trials have been adequately powered to demonstrate a difference in survival. In addition, the preoperative chemoradiotherapy and chemotherapy protocols used in these trials were not the current standards of care.

The German Phase III PreOperative therapy in Esophagogastric adenocarcinoma Trial (POET) is the most important one among these trials. Patients with resectable esophageal adenocarcinoma of the gastroesophageal junction were randomized to preoperative chemotherapy alone or induction chemotherapy followed by concomitant chemoradiotherapy (30 Gy in 15 fractions with cisplatin and etoposide). All end points were statistically significant with a trend for better overall survival for patients treated with preoperative chemoradiotherapy [35].

A recent meta-analysis of randomized trials comparing surgery alone to surgery with either preoperative chemoradiotherapy or preoperative chemotherapy for resectable esophageal cancer demonstrated a better survival trend with preoperative chemoradiotherapy compared to preoperative chemotherapy alone (HR, 0.88; 95% CI, 0.76–1.01; $p = 0.07$) [30].

The recently published phase III NEO-AEGIS trial compared preoperative chemotherapy with modified MAGIC or FLOT protocol, with preoperative chemoradiotherapy with CROSS protocol [38]. 377 patients with resectable adenocarcinoma of the esophagus or gastroesophageal junction were included in the trial. After a median follow-up of 24.5 months, there were 143 deaths, 70 in the preoperative CRT arm, and 73 in the preoperative CT arm, with 3-year survival probabilities of 56% and 57%, respectively (HR, 1.02), indicating no survival difference between the two modalities or noninferiority of preoperative chemotherapy with respect to preoperative chemoradiotherapy. However, all pathologic endpoints (pCR, N0, and R0 resection rates) favored preoperative chemoradiotherapy. Although this study suggests noninferiority of perioperative chemotherapy with respect to preoperative chemoradiotherapy, making perioperative chemotherapy another treatment option for patients with locoregional adenocarcinoma, the current standard should remain as preoperative chemoradiotherapy [18, 19, 38].

While the results of other prospective studies are awaited, more work remains to be done to improve the outcomes of preoperative chemoradiotherapy with the CROSS protocol. Among the parameters that may improve the results of preoperative chemoradiotherapy, radiation field size and radiation dose and the accompanying chemotherapy protocol are the most important ones [14, 39–41]. Muijs et al. demonstrated that 14% of the patients treated with the CROSS protocol had residual microscopic tumors after preoperative chemoradiotherapy outside the confines of the radiation fields. The radiation fields were intentionally reduced craniocaudally by the authors of the study to decrease the radiation toxicity [14, 39, 40]. This means that more efficient radiation field size and dose design can sterilize the tumor in more patients, thereby improve the results of preoperative chemoradiotherapy. Another method to improve the results of preoperative chemoradiotherapy may be administration of preoperative chemotherapy with FLOT followed by chemoradiotherapy, or administration of more potent chemotherapy combinations including FLOT or other oxaliplatin containing combinations concomitant with radiotherapy [41–43].

## 46.8 Response to Preoperative Therapy and Role of Postoperative Therapy

The pathologic complete response rates for patients with esophageal or gastric cancer who received preoperative treatment range from 15 to 40% (average 25%) after preoperative chemoradiotherapy, and 2–13% (average 5%) after chemotherapy alone [18, 22, 27, 30]. The most important prognostic factor associated with improved survival is the pathological complete response to neoadjuvant therapy [26, 34, 44–48]. Better overall survival has been demonstrated in the meta-analysis for patients who had pCR after neoadjuvant treatment [49]. Nodal status following neoadjuvant chemotherapy [47, 48, 50] or CRT [51–53] has also been demonstrated to be a prognostic factor for survival. Pathological involvement of lymph nodes was the strongest independent prognostic factor associated with risk of death for patients treated with preoperative chemotherapy in the MAGIC trial, (HR, 3.63; 95% CI, 1.88–7.0; $p < 0.001$) [48]. Pathological response to neoadjuvant therapy provides useful information for patients regarding the risk of recurrence. Patients with poor responses to preoperative therapy are at higher risk for recurrence, and ongoing trials investigate the use of novel adjuvant therapy regimens including chemotherapy or immunotherapy in these patients.

## 46.9 Nonsurgical Treatment: Definitive Chemoradiotherapy

Definitive concomitant chemoradiotherapy (CRT) is the principal treatment for patients with locoregionally advanced esophageal cancer or for patients who are not suitable for surgery due to medical reasons [54–57].

The Radiation Therapy Oncology Group (RTOG) 85-01 Trial was the principal trial which demonstrated survival benefit with definitive CRT (cisplatin, 5-FU, and

50.4 Gy) [58, 59]. Definitive CRT became the standard nonsurgical treatment of patients with locoregionally advanced esophageal cancer.

The improvement in survival with the definitive CRT is related to reduction in both local and distant recurrence rates. RTOG 85-01 reported a crude local persistence or recurrence rate of 44% in definitive CRT group and 64% in the radiotherapy alone group. The 2-year local failure rate was reduced from 68% to 43% ($p < 0.01$), and the rate of distant metastases was reduced from 70% to 25% ($p = 0.005$) with the addition of concomitant chemotherapy to radiotherapy [58, 59].

The high locoregional failures led to several subsequent trials. The aim of these trials was to decrease locoregional recurrences, either by induction chemotherapy (5-FU, cisplatin, Intergroup 0122 Trial) or by increasing radiation dose (5-FU, cisplatin, and 64.8 Gy, RTOG 94–05 Trial) [60, 61] or by integration of new generation chemotherapeutics, like paclitaxel (RTOG 0113 Trial) [62]. While none of those strategies resulted in better locoregional control rates or survival, they resulted in increased toxicity and treatment-related mortality [60–62]. The radiation dose and field design of these new generation trials were like that of the Intergroup 0123 Trial. Intergroup-0123 trial compared two different RT doses with the same concomitant chemotherapy regimen (fluorouracil and cisplatin) [60]. In this trial, 218 patients with either squamous cell carcinoma (85%) or adenocarcinoma (15%) (cT1–cT4, N0–1, M0) were randomized between 50.4 Gy or a higher dose of 64.8 Gy. There was no significant difference either in median survival (13 vs. 18 months) or in locoregional failure rates (56% vs. 52%) between 64.8 Gy and 50.4 Gy. Two more recent phase III trials (ARTDECO and CONCORDE [PRODIGE-26]) re-evaluated the role of dose escalation beyond 50 Gy to improve local control and survival [63, 64]. Unfortunately, these trials did not demonstrate any benefit with the use of radiation doses above 50 Gy for definitive chemoradiotherapy. However, radiation field design may be responsible for the failure of the trials. As we know from the CROSS trial, 14% of the patients with the current radiation field design have still residual disease outside the radiation fields [14, 39, 40].

Paclitaxel and carboplatin combination that became the most preferred chemotherapy combination after the CROSS Trial also became the preferred chemotherapy combination together with definitive radiotherapy due to better toxicity profile with respect to fluorouracil and cisplatin. Fluorouracil and oxaliplatin (FOLFOX) are another option for preoperative or definitive CRT. The efficacy and safety of FOLFOX combined with RT were evaluated in a phase II SWOG trial in 93 patients with clinically staged II or III esophageal adenocarcinoma [65]. Pathologic complete response rate was 28%, and median and 3-year OS were 28.3 months and 45.1%, respectively [65]. There is an ongoing randomized phase II (PROTECT) trial that will compare FOLFOX to paclitaxel and carboplatin concurrent with 41.4 Gy RT, in patients with resectable stage IIB–III squamous or adenocarcinoma of esophagus and EGJ [66]. This trial is a direct comparison of two standards of preoperative CRT in the setting of resectable, locally advanced esophageal or EGJ cancers. Both paclitaxel and carboplatin and FOLFOX combination chemotherapy can be better alternatives to fluorouracil and cisplatin during definitive radiotherapy.

## 46.10 Definitive CRT (Bimodality Therapy) vs. Preoperative CRT and Surgery (Trimodality Therapy)

Universally accepted radiation treatment fields and radiation doses used in the management of esophageal cancer are the two most important causes of residual tumor and locoregional recurrences in esophageal cancer after chemoradiotherapy [14]. Radiation doses around 50 Gy are only effective for controlling microscopic tumors in most tumors treated with radiotherapy in the adjuvant setting. Muijs et al. demonstrated insufficiency of the radiation treatment fields that are accepted as standards for the treatment of esophageal cancer [39]. They found that 14% of the patients had still residual tumors outside the radiotherapy target volume after preoperative CRT.

The major role of surgery in esophageal cancer treatment after preoperative or definitive CRT is to remove the residual tumor that remains viable after chemoradiotherapy either in the lymph nodes or in the primary tumor area [14, 18, 30, 39, 40, 67–73].

The role of preoperative CRT before surgery is to sterilize the tumors either in the lymph nodes or in the primary tumor area. Surgical removal of the tumor is not always easy due to its proximity to vital structures (circumferential resection margins). Anatomical difficulty to reach and resect involved lymph nodes is another problem in esophageal cancer surgery [14, 18, 30, 39, 40, 67–73]. While CRT compensates for the insufficiency of surgery, surgery compensates for the insufficiency of CRT [14].

Although preoperative CRT is very important in the surgical treatment of esophageal cancer, the role of surgery after definitive CRT is questionable. Two randomized trials searched the addition of surgery after definitive CRT [67, 74].

The German Esophageal Cancer Study Group and the FFCD 9102 trial compared preoperative CRT with surgery versus definitive CRT alone [67, 74].

In the FFCD 9102 trial, locally advanced esophageal squamous cell carcinoma patients who received two cycles of cisplatin and 5-FU concurrent with either 46 Gy at 2 Gy per day or split course 15 Gy at weeks 1 and 3 and had at least partial response to the treatment (259 patients) were randomized between surgery or continuation of CRT either 20 Gy at 2 Gy per day or split course 15 Gy [74]. Although there was no significant difference in 2-year survival (34% vs. 40%, $P = 0.44$) or median survival (17.7 vs. 19.3 months) in patients who underwent surgery or additional CRT, treatment-related mortality was high in operated patients. There were more locoregional recurrences in the CRT arm ($P = 0.03$).

In the German Trial, patients with squamous cell carcinoma were randomized between preoperative therapy (three cycles of 5-FU, etoposide, and cisplatin, followed by concurrent 40 Gy radiotherapy with etoposide and cisplatin) followed by surgery versus definitive CRT (the same chemotherapy but the radiation dose was increased to 60–65 Gy). Despite a decrease in 2-year local failure in operated patients (36% versus 58%, $P = 0.003$), there was no significant difference in 3-year survival rates (31% vs. 24%) [67]. These two randomized studies showed that role of surgery is negligible when radiation doses are increased above 50 Gy in the treatment of esophageal cancer with definitive CRT.

RTOG 0246 is a phase II trial that examined the role of surgery in locally advanced esophageal cancer patients treated with 50.4 Gy CRT [75, 76]. This study demonstrated that surgical resection is necessary only in patients that have still residual disease (selective surgery), or patients who had recurrence without distant metastasis (salvage surgery). Half (49%) of the patients in this study did not require esophageal resection, suggesting that watchful waiting is an organ-preserving approach for patients who achieve a clinical complete response to CRT [75, 76].

There are ongoing prospective trials evaluating the role of active surveillance and salvage surgery after definitive CRT. The Dutch Surgery As Needed in Oesophageal cancer (SANO) trial is a phase-III trial, randomizing patients who achieve clinical complete response after CRT either between active surveillance or planned esophagectomy [77].

There are several meta-analyses comparing bimodality (Definitive CRT) with trimodality (preoperative CRT with surgery) treatment in the management of locally advanced esophageal cancer [78, 79]. Based on the available data, the addition of surgery to chemoradiotherapy in locally advanced esophageal squamous cell carcinoma, provides little or no difference on overall survival. Adding esophagectomy may reduce locoregional recurrences, but this is not reflected in survival rates and may be associated with higher morbidity and mortality. It is unclear whether these results can be applied to the treatment of adenocarcinoma histology, tumors involving the distal esophagus and GEJ [78, 79].

## 46.11 Postoperative Treatment: Chemotherapy and Chemoradiotherapy

Studies investigating the role of adjuvant CT or CRT for resected squamous cell carcinoma of the esophagus are limited and mostly retrospective [80–82].

The effect of adjuvant chemotherapy on the survival of patients with esophageal squamous cell carcinomas is controversial. Patients with involved lymph nodes may benefit from adjuvant chemotherapy [83]. On the other hand, studies have suggested a survival benefit with adjuvant CRT for node-positive squamous cell carcinoma of the esophagus after surgery [78]. A National Cancer Database analysis that investigating the role of postoperative CRT in patients with locally advanced esophageal squamous or adenocarcinoma after surgical resection demonstrated a survival advantage [81].

Macdonald et al. have demonstrated the benefit of postoperative CRT for GEJ adenocarcinomas in the intergroup INT0116 Trial [84]. Although the trial included mostly gastric cancer patients, a total of 559 patients with nonmetastatic adenocarcinoma of the stomach or GEJ (20% of patients) after curative resection were randomized to either observation alone or postoperative CRT consisting of bolus 5-FU and 45 Gy concurrent radiation [84]. Patients who received postoperative CRT had a significant decrease in local failure and an increase in median survival (36 vs. 27 months), 3-year relapse-free survival (48% vs. 31%), and OS (50% vs. 41%, $P = 0.005$). Updated results, with more than 10 years of follow-up, showed the benefit in PFS and OS with adjuvant CRT [85].

While INT0116 Trial demonstrated a survival advantage with postoperative CRT in patients with gastric and GEJ adenocarcinomas, The CRITICS trial (Chemotherapy vs. chemoradiotherapy after surgery and preoperative chemotherapy for resectable gastric cancer) demonstrated no improvement with postoperative CRT with respect to the patients treated with perioperative CT [86]. 788 patients were included in the study, and they were randomized to either perioperative chemotherapy or preoperative chemotherapy with postoperative chemoradiotherapy, only 17% of the patients had GEJ tumors.

A recent meta-analysis consisting of 2165 patients with esophageal cancer investigated the role of different postoperative treatments including CT, RT, and CRT [87]. This meta-analysis showed that postoperative CRT significantly improved survival and significantly reduced the locoregional recurrences compared to other postoperative treatments (postoperative CT, postoperative RT, or observation) [87]. Although no difference was seen in the rate of distant metastases between these groups, postoperative CRT provided significant survival benefits and improved locoregional control with tolerable toxicity. Postoperative CRT is very important for patients who had involved surgical margins (R1 resected patients) after surgery. Salvage can be possible with postoperative CRT [29].

## 46.12 Postoperative Immunotherapy

Patients who are operated after preoperative CRT and had residual disease at pathologic examination have very high risk of recurrence despite R0 resection. CHECKMATE-577 Trial is a randomized phase 3 trial, comparing adjuvant 1 year of immunotherapy with nivolumab to placebo in patients operated with R0 resection but having residual disease. The trial included 794 patients, majority of them had adenocarcinoma (71%), with stage III disease (65%), and 72% tested for PD-L1 positive in the tumor [88]. Disease-free survival was significantly improved with the addition of adjuvant nivolumab compared to placebo (22.4 months to 11.0 months, $p < 0.0003$). This benefit was seen irrespective of histology, nodal, or PD-L1 status. These results led to a paradigm change and the approval of adjuvant nivolumab for esophageal cancer patients without complete pathological response after CRT and R0 resection by the European Medicines Agency (EMA) and FDA [88].

## 46.13 Palliative Radiotherapy

Palliative treatment is an important part of treatment for palliation of dysphagia, bleeding, and pain in patients with unresectable locally advanced, locally recurrent, or metastatic esophageal cancer. The main goal is to prevent and alleviate the symptoms arising from the presence of the disease and to maintain the best possible quality of life. Interventions undertaken to relieve major symptoms may result in a significant prolongation of life. Interdisciplinary approach to palliative care of the esophageal cancer patient is very important and should be encouraged [89, 90].

Chemotherapy together with best support care may not only increase survival but also improve quality of life and should be considered in patients with good performance status [89, 90].

Radiotherapy is necessary in one-third of the patients with advanced disease. Esophageal radiation may alleviate obstructive symptoms (dysphagia, odynophagia) and bleeding from esophageal tumors and is one of the most effective palliative treatments [89, 90].

Radiotherapy should be the first choice for palliation of dysphagia in patients with long life expectancy and good performance status. Stenting should be considered in patients with a short-term life expectancy and necessity of rapid resolution of symptoms [89]. Although radiotherapy and self-expanding metal stent placement are associated with prolonged dysphagia and better survival, the risk of major side effects such as perforation and fistula development should also be considered [89, 90]. Therefore, it is better to consider stent placement in patients who have failed prior radiotherapy.

Palliative radiotherapy may be administered with concomitant chemotherapy in patients with good performance and may provide better result.

## References

1. Practical guides in radiation oncology: gastrointestinal malignancies. 1st ed. Springer; 2018.
2. Radiation therapy for gastrointestinal cancers. 1st ed. Springer; 2017.
3. Siewert JR, Feith M, Werner M, et al. Adenocarcinoma of the esophagogastric junction: results of surgical therapy based on anatomical/topographic classification in 1,002 consecutive patients. Ann Surg. 2000;232(3):353–61.
4. Cancer AJCO. AJCC cancer staging manual. 8th ed. New York: Springer; 2016.
5. Mariette C, Balon JM, Piessen G, et al. Pattern of recurrence following complete resection of esophageal carcinoma and factors predictive of recurrent disease. Cancer. 2003;97(7):1616–23.
6. Katayama A, Mafune K, Tanaka Y, et al. Autopsy findings in patients after curative esophagectomy for esophageal carcinoma. J Am Coll Surg. 2003;196(6):866–73, 89.
7. Czito BG. Esophageal cancer. In: Halperin EC, Wazer DE, Perez CA, Brady LW, editors. Principles and practice of radiation oncology. 6th ed. Philadelphia: Lippincott, Williams & Wilkins; 2013. p. 995–1022.
8. Tachimori Y, Nagai Y, Kanamori N, et al. Pattern of lymph node metastasis of esophageal squamous cell carcinoma based on the anatomical lymphatic drainage system. Dis Esophagus. 2011;24:33–8.
9. Dresner SM, Lamb PJ, Bennett MK, et al. The pattern of metastatic lymph node dissemination from adenocarcinoma of the esophagogastric junction. Surgery. 2001;129:103–9.
10. Hosch SB, Stoecklein NH, Pichlmeier U, et al. Esophageal cancer: the mode of lymphatic tumor cell spread and its prognostic significance. J Clin Oncol. 2001;19:1970–5.
11. Akiyama H, Tsurumaru M, Kawamura T, et al. Principles of surgical treatment for carcinoma of the esophagus: analysis of lymph node involvement. Ann Surg. 1981;194:438–46.
12. Huang W, Li B, Gong H, et al. Pattern of lymph node metastases and its implication in radiotherapeutic clinical target volume in patients with thoracic esophageal squamous cell carcinoma: a report of 1077 cases. Radiother Oncol. 2010;95:229–33.
13. Katayama A, Mafune K, Tanaka Y, et al. Autopsy findings in patients after curative esophagectomy for esophageal carcinoma. J Am Coll Surg. 2003;196:866–73.

14. Gemici C, Yaprak G, Batirel HF, et al. Radiation field size and dose determine oncologic outcome in esophageal cancer. World J Surg Oncol. 2016;14:263–72.
15. Boshier PR, Anderson O, Hanna GB. Transthoracic versus transhiatal esophagectomy for the treatment of esophagogastric cancer: a meta-analysis. Ann Surg. 2011;254(6):894–906.
16. Biere SS, van Berge Henegouwen MI, Maas KW, et al. Minimally invasive versus open oesophagectomy for patients with oesophageal cancer: a multicentre, open-label, randomised controlled trial. Lancet. 2012;379:1887–92.
17. Nieman DR, Peters JH. Treatment strategies for esophageal cancer. Gastroenterol Clin N Am. 2013;42:187–97.
18. van Hagen P, Hulshof MC, van Lanschot JJ, et al. Preoperative chemoradiotherapy for esophageal or junctional cancer. N Engl J Med. 2012;366:2074–84.
19. Shapiro J, van Lanschot JJB, Hulshof M, et al. Neoadjuvant chemoradiotherapy plus surgery versus surgery alone for oesophageal or junctional cancer (CROSS): long-term results of a randomised controlled trial. Lancet Oncol. 2015;16:1090–8.
20. Mariette C, Dahan L, Mornex F, et al. Surgery alone versus chemoradiotherapy followed by surgery for stage I and II esophageal cancer: final analysis of randomized controlled phase III trial FFCD 9901. J Clin Oncol. 2014;32:2416–22.
21. Boonstra JJ, Kok TC, Wijnhoven BP, et al. Chemotherapy followed by surgery versus surgery alone in patients with resectable oesophageal squamous cell carcinoma: long-term results of a randomized controlled trial. BMC Cancer. 2011;11:181.
22. Cunningham D, Allum WH, Stenning SP, et al. Perioperative chemotherapy versus surgery alone for resectable gastroesophageal cancer. N Engl J Med. 2006;355(1):11–20.
23. Ychou M, Boige V, Pignon JP, et al. Perioperative chemotherapy compared with surgery alone for resectable gastroesophageal adenocarcinoma: an FNCLCC and FFCD multicenter phase III trial. J Clin Oncol. 2011;29(13):1715–21.
24. Schuhmacher C, Gretschel S, Lordick F, et al. Neoadjuvant chemotherapy compared with surgery alone for locally advanced cancer of the stomach and cardia: European Organisation for Research and Treatment of Cancer randomized trial 40954. J Clin Oncol. 2010;28(35):5210–8.
25. Alderson D, Cunningham D, Nankivell M, et al. Neoadjuvant cisplatin and fluorouracil versus epirubicin, cisplatin, and capecitabine followed by resection in patients with oesophageal adenocarcinoma (UK MRC OE05): an open-label, randomised phase 3 trial. Lancet Oncol. 2017;18(9):1249–60.
26. Cunningham D, Stenning SP, Smyth EC, et al. Peri-operative chemotherapy with or without bevacizumab in operable oesophagogastric adenocarcinoma (UK medical research council ST03): primary analysis results of a multicentre, open-label, randomised phase 2–3 trial. Lancet Oncol. 2017;18(3):357–70.
27. Al-Batran SE, Homann N, Pauligk C, et al. Perioperative chemotherapy with fluorouracil plus leucovorin, oxaliplatin, and docetaxel versus fluorouracil or capecitabine plus cisplatin and epirubicin for locally advanced, resectable gastric or gastro-oesophageal junction adenocarcinoma (FLOT4): a randomised, phase 2/3 trial. Lancet. 2019;393(10184):1948–57.
28. Allum WH, Stenning SP, Bancewicz J, et al. Long-term results of a randomized trial of surgery with or without preoperative chemotherapy in esophageal cancer. J Clin Oncol. 2009;27:5062–7.
29. Kelsen DP, Ginsberg R, Pajak TF, et al. Chemotherapy followed by surgery compared with surgery alone for localized esophageal cancer. N Engl J Med. 1998;339:1979–84.
30. Sjoquist KM, Burmeister BH, Smithers BM, et al. Survival after neoadjuvant chemotherapy or chemoradiotherapy for resectable oesophageal carcinoma: an updated metaanalysis. Lancet Oncol. 2011;12(7):681–92.
31. Walsh TN, Noonan N, Hollywood D, et al. A comparison of multimodal therapy and surgery for esophageal adenocarcinoma. N Engl J Med. 1996;335:462–7.
32. Bosset JF, Gignoux M, Triboulet JP, et al. Chemoradiotherapy followed by surgery compared with surgery alone in squamous-cell cancer of the esophagus. N Engl J Med. 1997;337:161–7.
33. Burmeister BH, Smithers BM, Gebski V, et al. Surgery alone versus chemoradiotherapy followed by surgery for resectable cancer of the oesophagus: a randomised controlled phase III trial. Lancet Oncol. 2005;6:659–68.

34. Urba SG, Orringer MB, Turrisi A, et al. Randomized trial of preoperative chemoradiation versus surgery alone in patients with locoregional esophageal carcinoma. J Clin Oncol. 2001;19:305–13.
35. Stahl M, Walz MK, Riera-Knorrenschild J, et al. Preoperative chemotherapy versus chemoradiotherapy in locally advanced adenocarcinomas of the oesophagogastric junction (POET): long-term results of a controlled randomised trial. Eur J Cancer. 2017;81:183–90.
36. Burmeister BH, Thomas JM, Burmeister EA, et al. Is concurrent radiation therapy required in patients receiving preoperative chemotherapy for adenocarcinoma of the oesophagus? A randomised phase II trial. Eur J Cancer. 2011;47:354–60.
37. Klevebro F, Alexandersson von Dobeln G, Wang N, et al. A randomized clinical trial of neoadjuvant chemotherapy versus neoadjuvant chemoradiotherapy for cancer of the oesophagus or gastro-oesophageal junction. Ann Oncol. 2016;27:660–7.
38. Reynolds JV, Preston SR, O'Neill B, et al. Neo-AEGIS (neoadjuvant trial in adenocarcinoma of the esophagus and esophago-gastric junction international study): preliminary results of phase III RCT of CROSS versus perioperative chemotherapy (modified MAGIC or FLOT protocol). (NCT01726452). J Clin Oncol. 2021;39:4004–4.
39. Muijs C, Smit J, Karrenbeld A, et al. Residual tumor after neoadjuvant chemoradiation outside the radiation therapy target volume: a new prognostic factor for survival in esophageal cancer. Int J Radiat Oncol Biol Phys. 2014;88:845–52.
40. Gemici C, et al. Residual tumor after neoadjuvant chemoradiation outside the radiation therapy target volume: a new prognostic factor for survival in esophageal cancer. Int J Radiat Oncol Biol Phys. 2014;90:715–7.
41. Lorenzen S, Biederstädt A, Ronellenfitsch U, et al. RACE-trial: neoadjuvant radiochemotherapy versus chemotherapy for patients with locally advanced, potentially resectable adenocarcinoma of the gastroesophageal junction—a randomized phase III joint study of the AIO, ARO and DGAV. BMC Cancer. 2020;20:886.
42. Conroy T, Yataghene Y, Etienne PL, et al. Phase II randomised trial of chemoradiotherapy with FOLFOX4 or cisplatin plus fluorouracil in oesophageal cancer. Br J Cancer. 2010;103:1349–55.
43. Lorenzen S, Brücher B, Zimmermann F, et al. Neoadjuvant continuous infusion of weekly 5-fluorouracil and escalating doses of oxaliplatin plus concurrent radiation in locally advanced oesophageal squamous cell carcinoma: results of a phase I/II trial. Br J Cancer. 2008;99:1020–6.
44. Alderson D, Cunningham D, Nankivell M, et al. Neoadjuvant cisplatin and fluorouracil versus epirubicin, cisplatin, and capecitabine followed by resection in patients with oesophageal adenocarcinoma (UK MRC OE05): an open-label, randomised phase 3 trial. Lancet Oncol. 2017;18:1249–60.
45. Poplin E, Fleming T, Leichman L, et al. Combined therapies for squamous-cell carcinoma of the esophagus, a southwest oncology group study (SWOG-8037). J Clin Oncol. 1987;5:622–8.
46. Bates BA, Detterbeck FC, Bernard SA, et al. Concurrent radiation therapy and chemotherapy followed by esophagectomy for localized esophageal carcinoma. J Clin Oncol. 1996;14:156–63.
47. Noble F, Lloyd MA, Turkington R, et al. Multicentre cohort study to define and validate pathological assessment of response to neoadjuvant therapy in oesophagogastric adenocarcinoma. Br J Surg. 2017;104:1816–28.
48. Smyth EC, Fassan M, Cunningham D, et al. Effect of pathologic tumor response and nodal status on survival in the medical research council adjuvant gastric infusional chemotherapy trial. J Clin Oncol. 2016;34:2721–7.
49. Tomasello G, Petrelli F, Ghidini M, et al. Tumor regression grade and survival after neoadjuvant treatment in gastro-esophageal cancer: a meta-analysis of 17 published studies. Eur J Surg Oncol. 2017;43:1607–16.
50. Davarzani N, Hutchins GGA, West NP, et al. Prognostic value of pathological lymph node status and primary tumour regression grading following neoadjuvant chemotherapy—results from the MRC OE02 oesophageal cancer trial. Histopathology. 2018;72:1180–8.
51. Philippron A, Bollschweiler E, Kunikata A, et al. Prognostic relevance of lymph node regression after neoadjuvant chemoradiation for esophageal cancer. Semin Thorac Cardiovasc Surg. 2016;28:549–58.

52. Gu Y, Swisher SG, Ajani JA, et al. The number of lymph nodes with metastasis predicts survival in patients with esophageal or esophagogastric junction adenocarcinoma who receive preoperative chemoradiation. Cancer. 2006;106:1017–25.
53. Gaca JG, Petersen RP, Peterson BL, et al. Pathologic nodal status predicts disease-free survival after neoadjuvant chemoradiation for gastroesophageal junction carcinoma. Ann Surg Oncol. 2006;13:340–6.
54. Steiger Z, Franklin R, Wilson RF, et al. Complete eradication of squamous cell carcinoma of the esophagus with combined chemotherapy and radiotherapy. Am Surg. 1981;47:95–8.
55. Lokich JJ, Shea M, Chaffey J. Sequential infusional 5-fluorouracil followed by concomitant radiation for tumors of the esophagus and gastroesophageal junction. Cancer. 1987;60:275–9.
56. Coia LR, Paul AR, Engstrom PF. Combined radiation and chemotherapy as primary management of adenocarcinoma of the esophagus and gastroesophageal junction. Cancer. 1988;61:643–9.
57. Leichman L, Herskovic A, Leichman CG, et al. Nonoperative therapy for squamous-cell cancer of the esophagus. J Clin Oncol. 1987;5:365–70.
58. Herskovic A, Martz K, Al-Sarraf M, et al. Combined chemotherapy and radiotherapy compared with radiotherapy alone in patients with cancer of the esophagus. N Engl J Med. 1992;326:1593–8.
59. Cooper JS, Guo MD, Herskovic A, et al. Chemoradiotherapy of locally advanced esophageal cancer: long-term follow-up of a prospective randomized trial (RTOG 85–01). Radiation Therapy Oncology Group. JAMA. 1999;281:1623–7.
60. Minsky BD, Pajak TF, Ginsberg RJ, et al. INT 0123 (Radiation Therapy Oncology Group 94-05) phase III trial of combined-modality therapy for esophageal cancer: high-dose versus standard-dose radiation therapy. J Clin Oncol. 2002;20:1167–74.
61. Minsky BD, Neuberg D, Kelsen DP, et al. Neoadjuvant chemotherapy plus concurrent chemotherapy and high-dose radiation for squamous cell carcinoma of the esophagus: a preliminary analysis of the phase II intergroup trial 0122. J Clin Oncol. 1996;14:149–55.
62. Ajani JA, Winter K, Komaki R, et al. Phase II randomized trial of two nonoperative regimens of induction chemotherapy followed by chemoradiation in patients with localized carcinoma of the esophagus: RTOG 0113. J Clin Oncol. 2008;26:4551–6.
63. Hulshof M, Geijsen ED, Rozema T, et al. Randomized study on dose escalation in definitive chemoradiation for patients with locally advanced esophageal cancer (ARTDECO study). J Clin Oncol. 2021;39(25):2816–24.
64. Crehange G, Bertaut A, Peiffert D, et al. Exclusive chemoradiotherapy with or without dose escalation in locally advanced esophageal carcinoma: the CONCORDE study (PRODIGE 26). J Clin Oncol. 2017;35(15_suppl):4037–7.
65. Leichman LP, Goldman BH, Bohanes PO, et al. A phase II clinical and prospective molecular trial with oxaliplatin, fluorouracil, and external-beam radiation therapy before surgery for patients with esophageal adenocarcinoma. J Clin Oncol. 2011;29:4555–60.
66. Messager M, Mirabel X, Tresch E, et al. Preoperative chemoradiation with paclitaxel-carboplatin or with fluorouracil-oxaliplatin-folinic acid (FOLFOX) for resectable esophageal and junctional cancer: the PROTECT-1402, randomized phase 2 trial. BMC Cancer. 2016;16:318.
67. Stahl M, Stuschke M, Lehmann N, et al. Chemoradiation with and without surgery in patients with locally advanced squamous cell carcinoma of the esophagus. J Clin Oncol. 2005;23:2310–7.
68. Oppedijk V, van der Gaast A, van Lanschot JJ, et al. Patterns of recurrence after surgery alone versus preoperative chemoradiotherapy and surgery in the CROSS trials. J Clin Oncol. 2014;32:385–91.
69. Pottgen C, Stuschke M. Radiotherapy versus surgery within multlmodality protocols for esophageal cancer: a metaanalysis of the randomized trials. Cancer Treat Rev. 2012;38:599–604.
70. Welsh J, Settle SH, Amini A, et al. Failure patterns in patients with esophageal cancer treated with definitive chemoradiation. Cancer. 2012;118:2632–40.

71. Amini A, Ajani J, Komaki R, et al. Factors associated with local-regional failure after definitive chemoradiation for locally advanced esophageal cancer. Ann Surg Oncol. 2014;1:306–14.
72. Thoen H, Ceelen W, Boterberg T, et al. Tumor recurrence and in-field control after multimodality treatment of locally advanced esophageal cancer. Radiother Oncol. 2015;115:16–21.
73. Neishaboori N, Wadhwa R, Nogueras-Gonzales GM, et al. Distribution of resistant esophageal adenocarcinoma in the resected specimens of clinical stage III patients after chemoradiation: its clinical implications. Oncology. 2015;89:65–9.
74. Bedenne L, Michel P, Bouché O, et al. Chemoradiation followed by surgery compared with chemoradiation alone in squamous cancer of the esophagus: FFCD 9102. J Clin Oncol. 2007;25(10):1160–8.
75. Swisher SG, Winter KA, Komaki RU, et al. A phase II study of a paclitaxel-based chemoradiation regimen with selective surgical salvage for resectable locoregionally advanced esophageal cancer: initial reporting of RTOG 0246. Int J Radiat Oncol Biol Phys. 2012;82(5):1967–72.
76. Swisher SG, Moughan J, Komaki RU, et al. Final results of NRG oncology RTOG 0246: an organ-preserving selective resection strategy in esophageal cancer patients treated with definitive chemoradiation. J Thorac Oncol. 2017;12(2):368–74.
77. Noordman BJ, Spaander MCW, Valkema R, et al. Detection of residual disease after neoadjuvant chemoradiotherapy for oesophageal cancer (preSANO): a prospective multicentre, diagnostic cohort study. Lancet Oncol. 2018;19(7):965–74.
78. Vellayappan BA, Soon YY, Ku GY, et al. Chemoradiotherapy versus chemoradiotherapy plus surgery for esophageal cancer. Cochrane Database Syst Rev. 2017;8(8):1–30.
79. Voeten DM, den Bakker CM, Heineman DJ, et al. Definitive chemoradiotherapy versus trimodality therapy for resectable oesophageal carcinoma: meta-analyses and systematic review of literature. World J Surg. 2019;43(5):1271–85.
80. Hsu PK, Huang CS, Wang BY, et al. Survival benefits of postoperative chemoradiation for lymph node-positive esophageal squamous cell carcinoma. Ann Thorac Surg. 2014;97:1734–41.
81. Wong AT, Shao M, Rineer J, et al. The impact of adjuvant postoperative radiation therapy and chemotherapy on survival after esophagectomy for esophageal carcinoma. Ann Surg. 2017;265:1146–51.
82. Pasquer A, Gronnier C, Renaud F, et al. Impact of adjuvant chemotherapy on patients with lymph node-positive esophageal cancer who are primarily treated with surgery. Ann Surg Oncol. 2015;22(suppl 3):S1340–9.
83. Zhang SS, Yang H, Xie X, et al. Adjuvant chemotherapy versus surgery alone for esophageal squamous cell carcinoma: a meta-analysis of randomized controlled trials and nonrandomized studies. Dis Esophagus. 2014;27:574–84.
84. Macdonald JS, Smalley SR, Benedetti J, et al. Chemoradiotherapy after surgery compared with surgery alone for adenocarcinoma of the stomach or gastroesophageal junction. N Engl J Med. 2001;345:725–30.
85. Smalley SR, Benedetti JK, Haller DG, et al. Updated analysis of SWOGdirected intergroup study 0116: a phase III trial of adjuvant radiochemotherapy versus observation after curative gastric cancer resection. J Clin Oncol. 2012;30:2327–33.
86. Cats A, Jansen EPM, van Grieken NCT, et al. Chemotherapy versus chemoradiotherapy after surgery and preoperative chemotherapy for resectable gastric cancer (CRITICS): an international, open-label, randomised phase 3 trial. Lancet Oncol. 2018;19:616–28.
87. Kang J, Chang JY, Sun X, et al. Role of postoperative concurrent chemoradiotherapy for esophageal carcinoma: a meta-analysis of 2165 patients. J Cancer. 2018;9:584–93.
88. Kelly RJ, Ajani JA, Kuzdzal J, et al. Adjuvant nivolumab in resected esophageal or gastroesophageal junction cancer. N Engl J Med. 2021;384(13):1191–203.
89. Murray LJ, Din OS, Kumar VS, et al. Palliative radiotherapy in patients with esophageal carcinoma: a retrospective review. Pract Radiat Oncol. 2012;2:257–64.
90. Tinusz B, Soós A, Hegyi P, et al. Efficacy and safety of stenting and additional oncological treatment versus stenting alone in unresectable esophageal cancer: a meta-analysis and systematic review. Radiother Oncol. 2020;147:169–77.

GPSR Compliance

*The European Union's (EU) General Product Safety Regulation (GPSR) is a set of rules that requires consumer products to be safe and our obligations to ensure this.*

*If you have any concerns about our products, you can contact us on ProductSafety@springernature.com*

In case Publisher is established outside the EU, the EU authorized representative is:

Springer Nature Customer Service Center GmbH
Europaplatz 3
69115 Heidelberg, Germany

**Batch number: 10732023**

Printed by Printforce, the Netherlands